Atlas of Spinal Operations

Edited by
R. Bauer, F. Kerschbaumer, and S. Poisel

with contributions by

R. Bauer
W. Dick
A. Härle
H.-J. Hehne
F. Kerschbaumer
R. Kotz
R. Louis
S. Poisel
H.-J. Reulen
H. Sauer
C. J. Wirth
K. Zielke

720 illustrations by G. Spitzer, S. Cull, D. Fabian, S. Russo, and H. Schimek

1993
Georg Thieme Verlag, Stuttgart · New York
Thieme Medical Publishers Inc., New York

Library of Congress Cataloging-in-Publication Data

Atlas of spinal operations / ed. by R. Bauer ... With contributions by R. Bauer ... Ill. by G. Spitzer ... [Transl. by Gerhard Sharon. Ed. and adapted by Joachim Löhr]. – Stuttgart ; New York : Thieme ; New York : Thieme Med. Publ., 1993

Einheitssacht.: Orthopädische Operationslehre <engl.>
NE: Bauer, Rudolf [Hrsg.]; Spitzer, Gerhard [Ill.]; EST

Translated by Gerhard Sharon
Edited and adapted by Joachim F. Loehr, M.D., FRCSC

1st French edition 1993
1st German edition 1991
1st Italian edition 1992

This book is an authorized and revised translation of the German edition published and copyrighted 1991 by Georg Thieme Verlag, Stuttgart, Germany.
Title of the German edition:
Orthopädische Operationslehre, Band I: Wirbelsäule

Important Note: Medicine is an ever-changing science undergoing continual development. Research and clinical experience are continually expanding our knowledge, in particular our knowledge of proper treatment and drug therapy. Insofar as this book mentions any dosage or application, readers may rest assured that the authors, editors and publishers have made every effort to ensure that such references are in accordance with the state of knowledge at the time of production of the book.

Nevertheless this does not involve, imply, or express any guarantee or responsibility on the part of the publishers in respect of any dosage instructions and forms of application stated in the book. Every user is requested to examine carefully the manufacturers' leaflets accompanying each drug and to check, if necessary in consultation with a physician or specialist, whether the dosage schedules mentioned therein or the contraindications stated by the manufacturers differ from the statements made in the present book. Such examination is particularly important with drugs that are either rarely used or have been newly released on the market. Every dosage schedule or every form of application used is entirely at the user's own risk and responsibility. The authors and publishers request every user to report to the publishers any discrepancies or inaccuracies noticed.

Rüdigerstrasse 14, D-70469 Stuttgart, Germany
Thieme Medical Publishers, Inc.,
381 Park Avenue South, New York, N.Y. 10016
Typesetting by Druckhaus Götz GmbH,
D-71636 Ludwigsburg
Printed in Germany by K. Grammlich,
D-72124 Pliezhausen, Germany

ISBN 3-13-114001-1 (GTV, Stuttgart)
ISBN 0-86577-496-X (TMP, New York) 1 2 3 4 5 6

Addresses

Bauer, R., Prof. Dr.
Head, Orthopädische Universitätsklinik,
Anichstr. 35, 6020 Innsbruck, Austria

Dick, W., Prof. Dr.
Felix Platter Spital
Burgfelder Str. 101, 4000 Basel, Switzerland

Härle, A., Prof. Dr.
Professor emeritus, Klinik und Poliklinik für Allgemeine Orthopädie der Universität,
Albert-Schweitzer-Str. 33, 48149 Münster, Germany

Hehne, H.-J., Prof. Dr.
Professor emeritus, Reha-Klinik Hausbaden,
Hausbadener Str. 1, 79410 Badenweiler, Germany

Kerschbaumer, F., Prof. Dr.
Head, Abteilung für Rheumaorthopädie,
Orthopädische Universitätsklinik,
Marienburgstr. 2, 60528 Frankfurt, Germany

Kotz, R., Prof. Dr.
Head, Orthopädische Universitätsklinik,
Währinger Gürtel 18, 1090 Vienna, Austria

Louis, R., Prof. Dr.
Hôpital Hôtel Dieu, 6, Place Daviel, 13224 Marseille,
Cedex 1, France

Poisel, S., Prof. Dr.
Institut für Anatomie der Universität,
Müllerstr. 59, 6010 Innsbruck, Austria

Reulen, H.-J., Prof. Dr.
Direktor der Neurochirurgischen Klinik, Klinikum Großhadern,
Marchioninistr. 15, 81377 Munich, Germany

Sauer, H., Prof. Dr.
Head, Universitätsklinik für Kinderchirurgie (Pediatric Surgery),
Heinrichstr. 31, 8010 Graz, Austria

Wirth, C. J., Prof. Dr.
Orthopädische Klinik III der MHH im Annastift,
Heimchenstr. 1–6, 30625 Hannover, Germany

Zielke, K., Dr.
Chairman emeritus, Werner-Wicker-Klinik, Dept. II
Zentrum für Wirbelsäulenchirurgie (Center for Spinal Surgery),
34537 Bad Wildungen-Reinhardshausen, Germany

Preface

Our first atlas, Operative Approaches in Orthopedic Surgery and Traumatology, was rewarded with high sales in its many editions (German, English, French, Italian, Japanese, Spanish) for its novel presentation of surgical procedures. Therefore, we planned a further title with the same concept: color illustrations with concise accompanying text.

We are aware that it is not easy to publish a comprehensive collection of operative procedures in a day and age when techniques can become outdated within a short time. Therefore, we have not aimed to produce an "encyclopedia" of spinal operations; the authors have limited themselves to the presentation of the most tried-and-true techniques and standard procedures, with the exception of traumatologic operations, which will be published in forthcoming volumes of the German series Chirurgische Operationslehre (Vols. 8–10).

The basis for this atlas was, in addition to the operative experience of the authors, the anatomic substrate. To make the atlas easier to use, we compiled all the approaches in the first chapter. Then, the operations are presented step by step, including the indications, pitfalls, and complications. This format will be especially helpful to the resident learning these techniques, but can also serve as a memory jogger for the more experienced surgeon.

We would like to thank the authors, without whose contributions this atlas would not have been possible. Then we would like to extend our thanks to Dr. G. Hauff, Mr. A. Menge, and the staff at Thieme for their cooperation and the high quality of their work. We are grateful to the graphic artists, Prof. G. Spitzer, Ms. S. Cull, Mr. D. Fabian, Dr. S. Russo, and Ms. H. Schimek, who turned their sketches from the operating room and dissection table into excellent illustrations. The dissection of the cadavers was done at the Institute for Anatomy at the University of Innsbruck, Austria, for which our thanks go to Prof. W. Platzer.

Autumn 1993

R. Bauer, Innsbruck
F. Kerschbaumer, Frankfurt
S. Poisel, Innsbruck

Table of Contents

1 Approaches ... 1

R. Bauer, F. Kerschbaumer, S. Poisel, A. Härle

Anterior Approaches ... 2
Cervical Spine and Cervicothoracic Junction ... 2
  Transoropharyngeal Approach C1–C2 (C3) ... 2
  Anterior Approach to the Cervical Spine C3–T2 ... 4
  Exposure of Cervical Vertebrae C2–C6 ... 6
  Exposure of Vertebrae C7–T2 ... 9

Thoracic Spine ... 13
  Transthoracic Approach to Thoracic Spine T4–T11 ... 13
Thoracolumbar Junction ... 24
  Transpleural-Retroperitoneal Approach to the Thoracolumbar Spine, T9–L5 (Hodgson) ... 24
  Retroperitoneal-Extrapleural Approach to the Thoracolumbar Spine, T11–L5 (Mirbaha) ... 37
Lumbar Spine and Lumbosacral Junction ... 42
  Retroperitoneal Approach to the Lumbar Spine L2–L5 ... 42
  Pararectal Retroperitoneal Approach to the Lower Lumbar Spine and the Sacral Cavity, L3–S2 ... 46
  Transperitoneal Approach to the Lumbosacral Junction, L4–S1 ... 52

Posterior Approaches ... 56
Cervical Spine ... 56
  Posterior Approach to the Cervical Spine with Occipitocervical Junction ... 56
Thoracic and Lumbar Spine ... 60
  Costotransversectomy T3–T10 ... 60
  Posterior Approach to the Thoracic and Lumbar Spine ... 64
  Paraspinal Approach to the Lumbosacral Junction According to Wiltse ... 70
  Short Posterior Approach to the Lumbar Spine for Laminotomy and Intervertebral Disk Removal ... 71

2 Scoliosis ... 73

R. Bauer

Halo Traction Techniques ... 74

Posterior Scoliosis Operations ... 80
Harrington Operation ... 80
Scoliosis Operations in Children ... 97
  Posterior Fusion in Situ ... 98
  Posterior Fusion with Instrumentation ... 98
  Convex-Side Epiphysiodesis with Posterior Convex-Side Spinal Fusion ... 99
  Subcutaneous Harrington Instrumentation ... 100
  Hemivertebra Resection ... 100
Operations for Scoliosis in the Adult ... 103
  Mobilizing Spinal Osteotomy ... 104
  Rib Resection on the Concave Side ... 108
  Resection of Rib Hump on the Convex Side ... 109
Luque Operation ... 114
  Lumbosacral Fixation ... 126
  Harrington Operation Combined with Sublaminar Luque Wires ... 129
    Cotrel-Dubousset Instrumentation ... 131

Anterior Scoliosis Operations ... 147
Mobilizing Anterior Osteotomy ... 147
Resection of Hemivertebrae, Wedge Resection ... 151
Complete Vertebrectomy ... 156
Epiphysiodesis ... 160
The Dwyer Operation ... 163
Ventral Derotation Spondylodesis (Zielke) ... 178

3 Kyphosis ... 187

R. Bauer

Anterior Strut Grafting (Free Graft) ... 189
  Fusion in Situ or Fusion with Minimal Intraoperative Correction ... 191
  Intraoperative Corection Followed by Fusion ... 192
Vascularized Rib Graft ... 194
  Replacing a Vertebral Body Using a Vascularized Rib Graft (Bradford) ... 196
  Anterior Spinal Cord Decompression ... 198
  Simple Kyphosis ... 199
  Kyphosis with a Scoliotic Component and Marked Vertebral Torsion ... 203
  Kyphoscoliosis with a Very Severe Rotatory Component ... 203
Congenital Kyphosis ... 205
Operation for Kyphosis in Myelomeningocele ... 207
  Correction of Kyphosis in Older Patients ... 208
Short-Arc Kyphosis ... 212
Long-Arc Kyphosis (Scheuermann's Kyphosis) ... 215
Thoracic Lordosis ... 223

4 Ankylosing Spondylitis 227
H.-J. Hehne, K. Zielke

Operations for Kyphotic Deformity 228
Zielke Technique (Polysegmental Lumbar Lordosation Spondylodesis) 228
Hsu-Yau-Leong Technique as Modified by Zielke (Monosegmental Lumbar Lordosation Spondylodesis) 236
Technique of Mason and Urist (Monosegmental Cervical Lordosation Spondylodesis) 241
Operations for Spondylodiscitis (Andersson Lesion) 248
Anterior Interbody Spondylodesis 248
Operations for Fractures 248

5 Fusion of the Cervical Spine 251
W. Dick

Anterior Fusion (Robinson) 252
Interbody Fusion with Anterior Plate, Monosegmental or Polysegmental 256
Posterior Fusion 263

6 Fusion of the Lumbar Spine 269
W. Dick

Anterior Monosegmental Fusion L5–S1 270
Anterior Monosegmental Fusion of the Other Lumbar Segments 275
Posterior Transpedicular Stabilization Techniques .. 279
Posterolateral Fusion ot the Lumbosacral Junction (Wiltse) 291

7 Spondylolisthesis 293
R. Louis

Reconstruction of the Isthmus (Pars Interarticularis) 294
Reduction Combined with Fusion 298
Posterior Decompression With or Without Arthrodesis 307

8 Neurosurgical Operations 309
H.-J. Reulen

Transoral Approach in Dens Elevation 310
Cervical Myelopathy in Spondylosis 314
Thoracic Disk Herniation 317
Anterolateral Transthoracic Approach 318
Posterolateral Approach After Costotransversectomy 321
Lumbar Disk Herniation 325
Extracanalicular Disk Herniation 337
Stenoses in the Lumbar Spinal Canal 340
Stenosis of the Lateral Recess (Superior Facet Syndrome) 340
Stenosis of Lumbar Spinal Canal 342

9 Rheumatoid Instability 347
F. Kerschbaumer

Posterior Operations 351
Posterior Occipitocervical Fusion 361
Anterior Transoral Operations 373

10 Spondylitis 377
A. Härle

11 Tumors of the Spine 391
R. Bauer, R. Kotz

12 Tumors of the Chest Wall 411
R. Kotz

Rib Resections 412

13 Deformities of the Chest Wall 421
H. Sauer

Funnel Chest 422
Rehbein Operation 423
Ravitch Operation 432
Pigeon Breast 436
Ravitch Operation 436
Superior Sternoschisis 438
Sabiston Operation 438
Poland's Syndrome 439
Haller Operation 439

14 Torticollis 441
C. J. Wirth

Caudal Sternoclavicular Subcutaneous Tenotomy of the Sternocleidomastoid Muscle (Strohmeyer, König) 442
Caudal Sternoclavicular Open Tenotomy (von Volkmann) 443
Cranial Mastoidal Open Tenotomy (Tillaux, F. Lange) 446
Biterminal Tenotomy (Hellstadius, Putti) 448
Total Extirpation of the Sternocleidomastoid Muscle (Mikulicz) 448

Index 451

1 Approaches

R. Bauer
F. Kerschbaumer
S. Poisel
A. Härle

Anterior Approaches

Cervical Spine and Cervicothoracic Junction

Transoropharyngeal Approach C1–C2 (C3)

Principal Indications

- Posttraumatic conditions, dens fracture, or pseudarthrosis
- Tumors
- Osteomyelitis
- Os odontoideum

Preparation of Patient, Positioning, Anesthesia, Incision

The problem intrinsic to this approach is that the surgery is performed in an area colonized by bacteria, and involves the opening of cancellous bone cavities. Thorough oral disinfection should therefore precede the operation; the procedure is carried out under antibiotic coverage, and antibiotics are applied topically before wound closure. The patient is placed in a supine position, with the head down and the cervical spine slightly overextended. The anesthesia team is positioned at the side of the patient, while the surgeon stands at the head, with the assistants on either side.

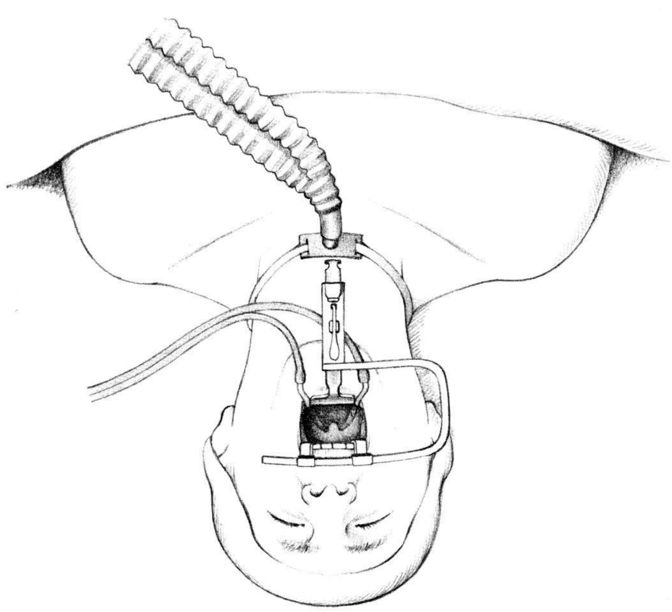

Fig. 1.**1** Transoropharyngeal approach. Status after tracheotomy. A mouth gag and tongue depressor have been introduced.

The transoral approach is facilitated by prior performance of a tracheostomy for anesthetic purposes. A tracheostomy is not absolutely necessary, however; the operation may also be performed with the aid of a transnasal or transoral tube, which is then retracted laterally using a long spatula. A mouth gag with a special blade to hold down the tongue is then inserted (Fig. 1.**1**). A retractor is used to pull up the soft palate.

Exposure of Vertebrae

The posterior pharyngeal wall is incised in the midline with a knife, the incision extending from the readily palpable anterior tubercle of the atlas to the level of C2 or C3. The length of the incision measures about 5–6 cm (Fig. 1.**2**). The long muscle of the neck is visualized (Fig. 1.**3**), and should be divided in the midline. Using an elevator, the soft tissues on the anterior side of C1 and C2 (possibly also C3) are retracted laterally, beginning at the midline. This brings into view the anterior tubercle, as well as the lateral mass of the atlas and the body of the axis. The operative field is visualized with flexible retractors; careful hemostasis is carried out by diathermy (Fig. 1.**4**). The atlas may be exposed to a maximum of 2 cm lateral to the midline, but the C2 and C3 vertebrae should not be exposed by more than 1 cm. The vertebral artery is at risk here, particularly at the inferior border of C2 (Fig. 1.**5**). Lateral to the lateral masses of the atlas, the elevator may penetrate the retromandibular fossa, and injuries to the ninth and twelfth cranial nerves may result.

Wound Closure

The wound closure is carried out in two layers, using resorbable interrupted sutures.

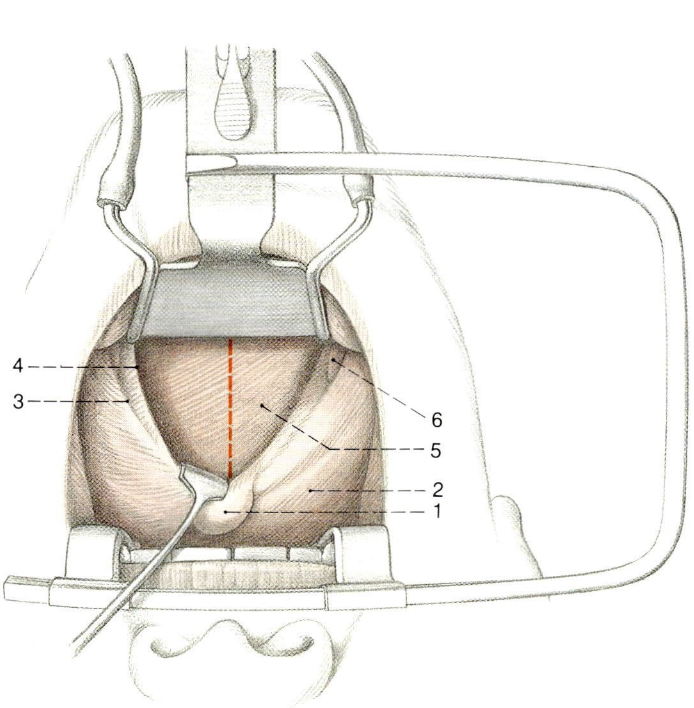

Fig. 1.**2** Retraction of the soft palate. Longitudinal incision of the posterior wall of the pharynx.

1 Uvula
2 Soft palate
3 Palatoglossal arch
4 Palatopharyngeal arch
5 Posterior pharyngeal wall with mucosa
6 Palatine tonsil

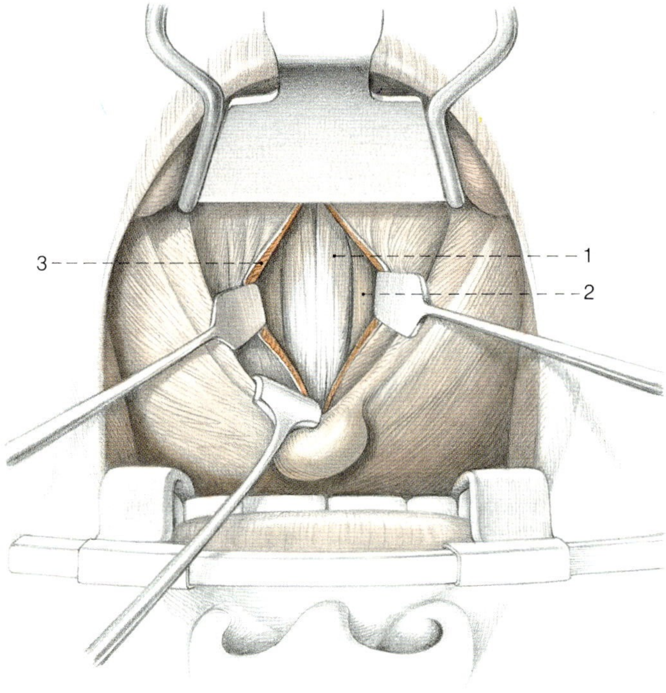

Fig. 1.**3** Status after splitting of the posterior pharyngeal wall.

1 Long muscle of the neck
2 Long muscle of the head
3 Superior constrictor muscle of the pharynx

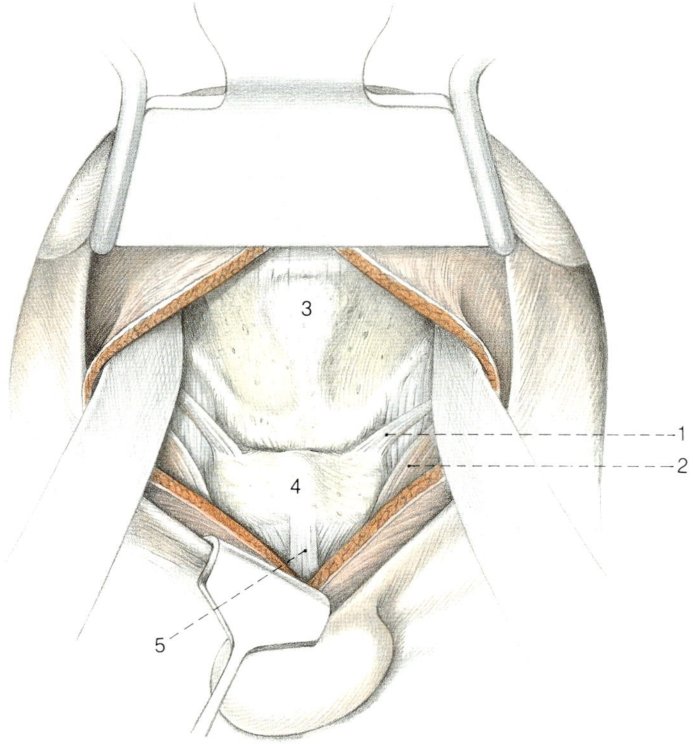

Fig. 1.**4** Exposure of the atlas and axis.

1 Long muscle of the neck
2 Long muscle of the head
3 Body of the axis
4 Anterior tubercle of the atlas
5 Anterior atlanto-occipital membrane

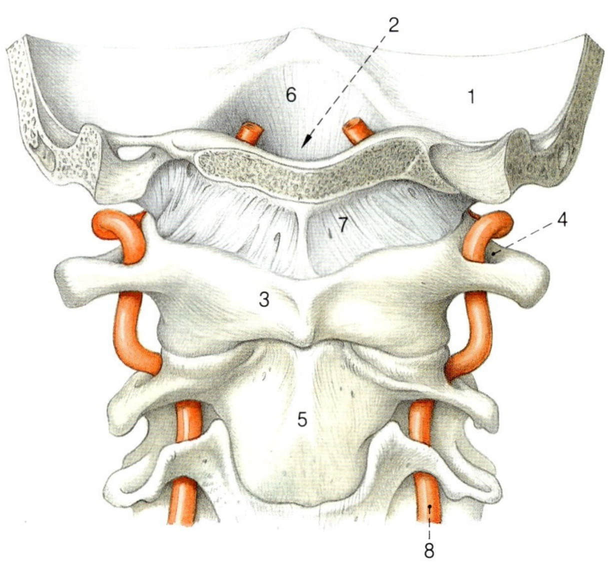

Fig. 1.**5** Anatomical site of C1 and C2 with the vertebral artery. Anterior view.

1 Occipital squama
2 Great foramen
3 Anterior tubercle of the atlas
4 Foramen of the transverse process
5 Body of the axis
6 Tectorial membrane
7 Anterior atlanto-occipital membrane
8 Vertebral artery

Anterior Approach to the Cervical Spine C3–T2

Principal Indications

- Trauma
- Degenerative changes
- Tumors
- Spondylitis

Choice of Side for the Approach

Approach from either side is possible for the middle and upper cervical spine. However, this depends on the side of the lesion. Right-handed persons generally prefer the right-sided approach. However, for exposure of the cervical spine from C6 downward, the left-sided approach is preferable so as to avoid injury to the recurrent laryngeal nerve, which has an irregular and higher course on the right side.

Positioning and Incision

The patient is placed in a supine position, usually without skeletal extension, except after recent trauma. A pad is placed between the scapulae; a rolled-up towel should be placed under the cervical spine if overextension is desired.

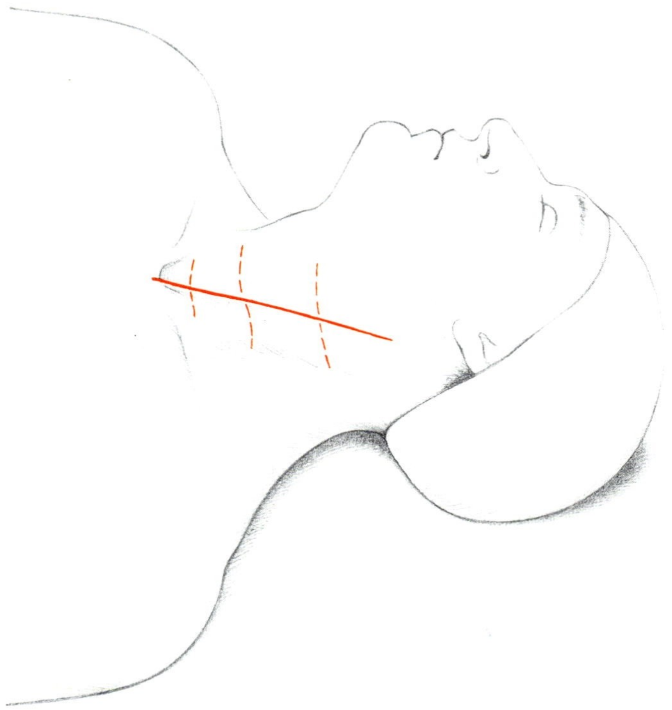

Fig. 1.**6** Anterior approach to the cervical spine. Longitudinal incision and possible alternative transverse incisions. Supine position, with the head turned and with the cervical spine slightly overextended.

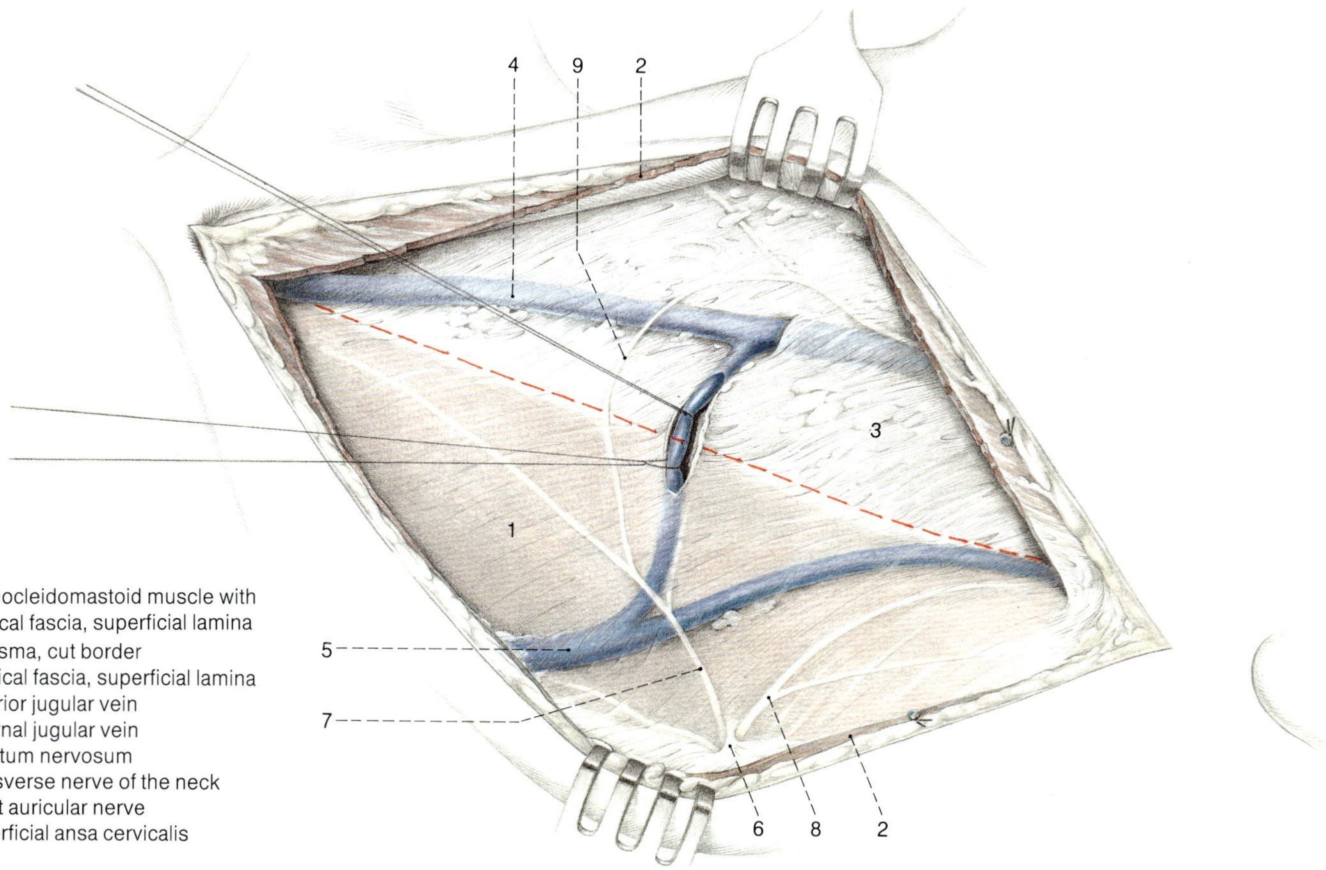

1 Sternocleidomastoid muscle with cervical fascia, superficial lamina
2 Platysma, cut border
3 Cervical fascia, superficial lamina
4 Anterior jugular vein
5 External jugular vein
6 Punctum nervosum
7 Transverse nerve of the neck
8 Great auricular nerve
9 Superficial ansa cervicalis

Fig. 1.**7** After longitudinal division of the subcutis and platysma, the anterior border of the sternocleidomastoid muscle is identified, and here the superficial cervical fascia is transected parallel to it. Transversely running veins and branches of the superficial ansa cervicalis are ligated.

Atlas of
Spinal Operations

The head is rotated slightly to the opposite side, and both shoulders are pulled downward with strips of adhesive tape. The operation is performed under endotracheal anesthesia.

The choice of incision depends on the amount of vertebral exposure needed. If it is sufficient to expose one or two segments only, a transverse skin incision parallel to the neck folds is advisable. The level of the transverse incision may be determined according to the following guidelines:

- Vertebrae C3 and C4: Incision two finger-breadths caudal to the mandible, at the level of the hyoid bone.
- Vertebrae C4 and C5: Incision at the level of the thyroid cartilage.
- Vertebrae C5 and C6: Incision at the level of the cricoid cartilage.
- Vertebrae C6 and T1: Incision two finger-breadths cranial to the clavicle.

For a broad exposure of several segments of the cervical spine, a longitudinal incision anterior to the sternocleidomastoid muscle is preferred. The skin incision begins at the level of the mandibular angle, and extends distally as far as the manubrium sterni (Fig. 1.**6**). The platysma is divided in the same direction, and is mobilized toward both sides for exposure of the superficial cervical fascia. This is divided in a longitudinal direction at the anterior border of the sternocleidomastoid muscle. This usually also requires ligating and transecting transversely coursing cervical veins and transecting branches of the transverse nerve of the neck (Fig. 1.**7**). The sternocleidomastoid musculature is retracted medially. The superior belly of the omohyoid muscle now runs transversely across the operative area (Fig. 1.**8**). It is undermined, divided between two ligatures, and retracted bilaterally. Further dissection is done bluntly with scissors, the middle layer of the cervical fascia being opened. In the depth, the cervical vertebrae are now digitally palpable. Often, veins crossing below the middle cervical fascia (middle thyroid vein) have to be cut between ligatures (Fig. 1.**9**). The middle cervical fascia is then bluntly dissected upward and downward, with transverse branches of the deep ansa cervicalis being sacrificed. Laterally, the pulse of the common carotid artery is palpable. The neurovascular bundle (common carotid artery, internal jugular vein, and vagus nerve) is cautiously retracted laterally, while the visceral structures (trachea, larynx, thyroid) and the sternohyoid and sternothyroid muscles are retracted medially (Figs. 1.**9**, 1.**10**).

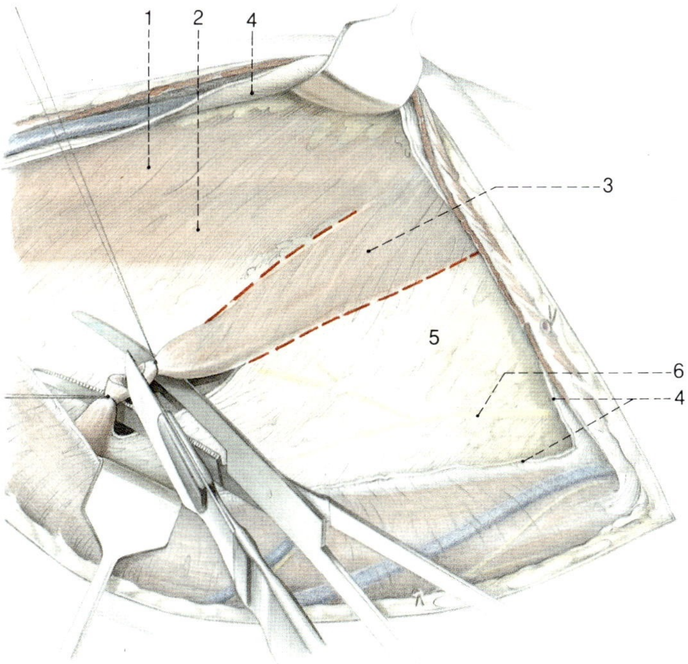

Fig. 1.**8** Undermining and division of the superior muscle belly of the omohyoid muscle between two ligatures.

1 Sternohyoid muscle
2 Sternothyroid muscle
3 Omohyoid muscle
4 Cervical fascia, superficial lamina
5 Cervical fascia, pretracheal lamina
6 Deep ansa cervicalis

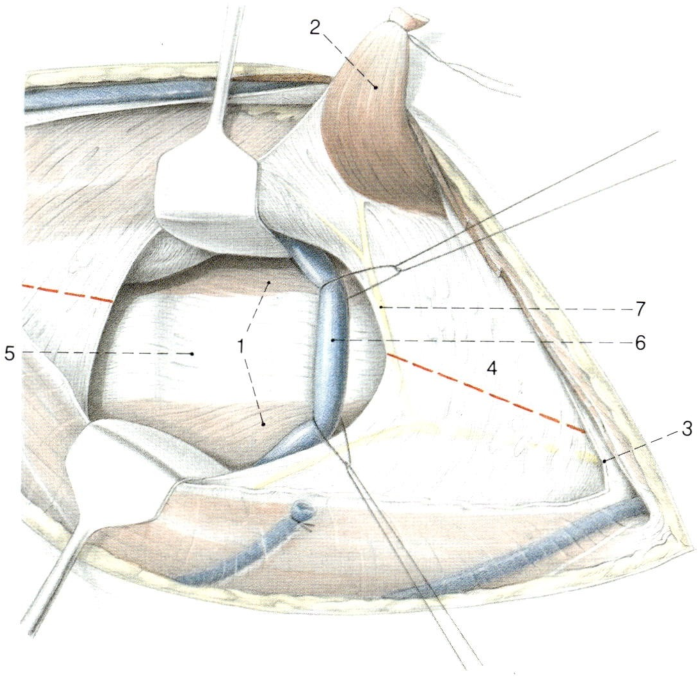

Fig. 1.**9** Blunt splitting of the middle cervical fascia, and ligation and transection of transversely coursing veins and branches of the deep ansa cervicalis. Application of blunt retractors and further dissection between the laterally situated neurovascular bundle and the medially positioned visceral structures.

1 Long muscle of the neck
2 Omohyoid muscle
3 Cervical fascia, superficial lamina
4 Cervical fascia, pretracheal lamina
5 Sixth cervical vertebra with deep cervical fascia
6 Middle thyroid vein
7 Deep ansa cervicalis

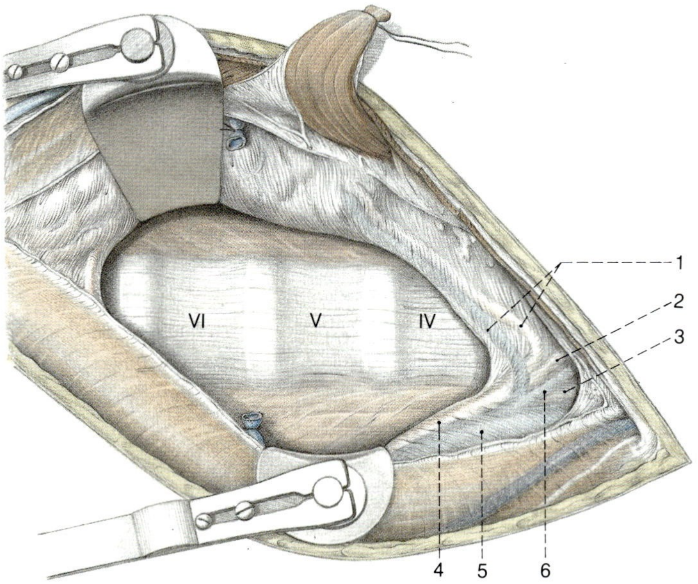

Fig. 1.**10** The deep cervical fascia and the anterior surfaces of the fourth, fifth, and sixth cervical vertebrae are exposed by retraction with Cloward retractors.

1 Superior thyroid artery and vein
2 Lingual artery
3 External carotid artery
4 Common carotid artery
5 Internal jugular vein
6 Facial vein
IV–VI Cervical vertebrae

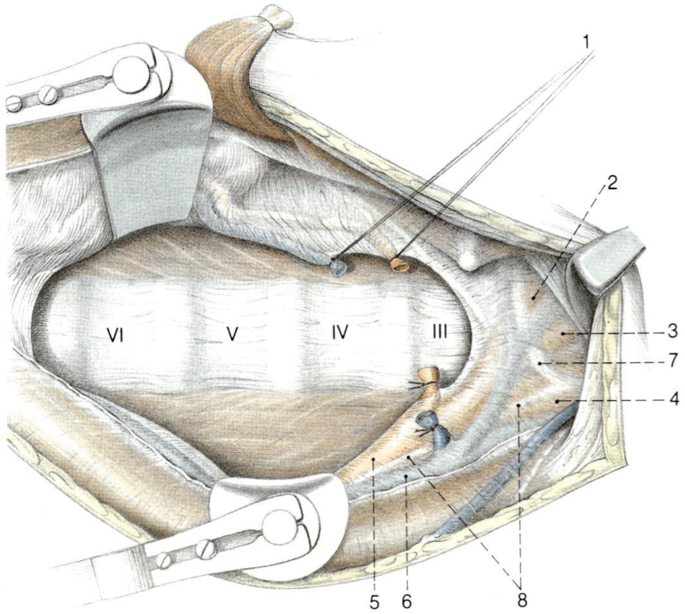

Fig. 1.**11** Exposure of the cervical vertebrae above C4 requires ligation and transection of the superior thyroid artery.

1 Superior thyroid artery and vein
2 Lingual artery
3 Facial artery
4 External carotid artery
5 Common carotid artery
6 Internal jugular vein
7 Hypoglossal nerve
8 Deep ansa cervicalis
III–VI Cervical vertebrae

Exposure of Cervical Vertebrae C2–C6

Further dissection medially and upward, between the deep cervical fascia covering the vertebrae, on one hand, and the esophagus and larynx, on the other, is best done with the finger. If additional dissection in a cranial direction for exposure of the third or second cervical vertebra is necessary, the superior thyroid artery has to be identified, ligated, and transected (Fig. 1.**11**).

Anatomical Site

(Figs. 1.**12a**, **b**)

The following anatomical structures have to be taken into consideration when exposing the proximal segments of the cervical spine: the superior thyroid artery, the lingual artery, and the facial artery, all of which arise from the external carotid artery and may be ligated if necessary. The hypoglossal nerve, which, coming from the cranial side, turns medially anterior to the external carotid artery, where it supplies the musculature of the tongue, has to be protected.

The superior laryngeal nerve, with its external and internal branches, originates from the vagus nerve and runs beneath the lingual and facial arteries to pass into the larynx. More cranially, the glossopharyngeal nerve, coursing medially from the base of the skull, passes into the superior constrictor muscle of the pharynx.

The irregularly coursing veins may be ligated if necessary (Fig. 1.**13**).

The approach routes are schematically represented in Figures 1.**14** and 1.**15**.

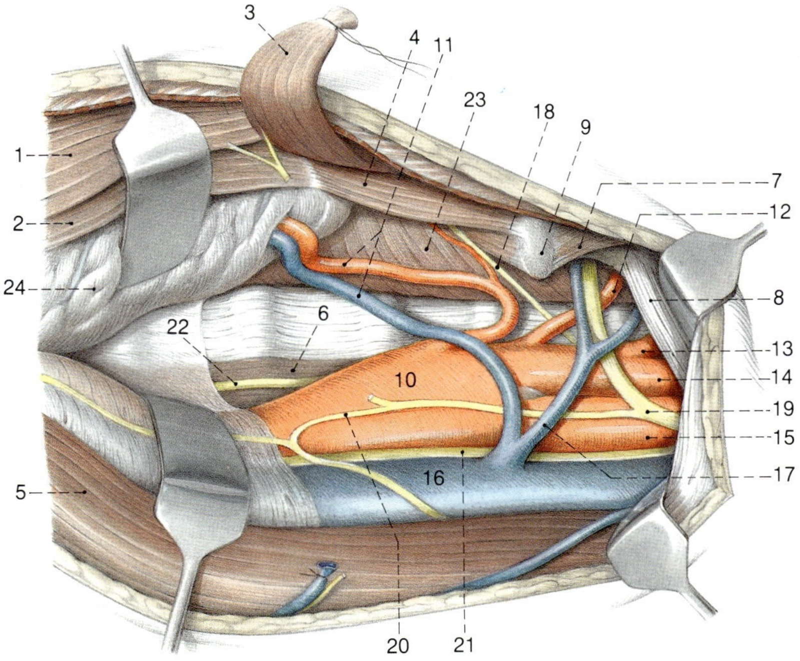

Fig. 1.**12a** Anatomical site of the upper cervical spine, as seen from the left.

1 Sternohyoid muscle
2 Sternothyroid muscle
3 Omohyoid muscle
4 Thyrohyoid muscle
5 Sternocleidomastoid muscle
6 Long muscle of the neck
7 Mylohyoid muscle
8 Digastric muscle
9 Hyoid bone, greater horn
10 Common carotid artery
11 Superior thyroid artery and vein
12 Lingual artery
13 Facial artery
14 External carotid artery
15 Internal carotid artery
16 Internal jugular vein
17 Lingual vein
18 Superior laryngeal nerve
19 Hypoglossal nerve
20 Deep ansa cervicalis
21 Vagus nerve
22 Sympathetic trunk
23 Middle constrictor muscle of pharynx
24 Thyroid gland

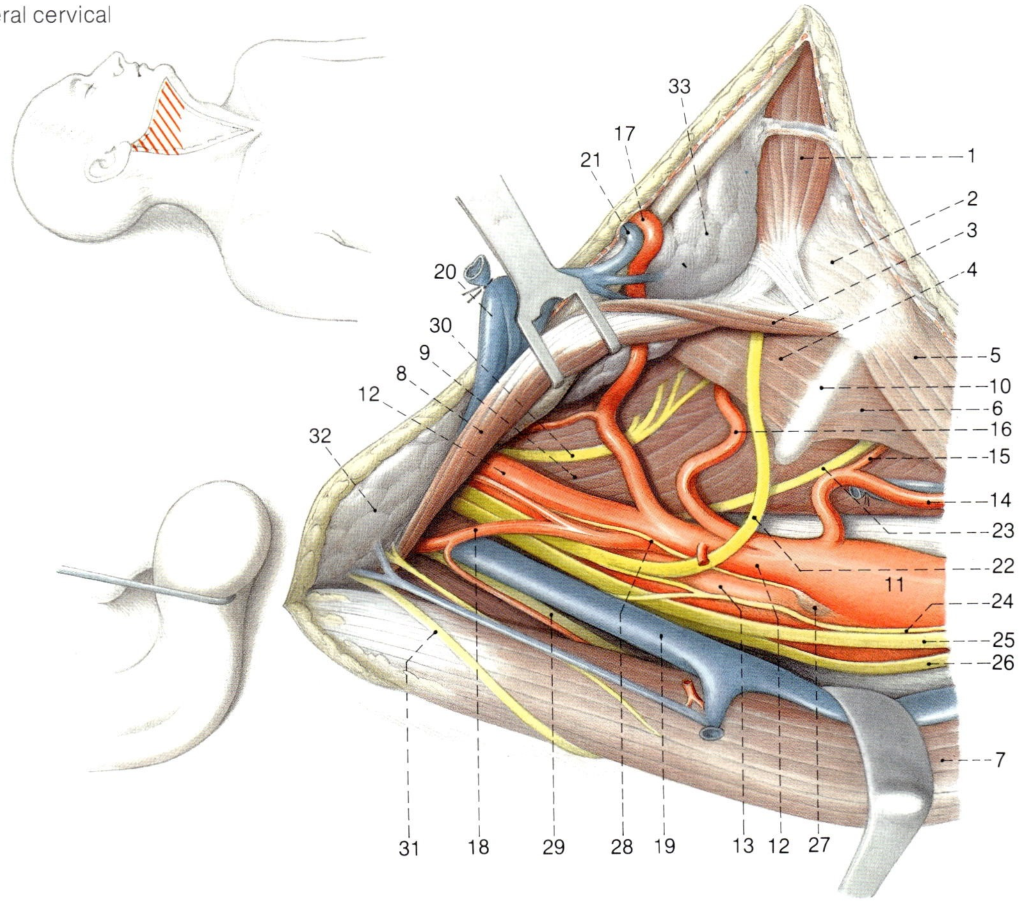

Fig. 1.**12b** Anatomical site of the lateral cervical region, as seen from the right.

1 Digastric muscle, anterior belly
2 Mylohyoid muscle
3 Stylohyoid muscle
4 Hyoglossal muscle
5 Omohyoid muscle, superior belly
6 Thyrohyoid muscle
7 Sternocleidomastoid muscle
8 Digastric muscle, posterior belly
9 Superior constrictor muscle of pharynx
10 Hyoid bone, greater horn
11 Common carotid artery
12 External carotid artery
13 Internal carotid artery
14 Superior thyroid artery
15 Superior laryngeal artery
16 Lingual artery
17 Facial artery
18 Occipital artery
19 Internal jugular vein
20 Retromandibular vein
21 Facial vein
22 Hypoglossal nerve
23 Superior laryngeal nerve
24 Deep ansa cervicalis
25 Vagus nerve
26 Sympathetic trunk
27 Carotid glomus
28 Carotid sinus branch
29 Accessory nerve
30 Glossopharyngeal nerve
31 Great auricular nerve
32 Parotid gland
33 Submandibular gland

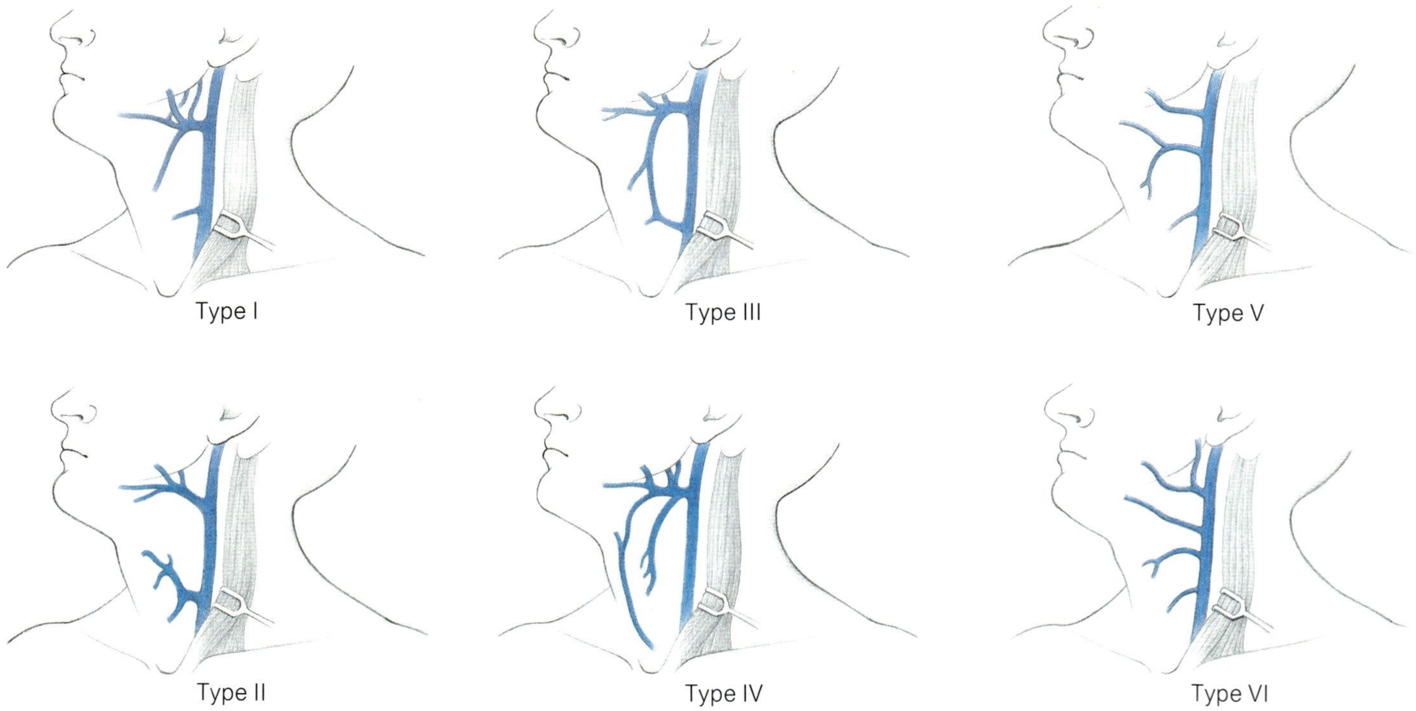

Fig. 1.**13** Variants of venous tributaries of the internal jugular vein.

Type I Thyrolinguofacial trunk (45%)
Type II Linguofacial trunk (9%)
Type III Linguofacial trunk with arcade (12%)
Type IV Thyrolinguofacial trunk with connection to anterior jugular vein (15%)
Type V Thyrolingual trunk (7%)
Type VI All three veins form independent tributaries (12%)

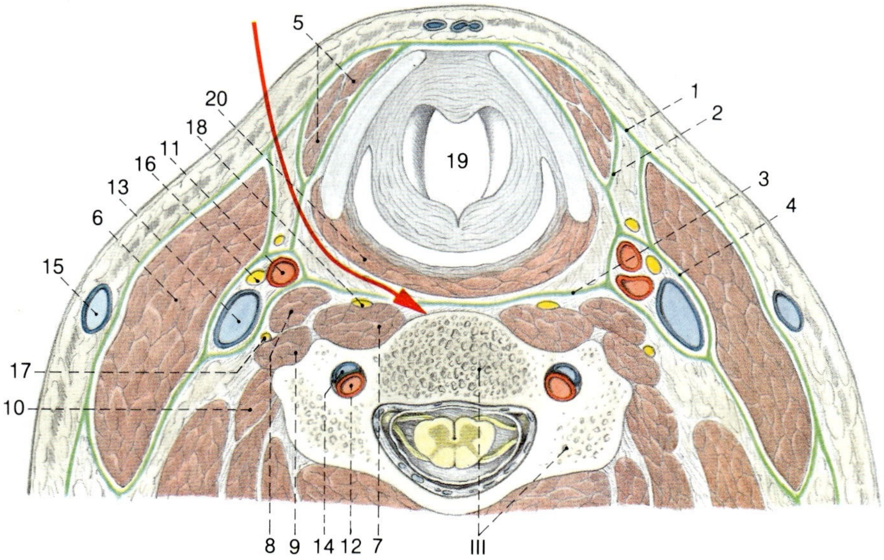

Fig. 1.**14** Anatomical cross-section at the level of the third cervical vertebra.

1 Cervical fascia, superficial lamina
2 Cervical fascia, pretracheal lamina
3 Cervical fascia, prevertebral lamina
4 Cervical fascia, vagina carotica
5 Infrahyoid muscles
6 Sternocleidomastoid muscle
7 Long muscle of the neck
8 Long muscle of the head
9 Anterior scalene muscle
10 Middle scalene muscle
11 Common carotid artery
12 Vertebral artery
13 Internal jugular vein
14 Vertebral vein
15 External jugular vein
16 Vagus nerve
17 Phrenic nerve
18 Sympathetic trunk
19 Larynx
20 Pharynx
III Cervical vertebra

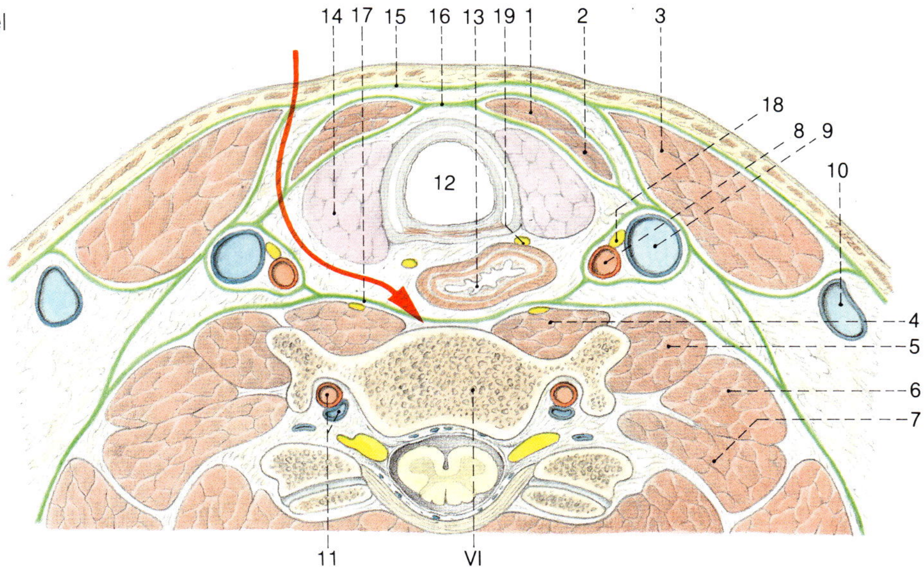

Fig. 1.**15** Anatomical cross-section at the level of the sixth cervical vertebra.

1 Sternohyoid muscle
2 Sternothyroid muscle
3 Sternocleidomastoid muscle
4 Long muscle of the neck
5 Anterior scalene muscle
6 Middle scalene muscle
7 Posterior scalene muscle
8 Common carotid artery
9 Internal jugular vein
10 External jugular vein
11 Vertebral vessels
12 Trachea
13 Esophagus
14 Thyroid gland
15 Cervical fascia, superficial lamina
16 Cervical fascia, pretracheal lamina
17 Cervical fascia, prevertebral lamina
18 Vagus nerve
19 Recurrent laryngeal nerve
VI Cervical vertebra

Exposure of Vertebrae C7–T2

When an exposure of the caudally situated cervical vertebrae and the two upper thoracic vertebrae is required, the inferior thyroid artery has to be identified and ligated. Further dissection of the middle cervical fascia inferiorly is performed bluntly with scissors, peanut swabs and, in part, digitally (Fig. 1.**16**).

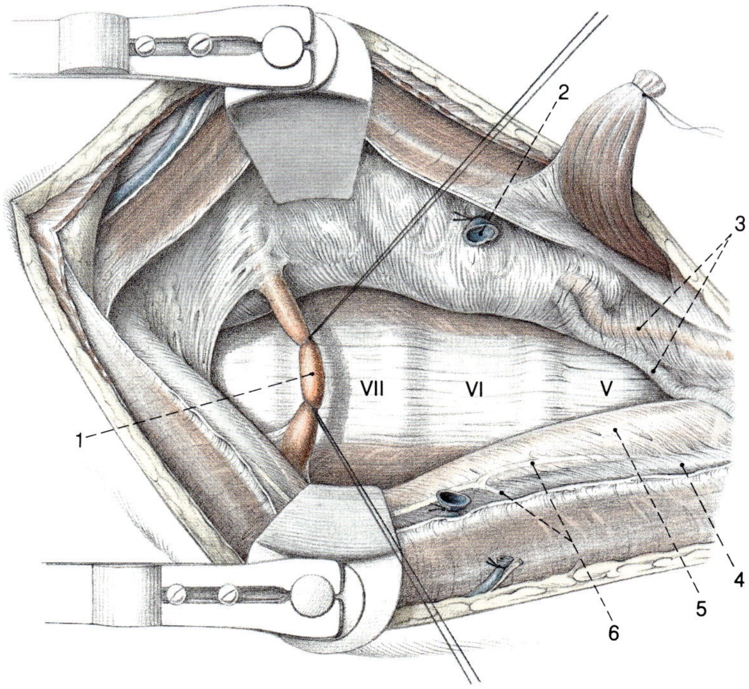

Fig. 1.**16** Exposure of the lower cervical spine and cervicothoracic junction (C6–T2). Ligation and transection of the inferior thyroid artery.

1 Inferior thyroid artery
2 Middle thyroid vein
3 Superior thyroid artery and vein
4 Internal jugular vein
5 Common carotid artery
6 Deep ansa cervicalis
V–VII Cervical vertebrae

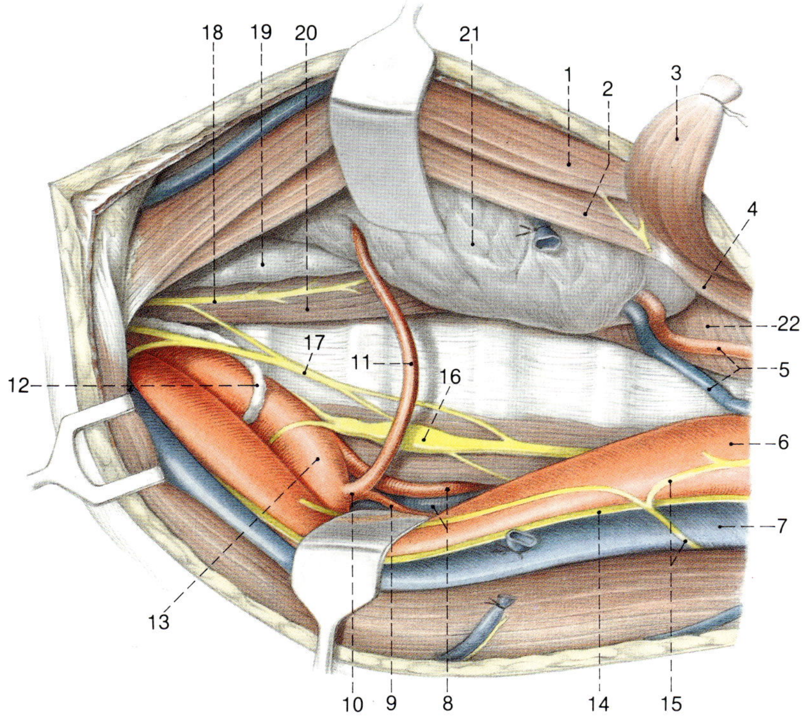

Fig. 1.**17** Anatomical site of the lower cervical spine, as seen from the left. Note the course of the recurrent laryngeal nerve and the thoracic duct.

1 Sternohyoid muscle
2 Sternothyroid muscle
3 Omohyoid muscle
4 Thyrohyoid muscle
5 Superior thyroid artery and vein
6 Common carotid artery
7 Internal jugular vein
8 Vertebral artery and vein
9 Ascending cervical artery
10 Thyrocervical trunk
11 Inferior thyroid artery
12 Thoracic duct
13 Subclavian artery
14 Vagus nerve
15 Deep ansa cervicalis
16 Stellate ganglion
17 Sympathetic trunk
18 Recurrent laryngeal nerve
19 Trachea
20 Esophagus
21 Thyroid gland
22 Pharynx

Anatomical Site

Descending from cranial, the anterior sides of the lower cervical and upper thoracic vertebrae are covered by the following structures:

On the left side (Figs. 1.**17** and 1.**18**): The inferior thyroid artery arises from the thyrocervical trunk or from the subclavian artery and runs transversely across the anterior surface of the vertebrae into the inferior pole of the thyroid gland. The sympathetic trunk with the stellate ganglion lies at approximately the same level, on the anterior surface of the long muscle of the neck, with the vertebral artery lateral to it. Located further caudally is the thoracic duct, which, arising from the thorax, travels anteriorly over the subclavian artery and then passes into the left angulus venosus. The cervical pleura lies approximately at the level of the first thoracic vertebra, between the long muscles of the neck and the subclavian artery. The recurrent laryngeal nerve, coming from the vagus nerve, courses on the left side behind the aortic arch and ascends further toward the

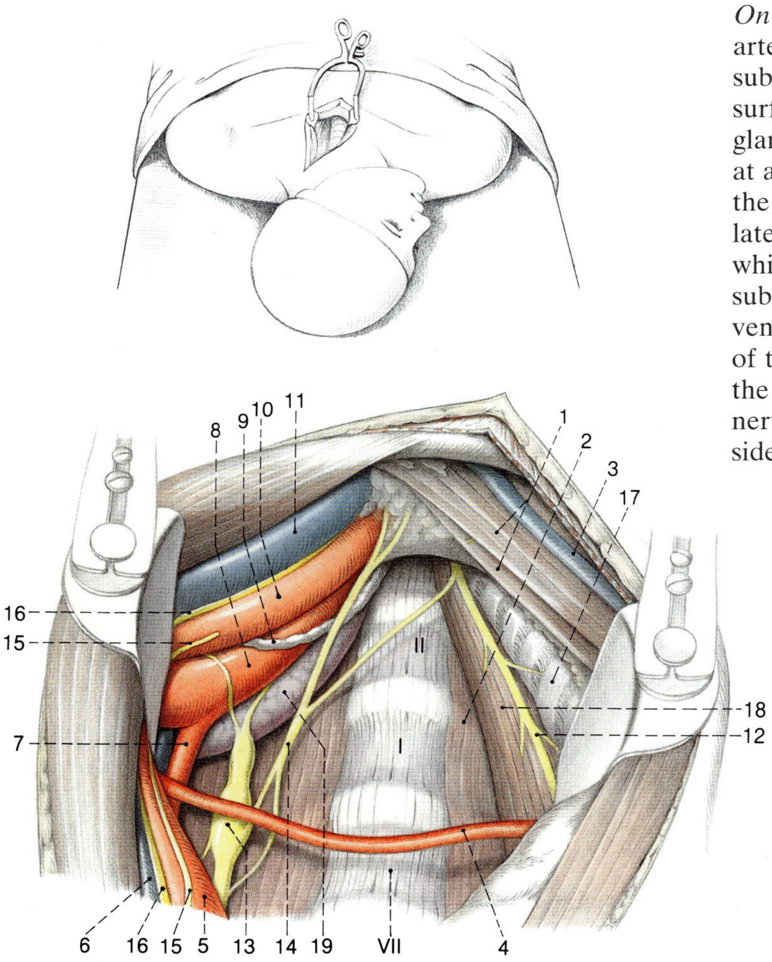

Fig. 1.**18** Anatomical site of the cervicothoracic junction, as seen from above left. Note the relation of the cervical pleura to the vertebrae.

1 Sternohyoid and sternothyroid muscles
2 Long muscle of the neck
3 External jugular vein
4 Left inferior thyroid artery
5 Common carotid artery
6 Internal jugular vein
7 Vertebral artery
8 Subclavian artery
9 Thoracic duct
10 Common carotid artery
11 Internal jugular vein
12 Recurrent laryngeal nerve
13 Stellate ganglion
14 Sympathetic trunk
15 Deep ansa cervicalis
16 Vagus nerve
17 Trachea
18 Esophagus
19 Cervical pleura
I–II Thoracic vertebrae
VII Cervical vertebra

larynx between the trachea and the esophagus. Of all the anatomical structures listed above, only the inferior thyroid artery may be ligated. All the nerves and the thoracic duct have to be spared, with the exception of small branches between the sympathetic trunk and the recurrent laryngeal nerve.

The deep prevertebral cervical fascia has to be divided in the midline and dissected laterally as far as the long muscle of the neck. Using a wide rasp, the long muscles of the neck are then elevated on both sides of the anterior longitudinal ligament as far back as the base of the transverse processes (Figs. 1.**19**, 1.**20**). The anterior surface of the cervical vertebrae may also be exposed subperiosteally by dividing the anterior longitudinal ligament in a longitudinal direction with the diathermy knife and then elevating it with the rasp. This method of dissection leads to bleeding from the nutrient foramina at the anterior surface of the cervical vertebrae, which can be stopped with bone wax. Identifying the correct level is most reliably accomplished during surgery by means of a C-arm or a lateral radiograph, using a needle inserted into the intervertebral disk as a marker. As a rule, the prominent transverse process of the sixth cervical vertebra (carotid tubercle, Chassaignac's tubercle) can be palpated easily lateral to the longus colli muscle. However, in less than ten percent of cases, the seventh cervical vertebra may also have a prominent transverse process if the vertebral artery enters the foramen of the transverse process at C7. Figure 1.**20** shows the operative site of the cervical spine from the left anterior approach from C3 to T2. Besides Cloward retractors, flexible, wide-bladed spatulas, which can be placed lateral to the base of the transverse processes, have been found satisfactory for a wide exposure of the spine.

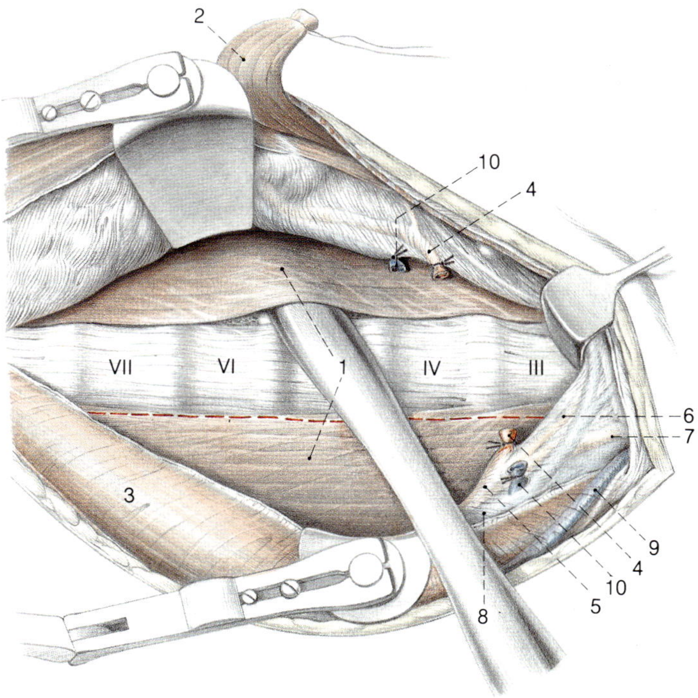

Fig. 1.**19** Status after division of the deep prevertebral cervical fascia; exposure of the vertebrae as far as the base of the transverse processes by bilateral stripping of the long muscles of the neck. Alternative method: subperiosteal exposure of the vertebrae by detachment of the anterior longitudinal ligament.

1 Long muscle of the neck
2 Omohyoid muscle
3 Sternocleidomastoid muscle
4 Superior thyroid artery
5 Common carotid artery
6 Lingual artery
7 External carotid artery
8 Internal jugular vein
9 External jugular vein
10 Superior thyroid vein
III–VII Cervical vertebrae

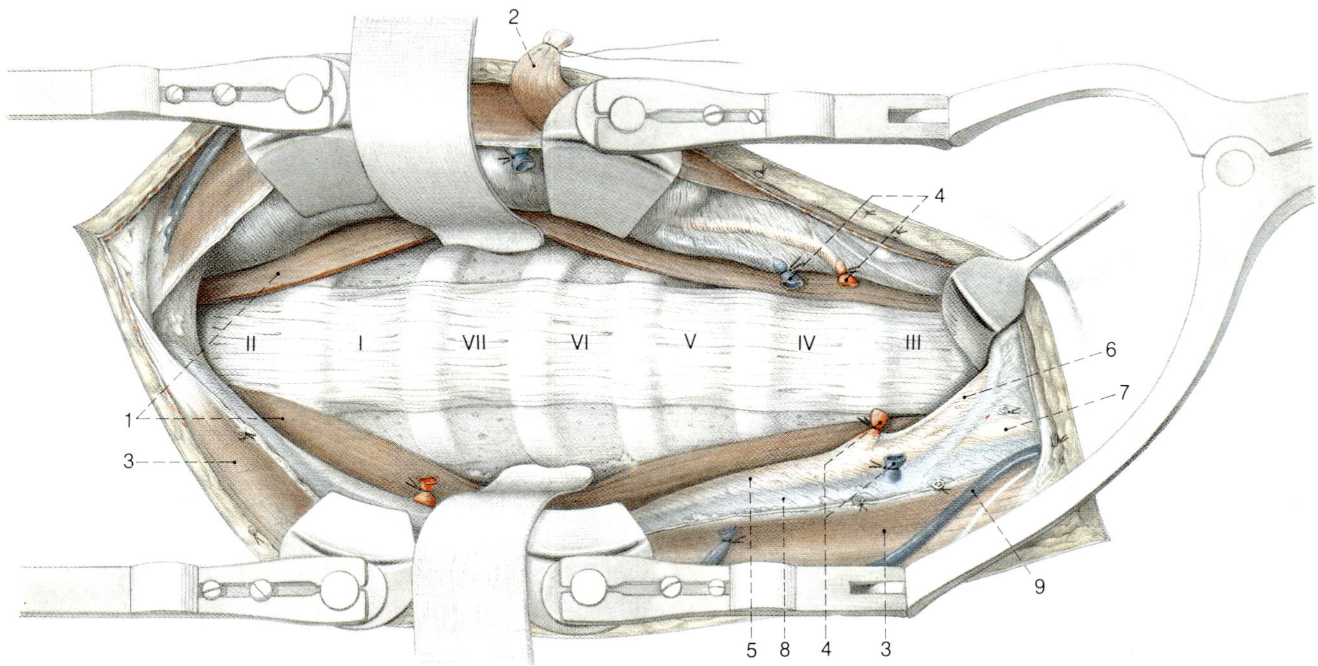

Fig. 1.**20** Exposure of the cervical spine from C3 to T2 by a left anterior approach, following bilateral mobilization of the longus colli muscle.

1 Long muscle of the neck
2 Omohyoid muscle
3 Sternocleidomastoid muscle
4 Superior thyroid vessels
5 Common carotid artery
6 Lingual artery
7 External carotid artery
8 Internal jugular vein
9 External jugular vein
III–VII Cervical vertebrae
I–II Thoracic vertebrae

On the right side: The right and left approaches differ mainly because of the different courses of the recurrent laryngeal nerve (Fig. 1.**21**). On the right side, this nerve may arise from the vagus nerve at different levels. It runs below the subclavian artery and then passes obliquely over the anterior side of the vertebra toward the groove between the trachea and the esophagus. Normally, the nerve runs behind the inferior thyroid artery, but on occasion it may lie in front of the artery, where it may be damaged by the retractors.

Wound Closure

Upon closure of the wound, the divided omohyoid muscle is reattached. Use of a Hemovac drain is recommended.

Pitfalls

Excessive traction on the visceral structures may lead to injuries of the thin-walled esophagus or to pharyngeal edema. Retractor pressure (beware of unduly short retractors!) can also cause damage to the recurrent laryngeal nerve, with resultant paresis of the vocal cord musculature. When exposing the cranial cervical vertebrae, the hypoglossal nerve may be injured, resulting in unilateral paralysis of the tongue musculature. A lesion of the superior laryngeal nerve, particularly in its external branch, can lead to disorders in the sensitivity of the laryngeal mucosa and to paralysis of the cricothyroid muscle. This may cause postoperative hoarseness and speech disturbances. A postoperative Horner syndrome may occur as a result of injuries to the sympathetic trunk, notably in the region of the stellate ganglion, if dissection has been performed too far laterally. The vertebral artery may be damaged if the elevators used for the dissection are too narrow, so that they may slip between the transverse processes. Exposure of the cervicoposterior junction by the anterior approach can result in injuries to the thoracic duct or the cervical pleura, which may lead to a chylothorax or pneumothorax.

Note

If there is adequate knowledge of the anatomy, the approach described is easy, and is associated with a low rate of complications. It therefore represents the standard approach for anterior exposure of the cervical spine. Further anterior and lateral approaches to the cervical spine have been described by Henry (1957), Whitesides and Kelly (1966), Verbriest (1969), Nanson (1957), Hodgson (1965a) and others. These approaches are especially developed for exposure of the spinal nerves, the vertebral artery, and the scalene compartments, and are less suitable for a clear anterior exposure of the cervical spine. For exposure of the upper cervical spine and the craniocervical junction in particular, Riley (1973) described an approach which, besides extensive dissection of the submandibular space, involves dislocation of the mandibular joint and removal of the submandibular gland.

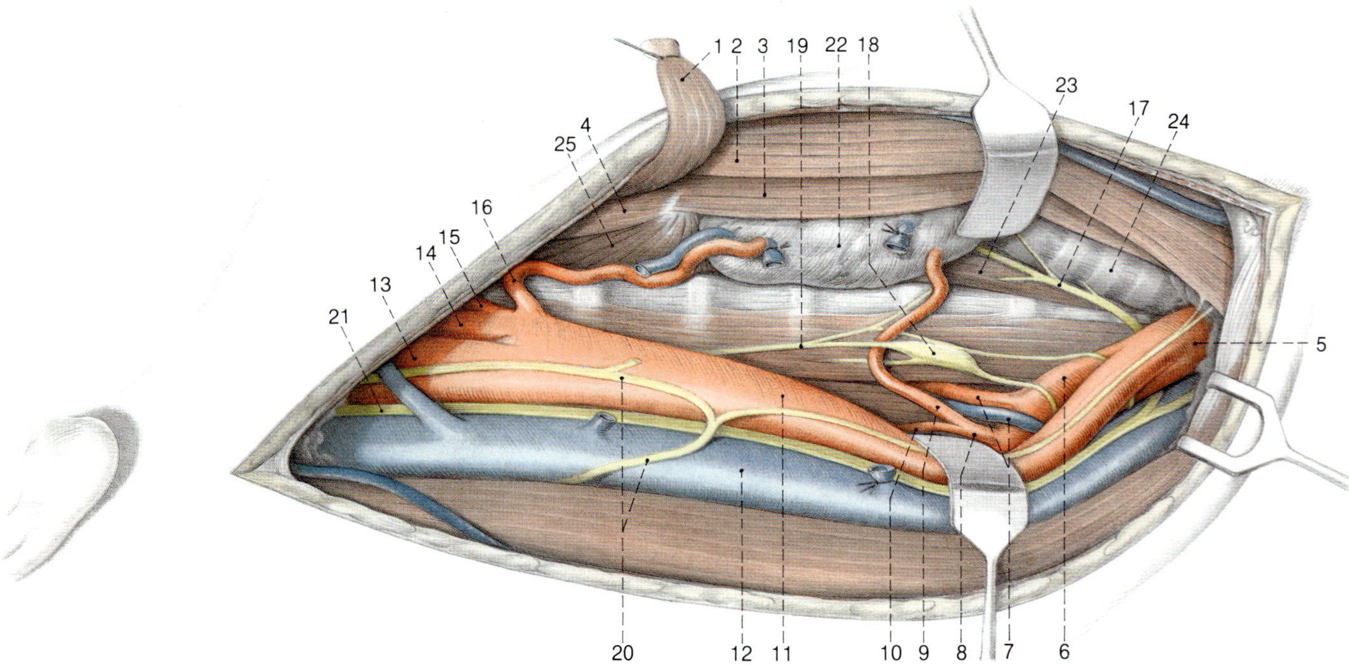

Fig. 1.**21** Anatomical site of the cervical spine, as seen from the right and front. Note the course of the recurrent laryngeal nerve.

1 Omohyoid muscle
2 Sternohyoid muscle
3 Sternothyroid muscle
4 Thyrohyoid muscle
5 Brachiocephalic trunk
6 Subclavian artery
7 Vertebral artery and vein
8 Thyrocervical trunk
9 Inferior thyroid artery
10 Ascending cervical artery
11 Common carotid artery
12 Internal jugular vein
13 Internal carotid artery
14 External carotid artery
15 Lingual artery
16 Superior thyroid artery
17 Recurrent laryngeal nerve
18 Stellate ganglion
19 Sympathetic trunk
20 Deep ansa cervicalis
21 Vagus nerve
22 Thyroid gland
23 Esophagus
24 Trachea
25 Pharynx

Thoracic Spine

Transthoracic Approach to Thoracic Spine T4–T11

Indications

- Kyphosis
- Scoliosis
- Vertebral fractures
- Tumors
- Spondylitis

Choice of Side of Approach

Generally speaking, the thoracic spine may be approached either by a right-sided or by a left-sided thoracotomy. If the indication does not dictate the use of one side, a right-sided thoracotomy seems appropriate, because of the vascular localization (left-sided course of the aorta). However, in cases of scoliosis, the thoracotomy is always performed on the side of the convexity.

Posterolateral Thoracotomy with Rib Resection

For an orthopedic indication, thoracotomy usually includes a rib resection. This gives better exposure in adult patients and in the presence of thoracic deformities associated with spinal deformities; in addition, the resected rib may be used as chip material for spinal fusion.

Choice of Rib to be Resected

As a rule, the approach is made two ribs higher than the center of the lesion. Due to the descending course of the ribs, it is easier to dissect caudally along the lower rib than proximally. When a rib that is situated too far caudally is chosen, it is difficult to reach the upper end of the deformity. In younger individuals with mobile ribs, it may be possible to reach the vertebra that corresponds to the resected rib. Should this prove difficult, the segment of the next higher rib that is close to the spine may be resected by the same approach. In favorable conditions, the following vertebrae can be reached:

- Resection of fifth rib: approach to T5–T11
- Resection of sixth rib: approach to T6–T12
- Resection of seventh rib: approach to T7–L1

There are exceptions to this rule. In patients with horizontally coursing ribs, resection of the sixth rib may permit exposure of vertebrae T5–T11. On the other hand, when the ribs slope steeply, resection of the fifth rib will only allow T6–T11 to be exposed. Finally, in patients with a severe curvature of the spine and commensurate thoracic deformities, it may be possible to reach no more than two or three vertebrae by rib resection and thoracotomy.

Positioning and Incision

The operation is performed with the patient in a lateral decubitus position. Good extension in the operative field can be obtained by raising the kidney rest or slightly tilting the operating table. The skin incision is slightly S-shaped and bypasses the scapula above the selected rib. It begins about four finger-breadths inferior to the spinous processes and moves anteriorly as far as the costochondral junction (Fig. 1.**22**). Hereafter, the latissimus dorsi muscle is completely divided in a direction transverse to that of the fibers (Fig. 1.**23**). Because of the neural supply (thoracoposterior nerve), this should be done as far caudally as possible. In the anterior region of the wound, the anterior serratus

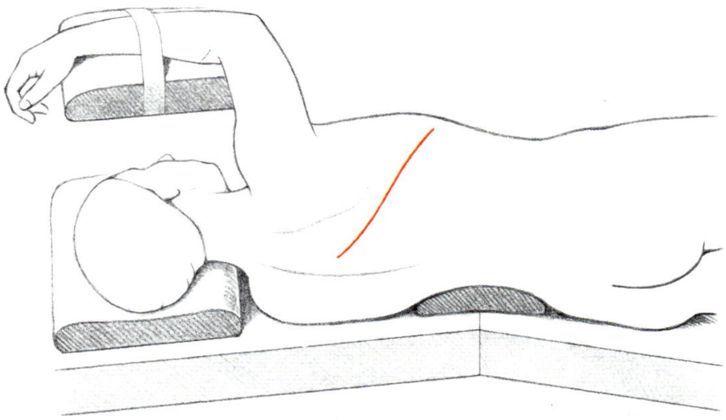

Fig. 1.**22** Positioning and incision.

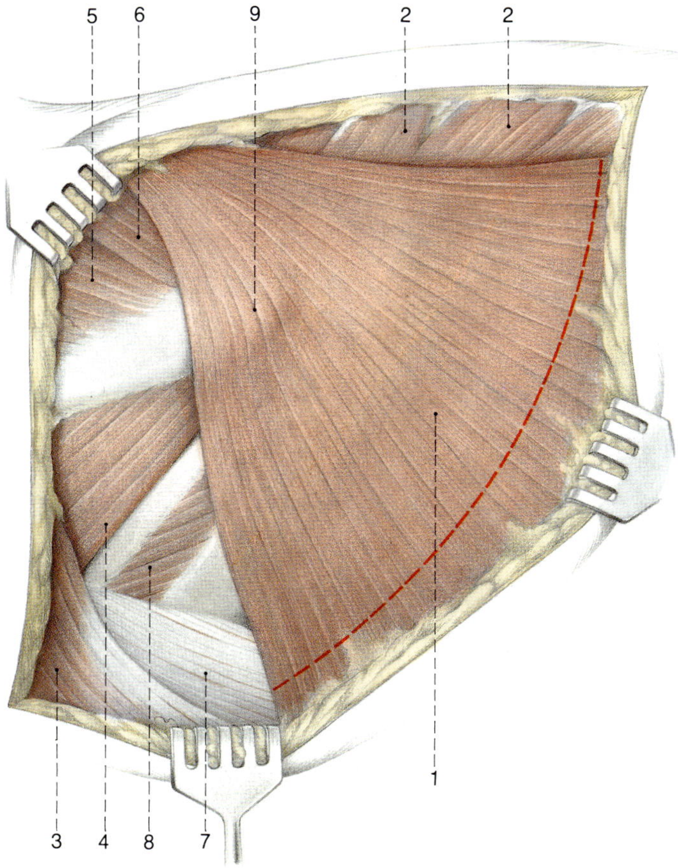

Fig. 1.**23** Anatomical exposure of the operative field after transection of the skin and subcutis. The muscular fasciae have been removed.

1 Latissimus dorsi muscle
2 Anterior serratus muscle
3 Trapezius muscle
4 Greater rhomboid muscle
5 Infraspinous muscle
6 Teres major muscle
7 Iliocostal muscle of the thorax
8 External intercostal muscle
9 Inferior angle of scapula

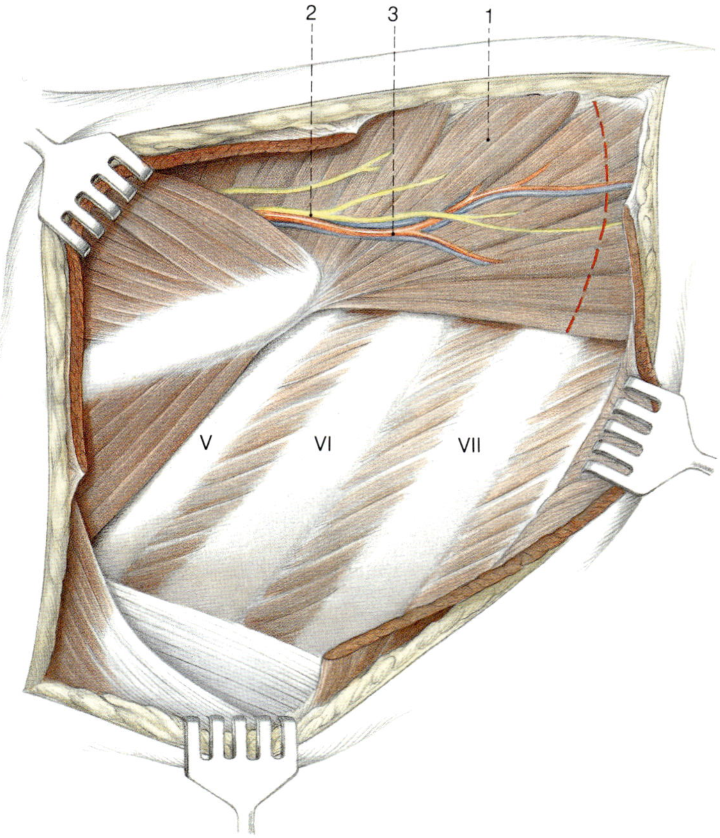

Fig. 1.**24** Anatomical exposure of the operative field after division of the latissimus dorsi muscle and before incision of the anterior serratus muscle. The appropriate incision site is identified by a dashed line.

1 Anterior serratus muscle
2 Long thoracic nerve
3 Lateral thoracic vessels
V–VII Ribs

muscle is exposed. It is now possible to pass a hand behind this muscle below the scapula and to count off the ribs from cranial to caudal. The first rib usually cannot be palpated, and the first palpable rib is therefore the second one. The anterior serratus muscle is likewise transected as far caudally as possible in order to spare the long thoracic nerve approaching from a superior direction as far as possible (Fig. 1.**24**). The periosteum of the selected rib is divided anteriorly with the diathermy knife as far as the costochondral boundary (Fig. 1.**25**) and is initially retracted with a straight elevator. At the superior margin of the rib, the dissection follows the course of the intercostal musculature from posterior to anterior; at the inferior margin, it proceeds from anterior to posterior. Complete exposure of the rib with the rib stripper follows (Fig. 1.**26**).

After the dissection, the rib is divided anteriorly at the costochondral border and raised; posteriorly, it is ablated with rib shears about two finger-breadths lateral to the costotransverse articulation. The thoracic cavity can now be opened in the bed of the resected rib (Fig. 1.**27**).

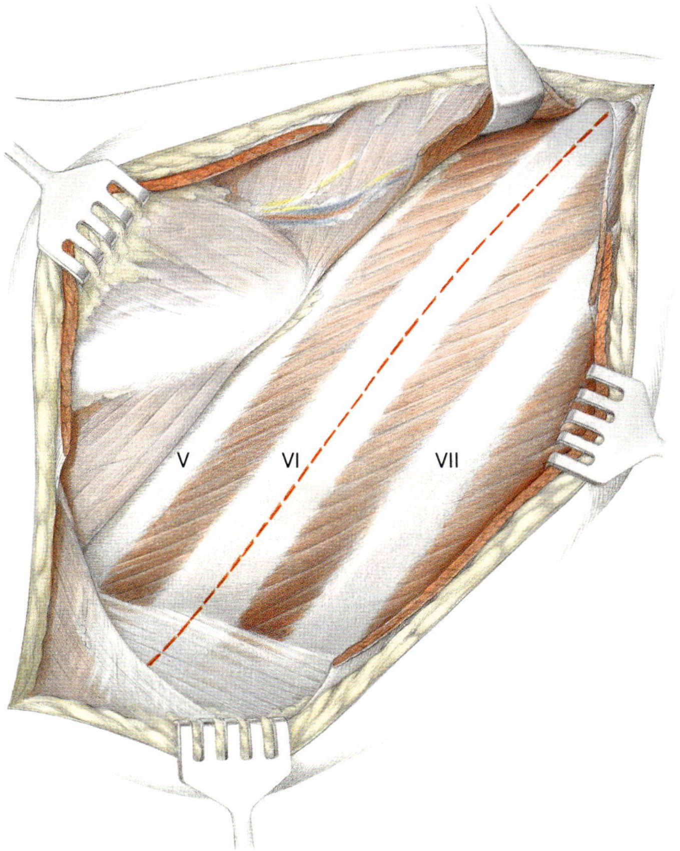

Fig. 1.**25** Operative site after division of the anterior serratus muscle. The periosteum is split over the sixth rib along the red dashed line.

V–VII Ribs

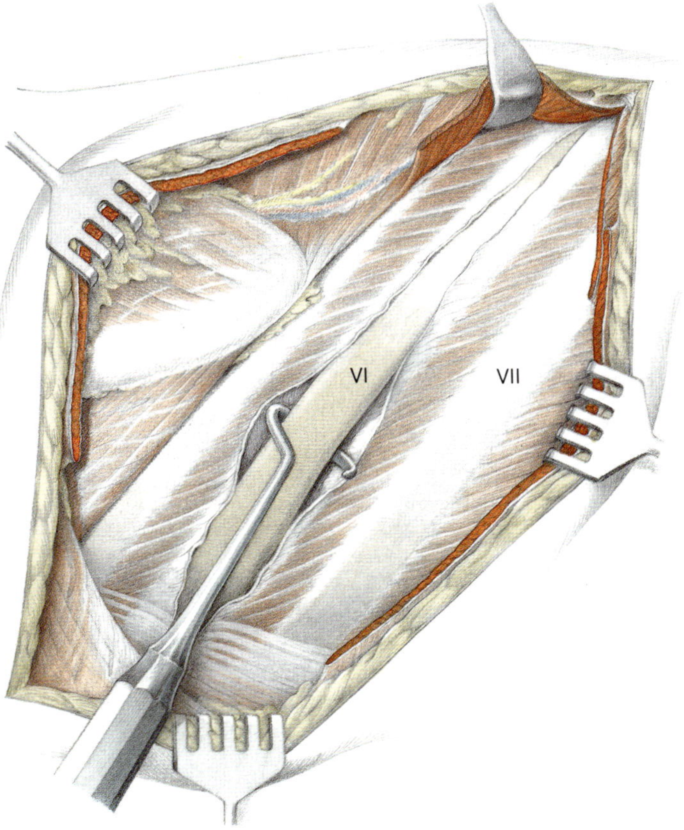

Fig. 1.**26.** Operative site after splitting of the periosteum and enucleation of the sixth rib with a rib stripper.

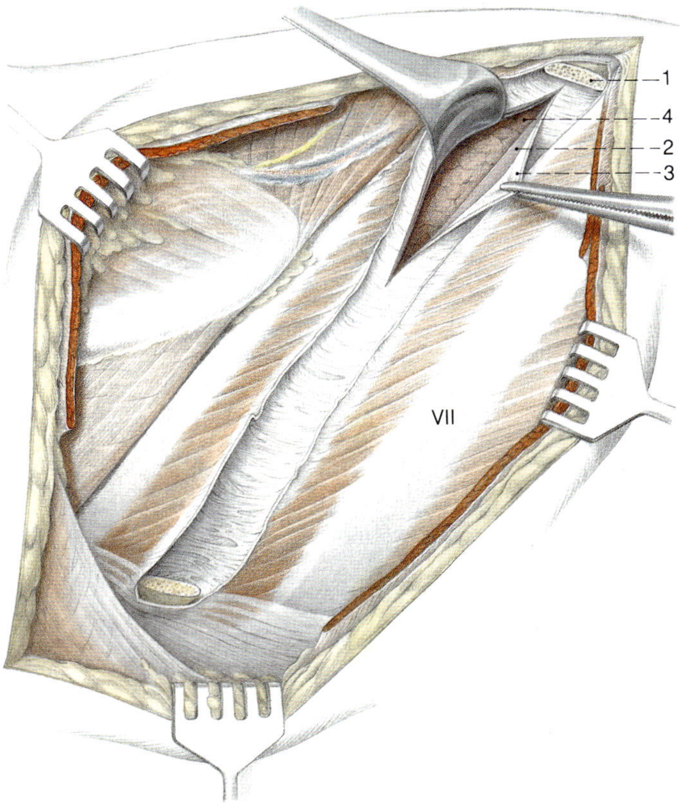

Fig. 1.**27** Operative site after rib resection and partial division of the periosteum and costal pleura.

1 Resection stump of the sixth rib
2 Costal pleura
3 Periosteum
4 Lung
VII Rib

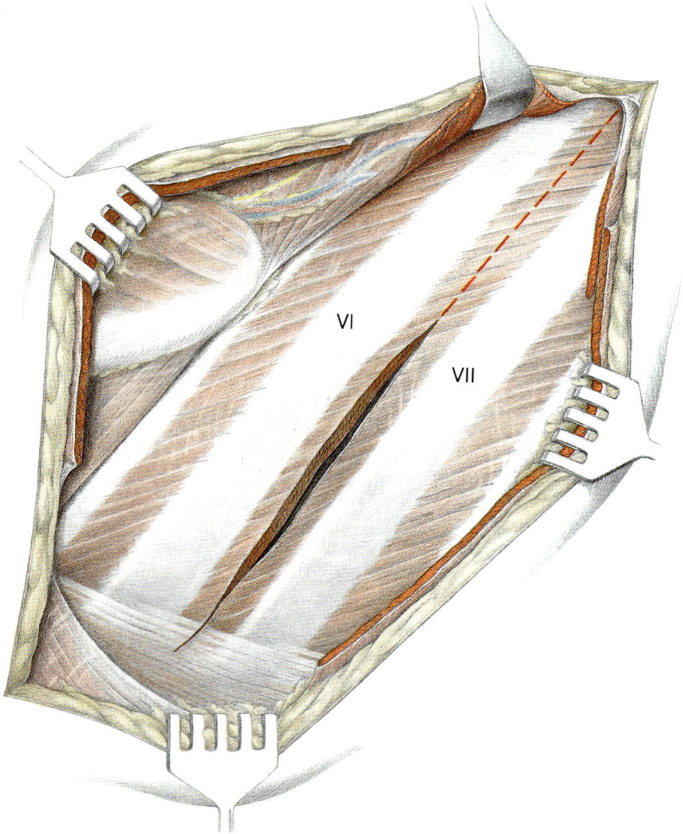

Fig. 1.**28** Intercostal approach to the pleural cavity. The intercostal muscles are divided between the sixth and seventh ribs. Care should always be taken to make the incision at the superior border of the lower rib, to avoid injury to the intercostal vessels and the intercostal nerve.

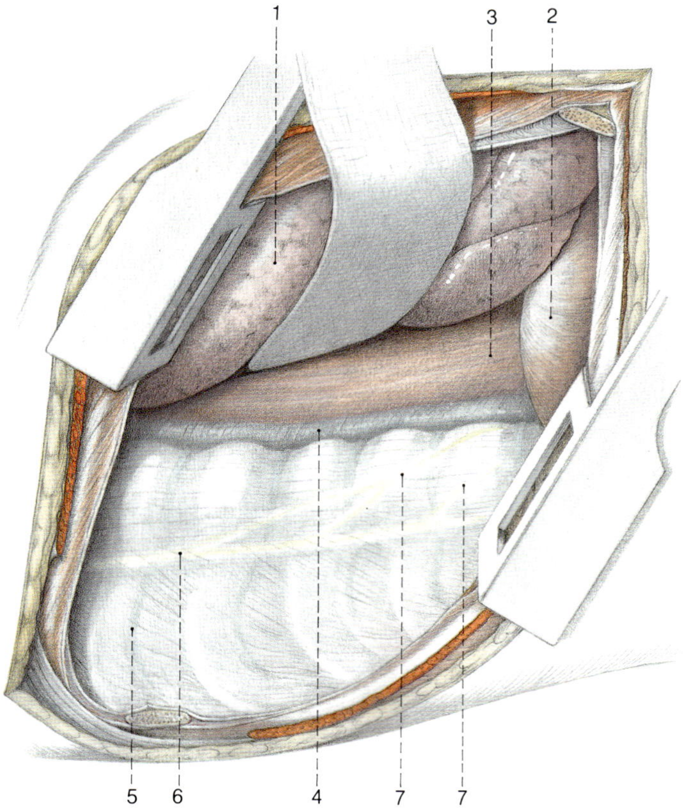

Fig. 1.**29** Operative site after opening of the pleural cavity. The parietal pleura (costal and mediastinal pleura) is preserved.

1 Right lung
2 Thoracic diaphragm
3 Esophagus
4 Azygos vein
5 Intercostal vessels
6 Sympathetic trunk
7 Greater splanchnic nerve

} Visible through the parietal pleura

Intercostal Thoracotomy

In children and adolescents with a mobile thorax, the thoracotomy may also be performed intercostally. This is indicated particularly if only a few vertebral bodies need to be exposed, and the rib is not needed for chips. The positioning and incision will be the same as for a posterolateral thoracotomy with rib resection. Division of the latissimus dorsi and anterior serratus muscles gives access to the selected intercostal space. As a rule, a plastic protector is inserted between the intercostal musculature and the parietal pleura, through which the intercostal musculature can then be divided with the diathermy knife (Fig. 1.**28**). The procedure following division of the parietal pleura conforms to thoracotomy with rib resection.

A thoracotomy spreader is used after complete transection of the pleura, and the thoracic cavity is opened. The lung is retracted anteriorly, and a good exposure is then obtained of the vertebrae covered by the parietal pleura (Fig. 1.**29**).

Anatomical Site

The anatomy of the posterior mediastinum and the retropleural space is shown in Figures 1.**30**–1.**32**. We shall briefly discuss the most important anatomical variations in structure in the posterior mediastinum (Figs. 1.**33**, 1.**34**). Injury to the thoracic duct during exposure of the vertebrae should be avoided if possible. A chylothorax may otherwise result. Figure 1.**33** shows variations in the course of the thoracic duct. It is evident that the thoracic duct follows the course of the aorta on the right side. Variations of the azygos and hemiazygos veins are shown in Figure 1.**34**. As a rule, the vertebrae can be accessed by a preferably median division of the intercostal veins, without violating the longitudinal venous systems.

Fig. 1.**30** Anatomical site of the posterior mediastinum and retropleural space, as seen from anterior.

1 Ascending aorta
2 Aortic arch
3 Brachiocephalic trunk
4 Left common carotid artery
5 Left subclavian artery
6 Intercostal arteries
7 Abdominal aorta
8 Celiac trunk
9 Superior vena cava
10 Entry of azygos vein
11 Right brachiocephalic vein
12 Left brachiocephalic vein
13 Accessory hemiazygos vein
14 Azygos vein
15 Hemiazygos vein
16 Intercostal veins
17 Thoracic duct
18 Right vagus nerve
19 Left vagus nerve
20 Esophageal plexus
21 Vagal trunks
22 Sympathetic trunk with ganglia
23 Greater splanchnic nerve
24 Lesser splanchnic nerve
25 Intercostal nerves
26 Subcostal nerve
27 Trachea
28 Esophagus
29 Thoracic diaphragm
V–XII Ribs

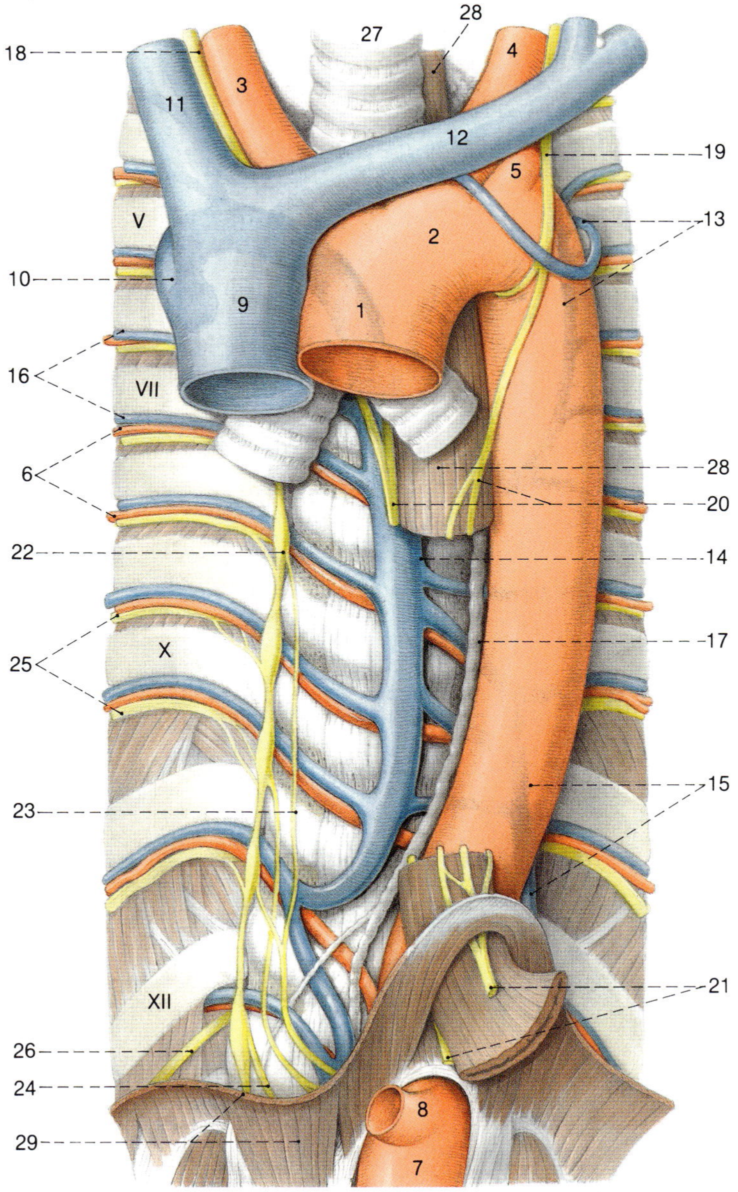

Fig. 1.**31** Anatomical site of the right half of the posterior mediastinum and right retropleural space.

1 Right lung
2 Esophagus
3 Cut border of parietal pleura
4 Esophageal plexus of vagus nerves
5 Thoracic diaphragm
6 Azygos vein
7 Intercostal vessels
8 Sympathetic trunk
9 Greater splanchnic nerve
10 Communicating branches
11 Intercostal nerve
I–X Ribs

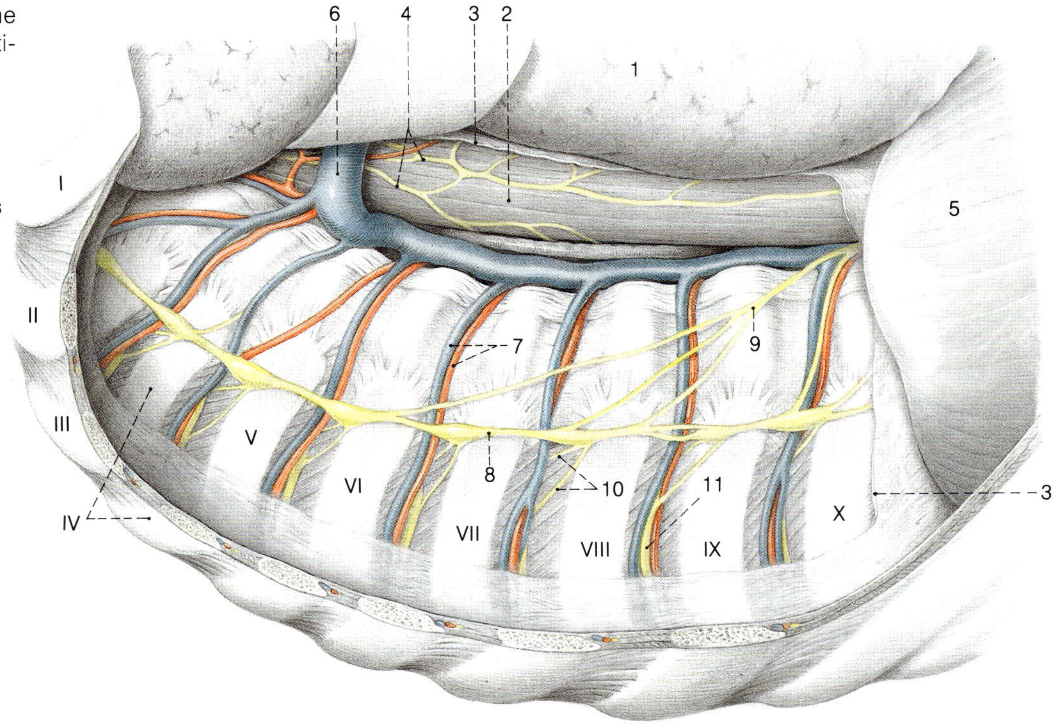

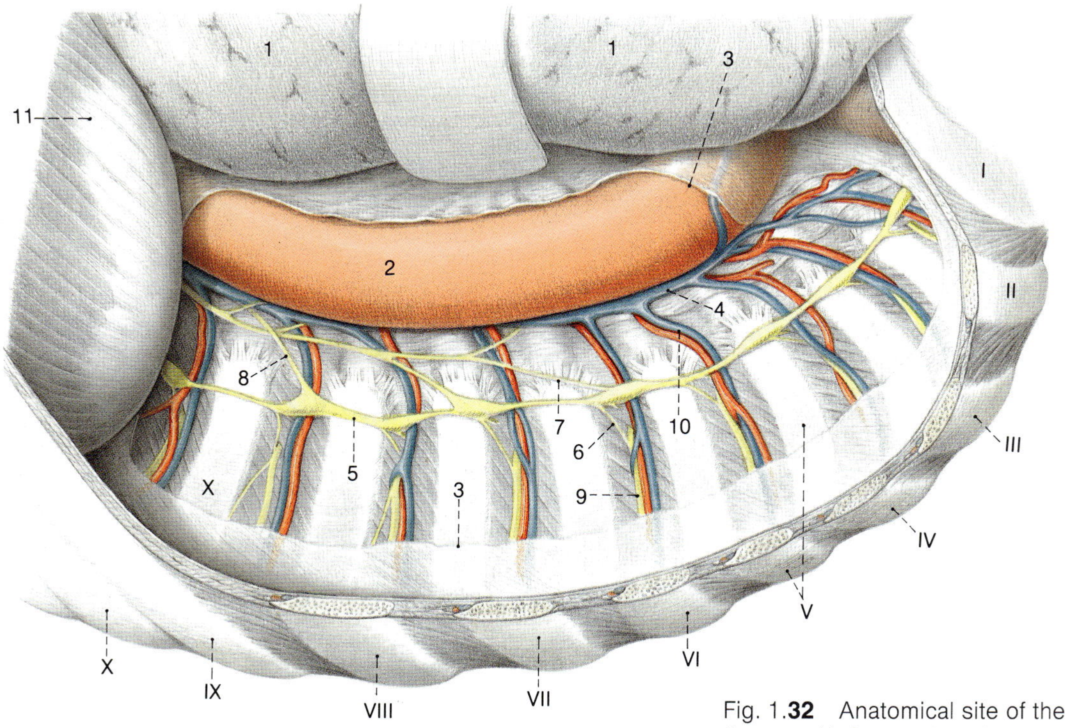

1 Left lung
2 Thoracic aorta
3 Cut border of parietal pleura
4 Accessory hemiazygos vein
5 Sympathetic trunk
6 Communicating branches
7 Greater splanchnic nerve
8 Lesser splanchnic nerve
9 Intercostal nerve
10 Intercostal vessels
11 Thoracic diaphragm
I–X Ribs

Fig. 1.**32** Anatomical site of the left half of the posterior mediastinum and left retropleural space.

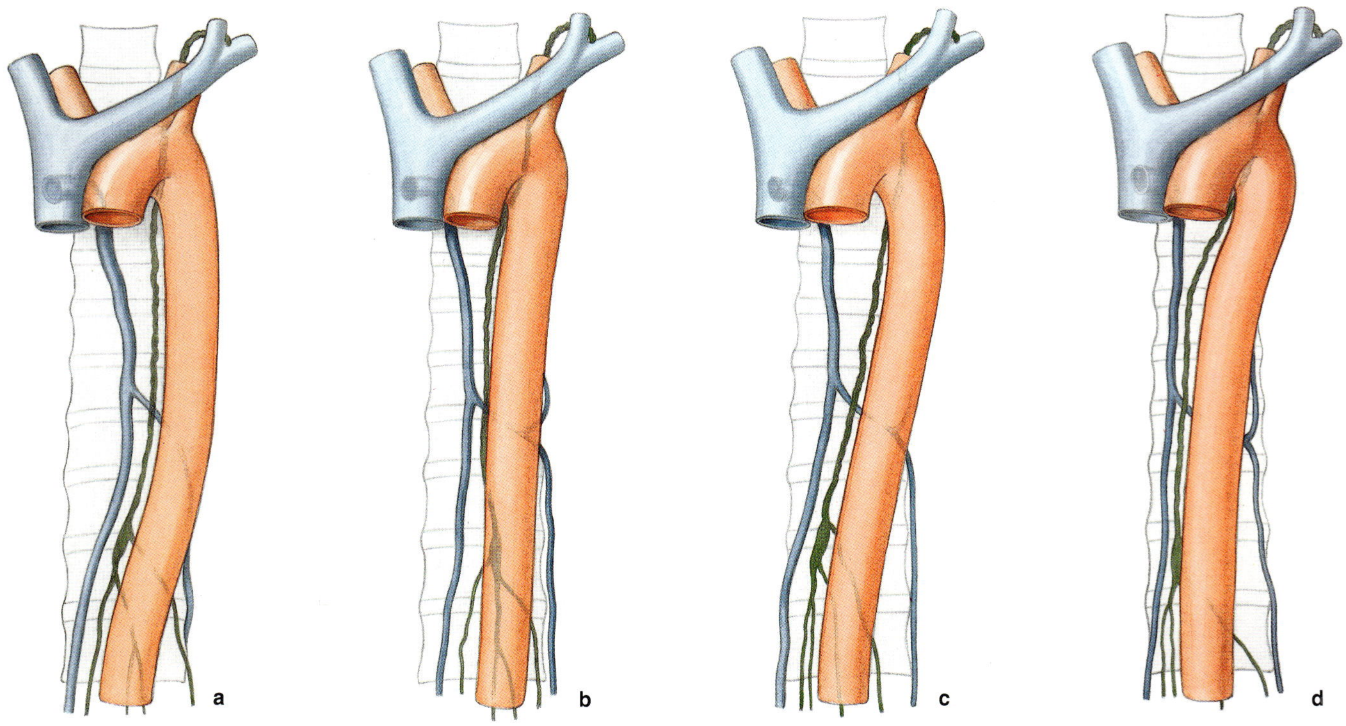

Fig. 1.**33** Positional variants of the thoracic aorta, azygos vein, and thoracic duct in relation to the thoracic spine (according to Kubik 1975). The left-sided position of the topographic unit of the thoracic duct–aorta–azygos vein may be considered an age-related displacement (83 percent of the individuals with left-sided position were over 70 years old).

a Left-sided position (36%)
b Middle position (20%)
c Oblique position (17%)
d Right-sided position (6%)

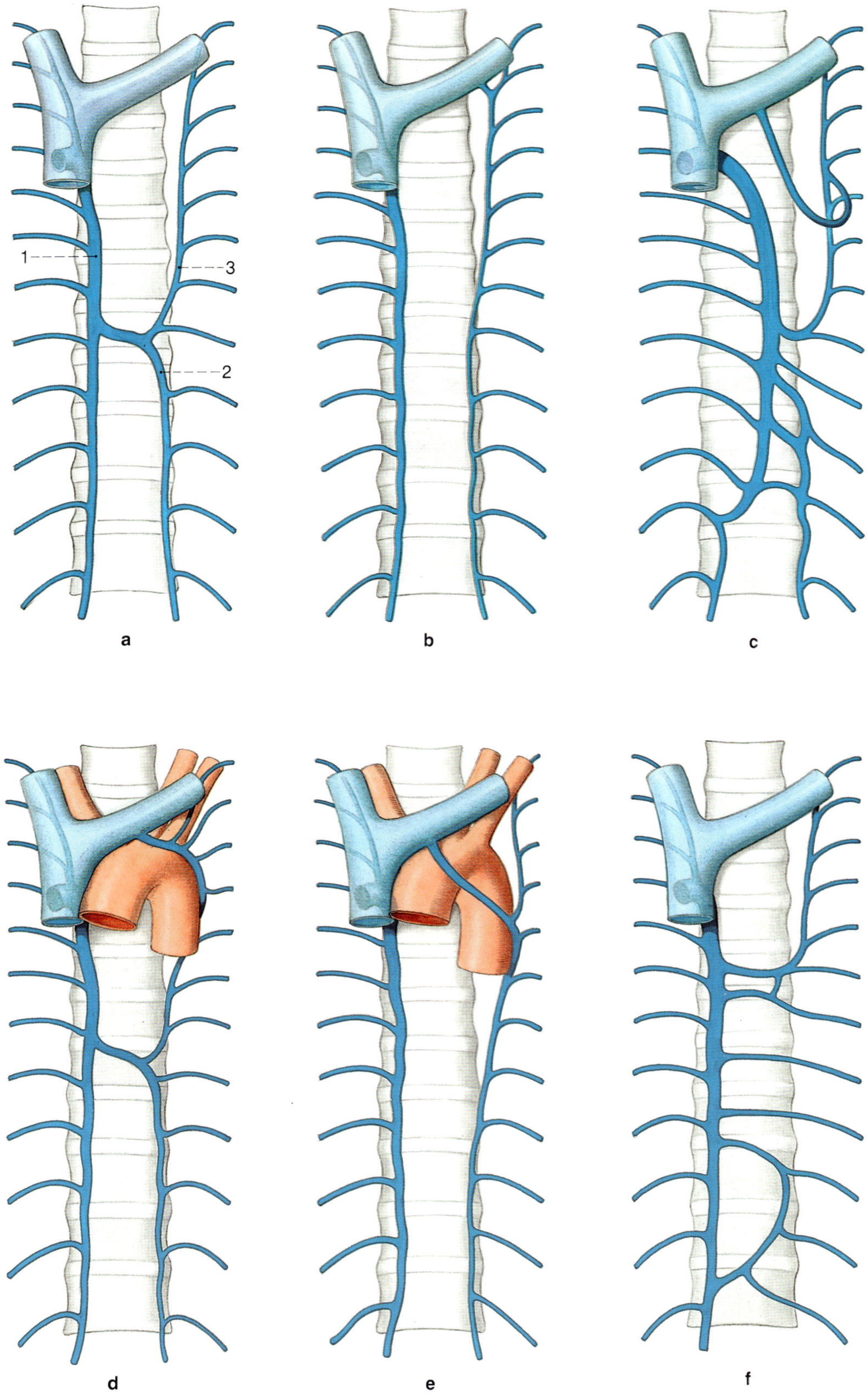

Fig. 1.**34** Variants in the shape and position of the azygos–hemiazygos venous system (according to Adachi 1931, Cordier et al. 1938, and our own observations).

a "Classic type"
1 Azygos vein
2 Hemiazygos vein
3 Accessory hemiazygos vein

b Absence of anastomosis between the azygos vein and the hemiazygos vein
c Multiple arcade formations and age-related arcuate leftward displacement of the azygos vein
d Cranioaortic arc of the hemiazygos vein
e Lateroaortic arc of the azygos vein and absence of an anastomosis between the azygos vein and the hemiazygos vein
f Multiple prevertebral anastomoses; absence of the hemiazygos vein.

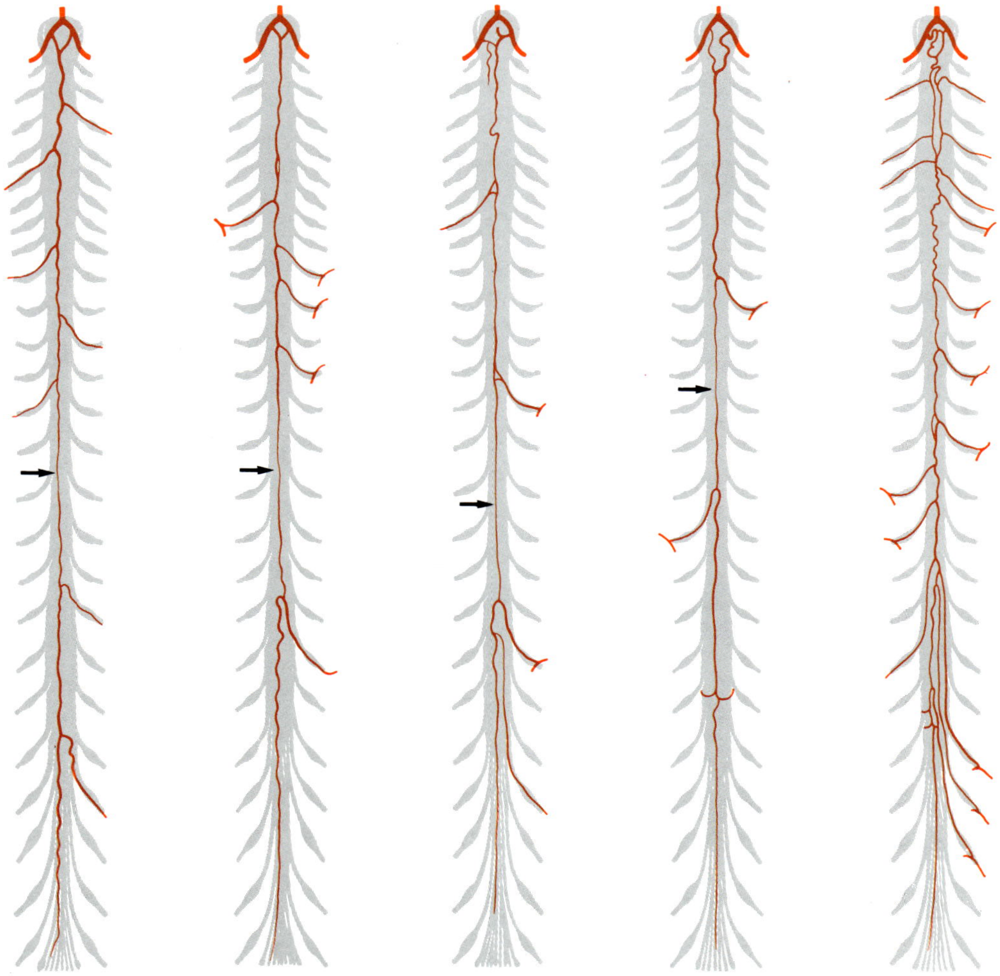

Fig. 1.**35** The segmental arterial tributaries of the spinal cord. "Critical supply zones" are indicated by arrows (after Dommisse 1974 and Kahle 1976).

Blood Supply of the Spinal Cord

The vascular supply of the spinal cord is of special importance in spinal surgery. We shall therefore briefly discuss the principal vascular supply here (Figs. 1.**35**, 1.**36**). The spinal cord is supplied by two different arterial systems: on the one hand by the vertebral arteries, which divide caudally into two posterior spinal arteries and one anterior spinal artery; and on the other by branches of the posterior intercostal arteries. With regard to the transthoracic approach to the spine, we shall consider only the latter; they are the spinal branches of the dorsal branches of the posterior intercostal arteries (Fig. 1.**36**). The segmental arteries, which reach the spinal cord via the interspinal foramina and anastomose with the anterior spinal artery, are variable in number and size, so that a classification does not seem feasible. At least two, and at most 16, spinal branches have been noted which approach the spinal cord at different levels and contribute to its blood supply (Dommisse 1974). The largest is the great radicular artery (Adamkiewicz artery), which in 80 percent of cases originates from a left posterior intercostal artery, at the level between the seventh thoracic and the fourth lumbar vertebrae, and here most commonly between the ninth and eleventh thoracic vertebrae.

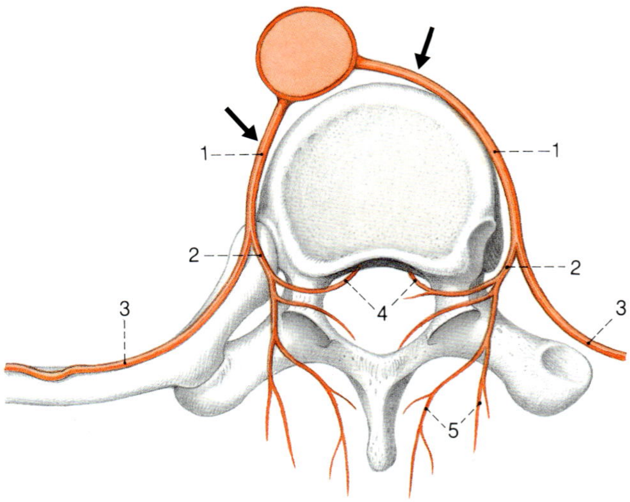

Fig. 1.**36** The blood supply of the vertebral canal and the spinal cord by a transverse section (according to Crock et al. 1977). The arrows show the appropriate ligature sites.

1 Posterior intercostal artery
2 Posterior branch
3 Anterior branch
4 Spinal branches
5 Muscular and cutaneous branches

Although it is important, it should be noted that the Adamkiewicz artery by itself is hardly sufficient to supply the caudal segments of the spinal cord alone. There are actually several medullary feeder arteries at different levels that are of major importance for maintaining the spinal cord supply. This also accounts for the experience of spinal surgeons who, especially while treating scoliosis, have ligated between four and 16 segmental arteries without causing any neurological deficits. It seems nevertheless necessary to spare the segmental arterial feeders to the spinal cord as far as possible.

The number and size of the cervical and lumbar medullary supply branches exceeds that in the area of the thoracic cord. The region of the thoracic medulla is also described as a watershed. The "critical supply zone" of the spinal cord generally lies between the fourth and ninth thoracic vertebrae, and operative measures in this zone require careful dissection.

When exposing the vertebrae by an anterior approach, it is imperative that the segmental arteries should be divided as far anteriorly as possible, and in addition, the vessels should be dissected free in the posterior direction over a short distance only (Fig. 1.**36**). In this manner, the arterial arcades that join the segmental arteries outside and within the vertebral canal are preserved. So as not to damage the spinal branches, one should not use electrocoagulation on the vessels in the vicinity of the intervertebral foramen.

Site of Thoracotomy in Scoliosis

(Figs. 1.**37**, 1.**38**)

In scoliosis, thoracotomy is always performed on the side of the convexity. Due to the severe vertebral torsion associated with scoliosis and the posterior rib hump on the convex side, contact is often made with the spine, which lies only a few centimeters below the resected rib, immediately following thoracotomy. The large thoracic vessels generally do not follow the line of the curvature, or do not follow it completely, and are therefore mostly found on the concave side. This means that in left-sided thoracotomy for left convex thoracic scoliosis, the aorta will generally be found on the right side of the spinal column.

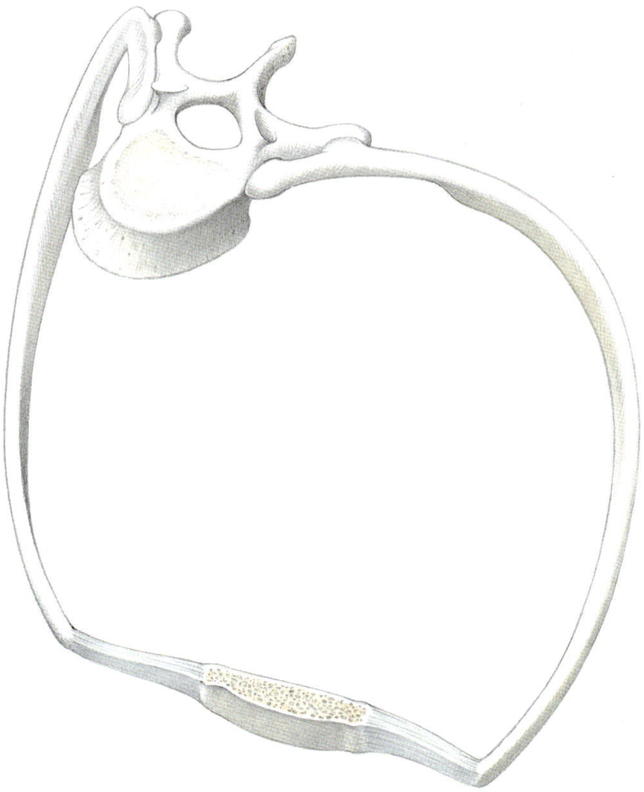

Fig. 1.**37** A vertebrocostal segment in severe right-sided scoliosis of the thoracic spine. The corpus of the right rib is nearly adherent to the thoracic vertebra.

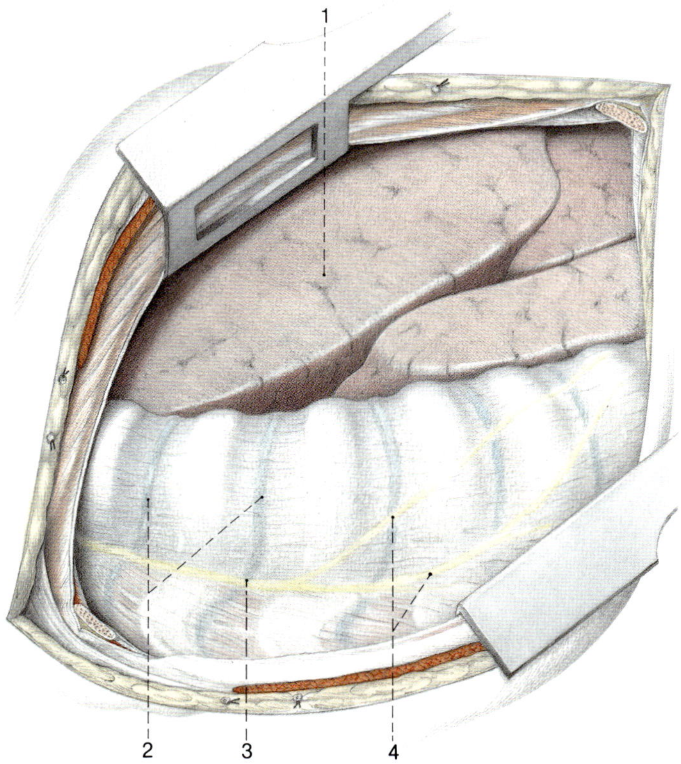

Fig. 1.**38** Operative site in right-sided convex scoliosis after opening of the pleural cavity. The vertebral pleura has not been split; the spine protrudes into the right pleural cavity, and the right lung has been displaced leftward.

1 Right lung
2 Intercostal vessels
3 Sympathetic trunk
4 Greater splanchnic nerve

Exposure of Individual Vertebrae

After thoracotomy, the vertebral pleura is preferably divided in the midline of the vertebrae, attention being paid particularly to vertebral torsion in scoliosis (see Fig. 1.**37**). The segmental vessels are exposed, ligated, and transected in the midline. After this, the entire anterior circumference of the vertebrae and intervertebral disks is accessible (Fig. 1.**39**).

Closure of Thoracotomy with Rib Resection

(Fig. 1.**40**)

A chest tube is placed. A rib approximator is applied, after which the pleura, periosteum, and intercostal musculature are, as a rule, readapted with a running suture (Fig. 1.**40**), followed by suturing of the anterior serratus and latissimus dorsi muscles (Fig. 1.**41**).

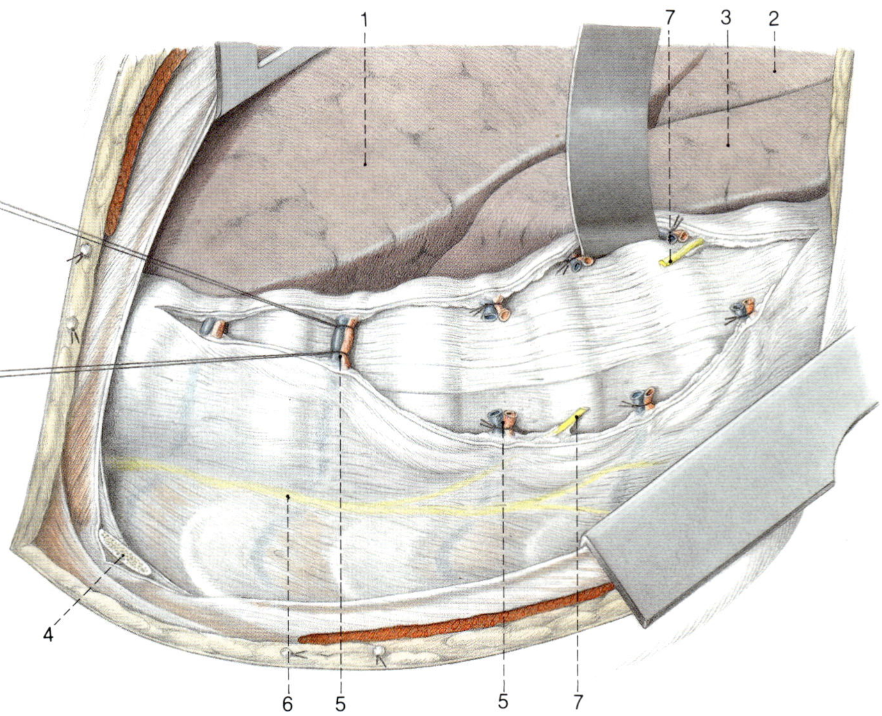

Fig. 1.**39** Operative site. The vertebral pleura has been split, and the intercostal vessels have been partly ligated or transected.

1 Superior lobe ⎫
2 Middle lobe ⎬ Right lung
3 Inferior lobe ⎭
4 Resection stump of the sixth rib
5 Intercostal vessels
6 Sympathetic trunk visible through the parietal pleura
7 Greater splanchnic nerve

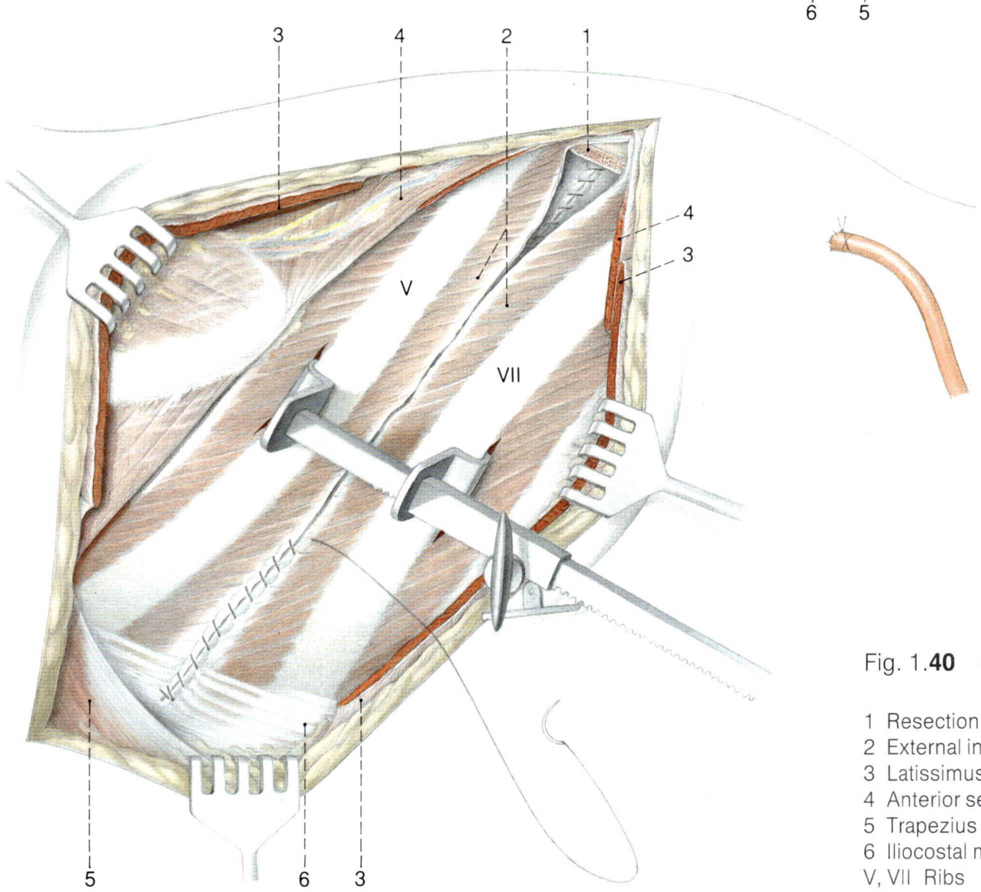

Fig. 1.**40** Closure of thorax with a rib approximator.

1 Resection stump of the sixth rib
2 External intercostal muscle
3 Latissimus dorsi muscle
4 Anterior serratus muscle
5 Trapezius muscle
6 Iliocostal muscle of the thorax
V, VII Ribs

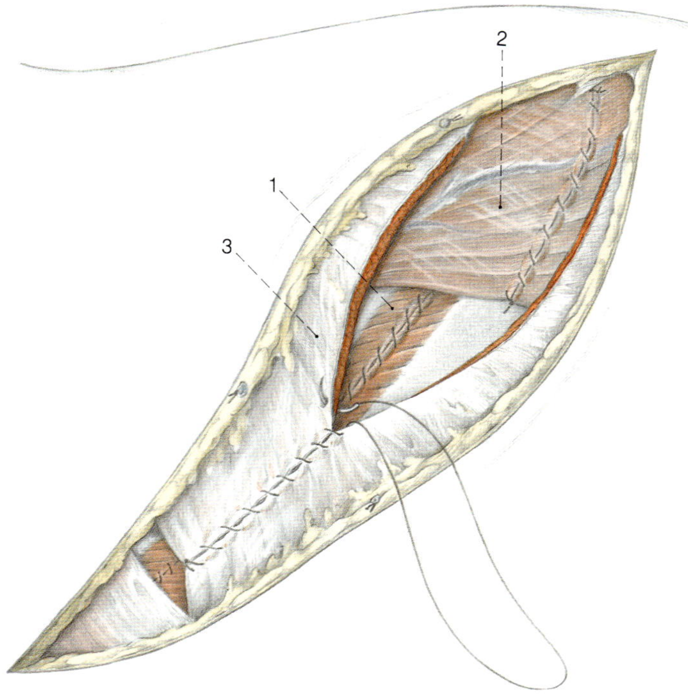

Fig. 1.**41** Suture of the extremity musculature of the thorax.

1 External intercostal muscle
2 Anterior serratus muscle
3 Latissimus dorsi muscle

Closure of Intercostal Thoracotomy

(Fig. 1.**42**)

Absorbable sutures are placed around the ribs. To avoid injury to the intercostal artery and bleeding, the insertion should not be made directly beneath the caudal rib. The pleura and intercostal musculature are readapted with the aid of the rib approximator, and the pericostal sutures are then tied. After this, closure is carried out in the same way as following thoracotomy with rib resection.

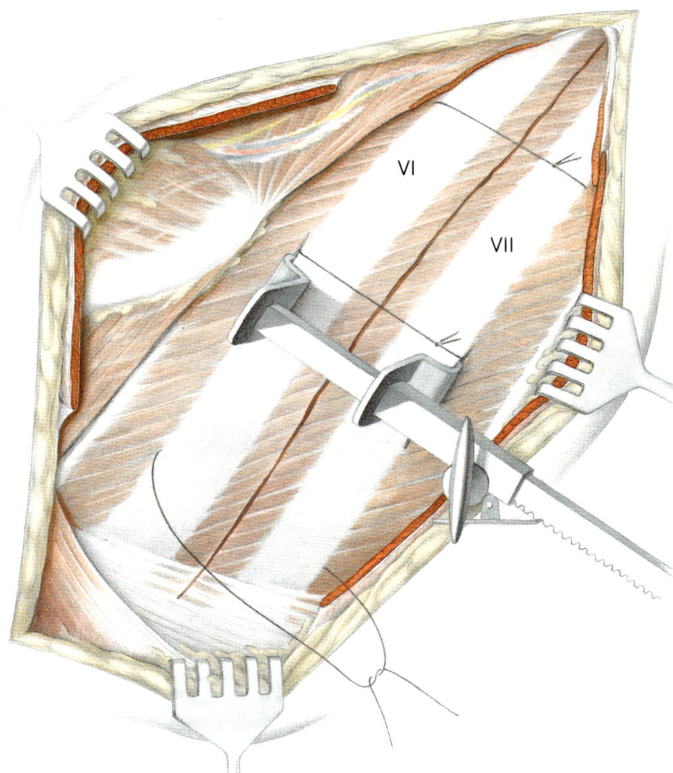

Fig. 1.**42** Closure of the thorax after intercostal thoracotomy.

VI, VII Ribs

Thoracolumbar Junction

Transpleural-Retroperitoneal Approach to the Thoracolumbar Spine, T9–L5 (Hodgson)

Principal Indications

- Scoliosis
- Kyphosis
- Vertebral fractures
- Tumors
- Spondylitis

Choice of Side of Approach

Generally speaking, exposure of the thoracolumbar junction is possible using a right-sided or a left-sided approach. If the indication does not mandate one or the other, the left-sided approach is preferable for anatomical reasons. The left subphrenic space is in a lower location, in addition to which right-sided exposure of the vertebrae is hampered by the liver and by the fragile inferior vena cava. In cases of scoliosis, entry on the convex side of the curvature is the rule.

Choice of Rib to be Resected

The standard approach with this technique, which is used mostly in the surgical treatment of scoliosis, is at the level of the ninth or tenth rib. Resection of the tenth rib gives access to the eleventh and possibly also the tenth thoracic vertebra, while choice of the ninth rib for the approach will naturally lead to the next more cranial segment. In younger patients, and in the presence of mobile ribs, it may be possible to reach the vertebral body corresponding to the resected rib. Should this prove difficult, the section of the next higher rib near the spine may be removed by the same approach. In favorable conditions, access is gained to the following vertebrae:

- Resection of the ninth rib: T9–L5
- Resection of the tenth rib: T10–L5

Positioning and Incision

(Fig. 1.**43**)

The patient is placed in a right lateral decubitus position. The skin incision begins posteriorly near the median line, follows the course of the tenth rib as far as the costal cartilage, and then continues obliquely downward on the upper and middle abdomen, following the direction of the segmental nerves (Fig. 1.**44**). It usually ends at a level between the umbilicus and the pubic symphysis. If only the thoracolumbar spinal junction needs to be exposed, the incision may be made shorter. After division of the skin, the dissection is continued with the diathermy knife. Thorough hemostasis is required during the operation. After this, the extremity musculature of the thorax is divided along the course of the tenth rib (Fig. 1.**45**). More distally, the internal oblique muscle of the abdomen is divided in the direction of the fibers, bringing into view the tenth rib (Fig. 1.**46**).

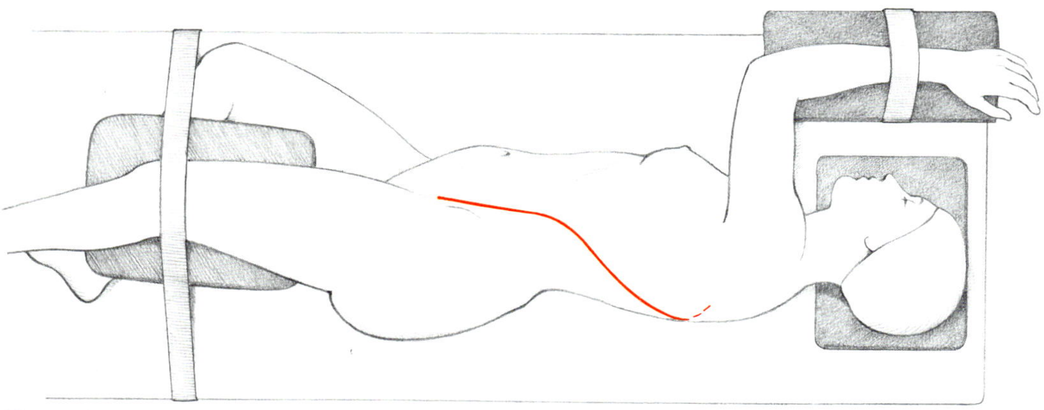

Fig. 1.**43** Approach to the thoracolumbar spine according to Hodgson. Positioning and incision.

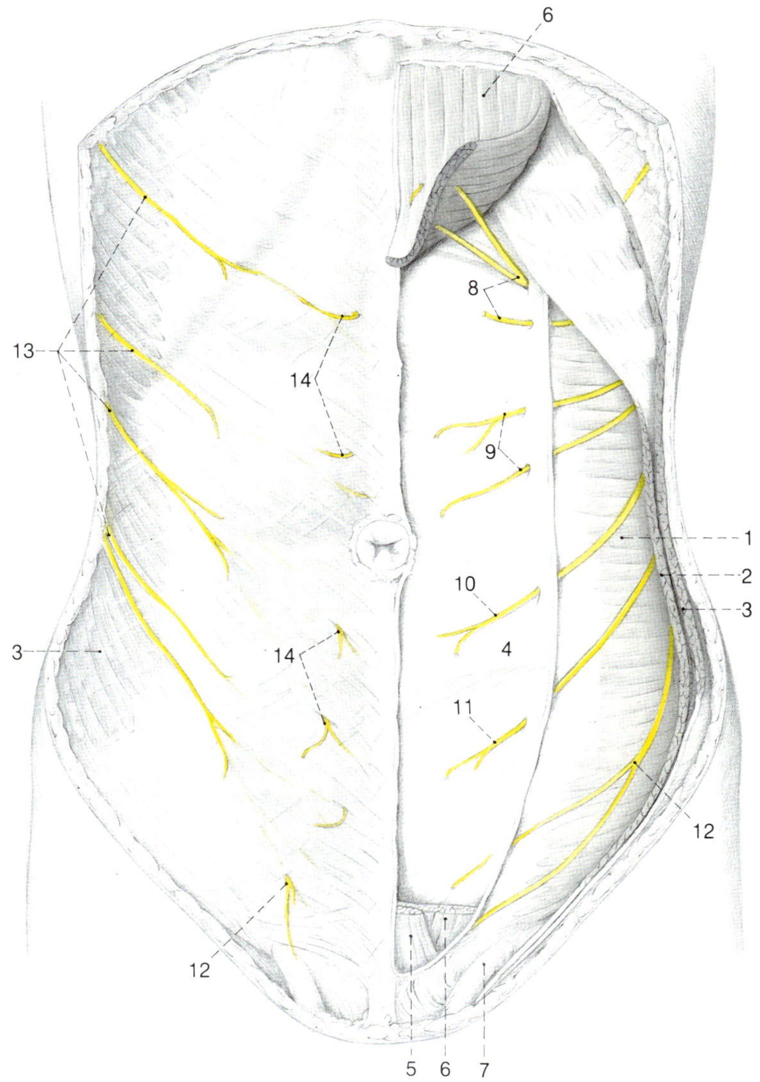

Fig. 1.**44** Exposure of the nerve supply of the anterior abdominal wall.

1 Transverse muscle of the abdomen
2 Internal oblique muscle of the abdomen
3 External oblique muscle of the abdomen
4 Sheath of the rectus abdominis muscle, posterior lamella
5 Pyramidal muscle
6 Rectus abdominis muscle
7 Spermatic cord
8 Ninth intercostal nerve
9 Tenth intercostal nerve
10 Eleventh intercostal nerve
11 Subcostal nerve
12 Iliohypogastric nerve
13 Lateral cutaneous branches
14 Anterior cutaneous branches

During the rest of the procedure, it proves advantageous to dissect the peritoneum first from the abdomen. The deep abdominal muscle layers (internal oblique and transverse muscles of the abdomen) are bluntly split with scissors, and two blunt retractors are inserted (Fig. 1.**46**). The peritoneum becomes visible in the depth and is now retracted medially from the lateral abdominal wall, using a swab on a stick. The deep abdominal muscle layers are further divided in the direction of the costal arch and parallel to the course of the neuromuscular bundle. This allows exposure of the upper lumbar spine retroperitoneally (Fig. 1.**47**). The peritoneum is then stripped from the inferior surface of the diaphragm.

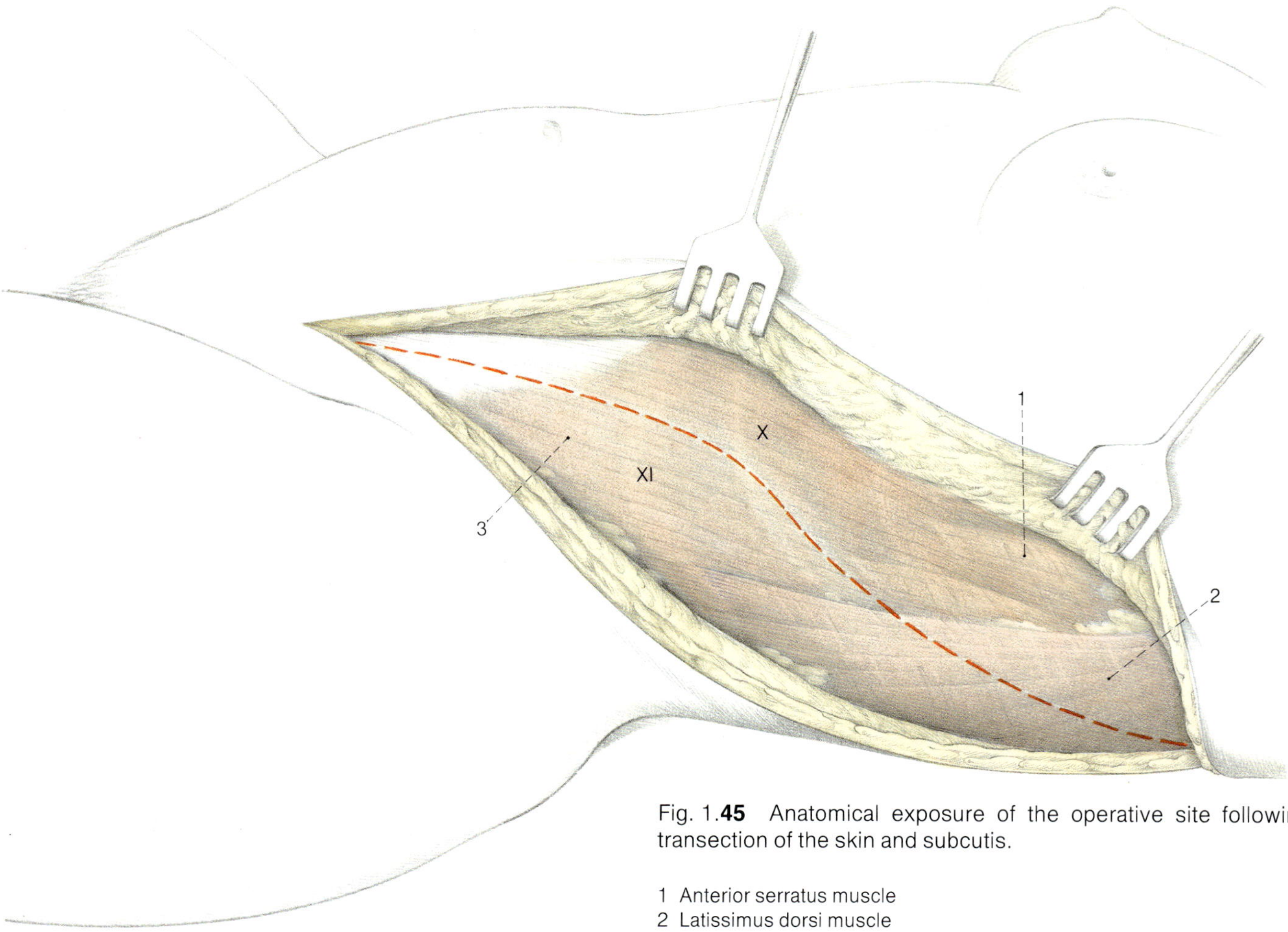

Fig. 1.**45** Anatomical exposure of the operative site following transection of the skin and subcutis.

1 Anterior serratus muscle
2 Latissimus dorsi muscle
3 External oblique muscle of the abdomen
X–XI Position of the ribs

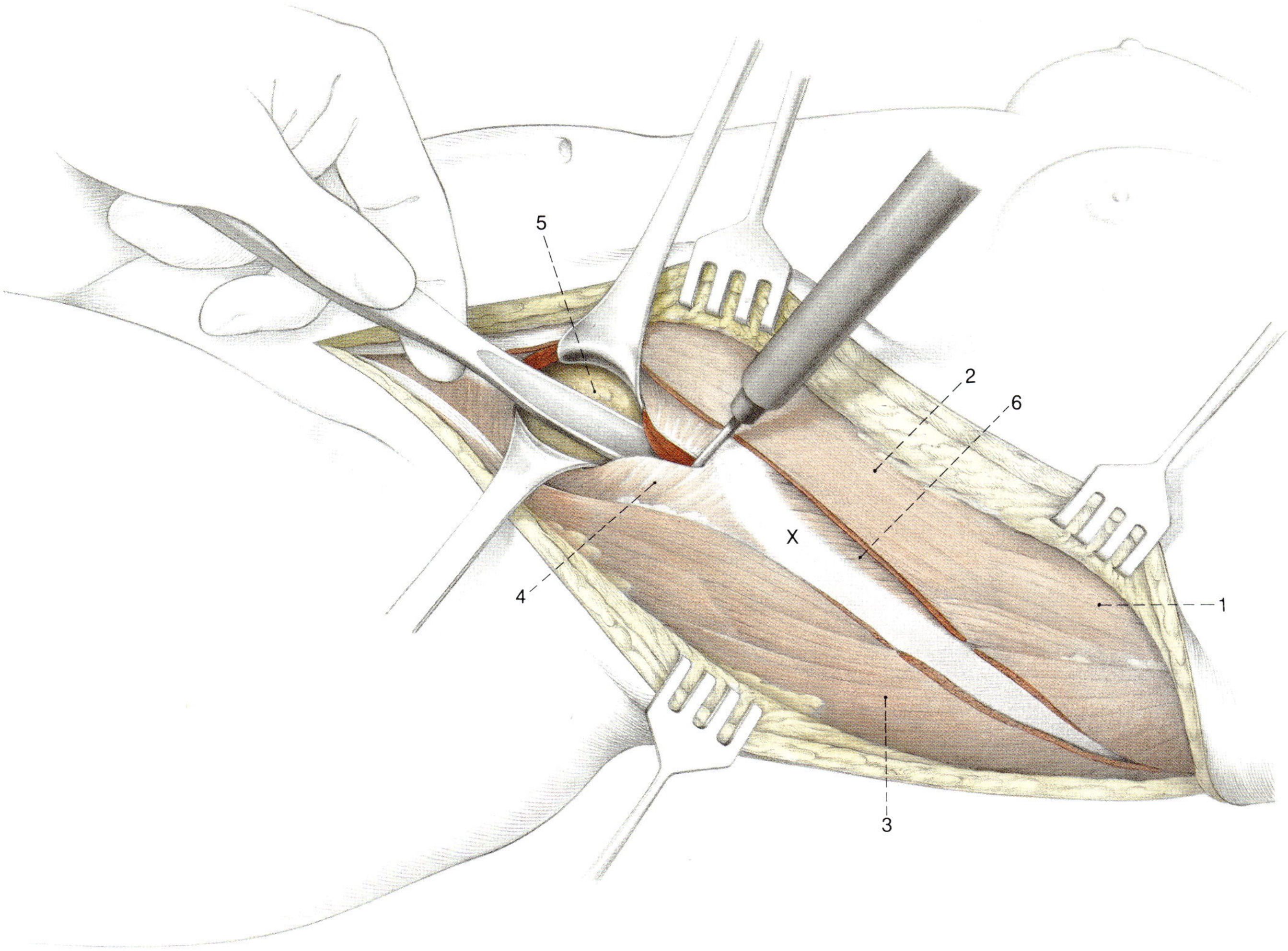

Fig. 1.**46** Operative site after division of the latissimus dorsi muscle, anterior serratus muscle, external oblique muscle of the abdomen, and of the deep abdominal muscle layers.

1 Anterior serratus muscle
2 External oblique muscle of the abdomen
3 Latissimus dorsi muscle
4 Internal oblique muscle of the abdomen and transverse muscle of the abdomen
5 Peritoneum with preperitoneal adipose tissue
6 External intercostal muscle
X Rib

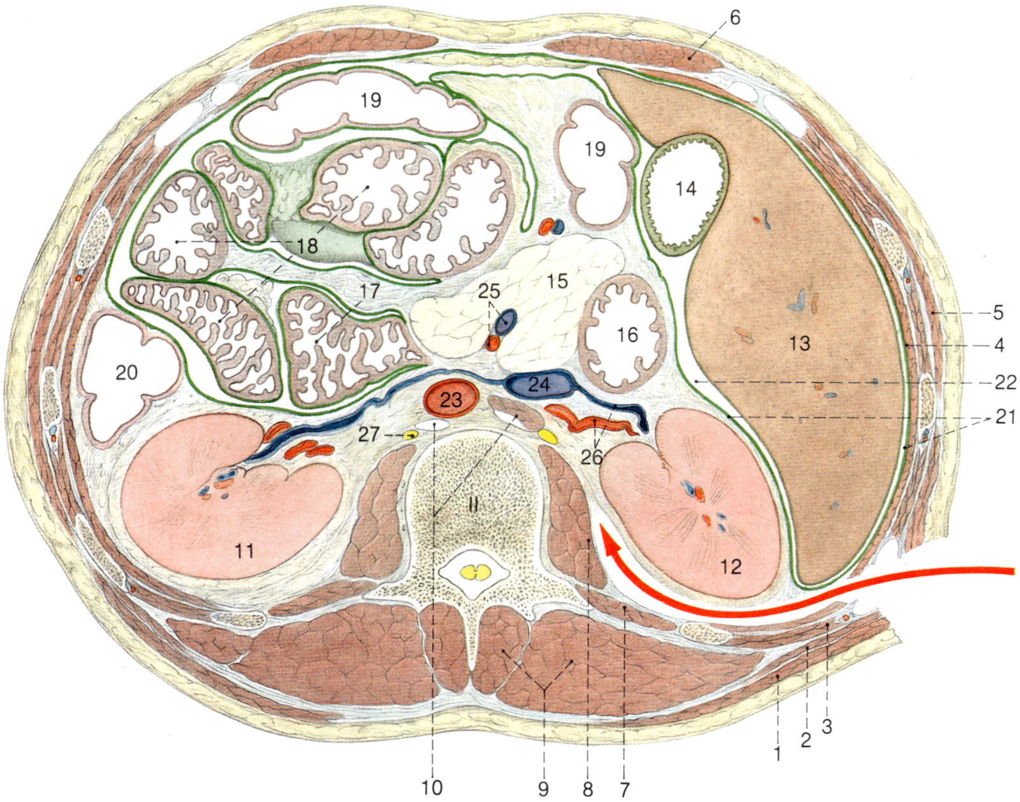

1 Latissimus dorsi muscle
2 Posterior inferior serratus muscle
3 Intercostal muscles
4 Thoracic diaphragm
5 Lateral abdominal musculature
6 Rectus abdominis musculature
7 Quadratus lumborum muscle
8 Greater psoas muscle
9 Intrinsic musculature of the back
10 Thoracic diaphragm, medial crus
11 Left kidney
12 Right kidney
13 Right lobe of the liver
14 Gallbladder
15 Pancreas
16 Descending part of the duodenum
17 Duodenal flexure
18 Jejunum
19 Transverse colon
20 Descending colon
21 Parietal peritoneum
22 Peritoneal cavity
23 Abdominal aorta
24 Inferior vena cava
25 Superior mesenteric vessels
26 Right renal vessels
27 Sympathetic trunk
II Lumbar vertebra

Fig. 1.**47** Transverse section at the level of the second lumbar vertebra. The approach for the retroperitoneal dissection is identified by an arrow (right-sided approach).

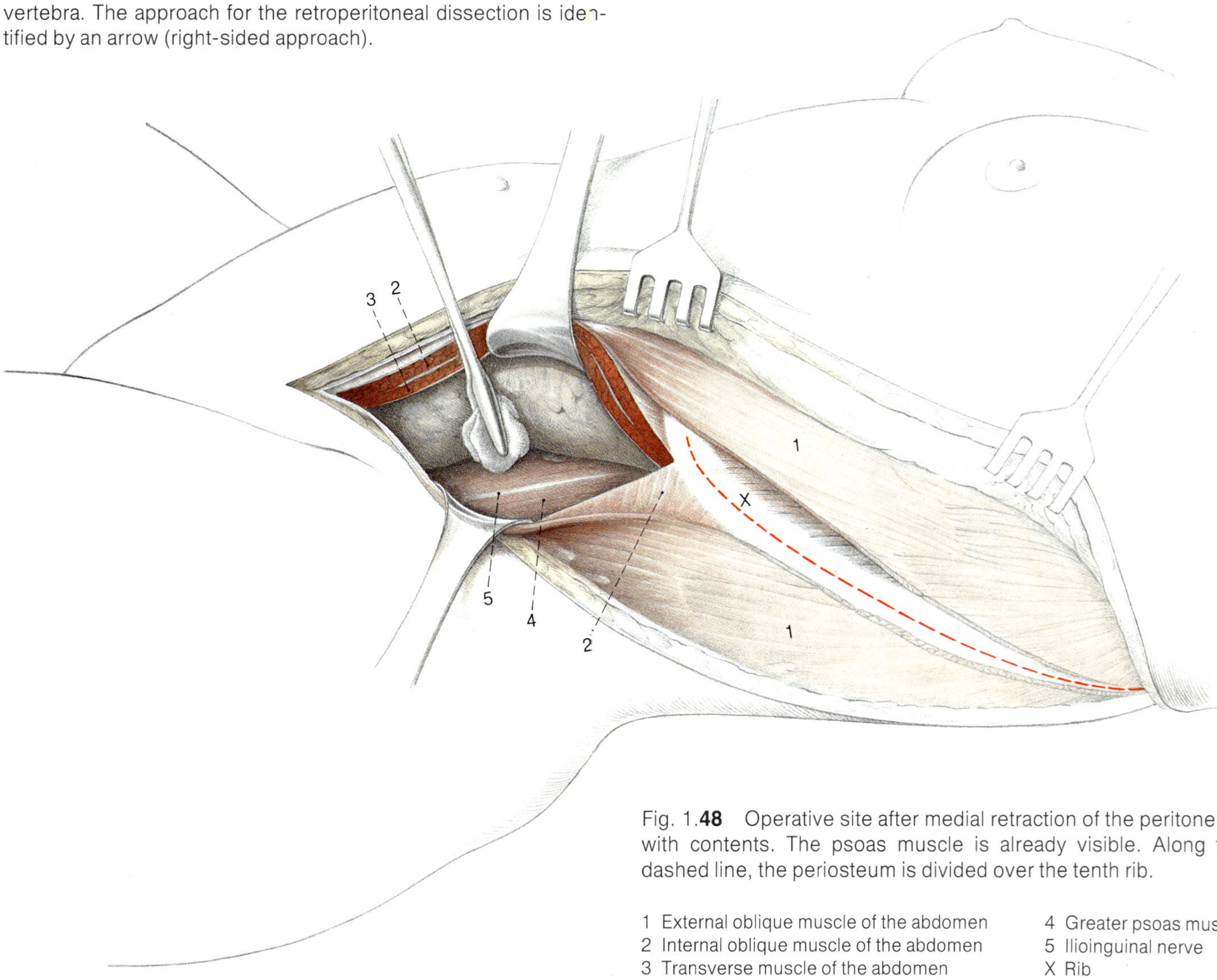

Fig. 1.**48** Operative site after medial retraction of the peritoneum with contents. The psoas muscle is already visible. Along the dashed line, the periosteum is divided over the tenth rib.

1 External oblique muscle of the abdomen
2 Internal oblique muscle of the abdomen
3 Transverse muscle of the abdomen
4 Greater psoas muscle
5 Ilioinguinal nerve
X Rib

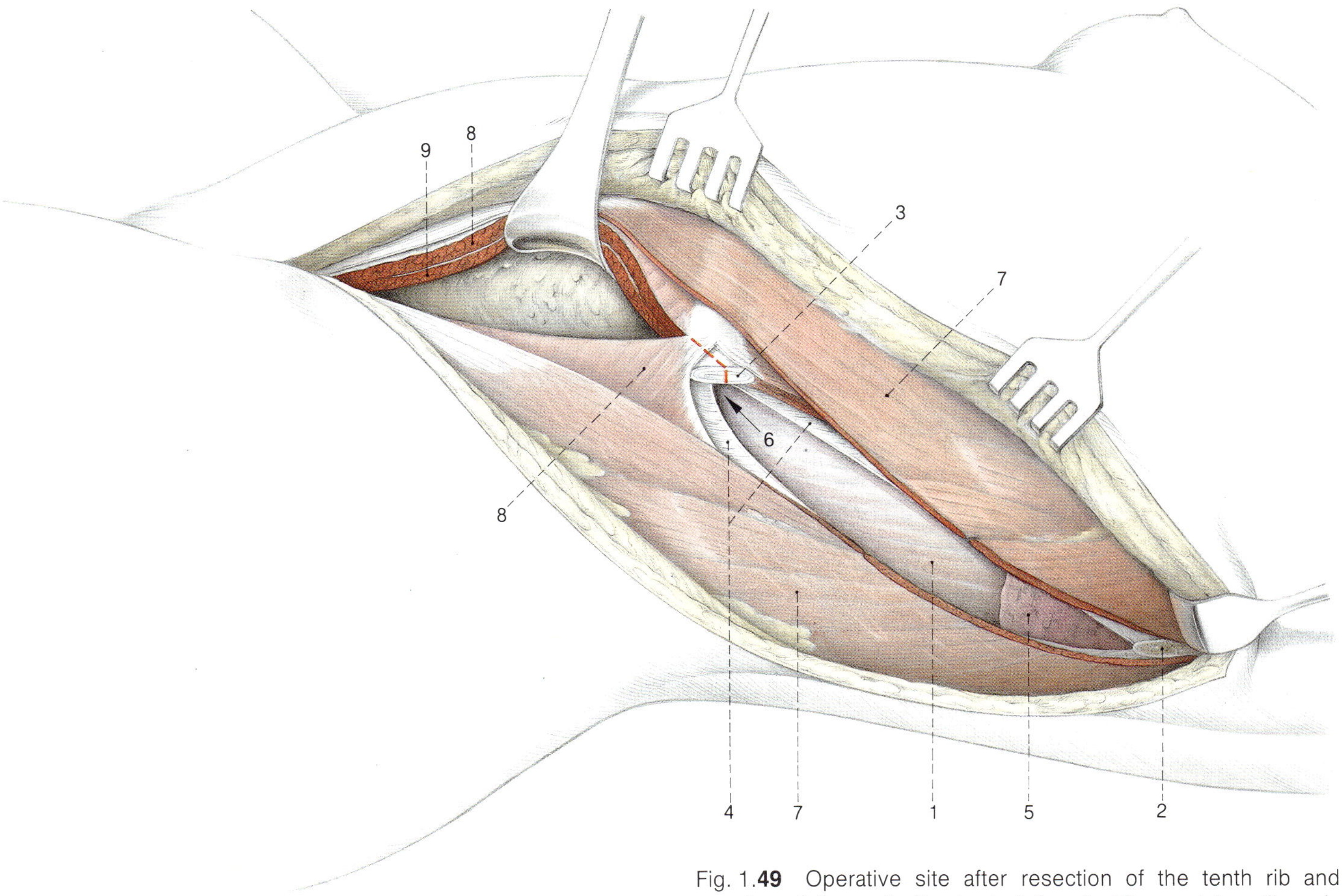

Fig. 1.**49** Operative site after resection of the tenth rib and opening of thorax in the bed of the rib. The costal cartilage is divided along the dashed line.

1 Thoracic diaphragm with diaphragmatic pleura
2 Stump of the tenth rib
3 Costal cartilage of the tenth rib
4 Costal periosteum and costal pleura
5 Left lung, inferior lobe
6 Costodiaphragmatic recess
7 External oblique muscle of the abdomen
8 Internal oblique muscle of the abdomen
9 Transverse muscle of the abdomen

The periosteum of the tenth rib is now transected with the electrocautery along its entire length (Fig. 1.**48**), after which the rib is exposed in the usual way with an elevator. This is done in the direction of the muscle fibers. The rib is dissected cranially from posterior to anterior, and caudally from anterior to posterior. Finally, the tenth rib is transversely resected with a knife at the costochondral margin, raised, resected posteriorly with rib cutters, and removed. The thorax is opened in the bed of the tenth rib by a longitudinal incision of the parietal pleura (Figs. 1.**25**–1.**27**). Through extension of the thoracotomy incision, the remaining posterior portion of the rib may be further exposed, if necessary, and resected afterwards with rib cutters near the costotransverse articulation. Enucleation of the head of the rib should be avoided, since it may cause severe bleeding. The costocartilage is then divided with a knife; it will later serve as a marker for wound closure (Fig. 1.**49**).

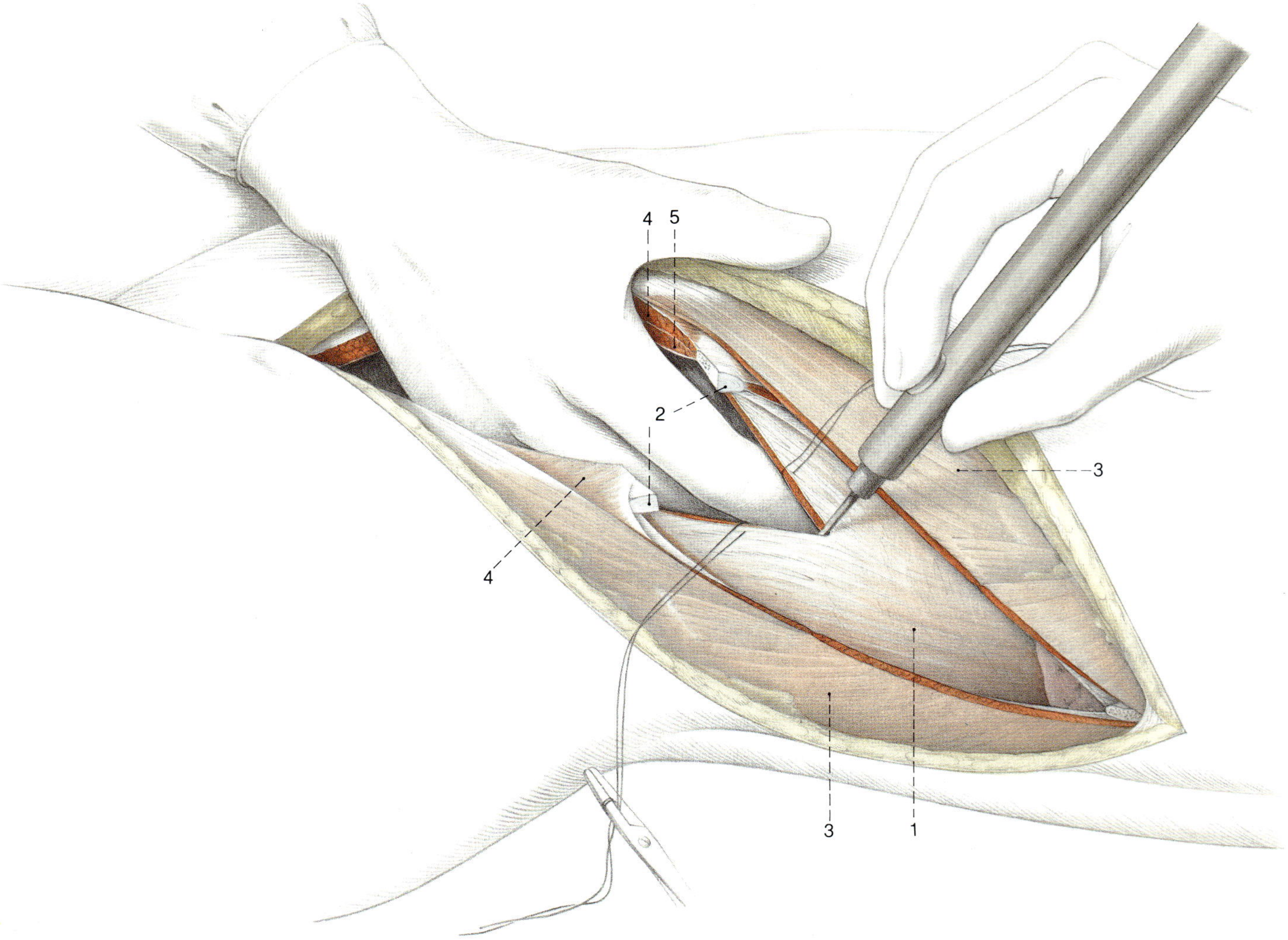

Fig. 1.**50** Operative site after thoracotomy. The diaphragm is divided with a curved incision with the electrocautery knife.

1 Thoracic diaphragm
2 Split costal cartilage of the tenth rib
3 External oblique muscle of the abdomen
4 Internal oblique muscle of the abdomen
5 Transverse muscle of the abdomen

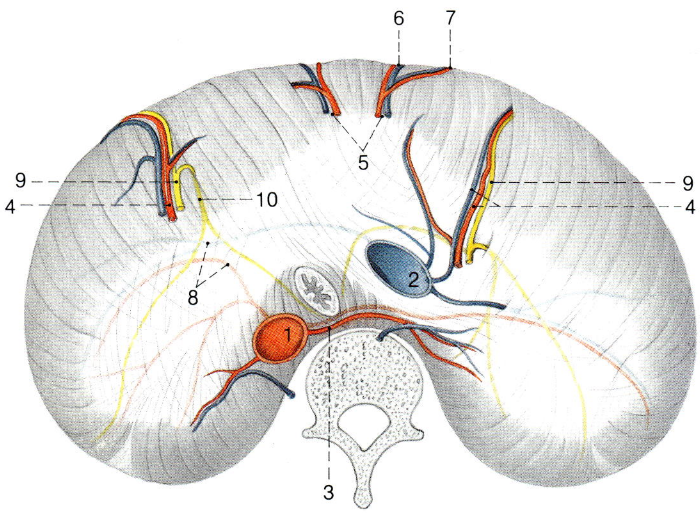

Fig. 1.**51** The diaphragm with the neurovascular supply, in a cranial view.

1 Aorta
2 Inferior vena cava
3 Superior phrenic artery
4 Pericardiacophrenic vessels
5 Internal thoracic vessels
6 Superior epigastric vessels
7 Musculophrenic vessels
8 Inferior phrenic vessels
9 Phrenic nerve

Once the peritoneum has been retracted from the underside of the diaphragm, the diaphragm may be transected under direct vision along a curved line about 2 cm from the rib insertion as far posterior as the spine (Fig. 1.**50**). Damage to the phrenic vessels and branches of the phrenic nerve can thus be avoided (Fig. 1.**51**).

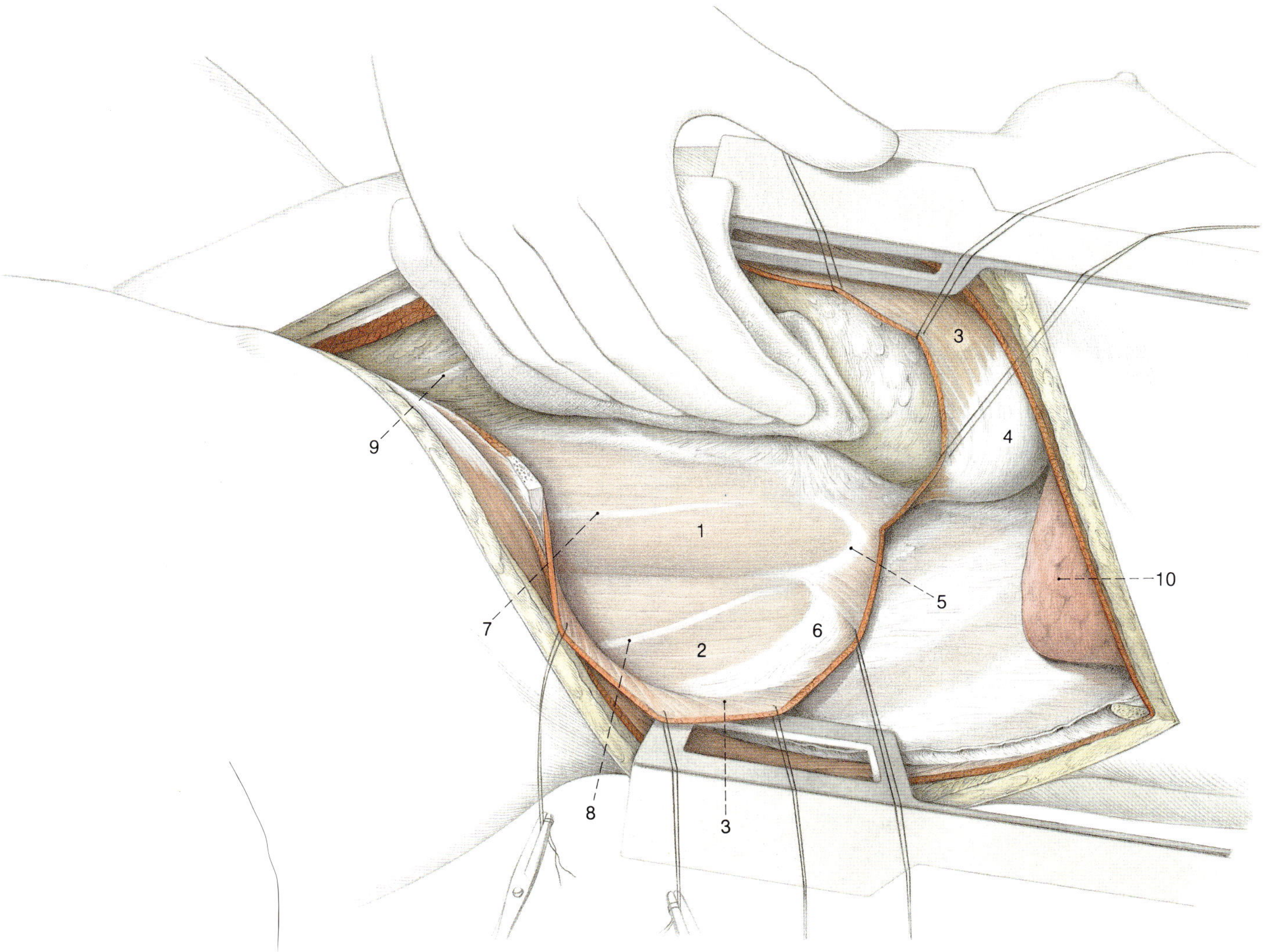

Fig. 1.**52** Operative site after thoracotomy and exposure of the left retroperitoneal space.

1 Greater psoas muscle
2 Quadratus lumborum muscle
3 Thoracic diaphragm
4 Thoracic diaphragm, tendinous center
5 Medial arcuate ligament
6 Lateral arcuate ligament
7 Ilioinguinal nerve
8 Iliohypogastric nerve
9 Ureter
10 Lung

It proves advantageous to place marking sutures from time to time to allow good approximation during later wound closure (Fig. 1.**52**). A chest spreader is inserted. The peritoneal contents and the lung are retracted by hand, or with the aid of suitable spatulas.

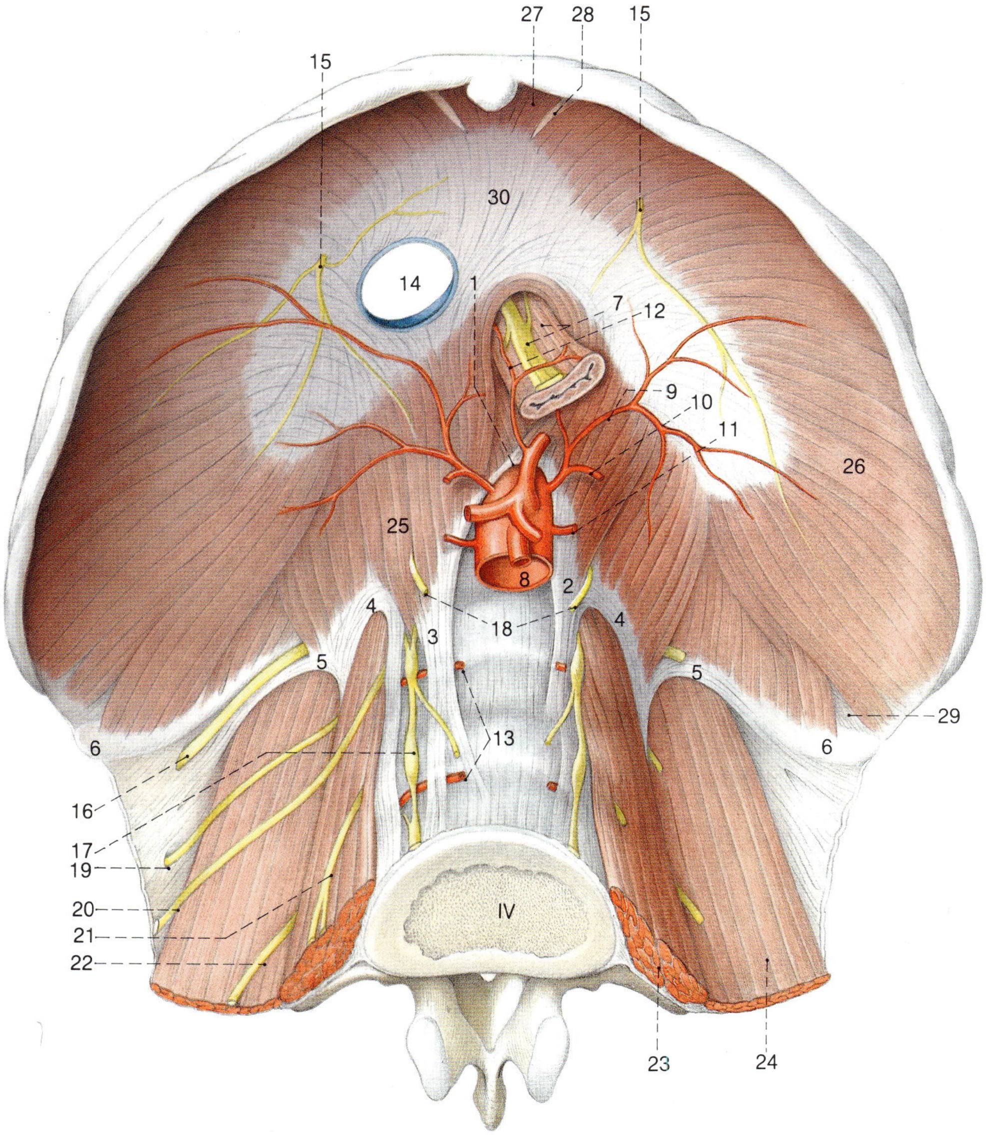

Fig. 1.**53** Anatomical exposure of the diaphragm and the structures passing through it.

1 Median arcuate ligament
2 Left medial crus
3 Right medial crus
4 Medial arcuate ligament
5 Lateral arcuate ligament
6 Twelfth rib
7 Esophagus and anterior vagal trunk
8 Aorta with celiac trunk and superior mesenteric artery
9 Inferior phrenic artery
10 Superior suprarenal artery
11 Middle suprarenal artery
12 Left gastric artery, esophageal branch
13 Lumbar arteries
14 Inferior vena cava
15 Phrenic nerve
16 Subcostal nerve
17 Sympathetic trunk
18 Greater splanchnic nerve
19 Iliohypogastric nerve
20 Ilioinguinal nerve
21 Genitofemoral nerve
22 Lateral cutaneous nerve of the thigh
23 Greater psoas muscle
24 Quadratus lumborum muscle
25 Thoracic diaphragm, lumbar part
26 Thoracic diaphragm, costal part
27 Thoracic diaphragm, sternal part
28 Sternocostal triangle
29 Lumbocostal triangle
30 Tendinous center
IV Lumbar vertebra

Next, the lumbar part of the diaphragm, with the left medial crus, is divided. Identification of the following structures is required at this point (Fig. 1.**53**): the greater thoracic splanchnic nerve, together with the ascending lumbar vein (or azygos vein), perforates the diaphragm between the medial crus and the intermediate crus and runs in a distal direction medial to the celiac plexus. Slightly laterally, the sympathetic trunk passes through the diaphragm between the intermediate and the lateral crus. The left diaphragmatic crus is dissected approximately 1.5 cm above the lateral or medial arcuate ligament. Preferably, a grooved director or a curved clamp is inserted into the aortic hiatus immediately below the diaphragmatic crus. The diaphragm is divided in the direction of the grooved director in such a way that the greater splanchnic nerve cranially, and the sympathetic trunk caudally, escape injury (Fig. 1.**54**). Occasionally, it becomes necessary to ligate and transect segmental vessels or branches of the ascending lumbar vein.

The retroperitoneal tissue overlying the spine or the parietal pleura is now raised with forceps and incised with scissors along the axis of the spine. The parietal pleura is then elevated bilaterally; the segmental vessels traversing the vertebral bodies are transected between ligatures (Fig. 1.**55**).

Fig. 1.**54** Operative site following complete transection of the left half of the diaphragm and the left medial diaphragmatic crus. Exposure of the vertebrae by division of the retroperitoneal tissue or the parietal pleura along the dashed line.

1 Thoracic diaphragm
2 Right medial crus
3 Left medial crus
4 Abdominal aorta
5 Lumbar vessels
6 Ascending lumbar vein
7 Sympathetic trunk
8 Greater splanchnic nerve

Fig. 1.**55** Operative site after division of the segmental vessels. Exposure of the vertebrae.

1 Greater psoas muscle, laterally retracted from the spint
2 Anterior longitudinal ligament
3 Lumbar vessels
4 Greater splanchnic nerve
5 Sympathetic trunk
II–IV Lumbar vertebrae

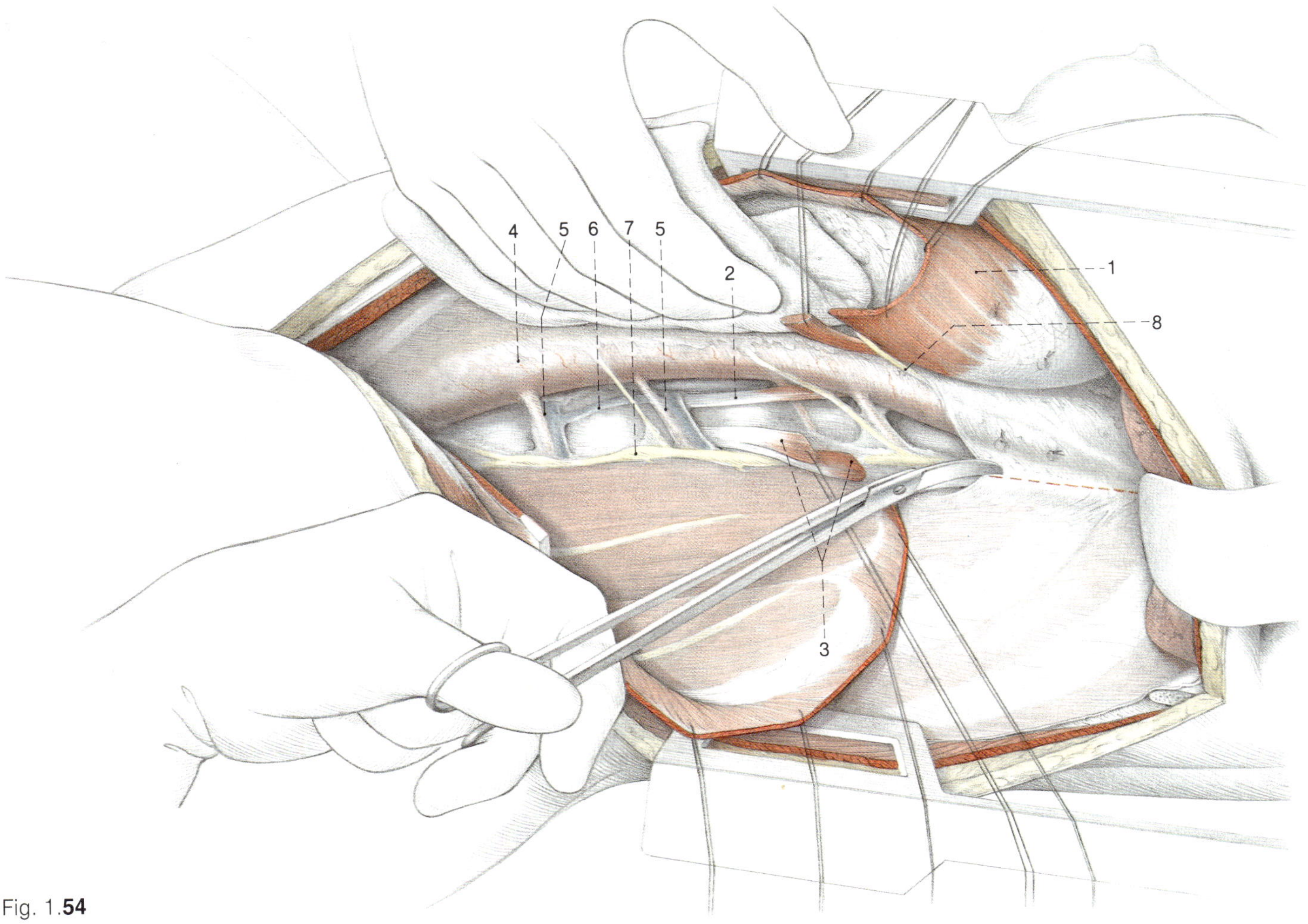

Fig. 1.**54**

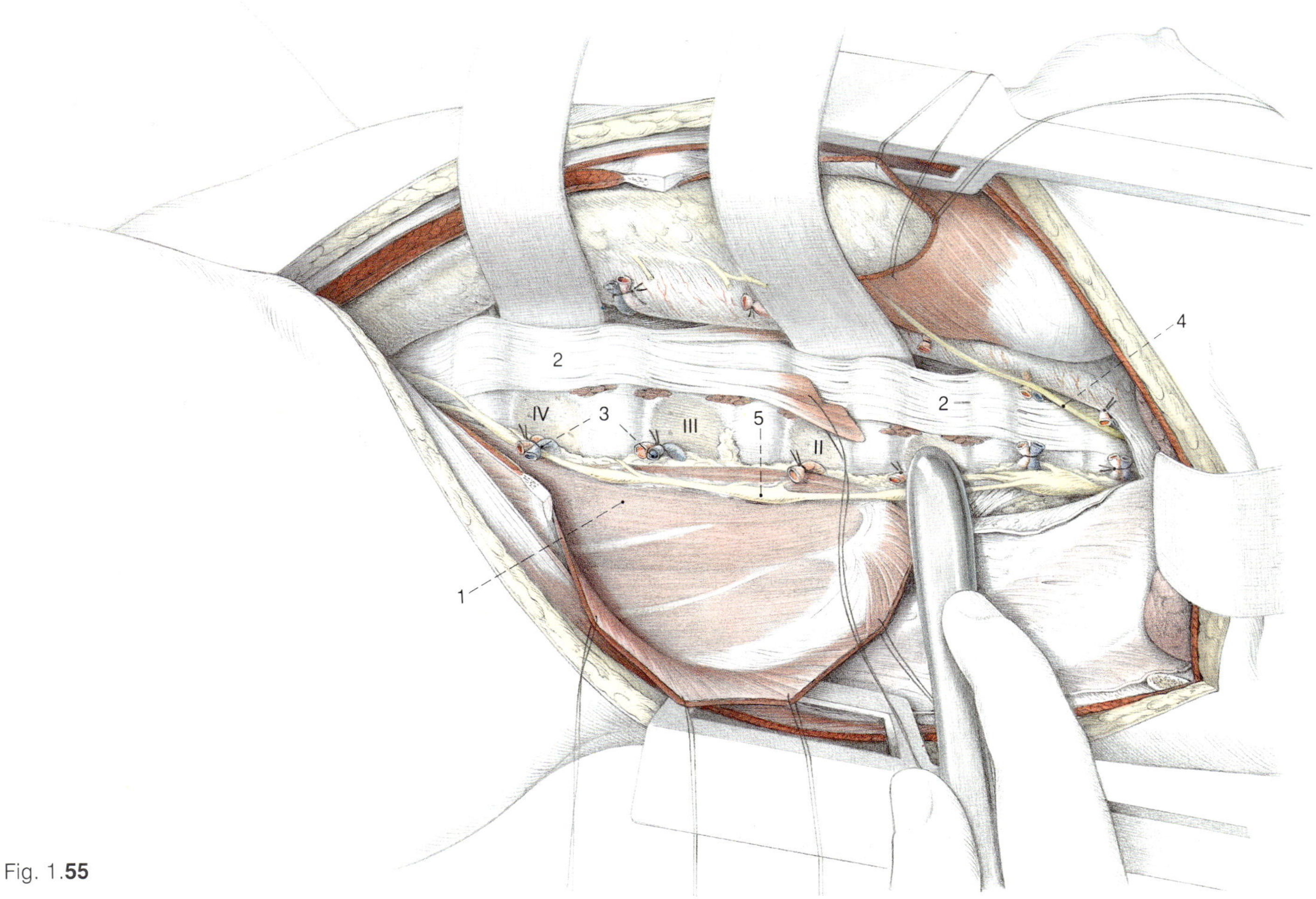

Fig. 1.**55**

Exposure of Individual Vertebrae

Exposure of the vertebrae now follows. Dissection is always begun over the intervertebral disks, which are the prominent landmarks, since no vessels are found in this area. Using a swab on a stick, the areolar tissues over the intervertebral disks or the vertebrae are elevated, and the tissues are retracted until the base of the transverse processes can be reached bilaterally. The sympathetic trunk is retracted laterally (Fig. 1.**55**). The origins of the psoas muscles are stripped from the intervertebral disks in the area of the lumbar spine so that they can be exposed as far as the intervertebral foramen. Figure 1.**56** shows the anatomical sites in this approach.

If the incision is long enough, this approach also gives access to the promontory and cranial portions of the sacrum (Fig. 1.**57**). Special importance should be placed on the exposure and ligation of the iliolumbar vessels.

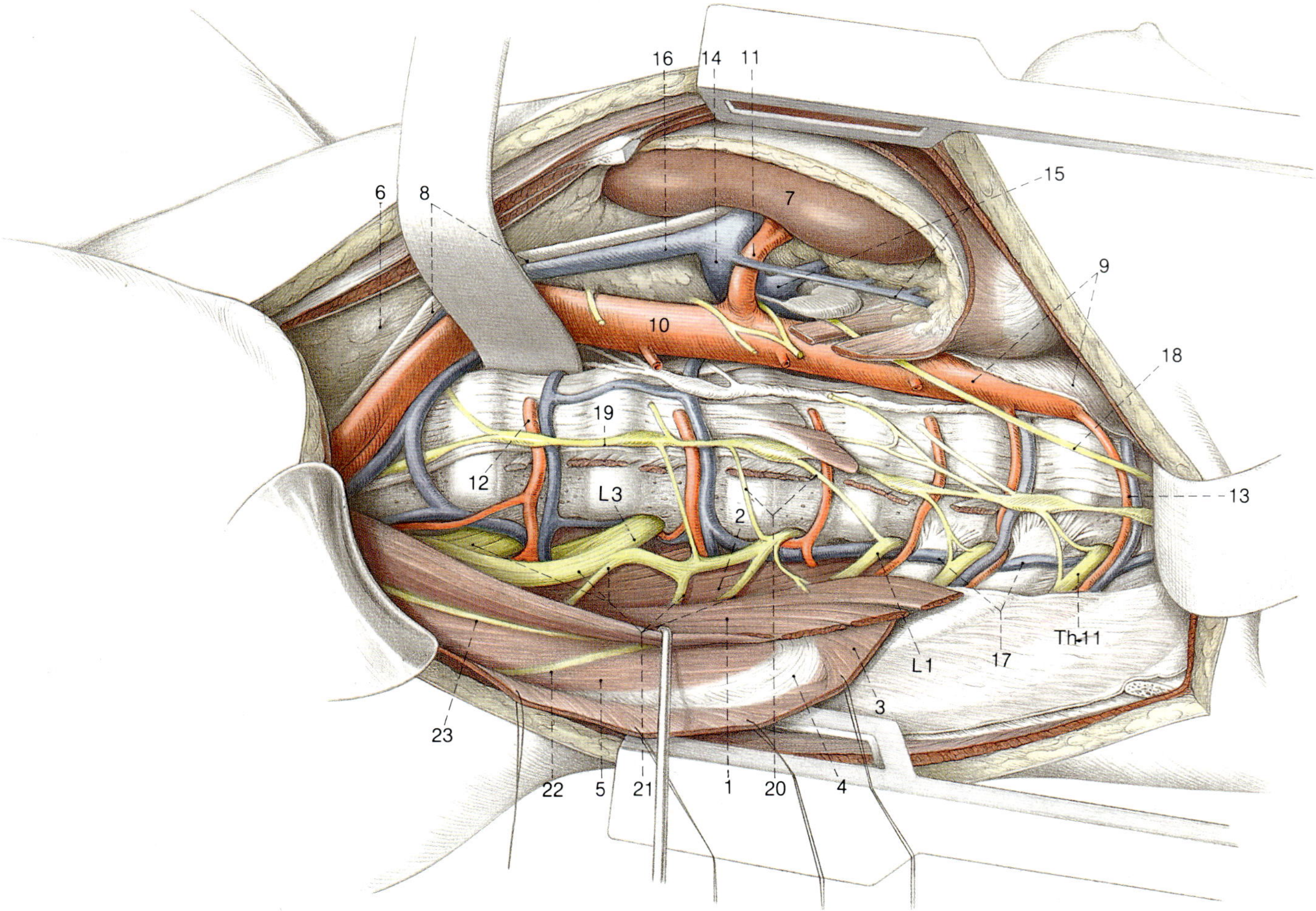

Fig. 1.**56** Anatomical site of the left retroperitoneal space and left retropleural space.

1 Greater psoas muscle, superficial origin
2 Greater psoas muscle, deep origin
3 Thoracic diaphragm
4 Lateral arcuate ligament
5 Quadratus lumborum muscle
6 Peritoneum
7 Left kidney
8 Ureter
9 Thoracic aorta
10 Abdominal aorta
11 Renal artery
12 Lumbar artery
13 Intercostal artery
14 Renal vein
15 Suprarenal veins
16 Ovarian vein
17 Ascending lumbar vein
18 Greater splanchnic nerve
19 Sympathetic trunk
20 Communicating branches
21 Lumbar plexus
22 Iliohypogastric nerve
23 Ilioinguinal nerve
T11, L1, L3 } Spinal nerves, anterior branches

Wound Closure

The psoas muscles are resutured to the area of their origin. Anatomical restoration of the left diaphragmatic crus is important (Fig. 1.**58**). In the thoracic region, the parietal pleura is closed over the spine by a running suture. Subsequently, the diaphragm is closed from medial posterior to lateral anterior, using single interrupted sutures that are tied extrathoracically. Finally, the cartilage of the tenth rib, that served as a marker, is sutured (Fig. 1.**59**). A chest tube is placed, a rib approximator is inserted, the parietal pleura is sutured in the bed of the resected rib, and the chest wall musculature (intercostal musculature, latissimus dorsi muscle, anterior serratus muscle) and abdominal musculature are closed in layers.

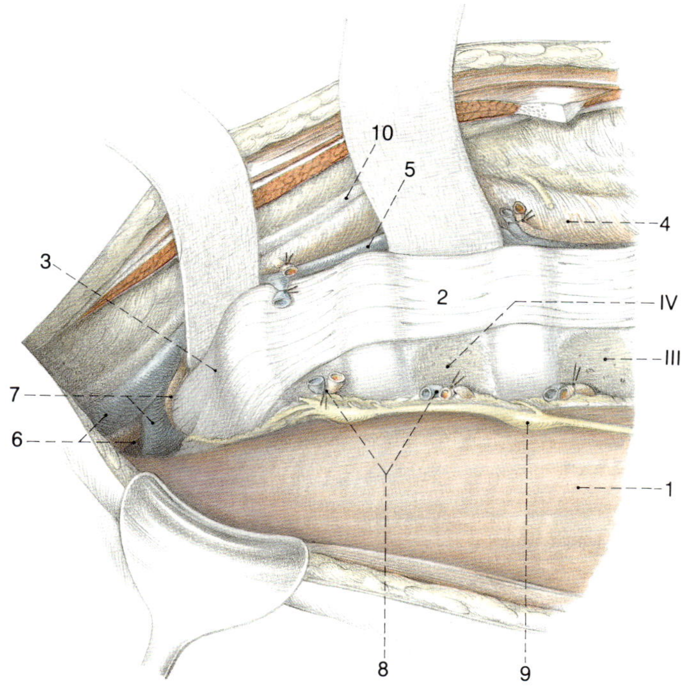

Fig. 1.**57** Operative site in exposure of the lumbosacral junction.

1 Greater psoas muscle
2 Anterior longitudinal ligament
3 Promontory
4 Abdominal aorta
5 Inferior vena cava
6 External iliac artery and vein
7 Internal iliac artery and vein
8 Lumbar artery and vein
9 Sympathetic trunk
10 Ureter
III–IV Lumbar vertebrae

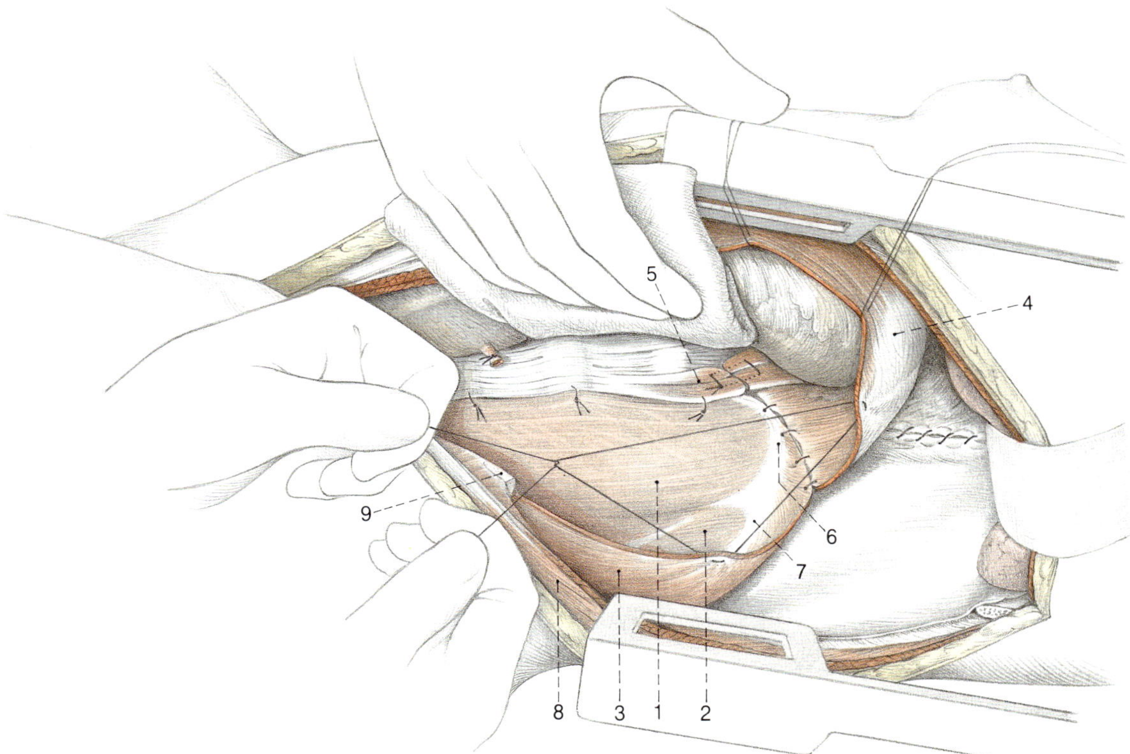

Fig. 1.**58** Reinsertion of the left diaphragmatic crus and suture of the diaphragm with interrupted stitches.

1 Greater psoas muscle
2 Quadratus lumborum muscle
3 Thoracic diaphragm, costal part
4 Thoracic diaphragm, tendinous center
5 Thoracic diaphragm, left medial crus
6 Thoracic diaphragm, medial arcuate ligament
7 Thoracic diaphragm, lateral arcuate ligament
8 External oblique muscle of the abdomen
9 Costal cartilage

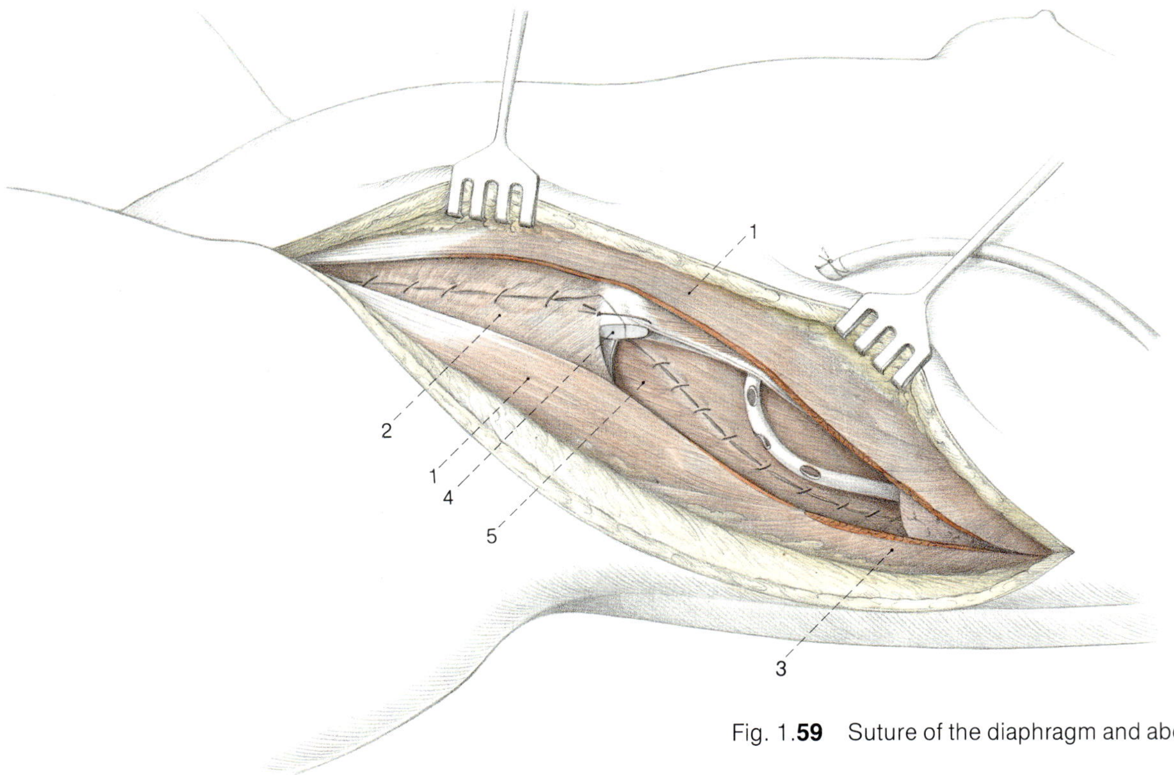

Fig. 1.**59** Suture of the diaphragm and abdominal musculature.

1 External oblique muscle of the abdomen
2 Internal oblique muscle of the abdomen
3 Latissimus dorsi muscle
4 Costal cartilage of the tenth rib
5 Thoracic diaphragm

Thoracolumbar Approach According to Hodgson From the Right

The operation is carried out in a similar way to the left-sided approach, except that the sides are reversed (Fig. 1.**47**). Differences arise mainly in the exposure from the side of the abdomen: the diaphragmatic surface of the right lobe of the liver is adherent to the right subphrenic space over an approximately palm-sized area. Therefore, only a relatively narrow portion of the diaphragm close to the rib can be exposed. In this region, the diaphragm is incised, and the liver is mobilized with the diaphragm step by step and retracted leftward. Difficulties may be caused by the inferior vena cava. Only after division of the right lumbar veins can the vena cava be retracted to the left.

Retroperitoneal-Extrapleural Approach to the Thoracolumbar Spine, T11–L5 (Mirbaha)

Principal Indications

- Kyphosis
- Tumors
- Spondylitis

As a rule, the transpleural approach according to Hodgson is preferred for clear exposure of several vertebrae in the area of the thoracolumbar junction. The extrapleural approach according to Mirbaha is chosen if only one to two spinal segments at the thoracolumbar junction need to be accessed.

This approach to the thoracolumbar junction is generally possible from the right as well as from the left. Whenever the side of the approach is not determined by the underlying disease (such as a scoliotic component of thoracolumbar kyphosis, tumor expansion, etc.), the left-sided approach will be chosen. As the transpleural retroperitoneal approach according to Hodgson was described from the left, the retropleural approach will now be presented from the right.

Positioning and Incision

(Fig. 1.**60**)

The patient is placed in a left lateral decubitus position, with the arm raised out of the operative field. The skin is incised along the spinous processes of T9–T11, and then anteriorly alongside the twelfth rib, to about a fingerbreadth above the anterior iliac spine. This gives an exposure as far as L2. If more inferior lumbar vertebrae need to be exposed in addition, the skin incision may be extended obliquely (segmental nerves!) caudad (Fig. 1.**44**).

The following muscles are divided (Fig. 1.**61**): the latissimus dorsi muscle and the external oblique muscle of the abdomen and, one layer below, the inferior posterior serratus muscle. After dissection—simple elevation may be sufficient in some cases—the iliocostal muscle, the lumbocostal ligament (Henle's ligament), a strong fascial band between the quadratus lumborum muscle, the psoas muscle, and the intrinsic musculature of the back, are exposed. The twelfth rib is now visualized. After this, the deep abdominal muscle layers (internal oblique and transverse muscles of the abdomen) are divided, bringing the peritoneum into view (Fig. 1.**62**). The peritoneum is now mobilized away from the lateral abdominal wall and retracted medially. This exposes the upper lumbar spine retroperitoneally. The peritoneum is then stripped from the undersurface of the diaphragm. Thick fascicles of Henle's ligament are detached from the costal process of L1, together with the uppermost portion of the quadratus lumborum muscle. Using a small peanut swab stick, the pleura is cautiously retracted proximally from the anterior side of the quadratus lumborum muscle (Fig. 1.**63**). The twelfth rib is exposed subperiosteally, and the medial portion is resected. Subsequently, the bed of the twelfth rib is incised in the middle, and the caudal half is retracted caudally together with the quadratus lumborum muscle (Fig. 1.**64**). The subcostal nerve should be spared. Using a peanut swab stick, the pleura is further mobilized craniad. When the pleura and the peritoneum have been freed (Fig. 1.**65**), the diaphragm is transected above the arcus lumbocostalis (medial arcuate ligament) in such a way as to permit readaptation later. The right medial crus of the diaphragm is also divided, following application of stay sutures (Fig. 1.**66**).

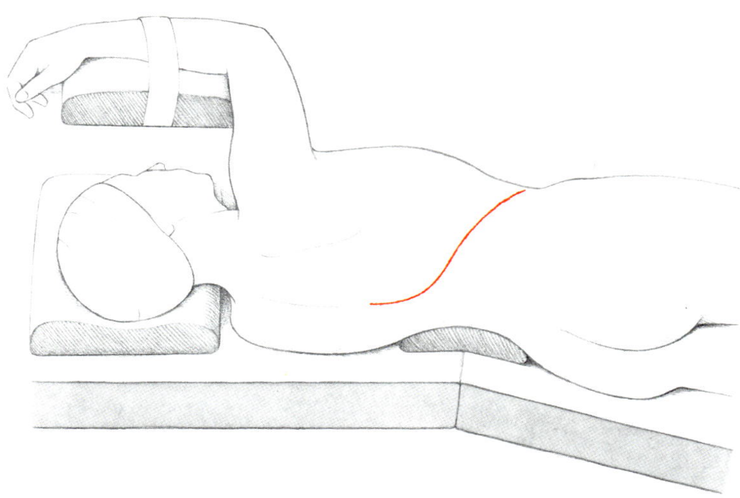

Fig. 1.**60** Extrapleural retroperitoneal approach according to Mirbaha. Positioning and incision.

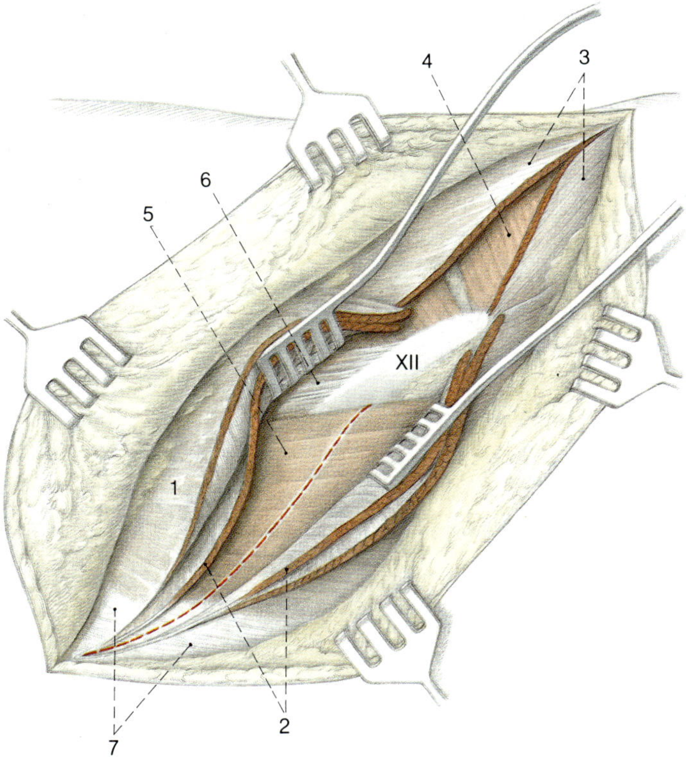

Fig. 1.**61** Operative site after division of the latissimus dorsi muscle, the external oblique muscle of the abdomen, and the inferior posterior serratus muscle. The iliocostal muscle (intrinsic musculature of the back) is divided along the dashed line.

1 Latissimus dorsi muscle
2 Posterior inferior serratus muscle
3 External oblique muscle of the abdomen
4 Internal oblique muscle of the abdomen
5 Iliocostal muscle
6 External intercostal muscle
7 Thoracolumbar fascia, superficial lamina
XII Rib

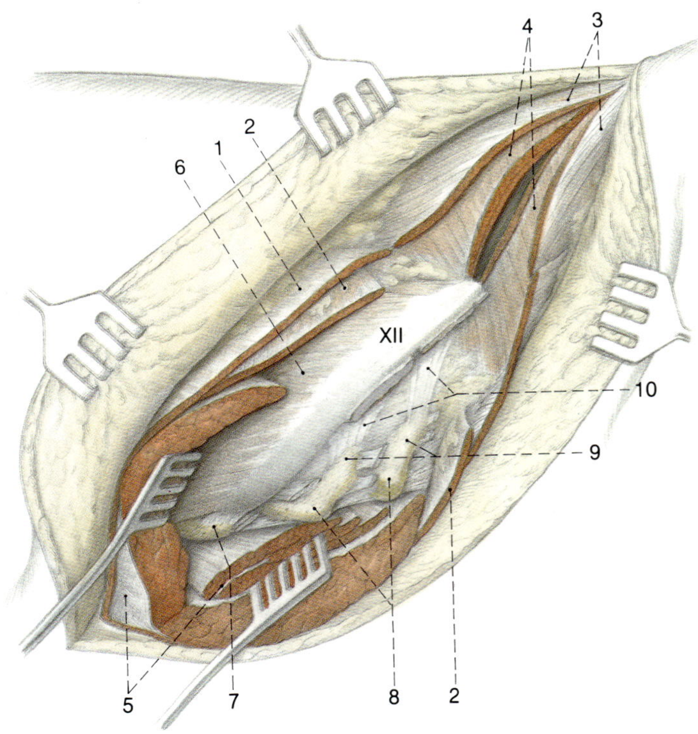

Fig. 1.**62** Operative site after division of the intrinsic musculature of the back and the deep abdominal muscle layers.

1 Latissimus dorsi muscle
2 Posterior inferior serratus muscle
3 External oblique muscle of the abdomen
4 Internal oblique muscle of the abdomen
5 Intrinsic musculature of the back
6 External intercostal muscle
7 Transverse process T12
8 Mamillary processes L1 and L2
9 Costal processes L1 and L2
10 Lumbocostal (Henle's) ligament
XII Rib

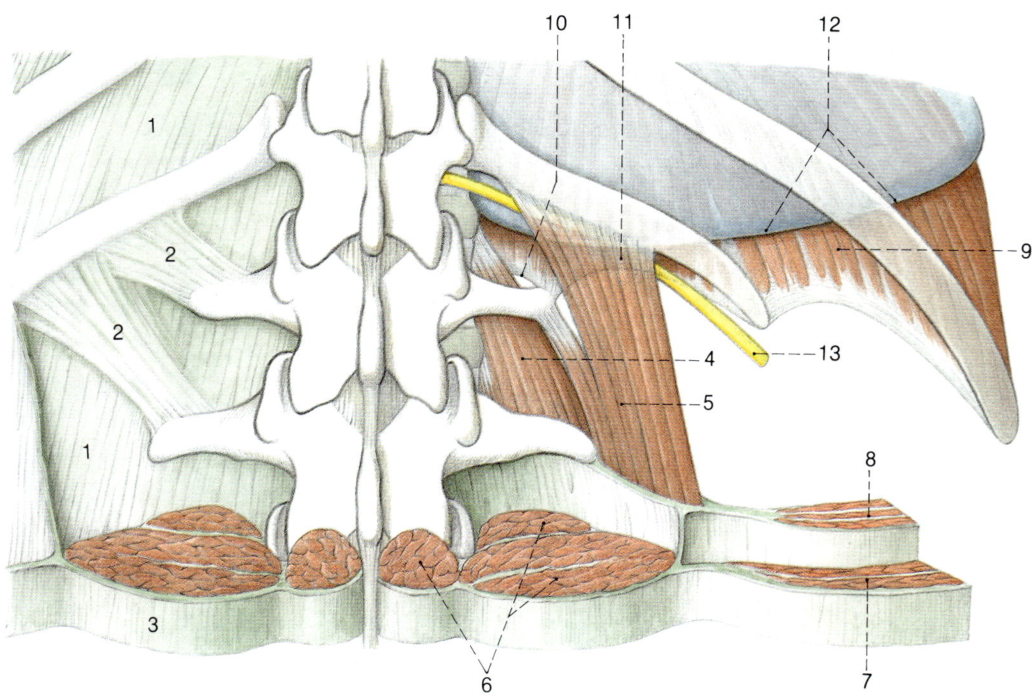

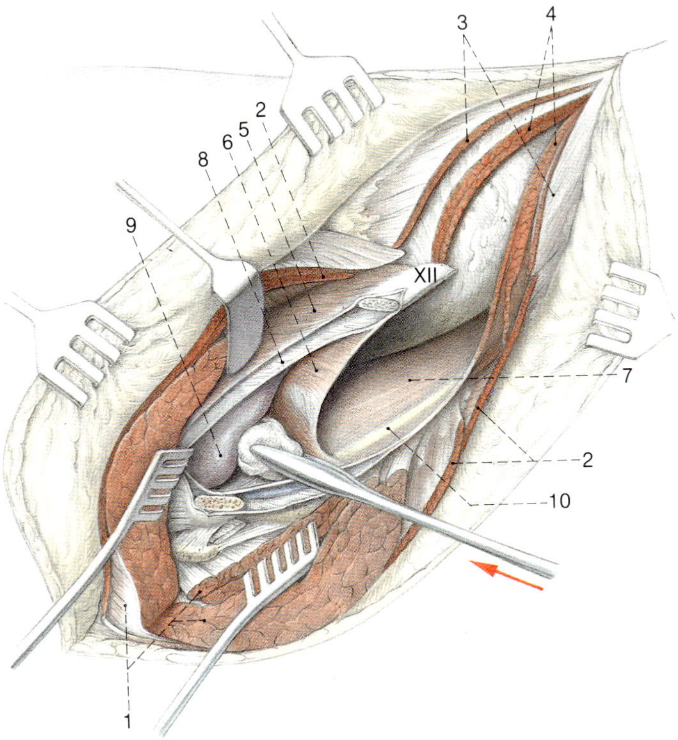

Fig. 1.**64** Operative site after partial resection of the twelfth rib. The parietal pleura is retracted further cranial with a sponge stick (see arrow).

1 Intrinsic musculature of the back
2 Latissimus dorsi muscle and posterior inferior serratus muscle
3 External oblique muscle of the abdomen
4 Internal oblique muscle of the abdomen and transverse muscle of the abdomen
5 External intercostal muscle
6 Thoracic diaphragm
7 Greater psoas muscle
8 Periosteum of the twelfth rib
9 Costodiaphragmatic recess with the lung
10 Subcostal nerve
XII Costal cartilage of the twelfth rib

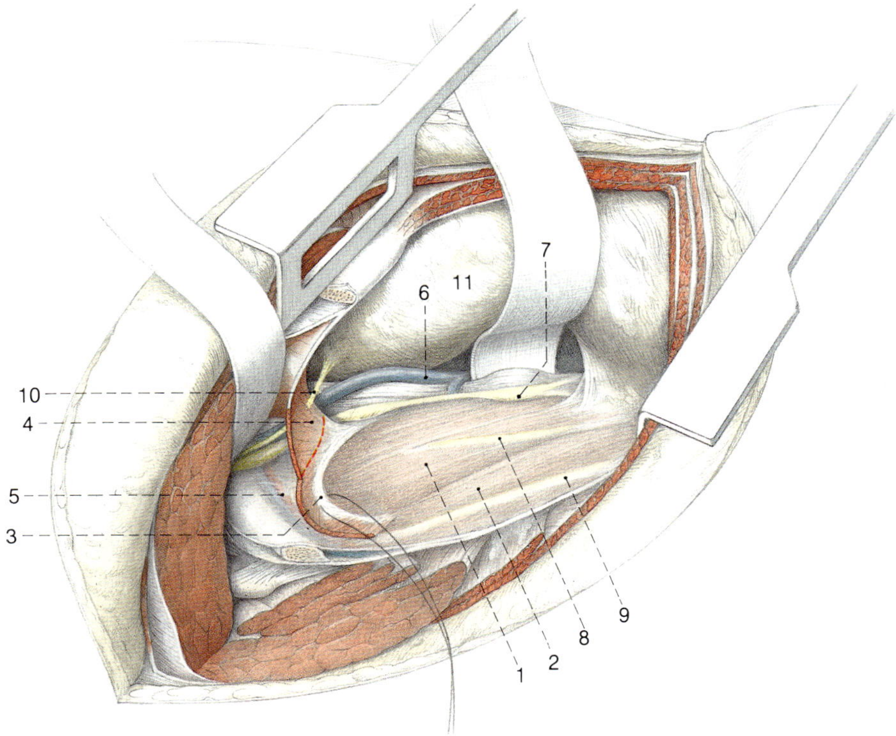

◀ Fig. 1.**63** The thoracolumbar junction, posterior view. Particular importance is attached to the relation between the following structures: twelfth rib, origins of the diaphragm, arcus lumbocostalis medialis and lateralis (medial and lateral arcuate ligaments), quadratus lumborum muscle, lumbocostal ligament, and pleural border.

1 Thoracolumbar fascia, deep lamina
2 Lumbocostal (Henle's) ligament
3 Thoracolumbar fascia, superficial lamina
4 Greater psoas muscle
5 Quadratus lumborum muscle
6 Intrinsic musculature of back
7 Trapezius muscle and inferior posterior serratus muscle
8 Lateral abdominal musculature
9 Thoracic diaphragm, costal part
10 Medial arcuate ligament
11 Lateral arcuate ligament
12 Costodiaphragmatic recess
13 Subcostal nerve

Fig. 1.**65** The right retroperitoneal space is exposed. The diaphragm is divided above the medial arcuate ligament along the dashed line.

1 Greater psoas muscle
2 Quadratus lumborum muscle
3 Medial arcuate ligament
4 Thoracic diaphragm
5 Subcostal vessels
6 Ascending lumbar vein
7 Sympathetic trunk
8 Genitofemoral nerve
9 Subcostal nerve
10 Greater splanchnic nerve
11 Parietal peritoneum with preperitoneal adipose tissue

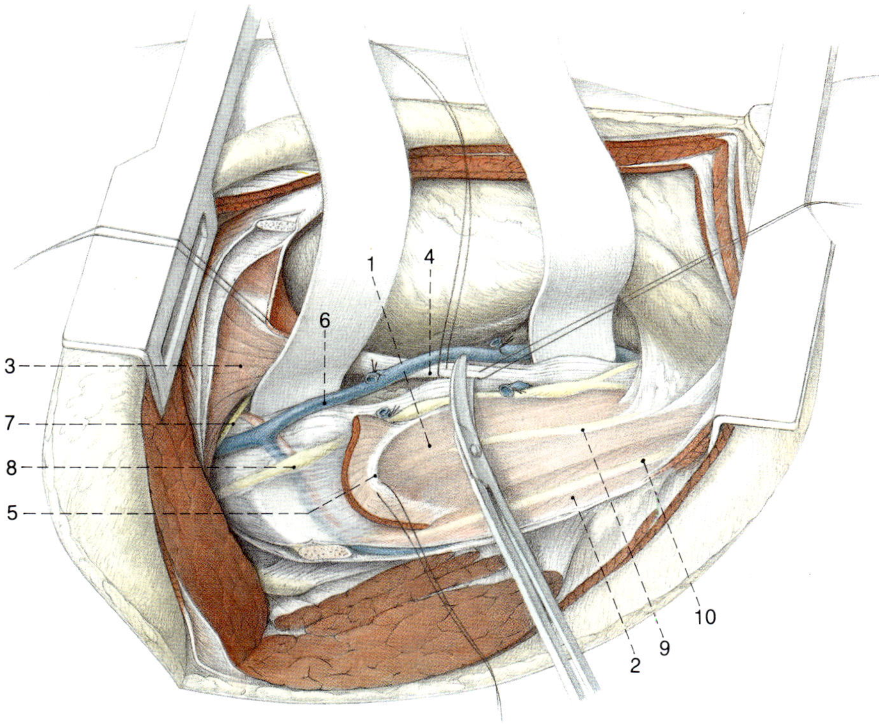

Fig. 1.**66** Operative site after division of the diaphragm. The right diaphragmatic crus is also transected following the placement of stay sutures.

1 Greater psoas muscle
2 Quadratus lumborum muscle
3 Thoracic diaphragm
4 Thoracic diaphragm, right medial crus
5 Medial arcuate ligament
6 Ascending lumbar vein
7 Greater splanchnic nerve
8 Sympathetic trunk
9 Genitofemoral nerve
10 Subcostal nerve

Exposure of Vertebrae

The vertebrae are exposed in the usual way. The retroperitoneal tissue and the parietal pleura, respectively, are split at the thoracolumbar junction, and the segmental vessels are exposed and transected after ligation. If a more cranial exposure is required, it is readily possible to retract the parietal pleura further in this direction and to resect the medial half of the eleventh rib (Fig. 1.**67**).

With a sufficiently long incision, this approach can give access to L5 or the cranial segment of the sacrum.

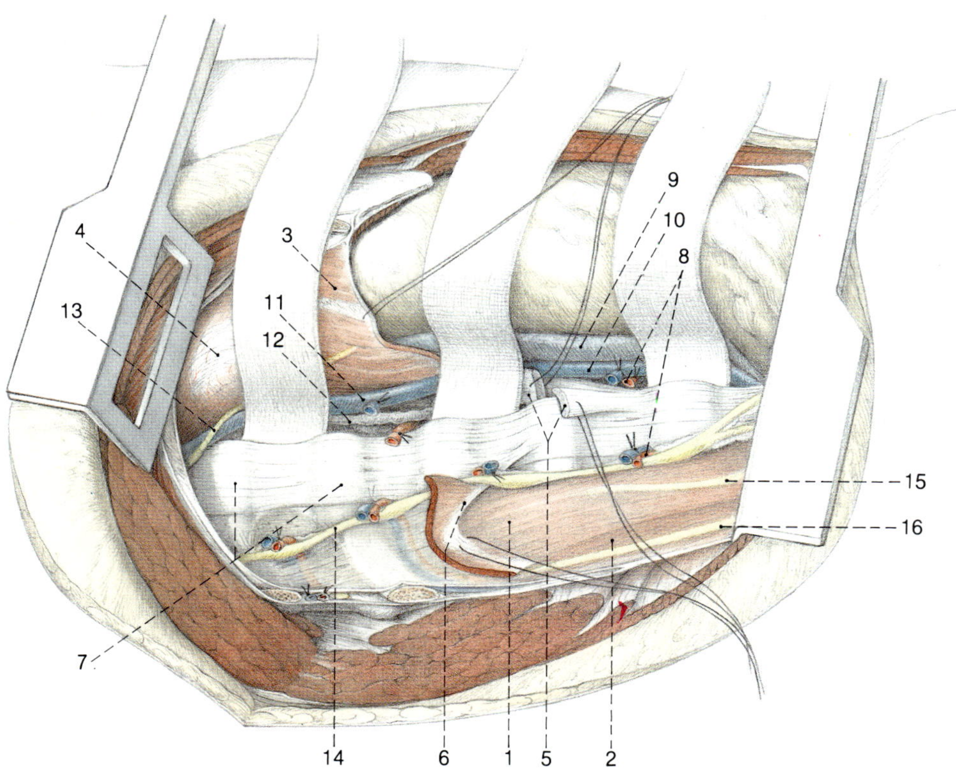

Fig. 1.**67** Operative site with exposure of vertebrae at the thoracolumbar junction after transection of the segmental vessels and additional resection of the eleventh rib.

1 Greater psoas muscle
2 Quadratus lumborum muscle
3 Thoracic diaphragm
4 Thoracic diaphragm, tendinous center
5 Thoracic diaphragm, right medial crus
6 Medial arcuate ligament
7 Anterior longitudinal ligament
8 Lumbar vessels
9 Inferior vena cava
10 Ascending lumbar vein
11 Azygos vein
12 Thoracic duct
13 Greater splanchnic nerve
14 Sympathetic trunk
15 Genitofemoral nerve
16 Subcostal nerve

Fig. 1.**68** Wound closure. After suture of the right diaphragmatic crus, the right half of the diaphragm is united by interrupted sutures that are tied extrapleurally.

1 Thoracic diaphragm
2 Thoracic diaphragm, right medial crus
3 Medial arcuate ligament

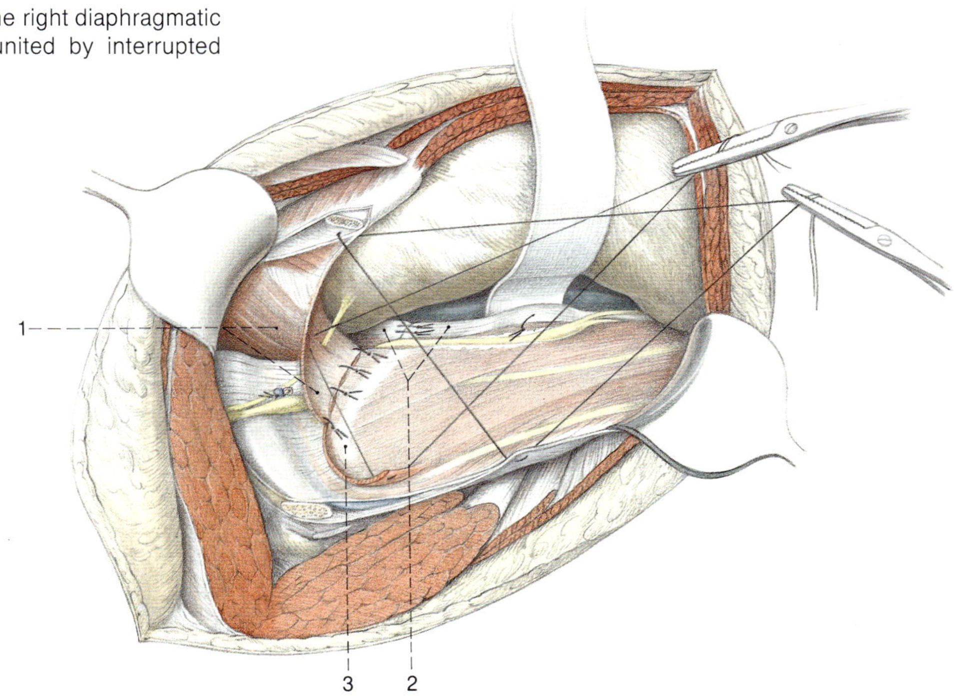

Wound Closure

The diaphragmatic crus is closed with interrupted sutures, and the diaphragm above the medial arcuate ligament is then sutured in the appropriate position. Corresponding stay sutures facilitate approximation (Fig. 1.**68**). Finally, the quadratus lumborum muscle is resutured to the cranial half of the periosteum of the twelfth rib; the abdominal musculature is closed in layers, and the iliocostal and inferior posterior serratus muscles, as well as the latissimus dorsi, are sutured (Fig. 1.**69**).

Fig. 1.**69** Suture of deep abdominal muscle layers and reinsertion of the quadratus lumborum muscle at the periosteum of the twelfth rib. Suture of the intrinsic musculature of the back.

1 Intrinsic musculature of the back
2 Latissimus dorsi muscle
3 Posterior inferior serratus muscle
4 External oblique muscle of the abdomen
5 Internal oblique muscle of the abdomen
6 Intercostal muscles
7 Intercostal vessels
XI–XII Ribs

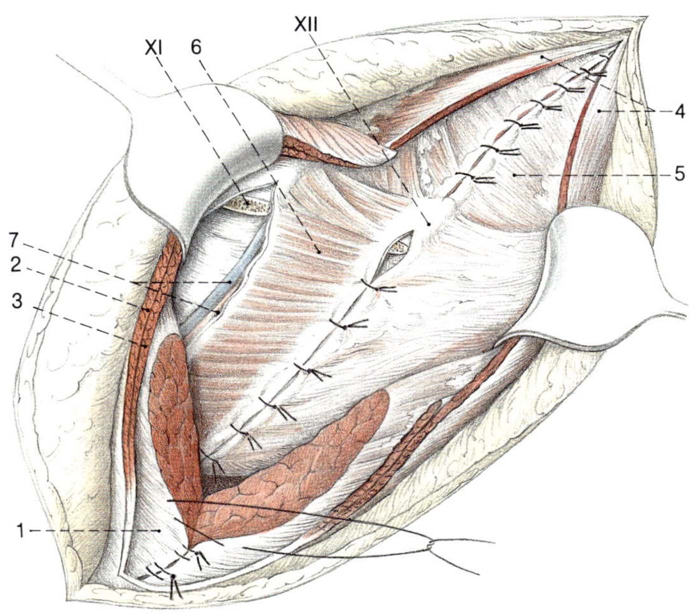

Lumbar Spine and Lumbosacral Junction

Retroperitoneal Approach to the Lumbar Spine L2–L5

Principal Indications

- Kyphosis
- Tumors
- Spondylitis

This approach to the lumbar spine can generally be made from the right as well as the left. If the side of the approach is not determined by the underlying disease (e.g., scoliotic component of thoracolumbar kyphosis, tumor expansion, etc.), the left-sided approach will be chosen.

Positioning and Incision

The patient is placed in a right lateral decubitus position; the table may be tilted in the lumbar region and a kidney rest provided, enlarging the distance between the costal arch and the iliac crest. To stabilize the position, the patient's right leg is flexed at the hip and knee, while the left leg remains relatively extended. To avoid pressure sores, a cushion is placed between the legs, and the patient is secured with straps (Fig. 1.**70**).

If access to L2 is required, it proves highly advantageous to resect the twelfth rib. The alternative would be a subcostal flank incision. The skin incision begins near the midline at the level of spinous process T11 and continues first along the twelfth rib, before running obliquely and anteriorly toward the vicinity of the rectus sheath. Depending on the exposure desired, the incision may be extended caudally lateral to the rectus sheath.

The latissimus dorsi muscle is now dissected transversely to the direction of the fibers, and the external oblique muscle of the abdomen is dissected in part parallel to its fibers (Fig. 1.**71**). At the next deeper level, the inferior posterior serratus muscle is divided in the posterior incision area and followed more anteriorly, together with the transverse muscle of the abdomen, by the internal oblique muscle of the abdomen (Fig. 1.**72**).

After division of the deep abdominal muscle layers, the retroperitoneal space is entered. The kidney and the ureter are retracted to the right, bringing into view the quadratus lumborum muscle (Fig. 1.**73**). The intrinsic back musculature is now divided at the level of the twelfth rib, as indicated by the dashed line; the periosteum is incised over the twelfth rib, and the peripheral portion of the rib is resected (Fig. 1.**74**). Opening the pleural cavity is thus avoided (Fig. 1.**75**; see also Fig. 1.**63**). After this, the periosteum of the rib bed is transected near the middle, and the cranial half, together with the diaphragm inserted here, is retracted superiorly. Care should be taken to spare the eleventh and twelfth (subcostal nerve) intercostal nerves. Finally, a chest spreader is used (Fig. 1.**76**). Figure 1.**77** shows the anatomical site.

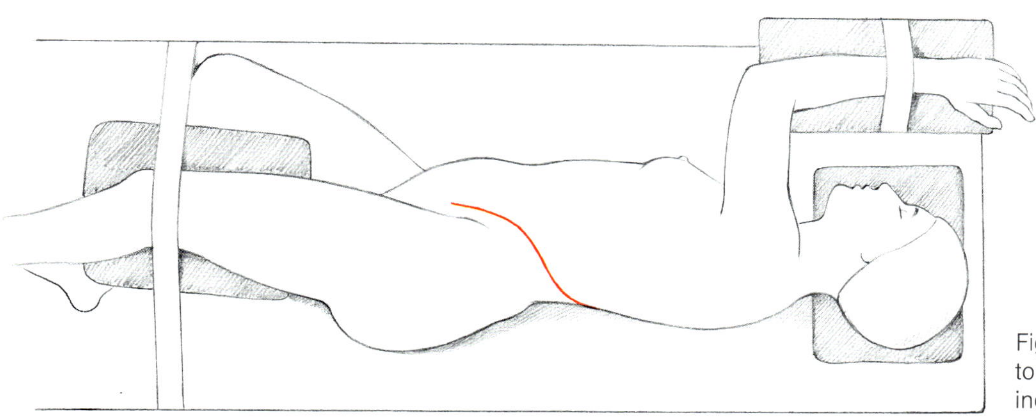

Fig. 1.**70** Retroperitoneal approach to the lumbar spine. Positioning and incision.

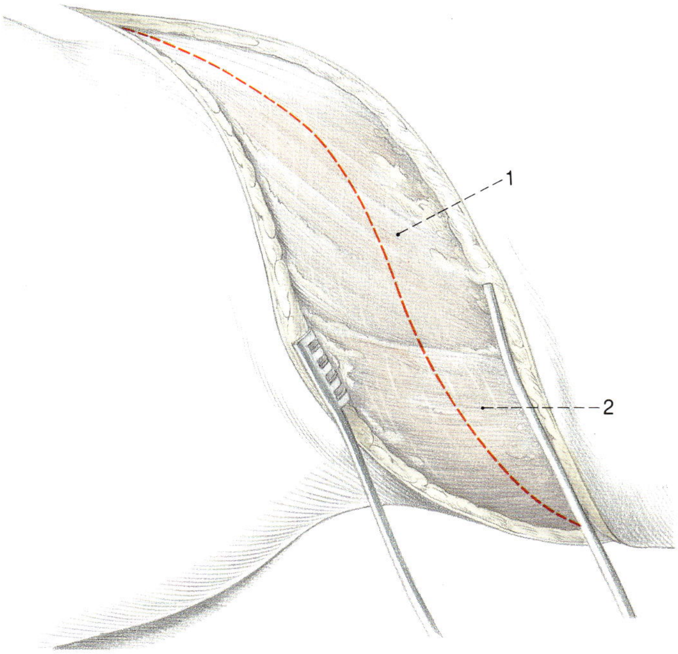

Fig. 1.**71** Division of the latissimus dorsi and external oblique muscle of the abdomen.

1 External oblique muscle of abdomen
2 Latissimus dorsi muscle

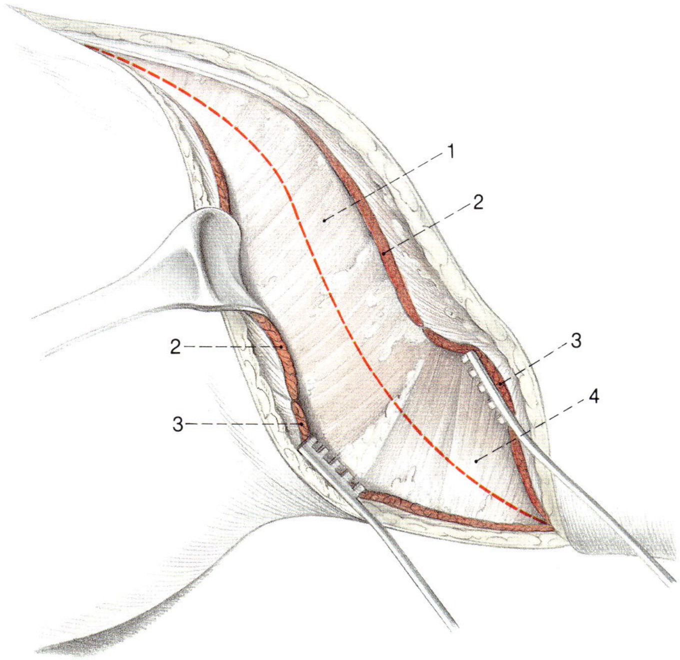

Fig. 1.**72** Division of the posterior inferior serratus muscle and of the deep abdominal muscle layers.

1 Internal oblique muscle of the abdomen
2 External oblique muscle of the abdomen
3 Latissimus dorsi muscle
4 Posterior inferior serratus muscle

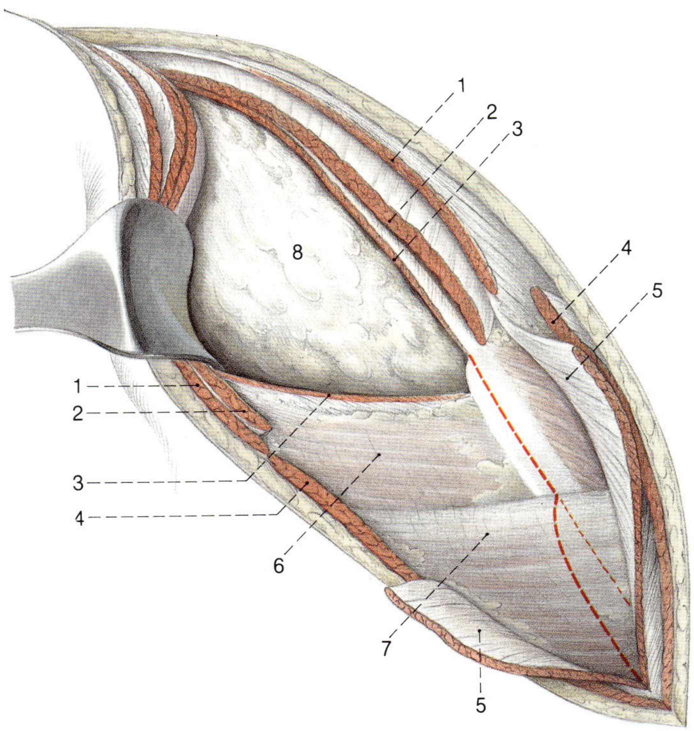

Fig. 1.**73** Status after division of the abdominal musculature. The iliocostal muscle is divided, and the periosteum of the twelfth rib incised (dashed line).

1 External oblique muscle of the abdomen
2 Internal oblique muscle of the abdomen
3 Transverse muscle of the abdomen
4 Latissimus dorsi muscle
5 Posterior inferior serratus muscle
6 Quadratus lumborum muscle
7 Iliocostal muscle
8 Preperitoneal adipose tissue

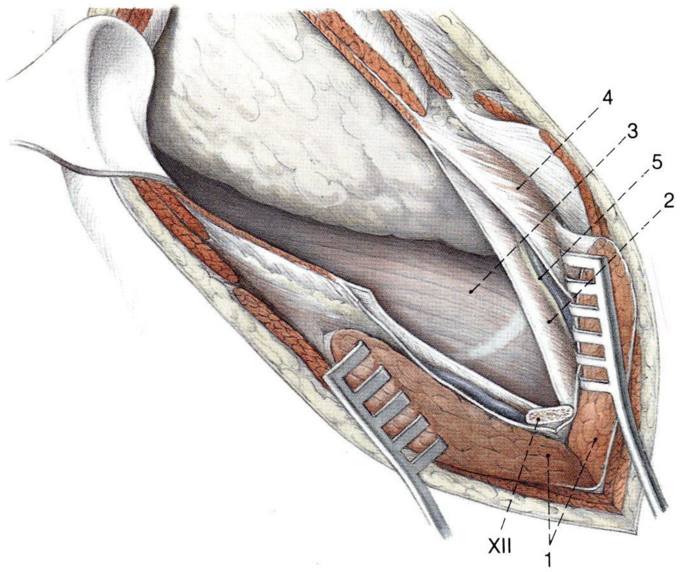

Fig. 1.**74** Status after resection of the twelfth rib and cleavage of the periosteal rib bed.

1 Iliocostal muscle
2 Thoracic diaphragm
3 Quadratus lumborum muscle
4 External intercostal muscle
5 Intercostal vein and nerve
XII Rib

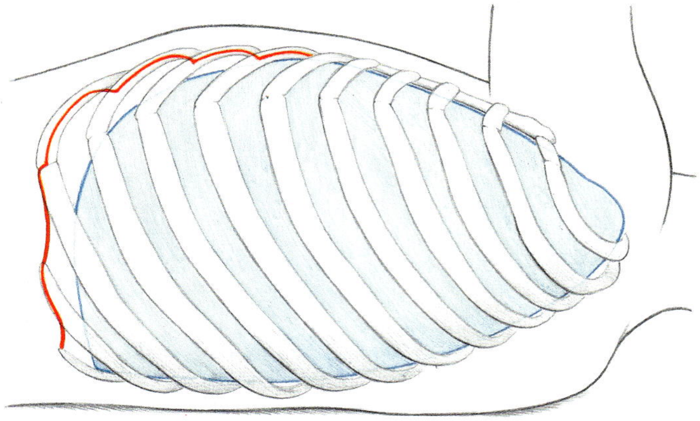

Fig. 1.**75** The pleural border (blue), origin of the diaphragm (red), and course of the ribs.

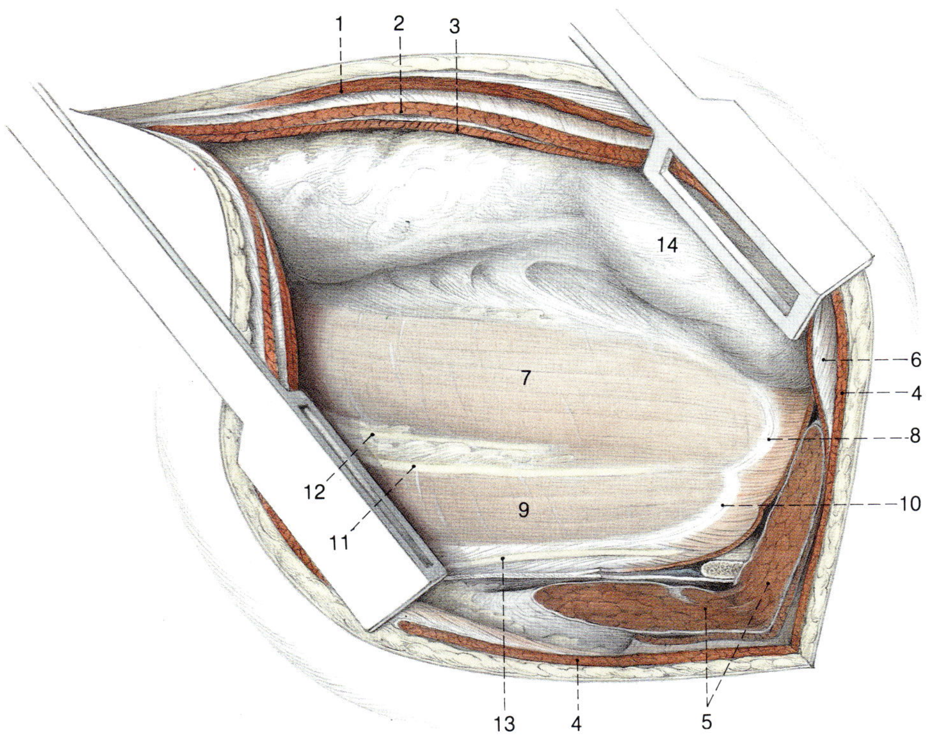

1 External oblique muscle of the abdomen
2 Internal oblique muscle of the abdomen
3 Transverse muscle of the abdomen
4 Latissimus dorsi muscle
5 Iliocostal muscle
6 Posterior inferior serratus muscle
7 Greater psoas muscle
8 Medial arcuate ligament
9 Quadratus lumborum muscle
10 Lateral arcuate ligament
11 Iliohypogastric nerve
12 Ilioinguinal nerve
13 Subcostal nerve
14 Adipose capsule of the kidney

Fig. 1.**76** Operative site after insertion of chest wall retractors.

Fig. 1.77 Anatomical site, retroperitoneal approach to the lumbar spine.

1 Greater psoas muscle
2 Quadratus lumborum muscle
3 Iliocostal muscle
4 Abdominal aorta
5 Lumbar artery and vein
6 Renal vein
7 Spermatic vessels
8 Inferior mesenteric artery
9 Subcostal nerve
10 Iliohypogastric nerve
11 Ilioinguinal nerve
12 Lateral cutaneous nerve of the thigh
13 Sympathetic trunk
14 Inferior mesenteric ganglion
15 Left kidney
16 Ureter
17 Adipose capsule of the kidney

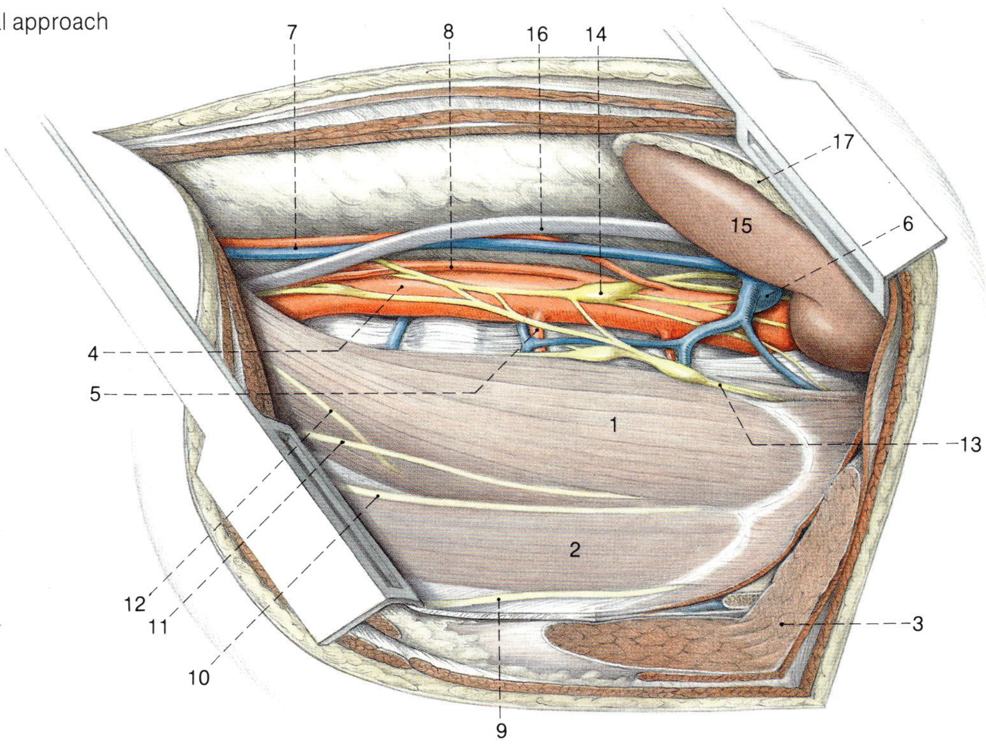

Exposure of Vertebrae

The retroperitoneal tissue over the lumbar spine is split longitudinally, the sympathetic trunk being left in place laterally. The segmental vessels are exposed in the usual way and, as far as possible, transected in the median line. After this, the vertebral bodies and intervertebral disks become accessible over their entire circumference (Fig. 1.**78**).

Wound Closure

To begin with, the rib bed (12) is reapproximated in the peripheral area. Further wound closure is performed in layers, largely following the procedure in the extrapleural retroperitoneal approach according to Mirbaha (see p. 37 and Fig. 1.**69**).

Fig. 1.**78** Operative site after transection of the segmental vessels.

1 Anterior longitudinal ligament
2 Subcostal nerve
3 Ilioinguinal nerve
4 Sympathetic trunk
5 Ureter
6 Right medial crus
7 Left medial crus
I–IV Vertebrae

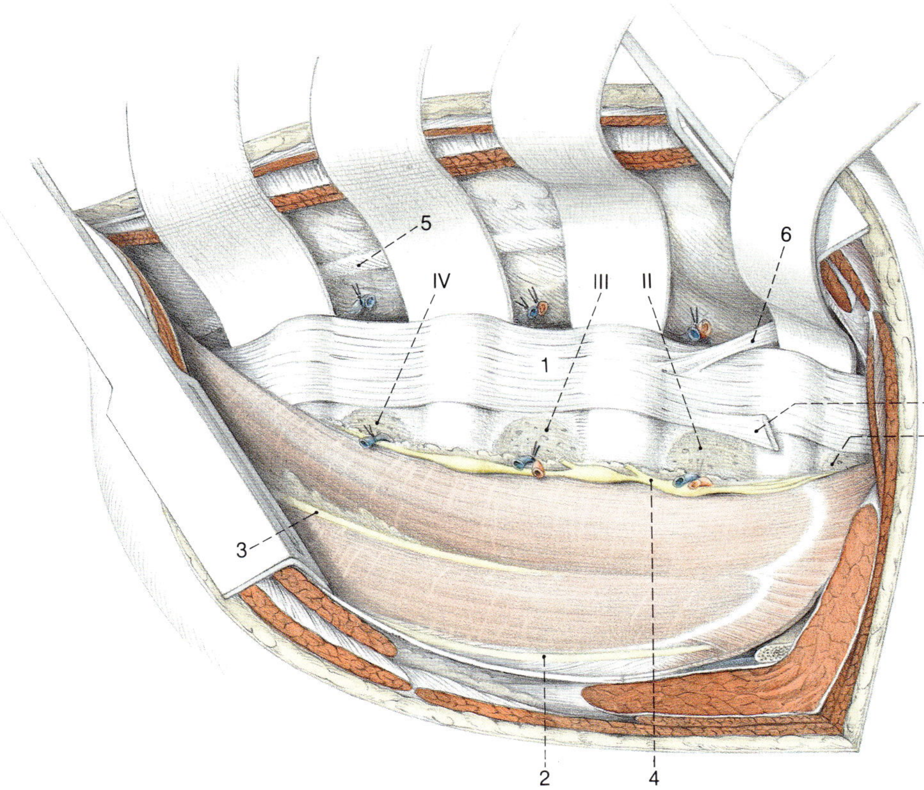

Pararectal Retroperitoneal Approach to the Lower Lumbar Spine and the Sacral Cavity, L3–S2

Positioning and Incision

The patient is placed in a supine position with the hip and knee joints flexed about 30 degrees, at a hip joint abduction of 15 degrees. Flexion in the hip joint relaxes the greater psoas muscle and the iliac vessels, so that the lower lumbar spine can be more easily exposed from anterolateral. Abduction of the hip permits an assistant to stand between the patient's legs. Flexion of the knee causes the lower legs to drop, thus reducing venous reflow. The skin incision is made in a curved line over the lateral border of the rectus muscle, from two to three finger-breadths above the umbilicus to three finger-breadths above the pubic symphysis (Fig. 1.**79**). The approach may generally be made from either side. Shown here is the approach from the right; however, for a unilateral approach, the left side is preferable, since the common iliac vein lies medial to the artery and thus does not need to be mobilized as far. Following dissection of the subcutaneous adipose tissue, the lateral border of the rectus muscle is identified. This contour can be palpated as a slight notch between the medially prominent rectus muscle and the lateral, flatter abdominal musculature. When incising the anterior sheath of the rectus, the superficial epigastric vessels should be ligated (Fig. 1.**80**). The caudal end of the incision runs medial to the superficial inguinal ring and therefore has to turn in a medial direction, following the outline of the rectus muscle.

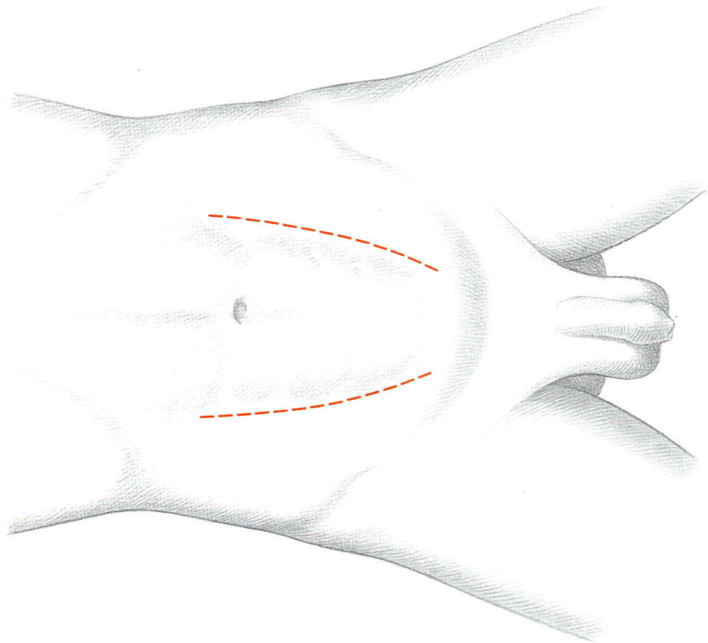

Fig. 1.**79** Positioning and skin incision in the pararectal approach. As a rule, a unilateral approach is sufficient; use of both approaches is recommended for sacral extirpation only.

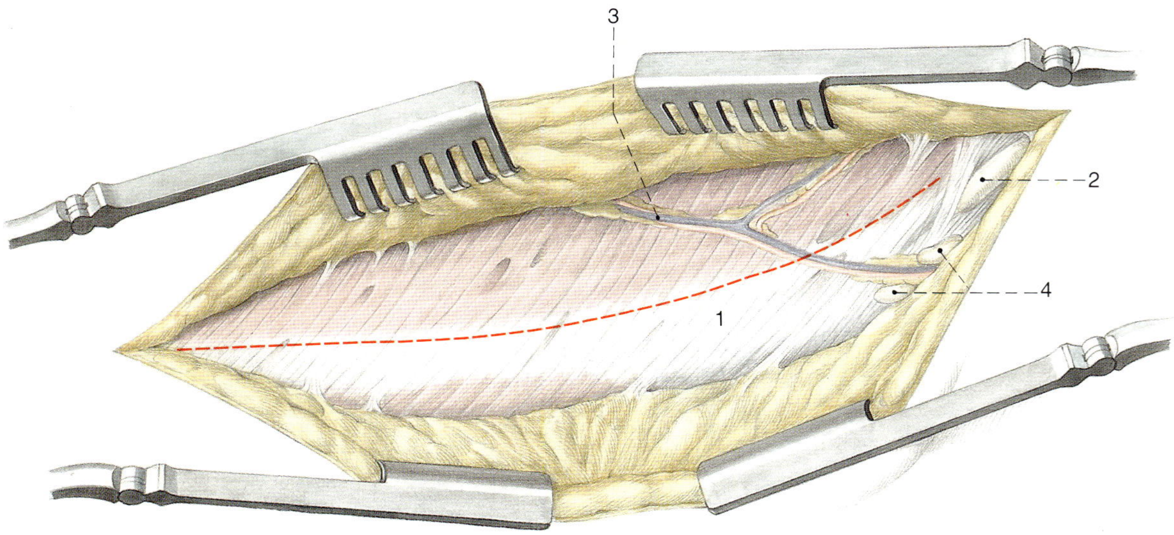

Fig. 1.**80** Exposure of abdominal fascia and incision of the rectus sheath.

1 Superficial abdominal fascia
2 Spermatic cord
3 Superficial epigastric artery and vein
4 Lymph nodes

Dissection in the Retroperitoneal Space

If the rectus sheath can be incised precisely at the union of the anterior and posterior layer, the preperitoneal space is entered at once; if the incision is carried out a little too far medially, the posterior layer of the rectus sheath is incised while being elevated with two forceps at the lateral border of the muscle (Fig. 1.**81**), avoiding injury to the peritoneum. Behind the posterior layer of the rectus sheath, the inferior epigastric vessels are exposed at the caudal border of the incision; these vessels generally need to be ligated if the lumbosacral junction is to be exposed (Fig. 1.**82**). Using a swab on a stick and digital dissection, the parietal peritoneum can then be retracted from the lateral abdominal wall. The longitudinally running psoas muscle with the overlying genitofemoral nerve is encountered first (Fig. 1.**83**). When the visceral sac is retracted to the other side, the common iliac artery and vein can be identified in the retroperitoneal fatty tissue, the artery running anterior to the vein. At the inferior margin of L4, the ureter crosses the common iliac artery from lateral to mediocaudal, accompanied by the testicular vessels. Coursing midway above the aortic bifurcation in a caudal direction is the superior hypogastric plexus, which fans out anteriorly to the promontory. This plexus is responsible for the sympathetic supply of the genitourinary system, and an attempt should always be made to preserve it, since injury in the male may lead to retrograde ejaculation. Subsequent dissection differs somewhat, depending on the intended operative field.

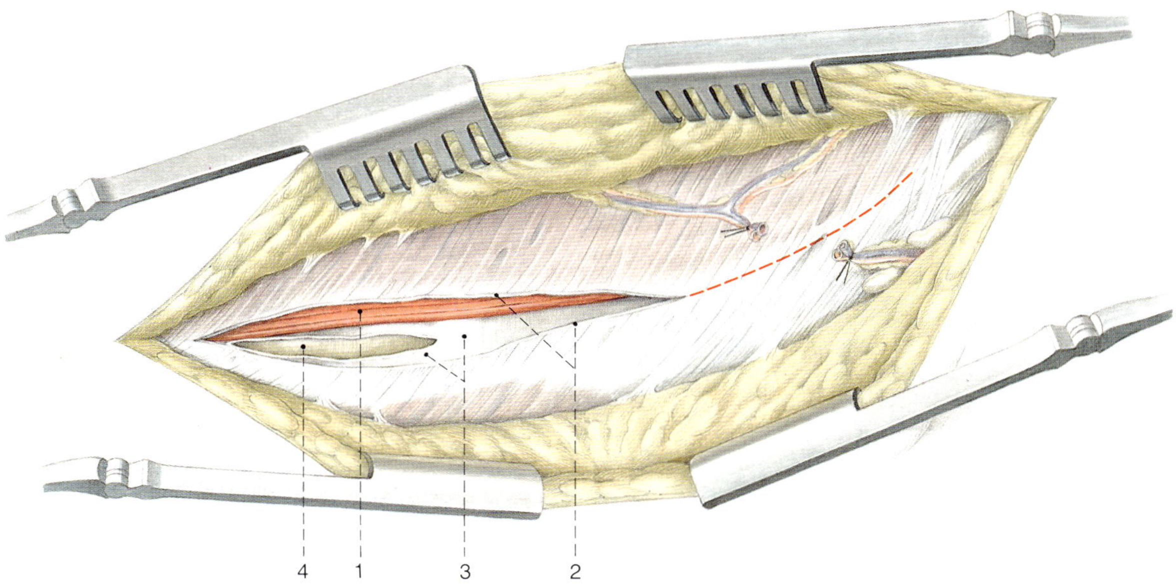

Fig. 1.**81** Division of the rectus sheath. The superficial epigastric vessels are ligated.

1 Rectus abdominis muscle
2 Anterior lamella of the rectus sheath
3 Posterior lamella of the rectus sheath
4 Peritoneum

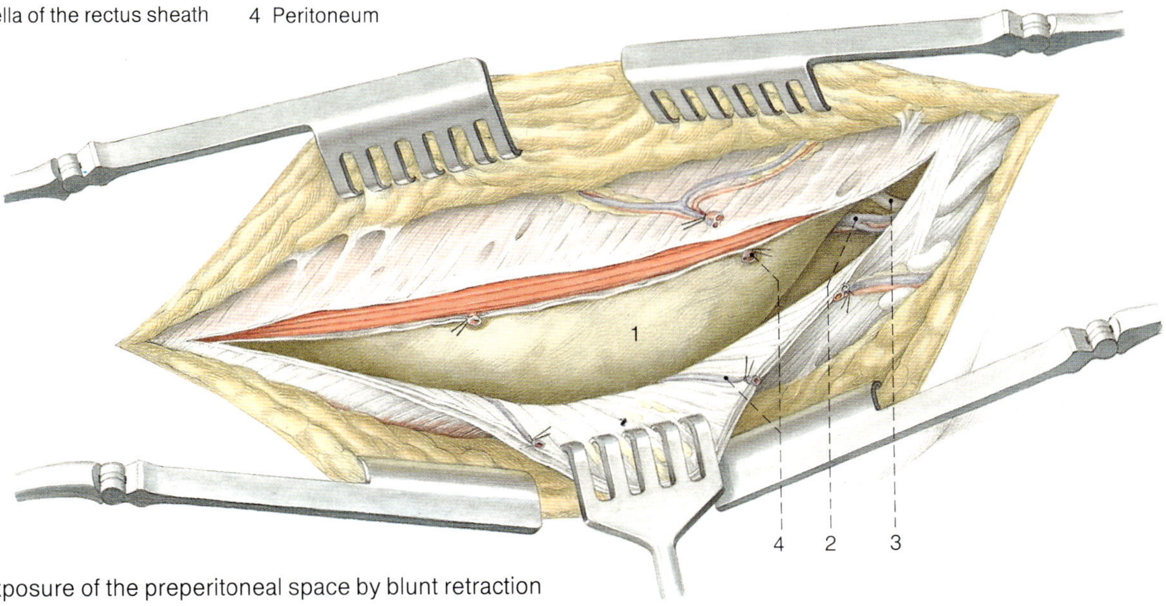

Fig. 1.**82** Exposure of the preperitoneal space by blunt retraction of the peritoneum.

1 Parietal peritoneum
2 Testicular artery and vein
3 Deferent duct
4 Inferior epigastric vessels

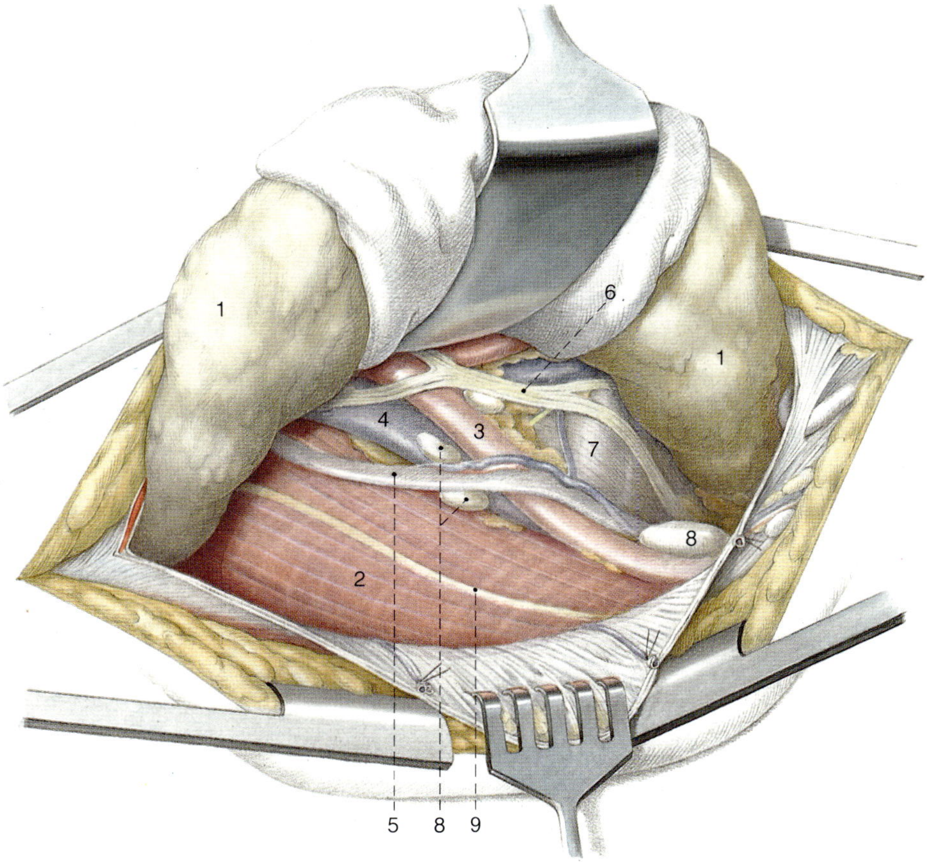

Fig. 1.**83** Exposure of the prevertebral space and iliac vessels by anterior and contralateral retraction of the parietal peritoneum.

1 Parietal peritoneum
2 Greater psoas muscle
3 Right common iliac artery
4 Right common iliac vein
5 Ureter with testicular vessels
6 Superior hypogastric plexus
7 Intervertebral disk L5–S1
8 Lymph node
9 Genitofemoral nerve

Exposure of the Middle and Lower Lumbar Spine

For exposure of the lower lumbar spine, as in spondylitis, for example, the psoas muscle is now cautiously detached from the medial side and retracted laterally. This exposes the segmental vessels and the relatively wide-caliber ascending lumbar vein (Fig. 1.**84**). Using this approach, the lumbar spine can be exposed from L3 to S1 without enlargement of the incision. Depending on the segment to be entered, the corresponding segmental vessels are exposed and ligated. Special caution has to be exercised with regard to the ascending lumbar vein, since damage to it can result in profuse bleeding. Prophylactic ligation of it, and of the segmental vessels, is therefore advisable in operations on the fourth lumbar vertebra and on the L4–L5 intervertebral disk (Fig. 1.**85**).

For exposure of the lumbar spine, the iliac vessels are now cautiously freed from the anterior longitudinal ligament and mobilized to the other side. This may prove difficult in the presence of inflammatory changes, since the common iliac vein may be firmly adherent to the spondylitic area. However, using the lateral entry it is nearly always possible to mobilize it far enough to permit the spinal segment involved to be approached from an anterolateral direction. If the common iliac vessels are mobilized to the other side, the sympathetic trunk is exposed; in operations above L5, it is retracted medially, and in operations below L5 laterally. Figure 1.**85** illustrates the anterolateral exposure of the vertebrae; if necessary, however, the entire anterior spinal region can be exposed as well.

Fig. 1.**84** Exposure of the anterolateral side of the prevertebral region by lateral retraction of the psoas muscle.

1 Internal iliac artery
2 Fourth lumbar artery and vein
3 Fifth lumbar artery and vein
4 Ascending lumbar vein
5 Promontory

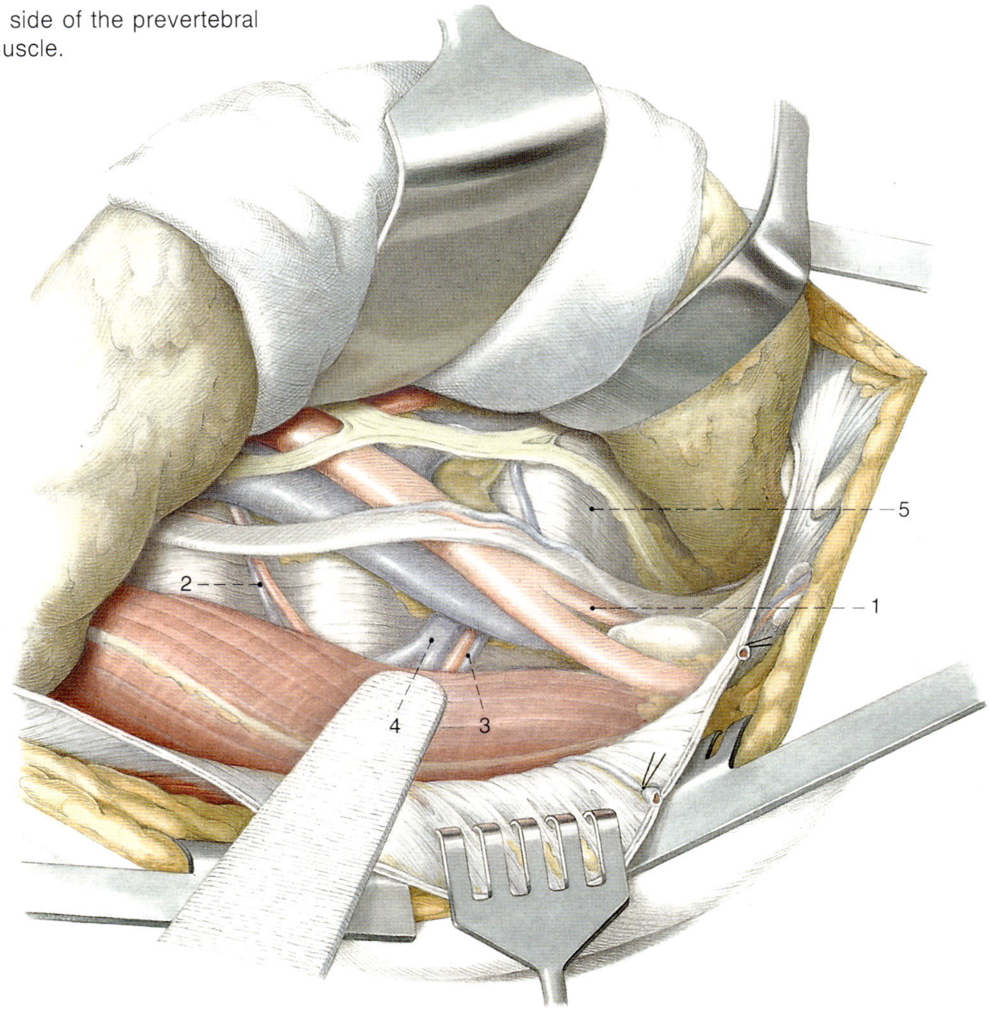

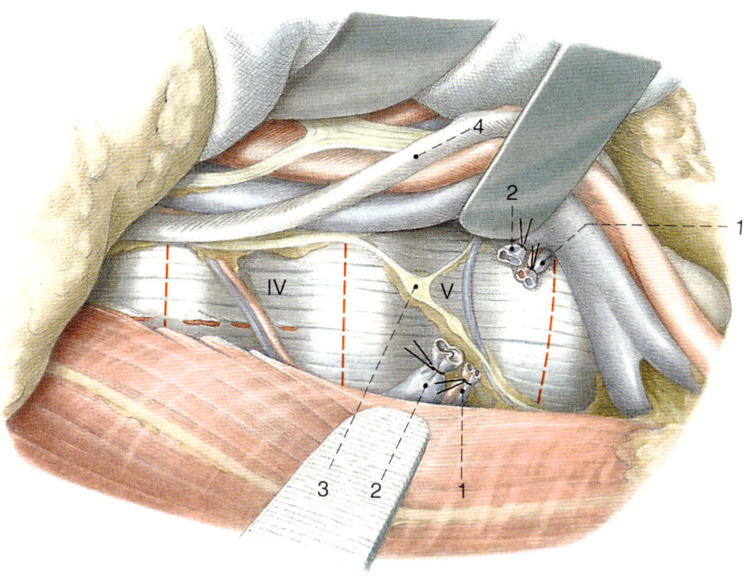

Fig. 1.**85** Anterolateral exposure of the lower lumbar spine, with ligation of the ascending lumbar vein and L5 segmental vessels.

1 Fifth lumbar artery and vein, transected
2 Ascending lumbar vein, transected
3 Sympathetic trunk with ganglion
4 Ureter

Exposure of the Promontory and Sacral Cavity

For exposure of the promontory, the sacral cavity, or the anterior side of the sacrum, the dissection proceeds as shown for the lumbar spine, up to Figure 1.**83**. It is advisable, however, to retract the urether with the visceral sac to the other side, to keep it out of the operative field (Fig. 1.**86**). To expose the promontory and the anterior side of the sacrum, the iliac vessels have to be mobilized so that they can be retracted medially (Fig. 1.**85**) as well as laterally (Fig. 1.**87**). During evacuations of the sacral cavity, the superior hypogastric plexus may remain untouched, but for exposure of the anterior side of the sacrum it has to be undermined and separated from the side. For removal of presacrally situated tumors originating in the sacrum, the internal iliac vessels are, as a first step, bilaterally ligated from anterior close to their origin from the common iliac artery and vein (Fig. 1.**87**). Besides reducing the blood supply to the tumor, this will greatly facilitate the subsequent posterior excision of the tumor, the principal vascular supply having already been excluded. Now the external iliac artery and vein, too, can be further retracted laterally for better exposure of the presacral structures. In particular, it is now possible to expose the first and second anterior sacral foramina. In the first session, we also carry out selective anterior osteotomy of the sacrum. The division may be done with a curved osteotome at any level between S1 and S2–S3. This has to be preceded by ligation of the middle sacral vessels, which should be effected, if at all possible, anteriorly to the promontory. In osteotomy at the level of the S1 foramen or above, it is often possible to spare the superior hypogastric plexus (Fig. 1.**88**). In order to prevent hemorrhages, the accompanying vessels of the first sacral root that emerge from the foramen in an anterior direction may be ligated as well.

Anatomical Site

(Fig. 1.**88**)

Together with the visceral sac, the ureter is retracted anteriorly and toward the other side; when the right-sided approach is used, the sigmoid colon, too, is lifted off anteriorly and to the left. A comparable site is afforded by the left-sided approach, since the sigmoid is relatively mobile and can readily be retracted in an anterior direction. The first anterior sacral foramen is exposed in order to perform a selective anterior osteotomy of the sacrum from the right iliosacral junction to the middle of the sacrum. Beneath the ligated internal iliac vein, the anterior branches of spinal nerves L4 and L5 can be identified, and these need to be retracted further laterally for the sacral

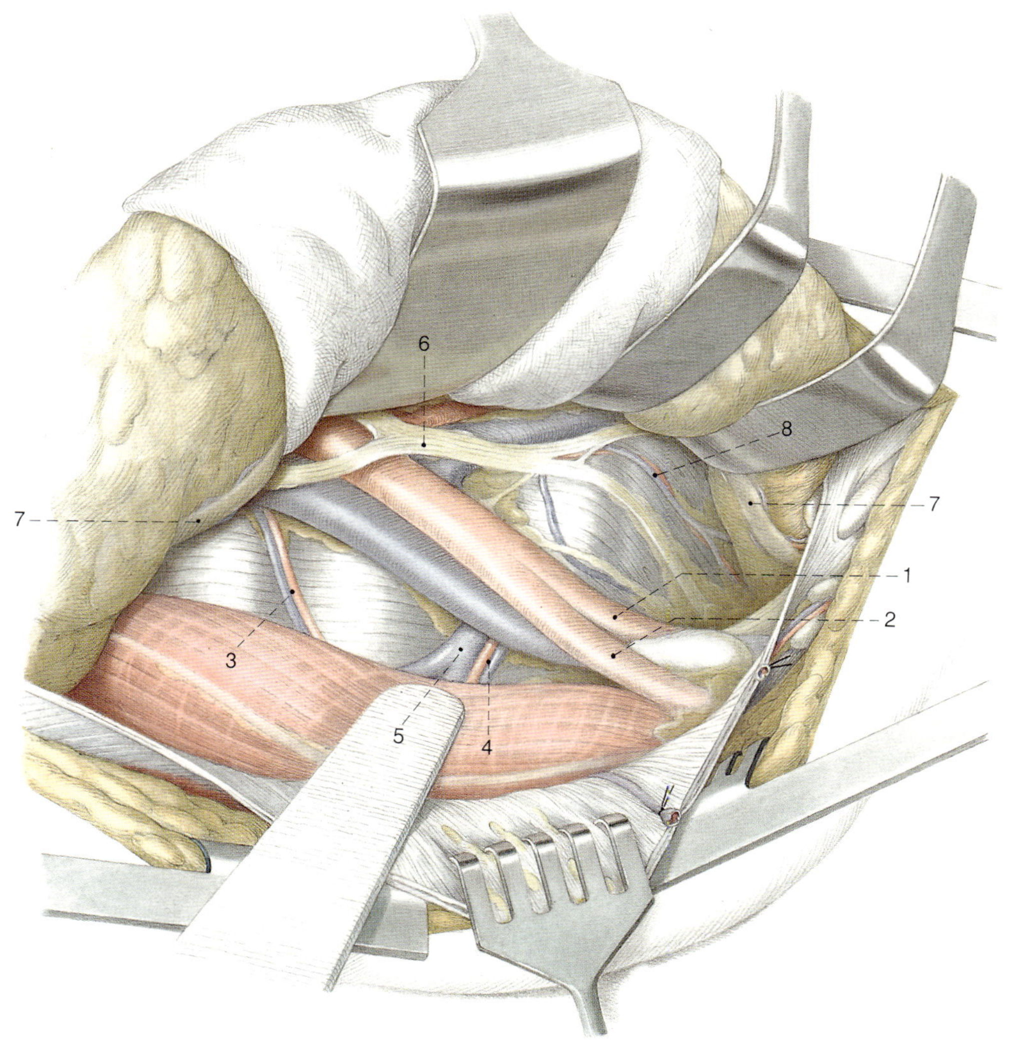

Fig. 1.**86** Exposure of the anterior lumbosacral junction, with retraction of the ureter.

1 Internal iliac artery
2 External iliac artery
3 Fourth lumbar artery and vein
4 Fifth lumbar artery and vein
5 Ascending lumbar vein
6 Superior hypogastric plexus
7 Ureter
8 Median sacral artery and vein

osteotomy. The superior hypogastric plexus and the sympathetic trunk may be lifted off the anterior side of the sacrum and retracted sufficiently to permit the sacral osteotomy to be performed without dividing them.

Wound Closure

Following application of a Hemovac drain or easy-flow drain to the lumbosacral junction, the wound is closed in a similar way for both exposures. The anterior and posterior rectus sheaths are joined to the lateral abdominal fascia with interrupted through-and-through sutures. Before this, however, it is necessary to look for any peritoneal injuries, which also require suturing. The anterior layer of the rectus sheath has to be sutured doubly to avoid diastasis of the rectus muscle. Suture of the subcutis and the skin follows.

Pitfalls

The greatest danger associated with exposure of the lumbosacral junction is injury to the iliac vessels, which can obstruct any view within seconds. Very tight adherence of the common or internal iliac vein to the anterior side of the vertebral body can be seen, particularly in the presence of inflammatory changes in the lower lumbar spine. The extremely difficult mobilization can, however, be accomplished more easily by dissection from the lateral rather than from the anterior side. If necessary, venous injuries, which generally occur on the posterior vessel wall, can also be repaired from lateral. In sacral osteotomy, the inferior lumbar nerve roots have to be isolated and retracted beforehand, to avoid inadvertently transecting them. Strong traction on Hohmann elevators can cause pressure damage, but in most cases this is completely reversible within a few weeks.

Note

The pararectal retroperitoneal approach facilitates exposure of the lumbosacral junction, since it allows the structures lying directly in front of the vertebrae to be bypassed. Anterolateral exposure is entirely sufficient for most operations, and may be completed by a contralateral approach. However, the main advantage is that the peritoneal cavity need not be opened, so that postoperative intestinal problems rarely occur. Damage to the superior hypogastric plexus, which is almost unavoidable in the anterior approach, can also easily be circumvented by this route.

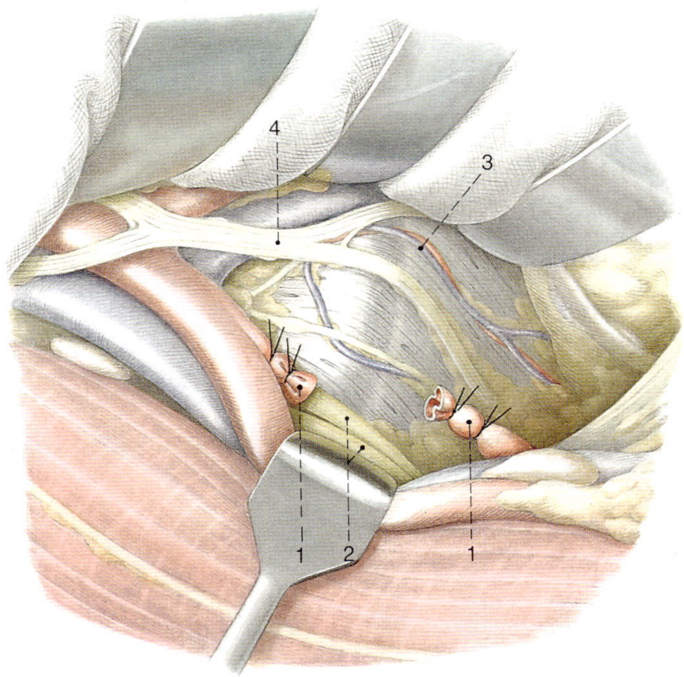

Fig. 1.**87** Exposure of the promontory by lateral retraction of the iliac vessels and transection of internal iliac artery and vein.

1 Internal iliac artery
2 Anterior branches of spinal nerves L4 and L5
3 Median sacral artery and vein
4 Superior hypogastric plexus

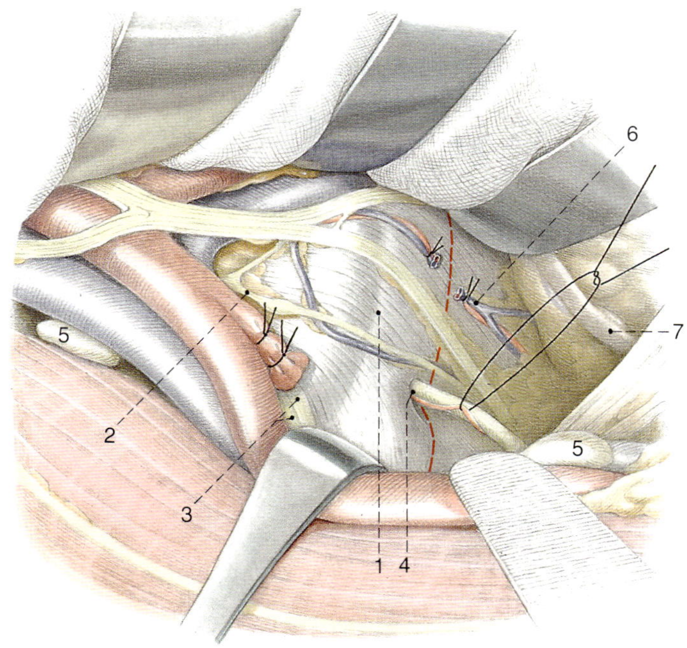

Fig. 1.**88** Exposure of the anterior aspect of the sacrum for sacral osteotomy at the level of the first sacral foramen.

1 Promontory
2 Sympathetic trunk with ganglion
3 Anterior branches of spinal nerves L4 and L5
4 First anterior sacral foramen with anterior branch
5 Lymph node
6 Median sacral artery and vein, ligated
7 Ureter

Transperitoneal Approach to the Lumbosacral Junction, L4–S1

Principal Indications

- Spondylolisthesis
- Presacral osteochondrosis
- Tumors

Positioning and Incision

The patient is placed in the supine position, with a roll under the lumbar spine. The operating table is angled in the middle to produce a hyperlordosis, which facilitates access to the promontory. At the same time, the position of the legs reduces venous reflux.

A median laparotomy is performed as usual, bypassing the umbilicus on the left (Fig. 1.**89**). The skin incision begins two to three finger-breadths above the umbilicus, and ends three finger-breadths above the symphysis.

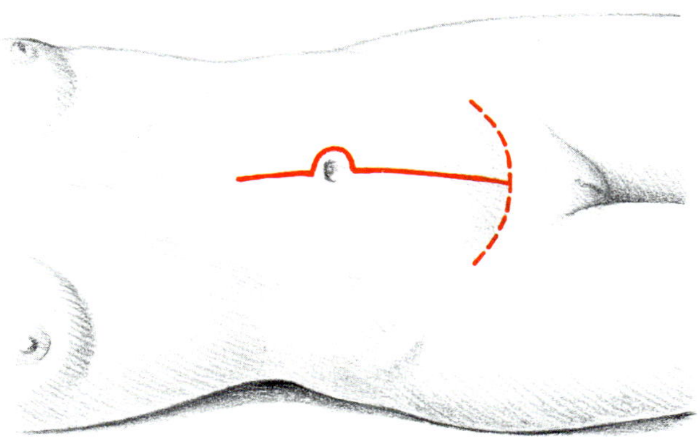

Fig. 1.**89** Transperitoneal approach to the lumbosacral junction. The skin incision may be made in the midline or, optionally, as a "Pfannenstiel" incision two finger-breadths above the symphysis.

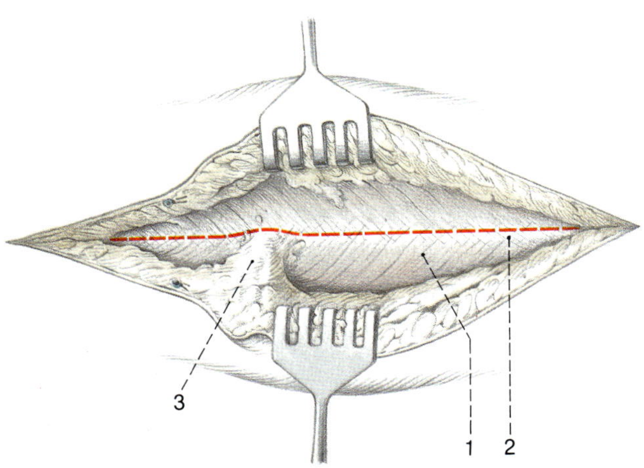

Fig. 1.**90** After transection of the skin and subcutis, the linea alba is incised with a knife in the midline.

1 Rectus abdominis muscle
2 Linea alba
3 Umbilicus

After dissection of the subcutis, the linea alba is exposed and transected in the midline with a scalpel. The subjacent peritoneum is then elevated with two forceps, incised with a scalpel, and split longitudinally with scissors (Figs. 1.**90**, 1.**91**).

Exposure of the Vertebrae

The wound is separated with large laparotomy hooks, and the greater omentum is retracted superiorly. The small bowel and the root of the mesentery are retracted superiorly using a bowel towel. The mesocolon on the right and left sides is also retracted with wet compresses, while the sigmoid situated caudally and on the left is retracted inferiorly with the aid of a spatula. The posterior peritoneal layer is incised about 2 cm to the right of the midline, from two finger-breadths proximal to the aortic bifurcation to two finger-breadths distal to the promontory (Fig. 1.**92**). When dividing the peritoneum, care should be taken not to injure branches of the subjacent superior hypogastric plexus. To facilitate dissection, saline solution may be infiltrated into the subjacent tissue prior to incision of the posterior peritoneal layer; this will cause the peritoneal layer to be lifted off, while the superior hypogastric plexus remains adherent to the vessels. Using blunt dissection and peanut swab sticks, the peritoneum is now bilaterally mobilized laterally and may be snared with one stay suture on each side. The retroperitoneal vessels and the superior hypogastric plexus are covered by a layer of fat and connective tissue, which should be bluntly opened over the right common iliac artery to the right of the midline. The tissue, with the superior hypogastric plexus, which runs inferiorly over the promontory and anterior to the aortic bifurcation, is now bluntly dissected free of the aortic bifurcation

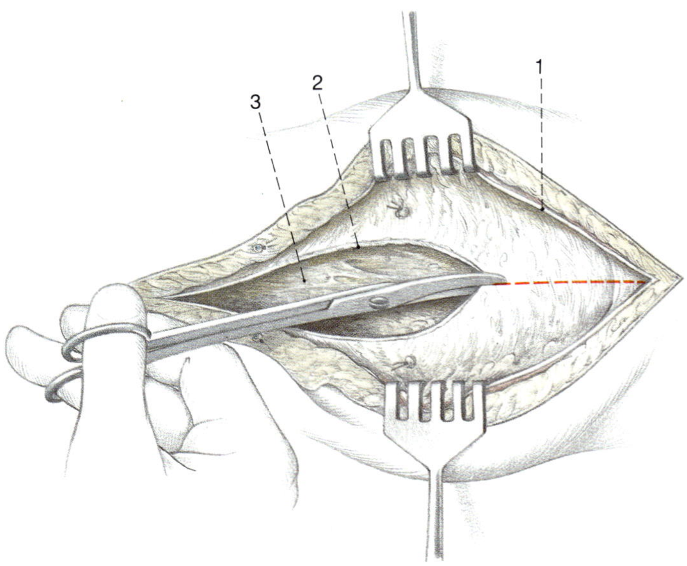

Fig. 1.**91** Division of the peritoneum with scissors.

1 Linea alba
2 Parietal peritoneum
3 Greater omentum

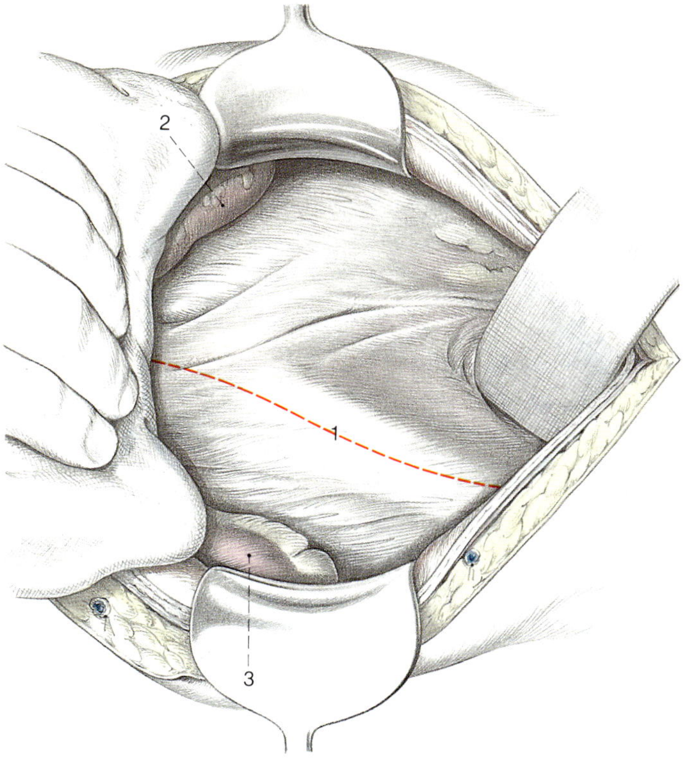

Fig. 1.**92** Operative site after opening of the abdomen. The posterior peritoneal layer is transected about 2 cm to the right of the midline, medial to the right ureter and above the right common iliac artery.

1 Parietal peritoneum
2 Sigmoid colon
3 Cecum

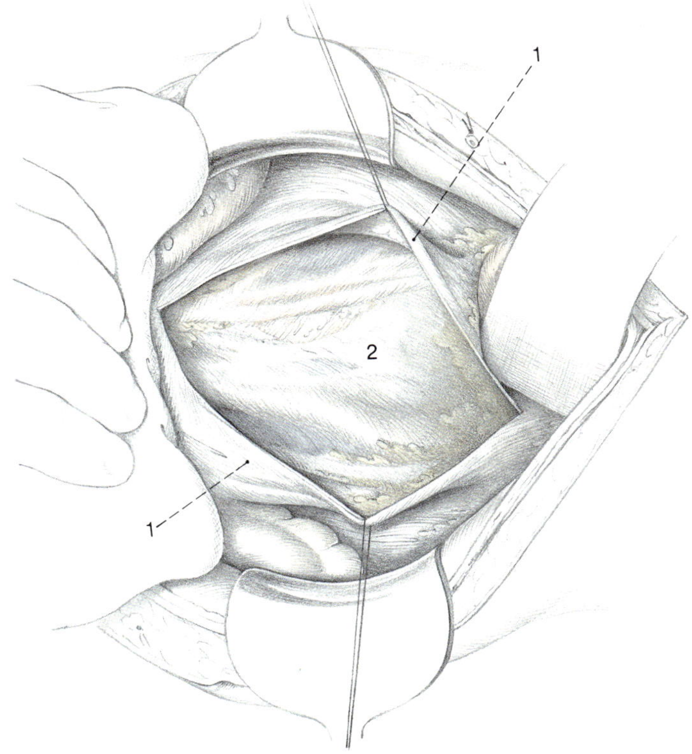

Fig. 1.**93** Blunt lateral dissection of peritoneum and securing with stay sutures. The superior hypogastric plexus is visualized.

1 Parietal peritoneum
2 Superior hypogastric plexus

toward the left, in one layer (Figs. 1.**92**, 1.**93**). The promontory is now readily visible, and the middle sacral artery as well as the middle sacral vein, which is not always present, may now be ligated. The aorta and the right and left common iliac arteries are mobilized with a vessel loop for better mobilization, if necessary. After this, the posteriorly situated vena cava and the left common iliac vein are cautiously retracted from the promontory superiorly. Flexible spatulas or Harmon retractors may then be used on both sides of the presacral intervertebral disk to protect the large pelvic vessels (Fig. 1.**94**).

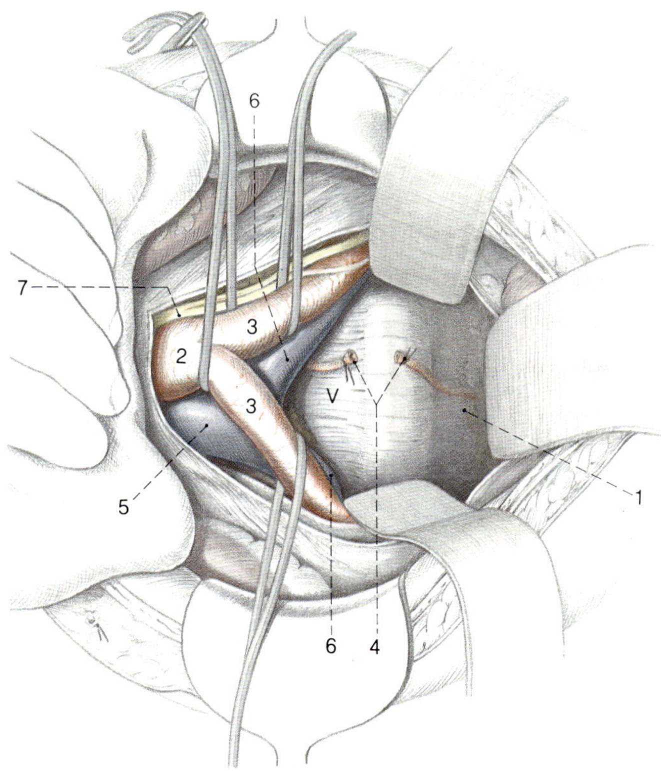

Fig. 1.**94** Exposure of the promontory and caudal half of the fifth lumbar vertebra, and the upper half of the first sacral vertebra after transection of the median sacral artery. The aorta and the right common iliac artery are secured, and the right and left common iliac veins are retracted.

1 Sacrum
2 Abdominal aorta
3 Common iliac artery
4 Medial sacral artery
5 Inferior vena cava
6 Common iliac vein
7 Superior hypogastric plexus
V Lumbar vertebra

This approach usually also permits exposure of the intervertebral disk L4–L5 if the left common iliac vein and the inferior vena cava are dissected with appropriate care. In case of a deeply localized aortic bifurcation or deep venous confluence, dissection between the aorta and the vena cava (Louis) has been found advantageous for exposure of the third and fourth intervertebral disks. In this case, it is first necessary to undermine and secure the aorta and retract it to the left, after which the fourth lumbar vascular bundle is ligated. The inferior vena cava can now be dissected free toward the right, using peanut swab sticks, so that the fourth and, if necessary, the third intervertebral disk, can be exposed between two Harmon retractors (Fig. 1.**95**).

Anatomical Site

(Fig. 1.**96**)

The following anatomical structures are found between the parietal peritoneum, on the one hand, and the fifth lumbar vertebra and the promontory, on the other hand: the superior hypogastric plexus forms a network overlying the anterior surface of the aorta, the promontory, and the left common iliac artery. It is responsible for the sympathetic nerve supply of the genitourinary system, and receives its main branches from the lumbar sympathetic trunk ganglia. The appearance and situation of this nerve plexus vary. Behind the nerve plexus, the aortic bifurcation is generally found at the level of the fourth lumbar vertebra or the L4–L5 intervertebral disk. Lying to the left of the aorta is the inferior mesenteric artery, which arises from the anterior side of the aorta, approximately at the level of the third lumbar vertebra. The two ureters cross the iliac arteries, descending from lateral to medial at the level of the origin of the internal iliac artery. The confluence of the left and right common iliac veins lies on the right caudally and posteriorly to the aortic bifurcation. In the majority of cases, the level of the venous confluence is above the fifth lumbar vertebra or the L4–L5 intervertebral disk. Exceptionally, the venous plexus may lie above the aortic bifurcation. The middle sacral artery lies in the midline above the promontory, and so, in most cases, does the middle sacral vein.

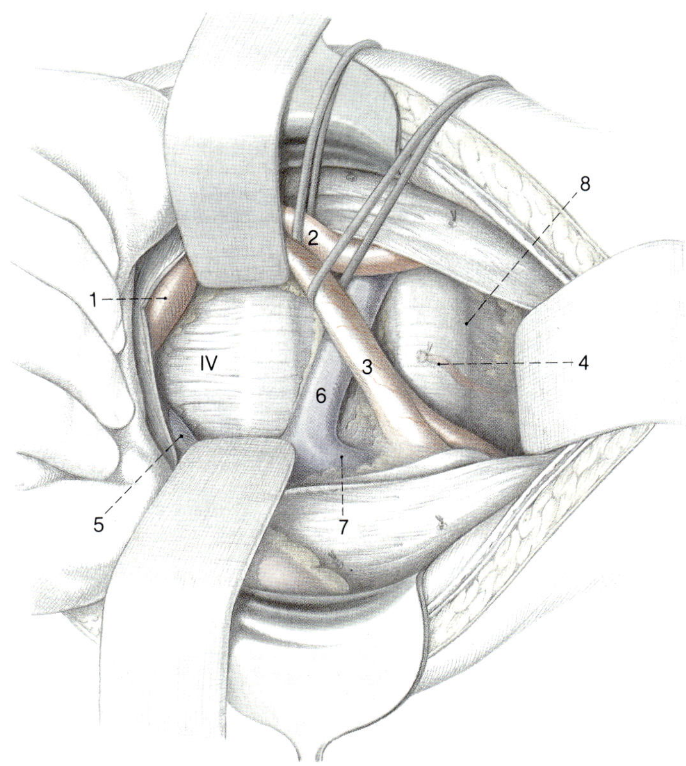

Fig. 1.**95** Exposure of the fourth lumbar vertebral body and of intervertebral disk L4–L5 between the aorta and the inferior vena cava following ligation and transection of the fourth segmental vascular bundle.

1 Abdominal aorta
2 Left common iliac artery
3 Right common iliac artery
4 Median sacral artery
5 Inferior vena cava
6 Left common iliac vein
7 Right common iliac vein
8 Promontory
IV Lumbar vertebra

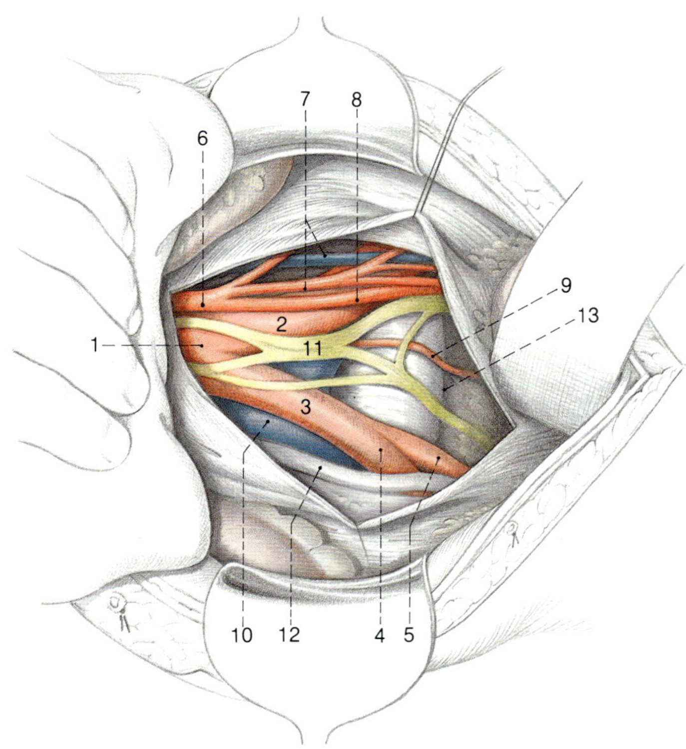

Fig. 1.**96** Anatomical site anterior to the fifth lumbar vertebra and the promontory.

1 Abdominal aorta
2 Left common iliac artery
3 Right common iliac artery
4 External iliac artery
5 Internal iliac artery
6 Inferior mesenteric artery
7 Sigmoid vessels
8 Superior rectal artery
9 Median sacral artery
10 Right common iliac vein
11 Superior hypogastric plexus
12 Right ureter
13 Promontory

Wound Closure

The parietal peritoneum is closed with a running suture with absorbable material. The wet bowel sponges are now removed, so that the small-bowel loops and the root of the mesentery resume their normal positions. Before the greater omentum is pulled down, care should be taken to ensure that no torsion of the mesenteric root has developed. The linea alba and the transverse fascia in the lower part of the wound are now grasped with Mikulicz clamps and raised, and the peritoneum is continuously sutured with absorbable material. After closure of the rectus sheath with nonabsorbable material, the subcutis and the skin are closed in the usual way.

Pitfalls

After opening of the parietal peritoneum, dissection of the aorta and the right and left common iliac arteries may cause injury to the superior hypogastric plexus. This injury may result in retrograde ejaculation in males. If dissection is carried too far laterally, there is a risk of injury to the ureters. They cross the iliac arteries at the level of the origin of the internal iliac artery. The ureter is usually adherent to the parietal peritoneum, and can be detected by showing contractions after digital palpation. Another danger is injury to the large vessels, notably the left common iliac vein and the inferior vena cava. Deep-seated ectopic kidneys or horseshoe kidneys can hinder or prevent a transperitoneal approach. Preoperative urography and computed tomography, in addition to angiography to define the level of the aortic bifurcation, are therefore recommended.

Note

If the patient is properly prepared (good bowel preparation and liquid diet preoperatively), the transperitoneal approach to the lumbosacral intervertebral disk can be carried out fairly rapidly. Since partial damage to the superior hypogastric plexus cannot be ruled out, even with careful dissection, this approach should be chosen in males only if a posterior or lateral extraperitoneal approach is not feasible.

Posterior Approaches

Cervical Spine

Posterior Approach to the Cervical Spine with Occipitocervical Junction

Principal Indications

- Occipitocervical instability
- Degenerative changes
- Trauma
- Tumors

Positioning and Incision

The patient is placed in prone position, with a cushion under the chest. The head is fixed in a slightly flexed position on a padded U-shaped tray (Fig. 1.**97**). Extension of the skull is possible if necessary (dislocation fractures, cervico-occipital instability in rheumatoid arthritis). Extensive shaving of the back of the neck and head is required. The median skin incision is begun two finger-breadths above the external occipital protuberance and continued as far as the tip of the spinous process of the seventh cervical vertebra (prominent vertebra).

After splitting of the subcutis, self-retaining retractors are applied and hemostasis is effected. Using a diathermy knife, the nuchal ligament is now approached via a midline incision of the cervical fascia. The trapezius muscle adherent to the fascia can then be mobilized bilaterally and a retractor placed in the next deeper plane (Fig. 1.**98**).

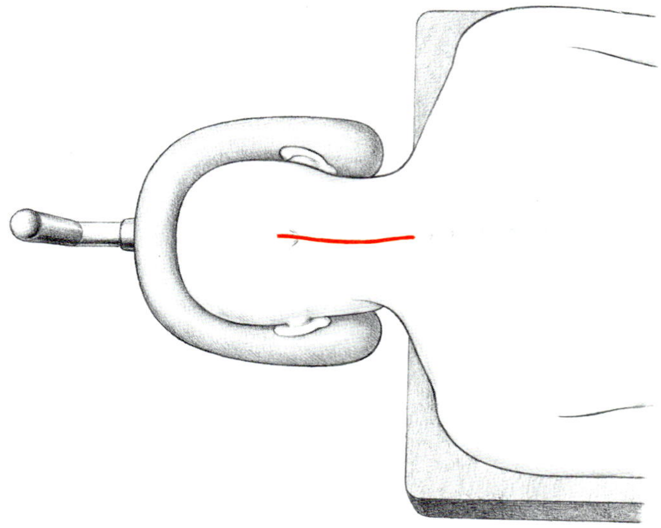

Fig. 1.**97** Posterior approach to the cervical spine with occipitocervical junction. Positioning and incision.

Exposure of the Spine

The nuchal ligament is divided in the midline and incised as far as the tips of the spinous processes. The muscle layer that has been divided in the midline is retracted to the side. After this, beginning at the spinous process of the second cervical vertebra, the deep muscle layer is stripped off the spinous processes close to the bone with the electrocautery, going from cranial to caudal. If necessary (as with

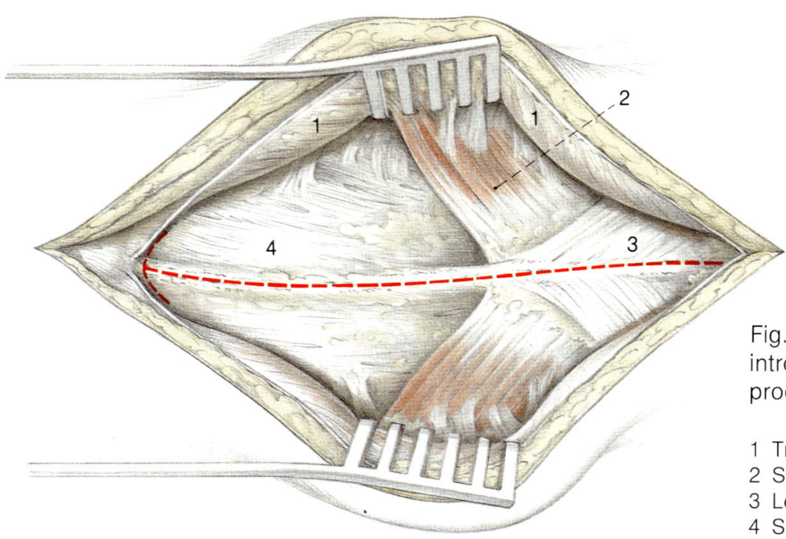

Fig. 1.**98** Operative site after division of the nuchal fascia and introduction of self-retaining retractors. The series of spinous processes is then approached in the midline (dashed line).

1 Trapezius muscle
2 Splenius capitis muscle
3 Lesser rhomboid muscle
4 Semispinalis capitis muscle

occipitocervical fusion), the musculature originating from, or attached to, the occiput (trapezius muscle, semispinalis capitis muscle) may be separated using a T-shaped dissection (Fig. 1.**99**). Beginning at the second spinous process and proceeding caudally, a sharp elevator is now used to strip the short rotator and multifidus muscles from the spinous processes and articular processes, and a subperiosteal dissection extending to the lateral boundary of the vertebral joints is carried out. Hemostasis is effected by insertion of rolled-up swabs. Subsequently, the part of the occipital squama that lies caudal to the external occipital protuberance is exposed subperiosteally with a sharp rasp. This invariably leads to bleeding from the suboccipital venous plexus, which can be stopped by electrocautery. The posterior tubercle of the atlas is now palpated with a fingertip in its deep, midline location. The musculature arising from it is detached on both sides and, using an elevator, the arch of the atlas is subperiosteally dissected for about 1.5 cm bilaterally (Fig. 1.**100**). The tip of the rasp must remain in constant contact with the bone to avoid damage to the vertebral artery. After passing through the foramen of the transverse process of the atlas, the vertebral artery bilaterally travels medially in the sulcus of the vertebral artery, the edge of which is visible and palpable after careful dissection (Fig. 1.**101**). More laterally, between the first and second cervical vertebrae, the posterior branch of the second spinal nerve arises, the main branch of which is the greater occipital nerve. This nerve should likewise be spared. The retractors are inserted into the deepest muscle layer and opened further. The vertebral arches, the yellow ligaments, and the atlanto-occipital membrane are exposed with curets and small dissectors. The interspinal ligaments are generally removed if posterior fusion is to be performed (Fig. 1.**102**).

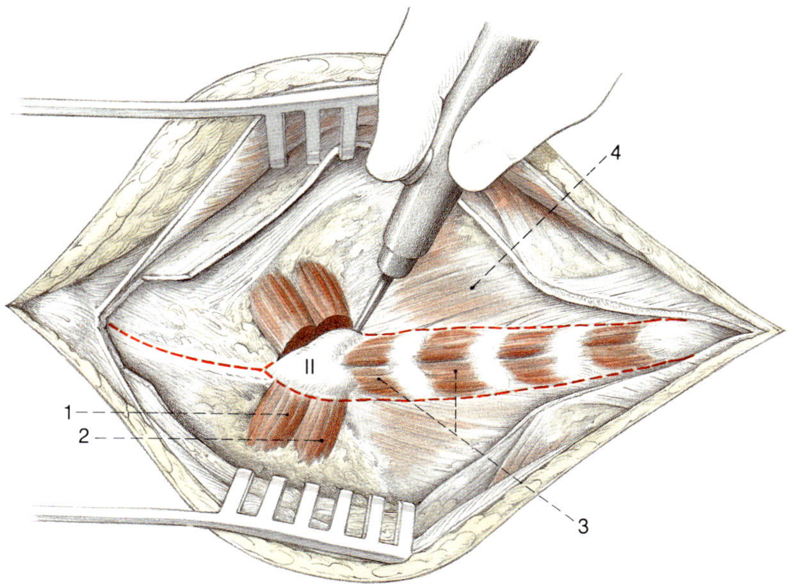

Fig. 1.**99** Dissection of the median and deep layers of the nuchal musculature near the bone, descending from the spinous process of the second cervical vertebra.

1 Greater posterior straight muscle of the head
2 Inferior oblique muscle of the head
3 Interspinal muscles
4 Semispinalis cervicis muscle
II Spinous process of the second cervical vertebra

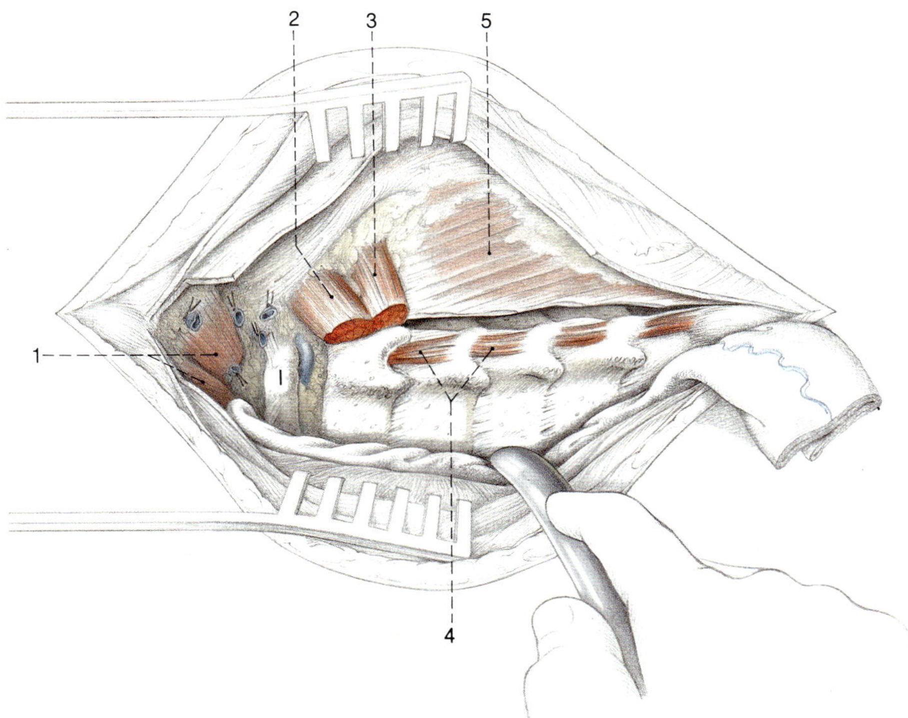

Fig. 1.**100** Subperiosteal retraction of the deep nuchal musculature, using an elevator, beyond the vertebral joints. Packing with gauze swabs. Ligation or electrocautery of the suboccipital venous plexus. Beware of subperiosteal dissection of the arc of the atlas more than 1.5 cm lateral to the midline, to avoid injury to the vertebral artery.

1 Smaller posterior straight muscle of the head
2 Greater posterior straight muscle of the head
3 Inferior oblique muscle of the head
4 Interspinal muscles
5 Semispinalis cervicis muscle
I Posterior tubercle of atlas

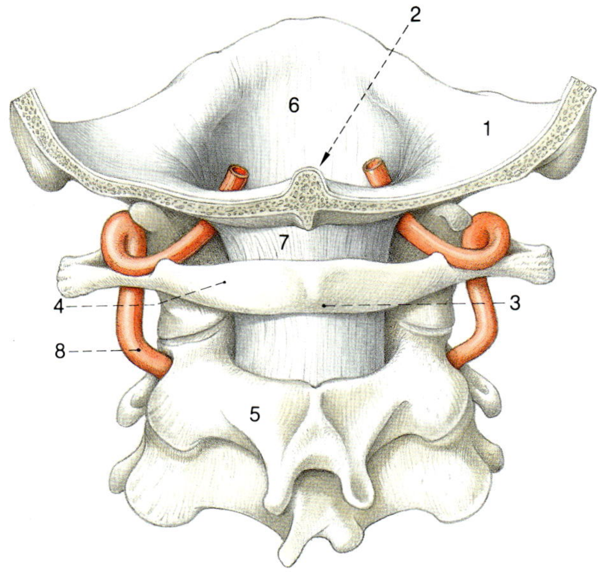

Fig. 1.**101** The occipitocervical junction from the rear, with the course of the vertebral artery.

1 Occipital squama
2 Great foramen
3 Posterior tubercle of the atlas
4 Posterior arch of the atlas
5 Spinous process of the axis
6 Tectorial membrane
7 Posterior atlanto-occipital membrane
8 Vertebral artery

Anatomical Site

(Figs. 1.**103**, 1.**104**)

The musculature of the neck is subdivided as follows:

- Trapezius muscle
- Lesser rhomboid muscle
- Intrinsic muscles of the back:
  Splenius capitis and cervicis muscles
  Semispinalis capitis and cervicis muscles
  Multifidus muscles
  Rotator muscles (variable); interspinal muscles
- Short nuchal muscles:
  Rectus capitis major and minor muscles
  Superior and inferior oblique muscles of the head

The posterior branch of the second spinal nerve (main branch: greater occipital nerve) runs in a posterior direction between the first and second cervical vertebrae. One finger-breadth distal to the tendinous arch between the trapezius and sternocleidomastoid muscles it runs subcutaneously, supplying the skin of the occiput. The posterior branch of the third spinal nerve courses posteriorly between the second and third cervical vertebrae. Its main branch, the third occipital nerve, is variable, and also supplies the skin of the occiput. The vertebral artery travels in a medial direction from the foramen of the transverse process of the atlas behind the atlanto-occipital articulation and then runs through the posterior atlanto-occipital membrane into the great foramen, and thus into the cranial cavity.

Pitfalls

Too extensive a dissection of the first and second vertebral arches in a lateral direction can cause injury to the vertebral artery or the suboccipital and greater occipital nerves. In rheumatoid arthritis, the posterior arch of the atlas is very thin, and it can be injured by excessive dissector pressure.

Wound Closure

Wound closure is accomplished by suturing the musculature and the nuchal ligament.

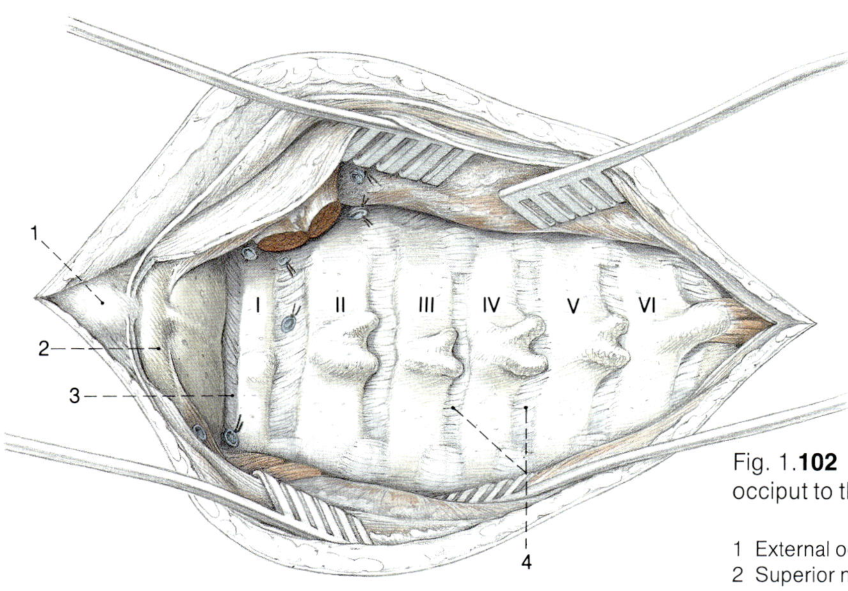

Fig. 1.**102** The cervical spine has been exposed from the occiput to the sixth cervical spine.

1 External occipital protuberance
2 Superior nuchal line
3 Posterior atlanto-occipital membrane
4 Yellow ligaments
I–VI Cervical vertebrae

Fig. 1.**103** Anatomical site of the superficial and median nuchal muscle layers.

1 Trapezius muscle
2 Semispinalis capitis muscle
3 Splenius capitis muscle
4 Lesser rhomboid muscle
5 Greater occipital nerve

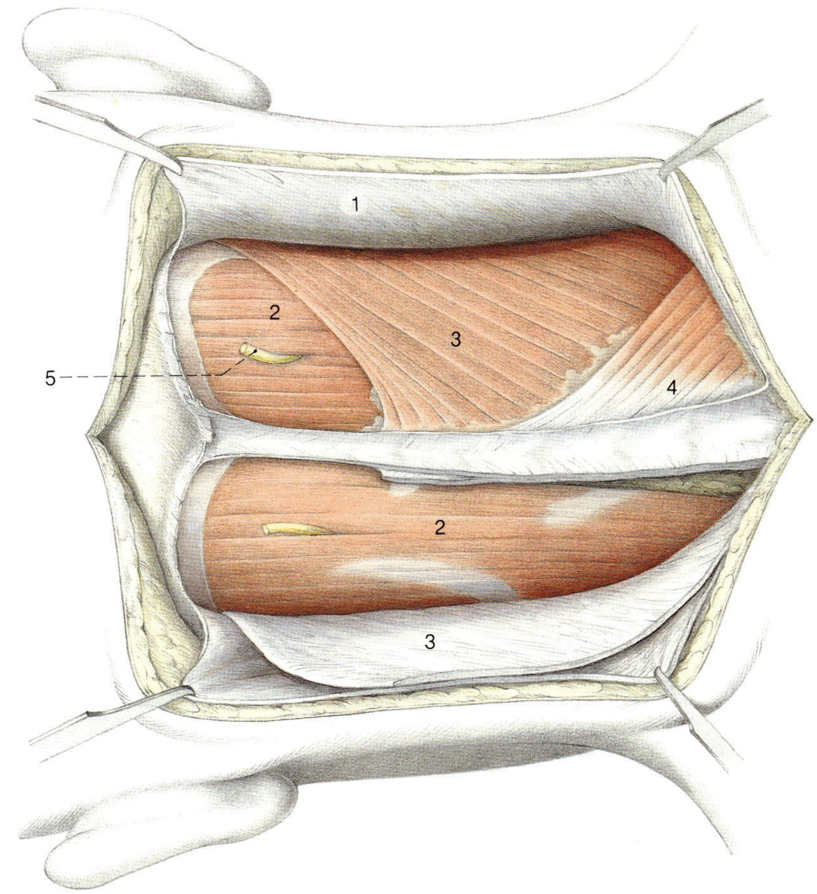

Fig. 1.**104** Anatomical site of the deep nuchal muscle layers.

1 Semispinalis capitis muscle
2 Semispinalis cervicis muscle
3 Superior oblique muscle of the head
4 Smaller straight muscle of the head
5 Greater straight muscle of the head
6 Inferior oblique muscle of the head
7 Posterior arch of the atlas
8 Zygapophyseal articulations
9 Vertebral artery
10 Occipital artery
11 Third occipital nerve
12 Greater occipital nerve
13 Suboccipital nerve

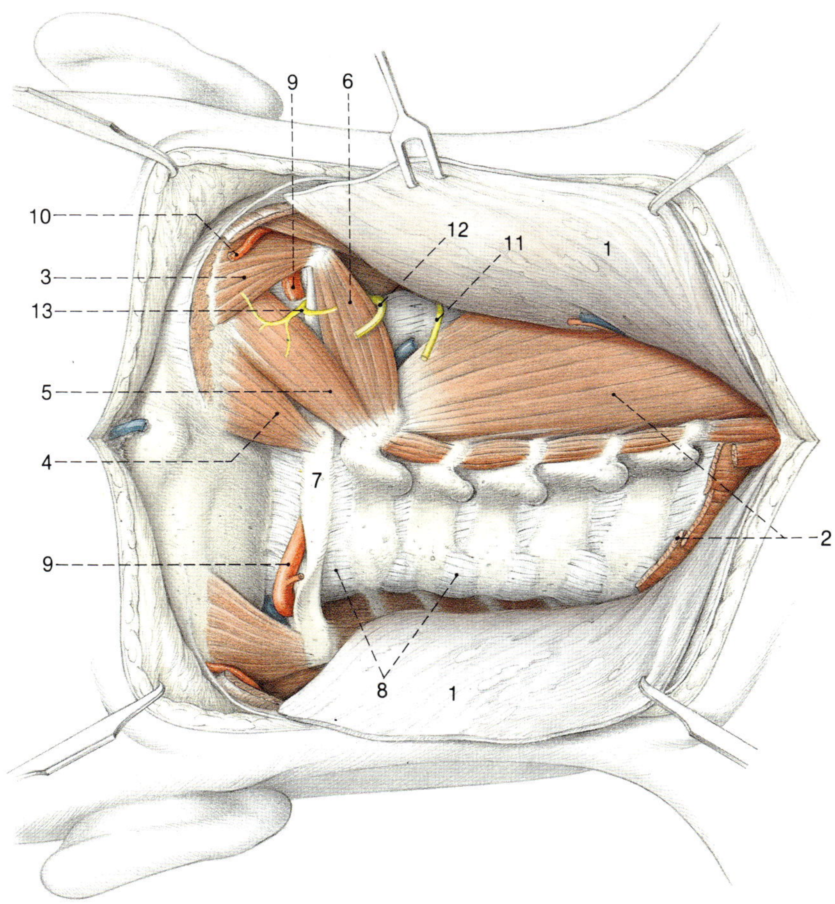

Thoracic and Lumbar Spine

Costotransversectomy T3–T10

Principal Indications

- Retropleural opening of abscess in spondylitis
- Biopsy
- Tumors
- Vertebral fractures

Choice of Side of Approach

The approach may be made from either side; the side chosen depends on the localization of the lesion.

Positioning and Incision

The operation may be performed with the patient in prone or semilateral position. If only the vertebrae are to be exposed, the semilateral position is preferable, since it provides a better view anteriorly. For approaches to the upper region of the thoracic spine, the arm on the affected side is maximally elevated in order to move the scapula as far away from the midline as possible (Fig. 1.**105**). Two types of skin incision are possible:

- A straight paramedian incision, approximately three finger-breadths beside the spinous processes.
- A T-shaped incision, which provides a better overview.

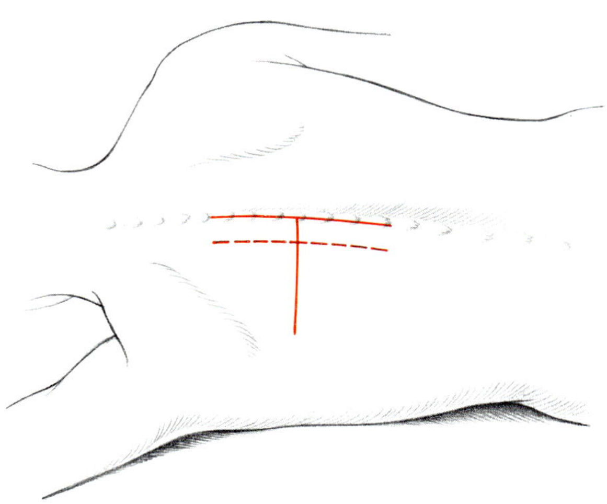

Fig. 1.**105** Costotransversectomy. Prone or semilateral position with elevated arm. T-shaped skin incision with the transverse limb over the involved vertebra, or three finger-breadths from the midline longitudinally (dashed line).

The transverse limb is at the level of the vertebra to be exposed (intraoperative identification using an image converter or radiograph). While the incision is made over the tip of the spinous processes and is about 15 cm long, transection of the skin and subcutis is followed by superior and inferior mobilization of the two skin flaps. The superficial muscle layer (trapezius muscle) is divided transversely (Fig. 1.**106**). Using an electrocautery knife, the intrinsic musculature of the back, in accordance with the skin incision, is now first separated from the spinous processes close to the bone. The intrinsic muscles of the back are dissected with a rasp from the vertebral arches and transverse processes above and below the transverse incision. After this, the longissimus muscle is transversely dissected and retracted superiorly and inferiorly (Fig. 1.**107**). The rib that leads to the involved vertebra is now identified. The periosteum over this rib is split with the electrocautery knife and cautiously retracted with the elevator. To begin with, the lower border of the rib is dissected subperiosteally from lateral to medial.

The upper border of the rib is dissected subperiosteally from medial to lateral until the entire circumference of the rib is subperiosteally exposed. A rib dissector is now applied, and the subperiosteal dissection is carried to the desired width in a lateral direction (8–10 cm). Medially, the subperiosteal exposure is continued as far as the costotransverse articulation. Using rib cutters, the rib is initially divided laterally; the costotransverse joint is then opened with a knife, and the transverse process is exposed subperiosteally as far as the lamina. The transverse process may subsequently be separated at its base with a narrow chisel and removed with a Luer bone rongeur. The laterally separated rib is lifted from the wound bed, and the periosteum below the rib is now cautiously stripped with an elevator as far as the costovertebral articulation, sparing the neurovascular bundle lying caudal to the rib. Removal of the rib is accomplished with rotatory movements on the rib and simultaneous retraction of the costovertebral joint capsule. Careless manipulation can lead to hemorrhages from the segmental vessels. As a rule, three ribs need to be resected.

Fig. 1.**106** Operative site after transection of the skin and subcutis. T-shaped incision of the musculature of the back (dashed line).

1 Trapezius muscle, transverse part
2 Trapezius muscle, ascending part

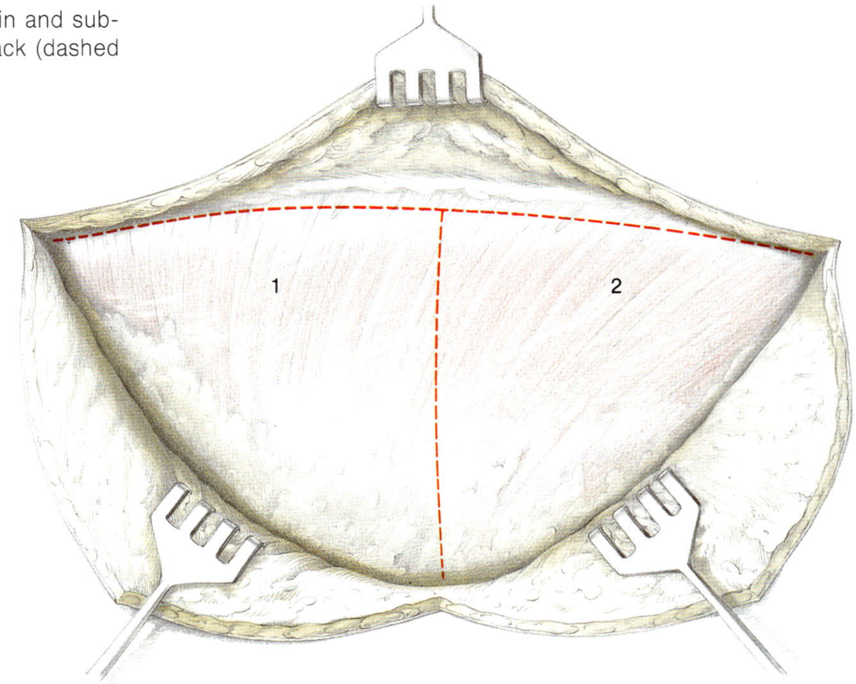

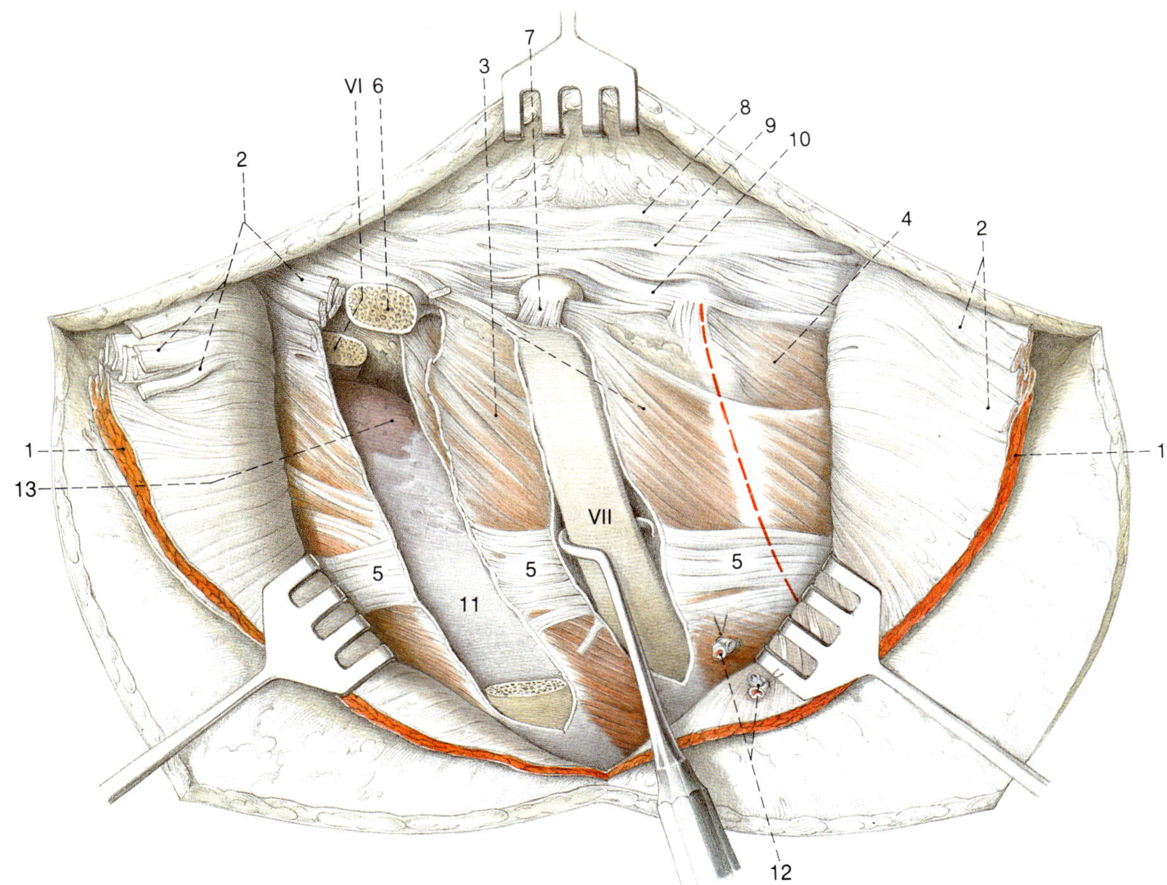

Fig. 1.**107** After cranial and caudal dissection of the muscle flaps, the rib periosteum is divided, and the rib is exposed subperiosteally over a length of 8–10 cm. Following opening of the costotransverse joint capsule and removal of the transverse process at the base, the rib is laterally divided with rib shears, lifted out of the wound, and exarticulated after careful detachment of the costovertebral joint capsule.

1 Trapezius muscle
2 Longissimus muscle
3 External intercostal muscles
4 Semispinalis muscle
5 Iliocostal muscle
6 Transverse process of the sixth thoracic vertebra
7 Costotransverse ligament
8 Supraspinal ligament
9 Interspinal ligament
10 Intertransverse ligament
11 Periosteum of the fifth rib
12 Intercostal vessels, lateral cutaneous branches
13 Parietal pleura
VI–VII Ribs

Exposure of Vertebrae

Using peanut sponge sticks, the endothoracic fascia beneath the rib periosteum as well as the parietal pleura is cautiously retracted from the anterior side of the vertebrae and the intervertebral disks, sparing the neurovascular bundles. The remnants of the intercostal muscles lying between the resected ribs are dissected off the segmental vessels (Fig. 1.**108**). If necessary, the intercostal vessels may be ligated and transected anterior to the vertebral body, but the segmental nerves should be preserved if possible, since these nerves, starting at T6, innervate the abdominal muscles. Following retraction of the parietal pleura from the anterior side of the vertebrae, flexible spatulas may now be inserted, so that two to three vertebrae are laterally visualized from behind (Fig. 1.**109**).

Wound Closure

Prior to wound closure, positive-pressure breathing should be used to make certain that the parietal pleura has not been injured. Injury would require insertion of a chest tube. Wound closure is effected by reapproximating the divided musculature in layers.

Note

Costotransversectomy was formerly considered a standard approach, particularly for surgical treatment of tuberculous spondylitis. Today, this approach has been largely superseded by thoracotomy, which provides a better overview. Costotransversectomy is especially indicated when thoracotomy is precluded by medical or technical factors, or when certain tumors affecting both the posterior vertebral elements and the vertebral body have to be resected in a single session. This approach has also been described for osteosyntheses of vertebral fractures, in cases in which anterior decompression of the vertebral canal was required at the same time.

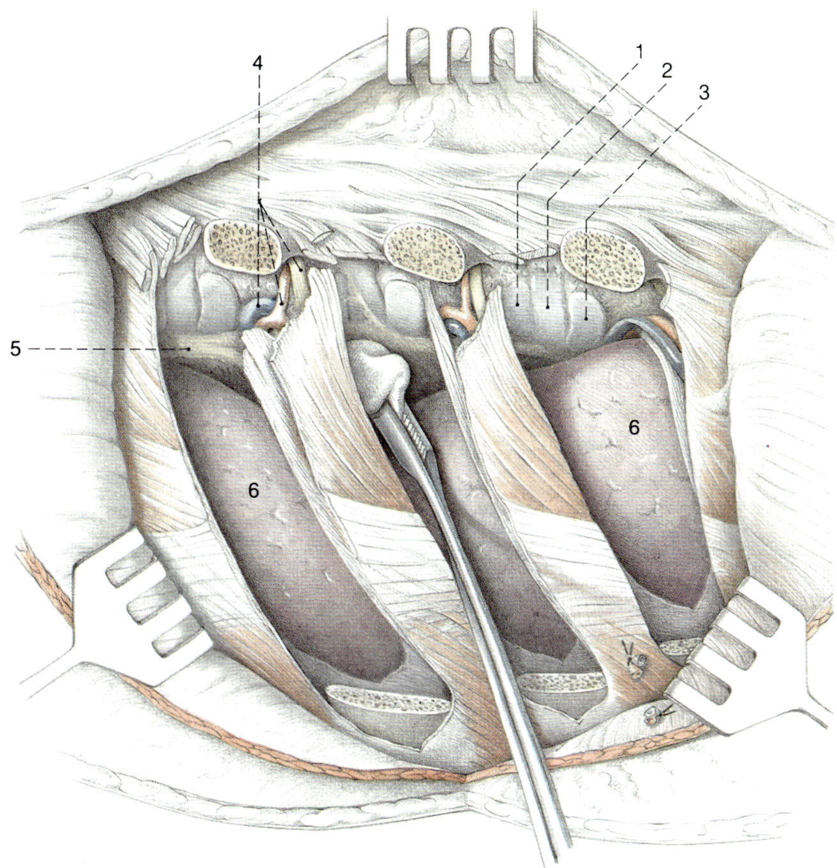

Fig. 1.**108** Blunt dissection of the endothoracic fascia lying under the rib bed, with the parietal pleura, from the lateral and anterior portions of the thoracic vertebrae, as well as from the intervertebral disks.

1 Inferior costal fovea
2 Intervertebral disk
3 Superior costal fovea
4 Intercostal artery, vein, and nerve
5 Sympathetic trunk
6 Lung with parietal pleura

Fig. 1.**109** Exposure of the intercostal neurovascular bundles by dissection of the intercostal musculature. If necessary, the intercostal vessels may be ligated and transected. The intercostal nerves should be spared.

1 Intercostal vessels
2 Greater splanchnic nerve
3 Sympathetic trunk
4 Communicating branch
5 Intercostal nerve

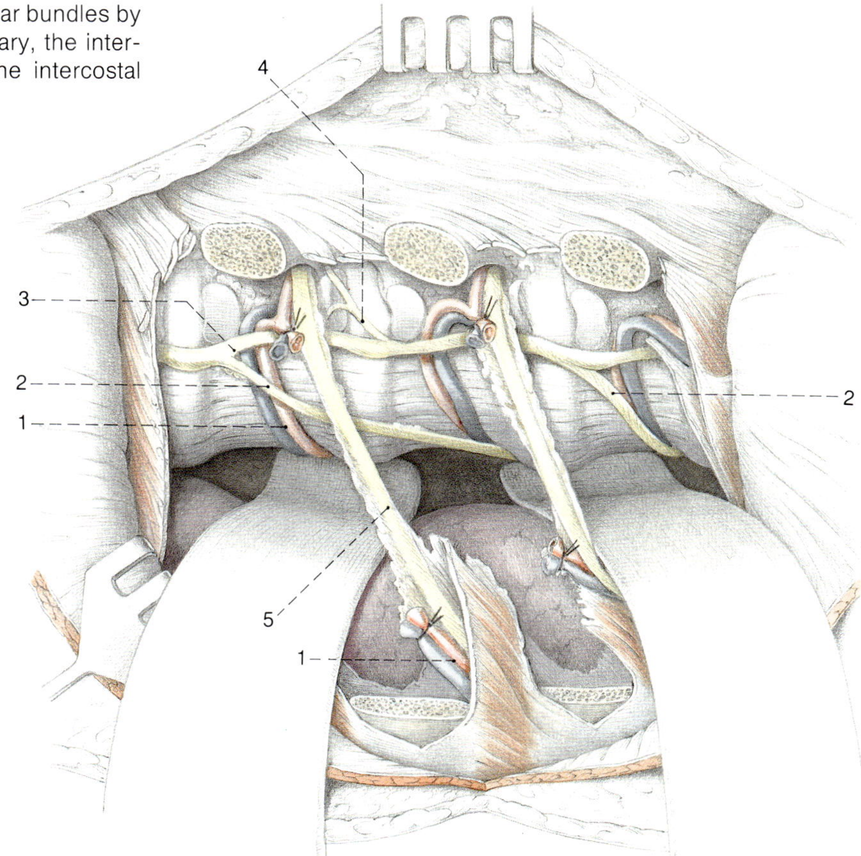

Posterior Approach to the Thoracic and Lumbar Spine

Principal Indications

- Scoliosis
- Kyphosis
- Fractures
- Tumors

Positioning and Incision

The patient is placed in a prone position, with cushions under the chest and under both iliac crests or on special supports, such as the Relton–Hall frame (Fig. 1.**110**). Care should be taken not to compress the abdomen, so as to prevent venous reflux and, consequently, increased venous bleeding during the operation. In scoliosis, too, the skin incision runs straight in the midline; for fusion operations, it should be one to two segments longer than the planned length of the fusion (Fig. 1.**111**). After this, the subcutis is divided as far as the fascia. Retractors are applied.

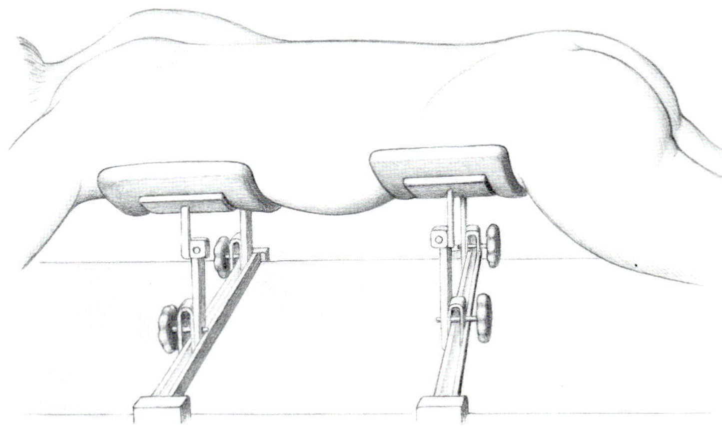

Fig. 1.**110** Posterior approach to the thoracic and lumbar spine. Positioning on Relton–Hall frame.

Exposure of the Thoracic Spine

In children and adolescents, the cartilaginous spinous process apophyses are split in the midline together with the interspinal ligaments (Fig. 1.**112**). The apophyses with the adherent periosteum can easily be retracted with a Cobb elevator to the base of the spinous processes or to the vertebral arches. In adult patients, the fascia has to be stripped near the bone with the electrocautery on both sides of the spinous process. In operations for scoliosis, retraction of the musculature is generally begun on the concave side (Fig. 1.**113**). Dissection is carried from caudal to cranial.

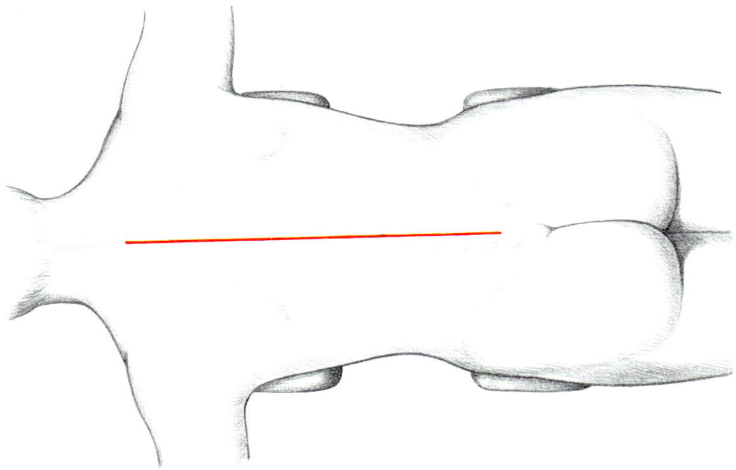

Fig. 1.**111** Incision.

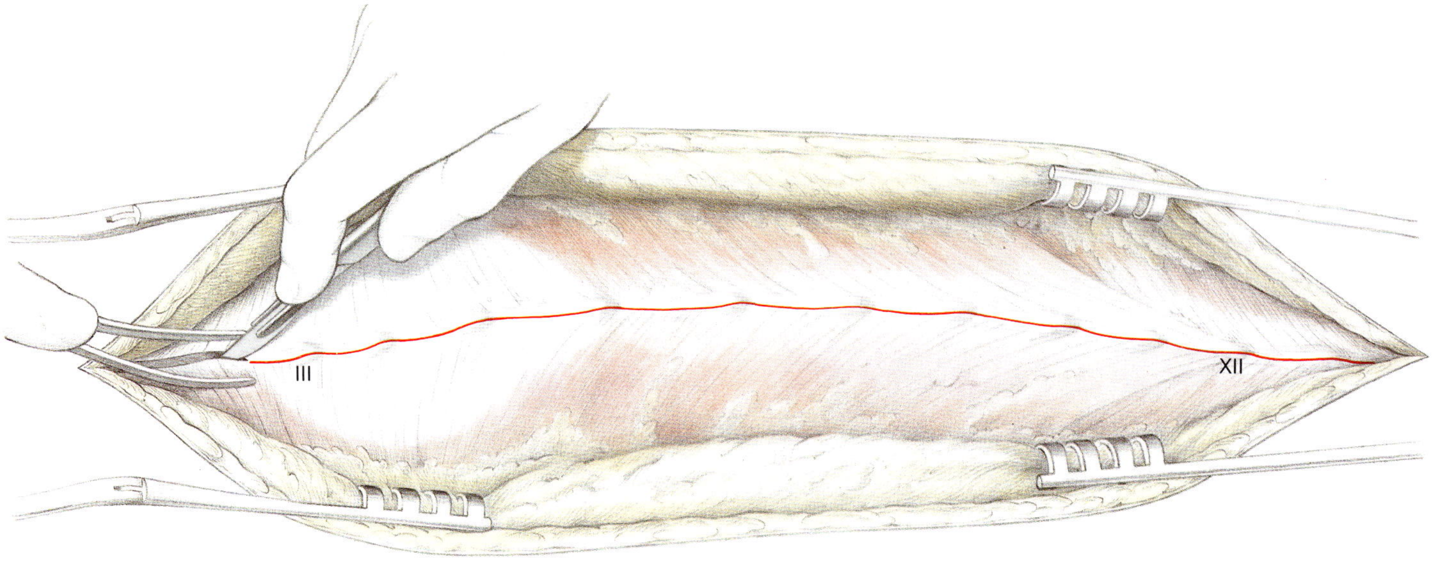

Fig. 1.**112** In adolescents and children, the cartilaginous spinous-process apophyses and the interspinal ligaments are incised in the midline and laterally retracted together with the periosteum.

III–XII Spinous processes of the thoracic vertebrae

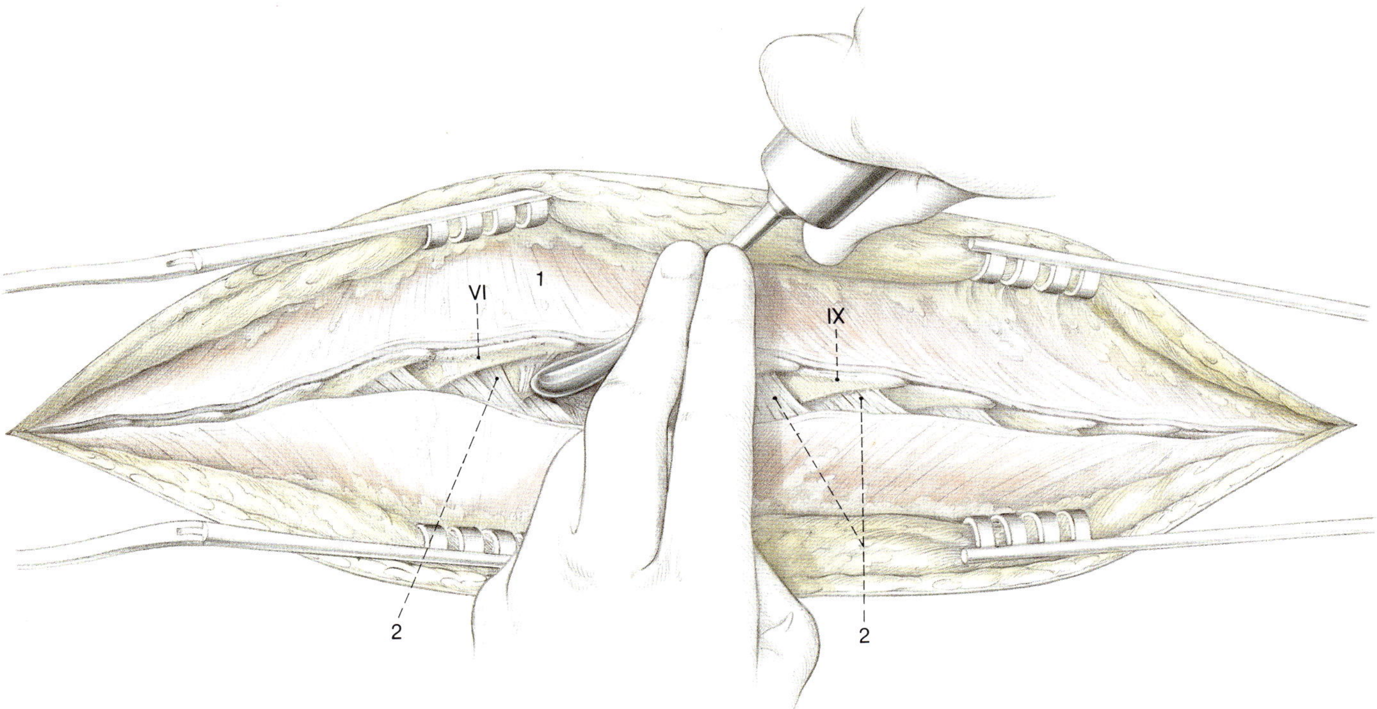

Fig. 1.**113** Subperiosteal dissection with an elevator as far as the base of the spinous processes.

1 Trapezius muscle
2 Multifidus muscles
VI, IX Spinous processes of the thoracic vertebrae

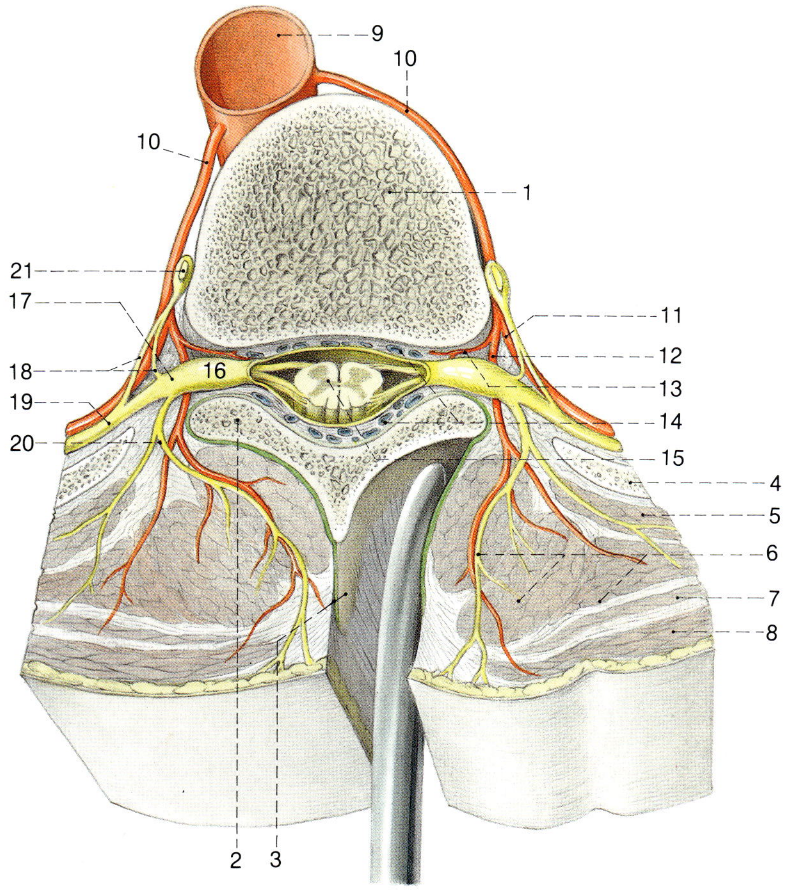

Fig. 1.**114** Cross-section through the area of the thoracic spine. Subperiosteal dissection.

1 Vertebral body
2 Lamina of vertebral arch
3 Spinous process
4 Rib
5 External oblique muscle of the abdomen
6 Intrinsic musculature of the back
7 Posterior inferior serratus muscle
8 Trapezius muscle
9 Thoracic aorta
10 Posterior intercostal arteries
11 Posterior branch
12 Collateral branch
13 Spinal branch
14 Anterior and posterior internal vertebral venous plexuses
15 Spinal medulla
16 Spinal ganglion
17 Spinal nerve
18 Communicating branches
19 Anterior branch
20 Posterior branch
21 Sympathetic trunk

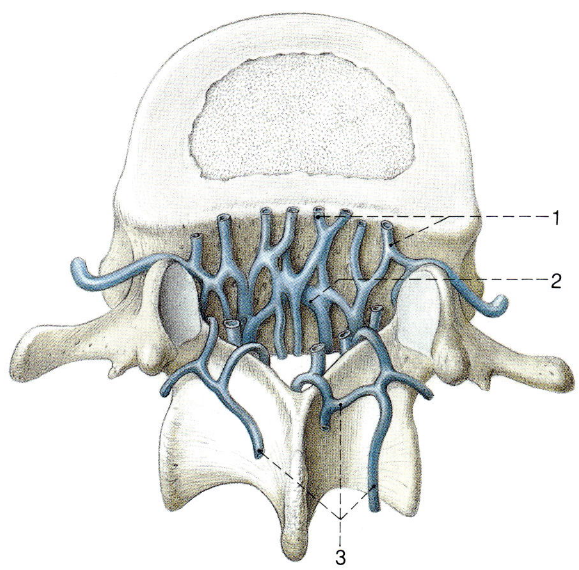

Fig. 1.**115** The vertebral venous plexus.

1 Anterior internal vertebral venous plexus
2 Basivertebral vein
3 Posterior external vertebral venous plexus

The dissection has to be strictly subperiosteal, so that the vascular and neural supply to the musculature may be spared and hemorrhages avoided (Fig. 1.**114**).

There may be severe bleeding from the posterior external vertebral venous plexus (Fig. 1.**115**), which has to be stopped by electrocautery or packing.

The subperiosteal dissection is extended laterally to the ends of the transverse processes. Once the concave side has been exposed, it is packed with large swabs; the same procedure is subsequently applied to the contralateral side.

Following detachment of the spinalis and semispinalis muscles, the multifidus and rotator muscles are dissected, particularly in adult patients, and use of the knife is necessary for sharp dissection of the tendons (Figs. 1.**116**, 1.**117**).

If spinal fusion is planned, the joint capsules of the segments in question need to be removed, together with all the remnants of the tendon insertions between the spinous processes and the interspinal ligaments. The capsules of the vertebral joints are dissected with a Cobb elevator from cranial medial to caudal lateral (Fig. 1.**118**).

To determine the level, the twelfth thoracic and first lumbar vertebrae are preferably used as landmarks. The twelfth thoracic vertebra has an involuted transverse process, which overlies the readily movable twelfth rib. The first lumbar vertebra has a nonmobile costal process. The joint between the eleventh and twelfth thoracic vertebrae is positioned frontally, similarly to the other thoracic vertebral joints, whereas the T12–L1 joint is aligned sagittally, similarly to the lumbar vertebral joints. This aid to localize the correct level is applicable in approximately 90 percent of cases. In the presence of malassimilation or lack of definition (lumbar ribs!), lateral radiographs taken intraoperatively will help to identify the level.

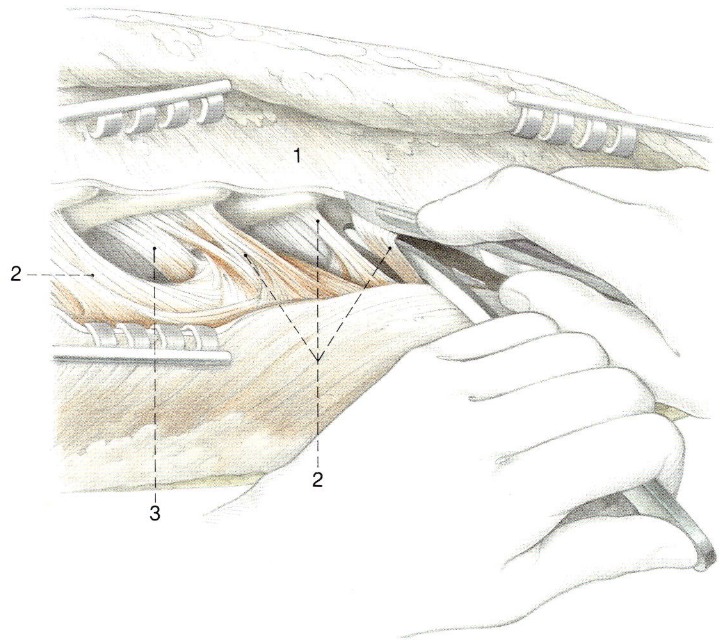

Fig. 1.**116** Dissection of the semispinalis and multifidus muscles from the inferior border of the spinous processes. Partially this dissection is done sharply with a knife.

1 Trapezius muscle
2 Semispinalis muscle
3 Multifidus muscles

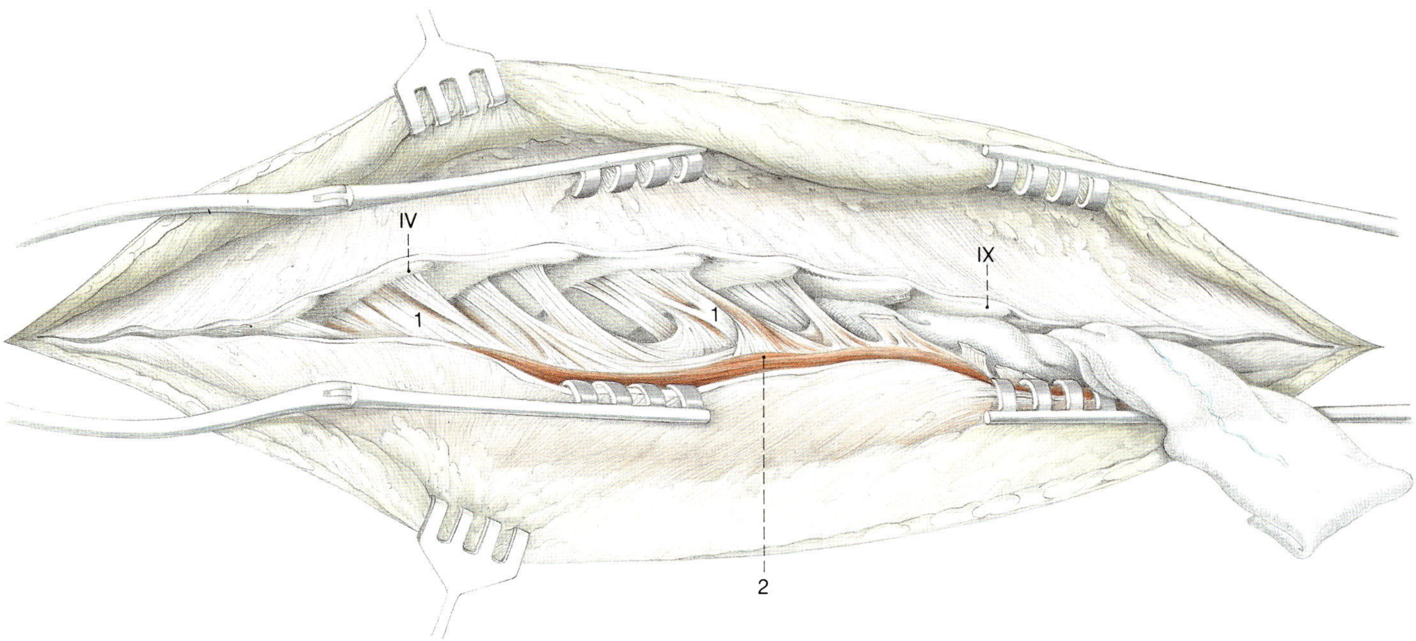

Fig. 1.**117** Packing the wound with gauze swabs, and insertion of retractors into the musculature. Dissection at the thoracic spine goes from inferior to superior.

1 Multifidus muscles
2 Spinal muscle
IV–IX Spinous processes of the thoracic vertebrae

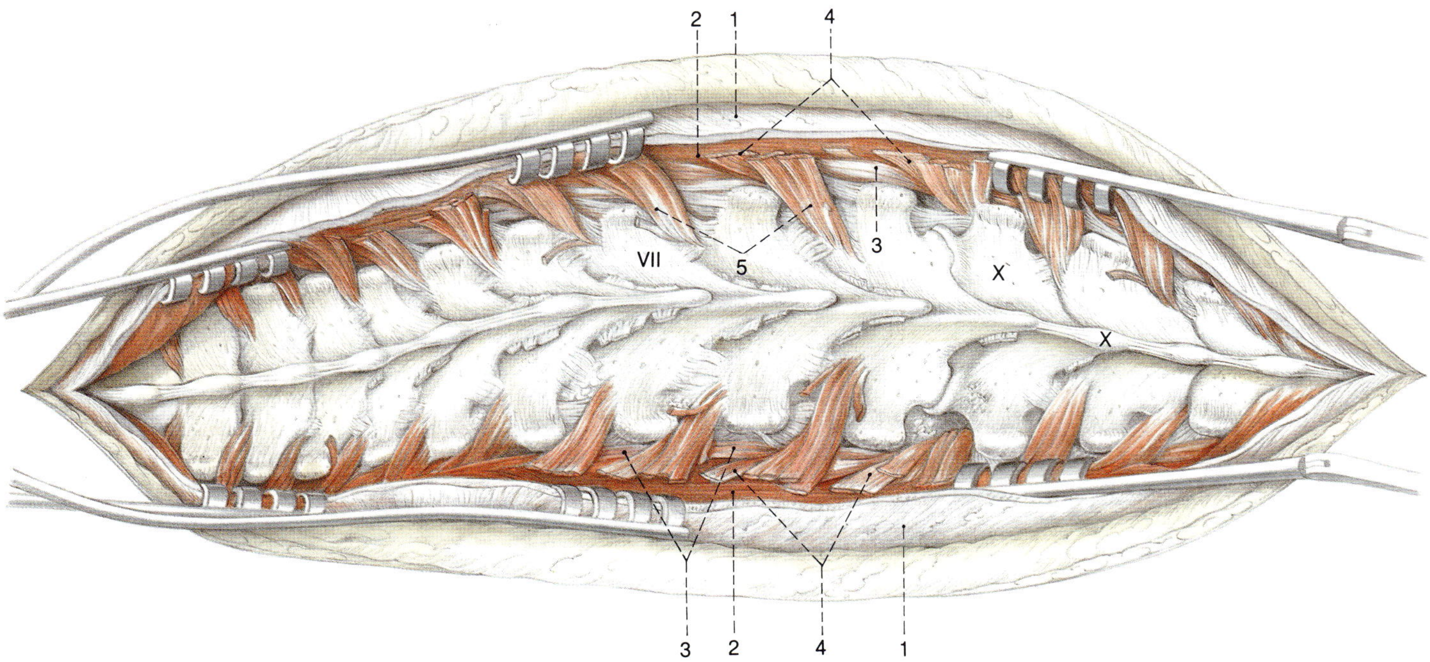

Fig. 1.**118** Operative site after subperiosteal exposure of the posterior vertebral elements. At the level of the ninth and tenth thoracic vertebrae, the capsules of the vertebral joints are bilaterally removed.

1 Trapezius muscle
2 Spinal muscle
3 Semispinalis muscle
4 Multifidus muscles
5 Rotator muscles
VII, X Thoracic vertebrae

Exposure of the Lumbar Spine

(Fig. 1.**119**)

Posterior exposure of the lumbar spine is carried out in the same way as exposure of the thoracic spine, except that dissection is performed from cranial to caudal. The muscles and tendons are likewise stripped from the spinous processes as subperiosteally as possible; in children and younger patients, the joint capsules may be dissected in the same plane.

Lying lateral and somewhat anterior and caudal to the upper articular process is the costal process, to which the dissection should be extended. Retraction of the musculature in this region requires more force than at the thoracic spine. The dissection may be facilitated by using the tip of the intact spinous process as a lever-type support for the Cobb elevator. The muscle remnants are retracted from the transverse processes with a sponge stick. The retractors are now placed in a deeper position and separated until the posterior vertebral elements are exposed as far as the ends of the costal processes. This is followed by clearing the lower borders of the spinous processes, in particular, of soft tissue and by removing the joint capsules, which is best done sharply with a knife and forceps (Fig. 1.**120**). Level determination at the lumbar spine is easy: caudal to S1 there is no yellow ligament (except in case of malassimilation). The spinous process of L5 is distinctly larger than that of S1, and as a rule the lumbosacral joint is the last vertebral joint.

In the presence of spina bifida or vertebral fractures, careless dissection may cause the elevator to enter the vertebral canal.

Wound Closure

Wound closure is effected in two layers by suture of the paraspinal musculature and the overlying fascia. In children and adolescents, the split spinous-process apophyses are readily united by sutures.

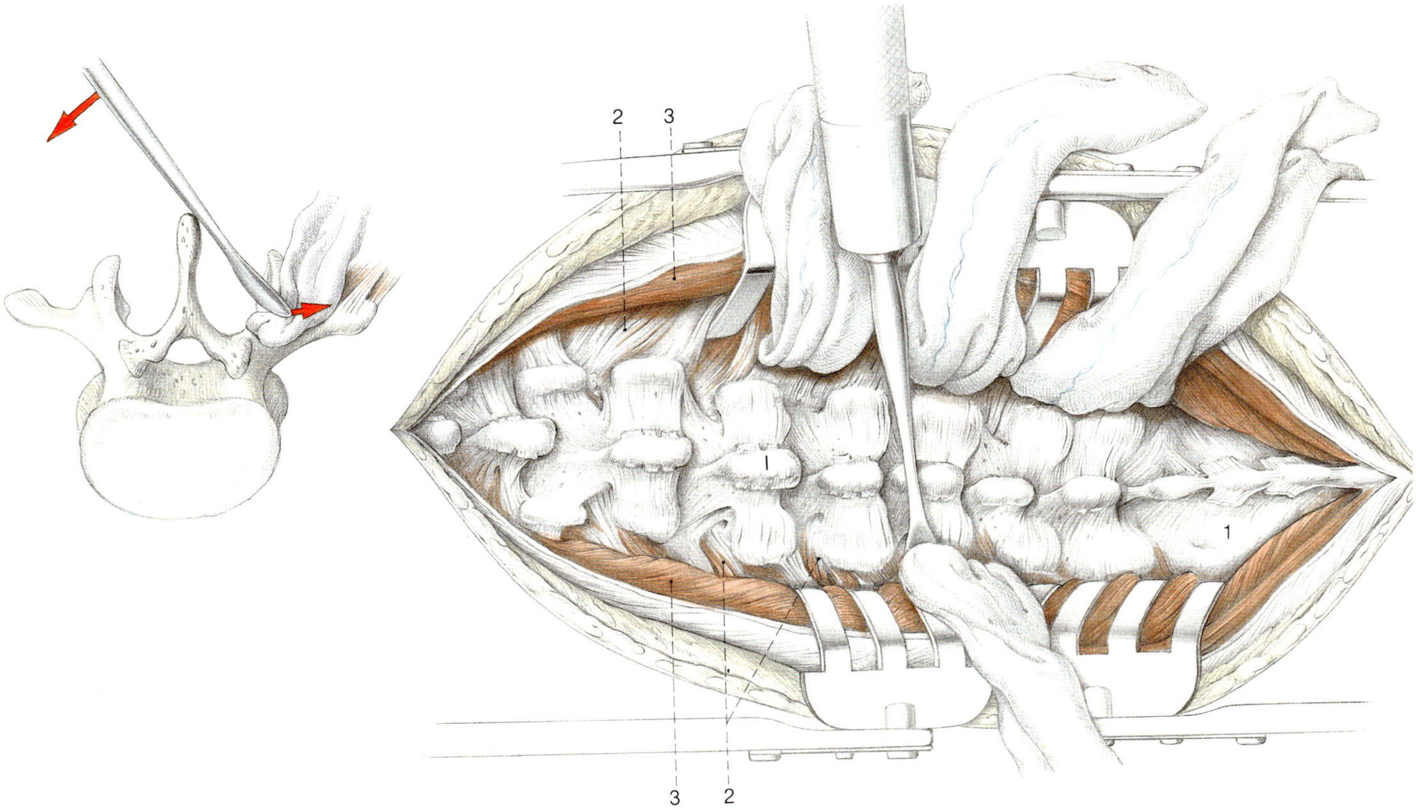

Fig. 1.**119** Posterior exposure of the lumbar spine. The spinous processes and vertebral arches are subperiosteally dissected beyond the joints to the base of the costal processes. At this point, sponges are introduced to complete the dissection as far as the tips of the costal processes (inset).

1 Sacrum
2 Multifidus muscles
3 Longissimus muscle
4 Spinous process

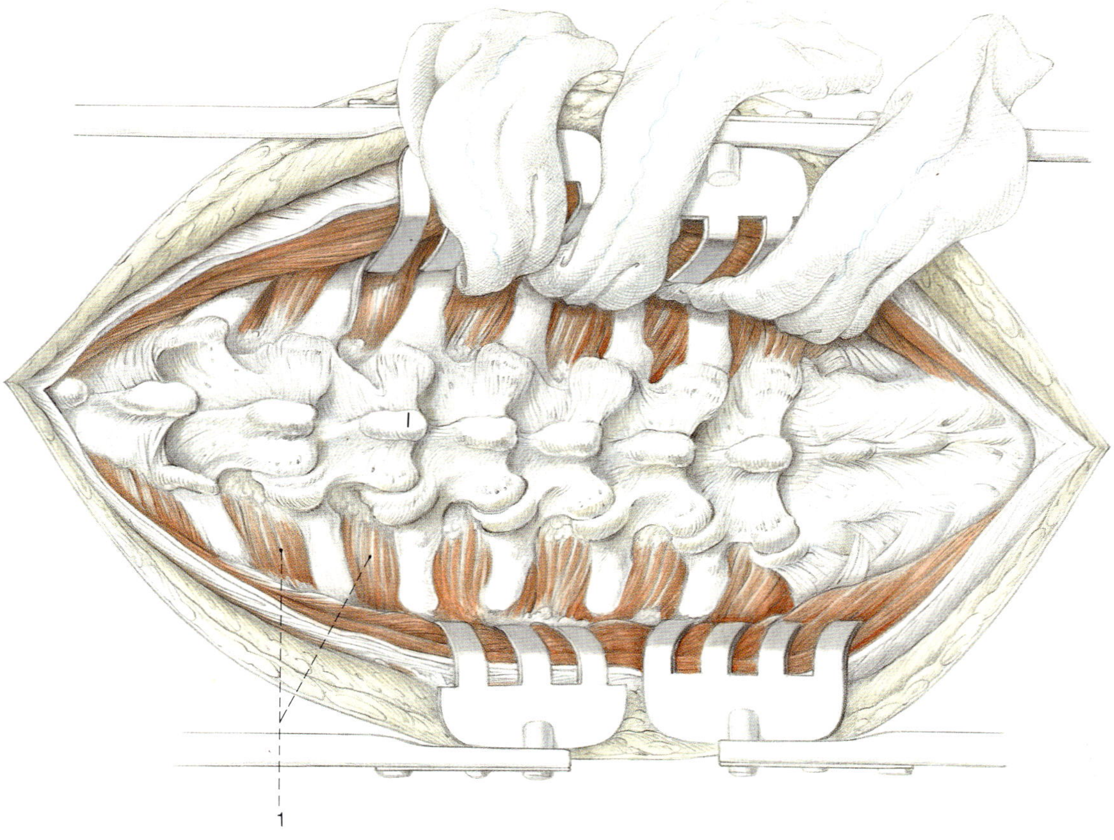

Fig. 1.**120** Posterior exposure of the lumbar spine and lumbosacral junction.

1 Multifidus muscles
I Lumbar vertebra

Paraspinal Approach to the Lumbosacral Junction According to Wiltse

Principal Indication

Spondylolisthesis.

Positioning and Incision

(Fig. 1.**121**)

The patient is placed in prone position on the Relton–Hall frame (Fig. 1.**110**).

A longitudinal midline incision is made, the skin being mobilized laterally by about two finger-breadths on both sides. The thoracolumbar fascia is incised lengthwise 2 cm lateral to the series of spinous processes.

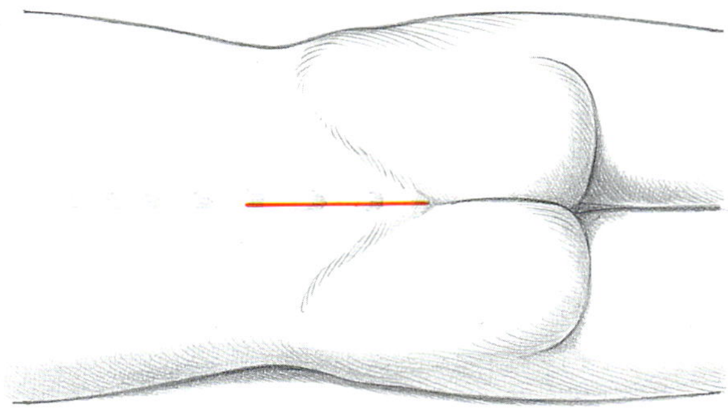

Fig. 1.**121** Paraspinal approach to the lumbar spine according to Wiltse. Skin incision.

Exposure of Posterolateral Vertebral Elements

(Fig. 1.**122**)

Between the lateral tract of the intrinsic musculature of the back (iliocostal and longissimus muscles) and the medial tract (multifidus muscles) there is a natural groove. Between these two layers the palpating finger reaches the vertebral joint L4–L5. After blunt separation of the two muscle groups, retractors are applied. Distal to them, the course of the multifidus muscle fibers becomes increasingly flat. These fibers have to be transected sharply with a knife or by diathermy. The L5–S1 joint is exposed by medial and lateral retraction of the musculature with a Cobb rasp. The musculature is split further in a superior or inferior direction as needed. After this, the sacral alae, the inferior and superior articular processes of L5, and the costal process of L5, are subperiosteally exposed. If necessary, the vertebral arch of L5, which is usually quite mobile in spondylolysis, and the yellow ligament, may be further exposed after medial retraction of the musculature. This also makes a laminectomy or foraminotomy possible. In spondylolysis, fibrous scar tissue, which may have to be removed sharply, is found in the area of the interarticular portion. In a posterolateral fusion of L5–S1 according to Wiltse, care should be taken to avoid opening the L4–L5 vertebral joint.

Too deep a dissection between the sacral alae and the costal process of L5 may lead to injury of the fifth lumbar spinal nerve.

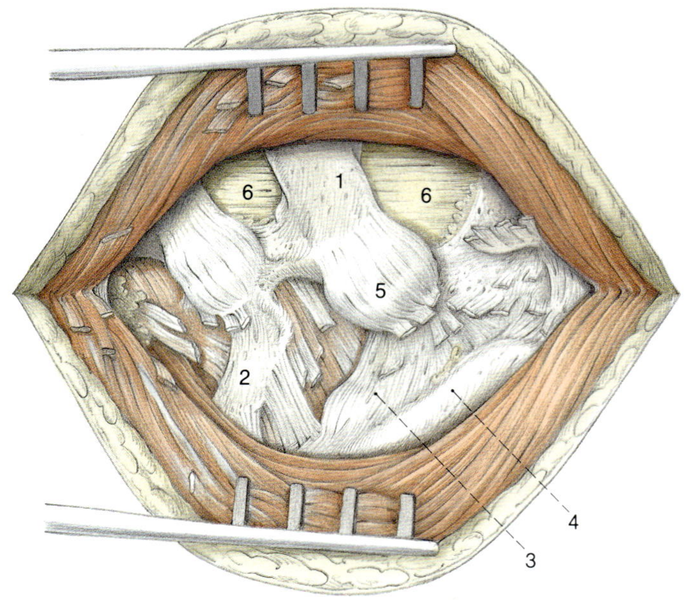

Fig. 1.**122** Status after longitudinal division of fascia and musculature. Exposure of vertebral joints L4–L5 and L5–S1, as well as of the costal process of the fifth lumbar vertebra and the ala sacralis. The soft tissues overlying the yellow ligament have been removed.

1 Lamina of the fifth lumbar vertebral arch
2 Costal process of the fifth lumbar vertebra
3 Ala sacralis
4 Iliac crest
5 Zygapophyseal articulation L5–S1
6 Yellow ligaments

Wound Closure

The wound is closed by suture of the intrinsic back musculature and the thoracolumbar fascia.

Short Posterior Approach to the Lumbar Spine for Laminotomy and Intervertebral Disk Removal

Principal Indications

- Disk herniation
- Spinal stenosis

Positioning and Incision

The operation may be performed with the patient in a lateral position, or in a knee–chest position with kyphosis of the lumbar spine (Fig. 1.**123**). The cutaneous incision is generally made over the fourth and fifth spinous processes to a length of approximately 10 cm (Fig. 1.**124**). The thoracolumbar fascia is opened in the midline with the diathermy knife, and the paraspinal musculature is then retracted with a rasp, as far subperiosteally as possible, over the vertebral joints. After hemostasis and tamponade with sponges, self-retaining retractors are applied. All soft tissues overlying the ligamentum flavum are now removed (Fig. 1.**125**).

Exposure of the Spinal Canal

The inferior margin of the next higher vertebral arch is removed with Leksell forceps or a Hajek punch. Subsequently, the ligamentum flavum is grasped with forceps and incised with a knife in the midline from superior to inferior, separated from the superior edge of the next vertebra, and removed (Fig. 1.**126**). The epidural fat is removed with the aid of a dissector and blunt dissection with a gauze swab; the dura and the nerve root are exposed. The nerve root may be cautiously retracted in a medial direction with a root retractor, so that the posterolateral aspect of the intervertebral disk is brought into view (Fig. 1.**127**).

Wound Closure

Wound closure is effected by suturing the elevated musculature and the fascia.

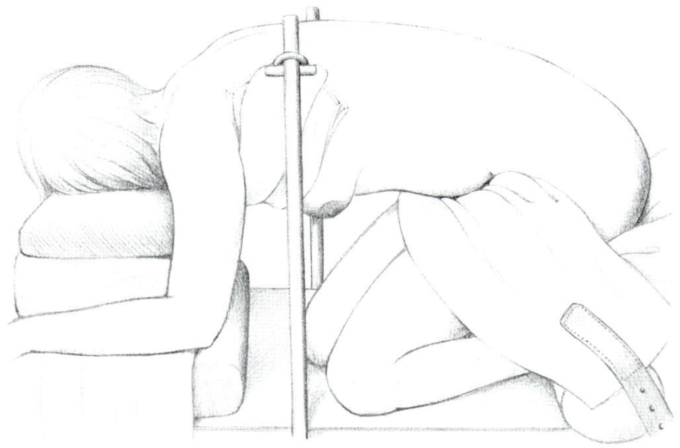

Fig. 1.**123** Short posterior approach to the lumbar spine (laminotomy). Knee–chest position.

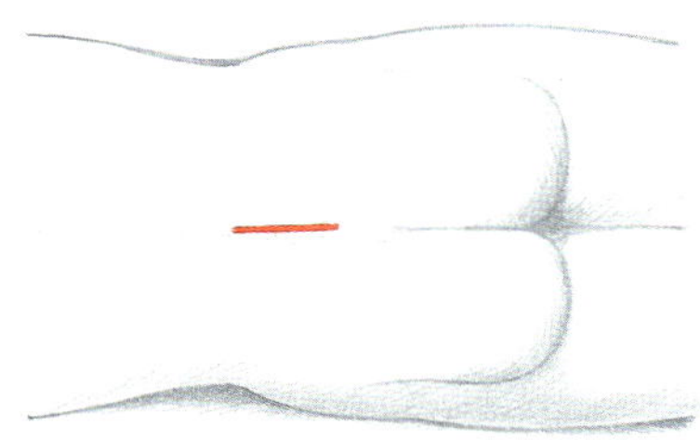

Fig. 1.**124** Skin incision 10 cm long in the midline.

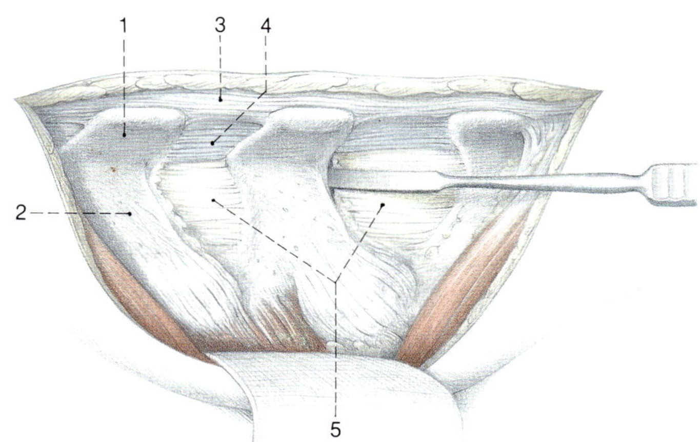

Fig. 1.**125** Operative site after retraction of the paraspinal musculature and exposure of the vertebral arches, ligamentum flavum, and vertebral joints. Retraction of the yellow ligament from the vertebral arch.

1 Spinous process
2 Lamina of the vertebral arch
3 Supraspinal ligament
4 Interspinal ligament
5 Yellow ligaments

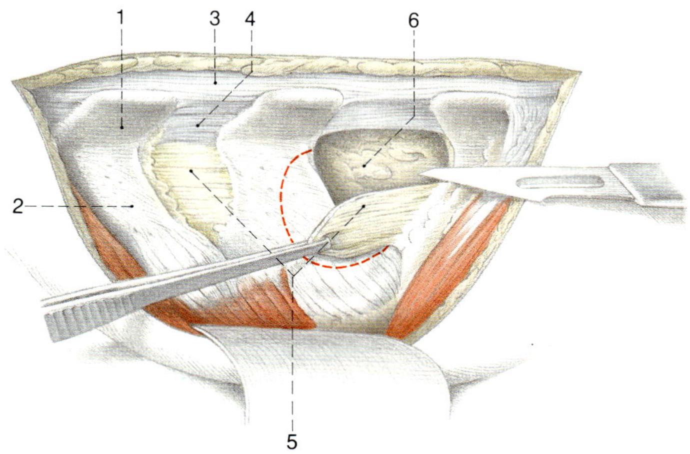

Fig. 1.**126** Resection of the ligamentum flavum. The extent of the laminotomy is shown by the dashed line.

1 Spinous process
2 Lamina of vertebral arch
3 Supraspinal ligament
4 Interspinal ligament
5 Yellow ligaments
6 Epidural adipose tissue

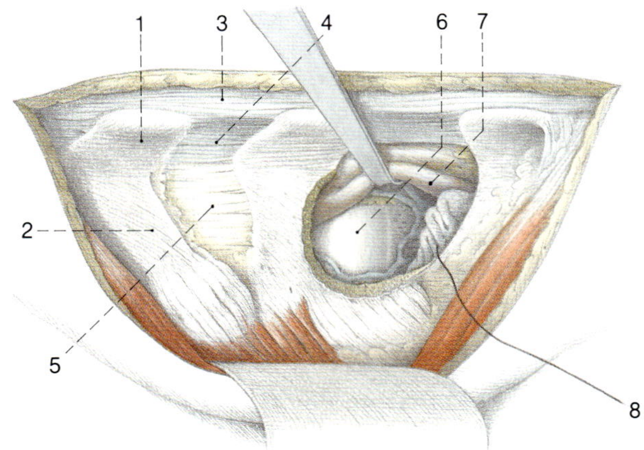

Fig. 1.**127** Operative site after laminotomy. Removal of the ligamentum flavum and the medial third of the vertebral joint for exposure of the nerve root, lateral recess, and intervertebral disk.

1 Spinous process
2 Lamina of the vertebral arch
3 Supraspinal ligament
4 Interspinal ligament
5 Yellow ligaments
6 Intervertebral disk
7 Root of the spinal nerve
8 Swab

Further Reading

Adachi B. Das Arteriensystem der Japaner, vol. 2. Kyoto, 1931.

Bauer R. Die operative Behandlung der Skoliose. Berne: Huber, 1979.

Bauer R. Der vordere Zugang zur Wirbelsäule. Stuttgart: Thieme, 1983.

Colletta AJ, Mayer PJ. Chylothorax: an unusual complication of anterior thoracic interbody spinal fusion. Spine 1982;7:46.

Cordier P, Devos L, Delcroix A. Essai de classification des variations du système azygos intrathoracique. CR Assoc Anat 1983;33:100-18.

Crock HV, Yoshizawa H. The blood supply of the vertebral column and the spinal cord in man. Berlin: Springer, 1977.

Denck H. Eingriffe an der Brustwand. In: Breitner B, Chirurgische Operationslehre. Munich: Urban and Schwarzenberg, 1981.

Dommisse GF. Some factors in the management of fractures and fracture dislocation of the spine at the lumbodorsal level: the significance of the blood supply to the spine. Reconstr Surg Traumatol 1972;13:108.

Dommisse GF. The blood supply of the human spinal cord: a critical vascular factor in spinal surgery. J Bone Jt Surg 1974;56-B:225.

Dwyer AF. Experience of anterior correction of scoliosis. Clin Orthop 1973;93:191.

Dwyer AF, Newton NC, Sherwood AA. An anterior approach to scoliosis: a clinical report. Clin Orthop 1969;62:192.

Eisenstein S, O'Brien JP. Chylothorax: a complication of Dwyer's anterior instrumentation. Br J Surg 1977;74:339.

Fang HSY, Ong GB. Direct anterior approach to the upper cervical spine. J Bone Jt Surg 1962;44-A:1588.

Fey B. L'abord du rein par voie thoracoabdominale. Arch Urol 1925;5:169.

Freebody D, Bendall R, Taylor RD. Anterior transperitoneal lumbar fusion. J Bone Jt Surg 1971;53-B:617.

Goldstein LA, Dickerson RC. Atlas of orthopaedic surgery. St. Louis: Mosby, 1981.

Hellinger J. Der transoropharyngeale Zugang zu C1 und C2. Beitr Orthop Traumatol 1981;28:25.

Henry AK. Extensile exposure. 2nd ed. Edinburgh: Livingston, 1957.

Hodge WA, DeWald RL. Splenic injury complicating the anterior thoracoabdominal surgical approach for scoliosis. J Bone Jt Surg 1983;65-A:396.

Hodgson AR. Approach to the cervical spine C3–C7. Clin Orthop 1965a;39:129.

Hodgson AR. Correction of fixed spinal curves. J Bone Jt Surg 1965b; 47-A:1221.

Hodgson AR, Stock FE. Anterior spinal fusion: preliminary communication on the radical treatment of Pott's disease and Pott's paraplegia. Br J Surg 1956;44:266.

Hodgson AR, Yau ACMC. Anterior surgical approaches to the spinal column. In: Apley AG, ed. Recent advances in orthopedics. London: Churchill, 1969:289–323.

Hughes FA. Resection to the twelfth rib in the surgical approach to the renal fossa. J Urol 1949;61:159.

Kahle W, Leonhardt H, Platzer W. Taschenatlas der Anatomie. 5th ed. Vol. 1: Bewegungsapparat. Stuttgart: Thieme, 1986.

Kirkaldy-Willis WH, Thomas DG. Anterior approaches in the diagnosis and treatment of infections to the vertebral bodies. J Bone Jt Surg 1965;47-A:87.

Kubik S. Lagevarianten, Lage- und Formveränderungen der Pars thoracalis des Ductus thoracicus. Fortschr Röntgenstr 1975;122:1-5.

Mirbaha MM. Anterior approach to the thoraco-lumbar junction of the spine by a retroperitoneal-extrapleural technic. Clin Orthop 1973;91:41.

Moe JH, Winter RB, Bradford DS, Lonstein JE. Scoliosis and other spinal deformities. Philadelphia: Saunders, 1978.

Nagamatsu G. Dorsolumbar approach to the kidney and adrenal with osteoplastic flap. J Urol 1950;63:569.

Nanson EM. The anterior approach to upper dorsal sympathectomy. Surg Gynecol Obstet 1957;104:118.

Platzer W. Atlas der topographischen Anatomie. Stuttgart: Thieme, 1982.

Riley L. Surgical approaches to anterior structures of the cervical spine. Clin Orthop 1973;91:16.

Riseborough EJ, Herndon JH. Scoliosis and other deformities of the axial skeleton. Boston: Little, Brown, 1975.

Salcman M, Jamaris J, Leveque H, Ducker TB. Transoral cervical corpectomy with the aid of the microscope. Spine 1979;4:209.

Seddon HK. Pott's paraplegia. In: Platt H, ed. Modern trends in orthopedics. London: Butterworth, 1956.

Southwick WO, Robinson RA. Surgical approach to the vertebral bodies in the cervical and lumbar regions. J Bone Jt Surg 1957;39-A:631.

Verbiest H. Anterolateral operations for fractures and dislocations in the middle and lower parts of the cervical spine. J Bone Jt Surg 1969; 51-A:1489.

Whitesides Jr TE, Kelly RP. Lateral approach to the upper cervical spine for anterior fusion. South Med J 1966;59:879.

Wiltse LL, Spencer CW. New uses and refinements of the paraspinal approach to the lumbar spine. Spine 1988;13:696.

Wiltse LL, Batemann JG, Hutchinson RH, Nelson WE. Paraspinal sacrospinalis-splitting approach to the lumbar spine. J Bone Jt Surg 1968;50-A:919.

2 Scoliosis

R. Bauer

Halo Traction Techniques

Indication

As a general rule, a halo cast or halo vest may be used for stabilization, especially of the cervical spine. The halo technique can also be used in various ways (halo–gravity traction, halo–wheelchair traction, halo–pelvic traction) to correct spinal deformities. The effectiveness of halo traction in the preoperative correction of scoliosis is a matter of controversy. An important indication for these techniques is the correction of spinal deformities between operative sessions, e.g., after a mobilizing spinal osteotomy.

Operative Technique

Application of Halo

(Fig. 2.**1**)

The halo is applied either under local anesthesia or under general anesthesia (the latter particularly if surgery is to be performed afterwards). The patient is placed in a supine position, with the head extending over the edge of the table. The head is either held by an assistant, or the occiput is placed on a narrow metal support. Before application of the halo ring, the patient's hair is shampooed for some time with disinfectant soap. When the pins are applied to the selected sites, the hair is merely retracted; shaving, even of small areas, is unnecessary.

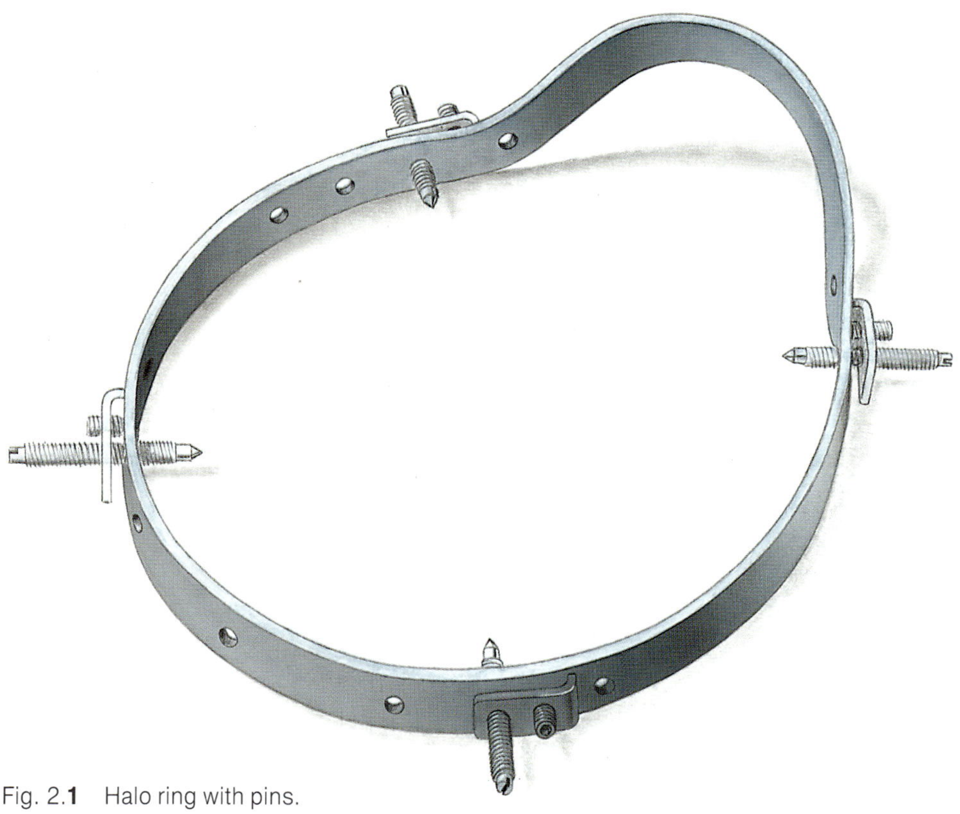

Fig. 2.**1** Halo ring with pins.

A halo ring of suitable size is chosen; the distance from the head should be approximately 1 cm, and not more than 2 cm (Fig. 2.**2**). The halo ring is positioned 1–2 cm above the ear or eyebrow. Appropriate holes in the ring are selected for positioning of the pins: the posterior pins should be placed at about the 5-o'clock and 7-o'clock positions, and the anterior pins over the lateral two-thirds of the eyebrows (Fig. 2.**7**). In this position, injury to the supraorbital nerve or penetration of the frontal sinus is avoided. The pins are applied under sterile conditions. It may be easier to apply them by using so-called positioning templates (one on the forehead and two posterolaterally, Fig. 2.**2**). The pins are then attached, using a torque screwdriver, without prior skin incision, either under local anesthesia following infiltration, or under general anesthesia. It is important that the ring should not be displaced during fixation of the pins. Two pins each are applied diagonally and are then slowly tightened simultaneously until the screw tip, after piercing the skin, penetrates the outer cortical substance. The pins are then alternately tightened until a torque of about 6 inch-pounds (ca. 0.7 newton meters) is reached. Finally, the pins are locked with a small screwplate. Additionally, pulleys are applied, as well as the extension set-up.

In the event of screw infection, local pin care and, possibly, the use of antibiotics based on antibiotic sensitivity testing are required. If the infection should not cease, the pin has to be reapplied at a different site.

Repeated tightening of the screws may lead to penetration of the internal table of the cranial bone. This is manifested by a sudden loss of pressure under the torque screwdriver. If this happens, the pin has to be removed and reapplied at a different site.

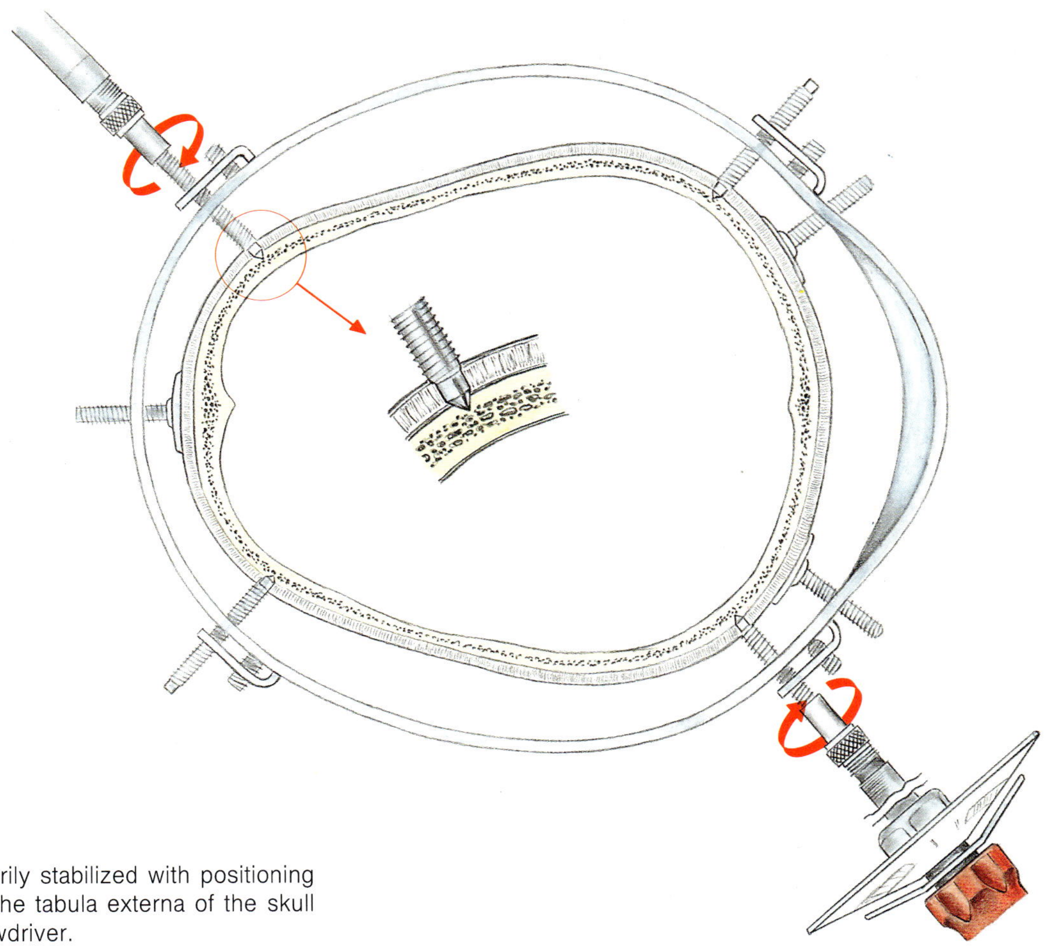

Fig. 2.**2** The halo ring is temporarily stabilized with positioning plates; the pins are inserted into the tabula externa of the skull bone (see inset) with a torque screwdriver.

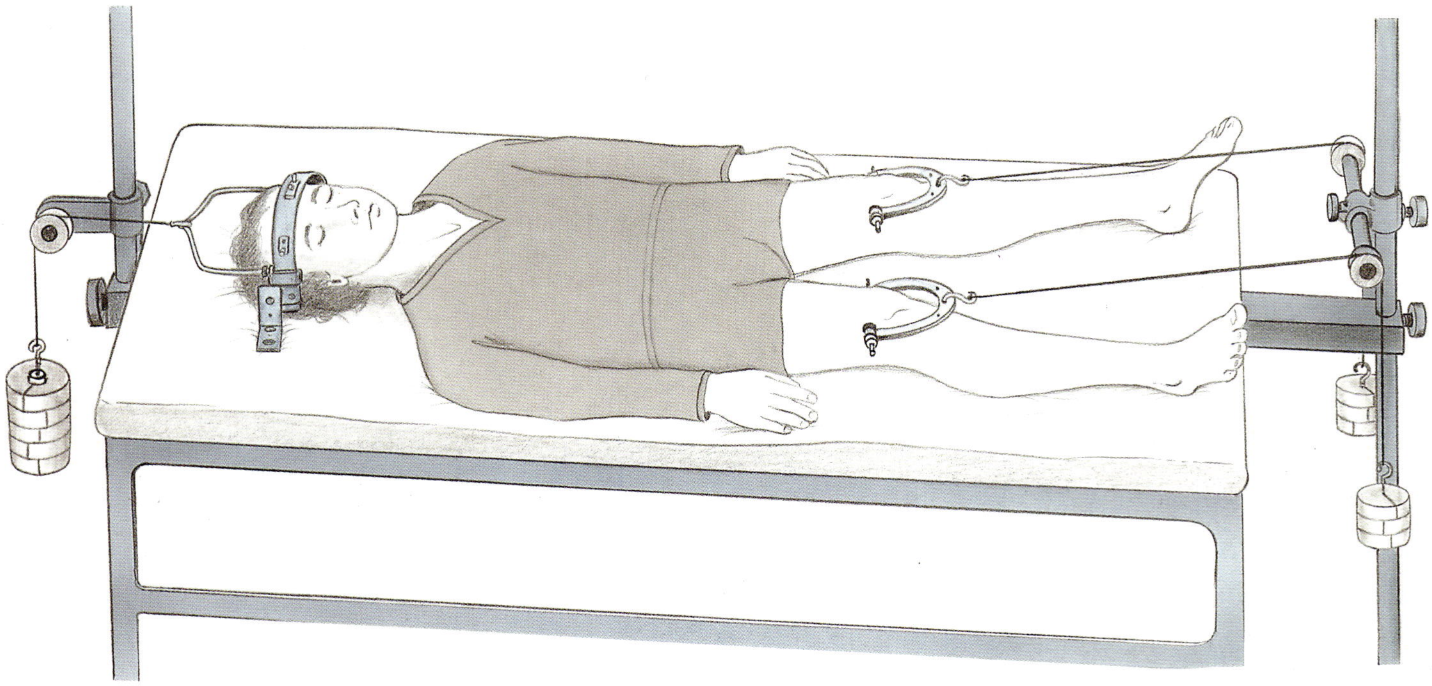

Fig. 2.**3** Halo–femoral traction.

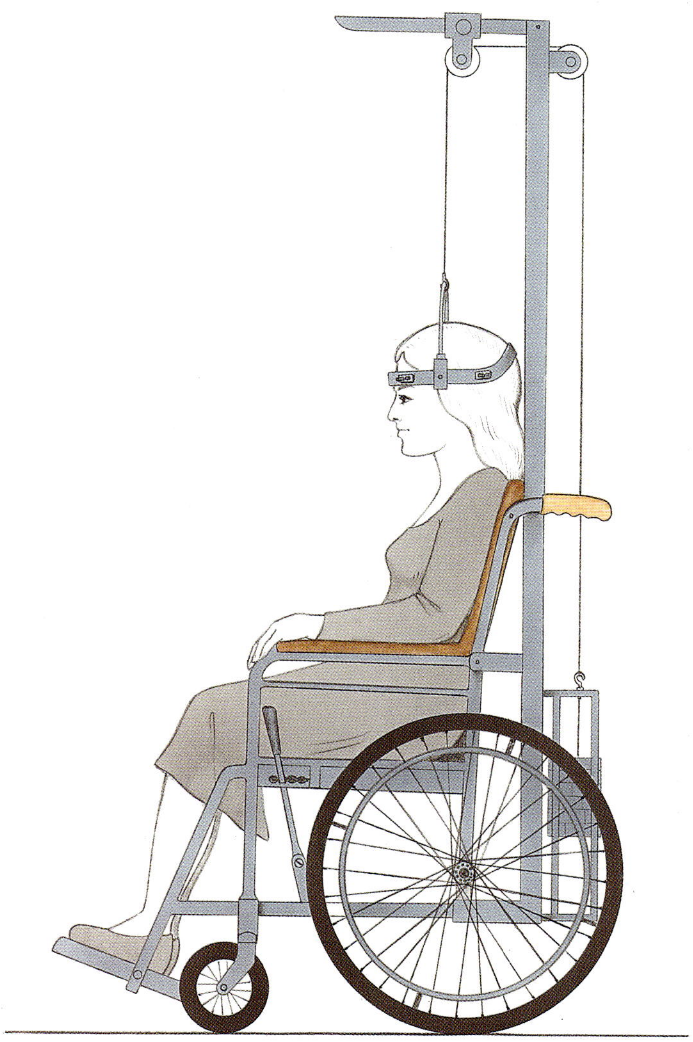

Fig. 2.**4** Halo–gravity traction in a wheelchair.

Halo–Femoral Traction

This involves a combination of halo traction with supracondylarly placed Steinmann nails (Fig. 2.**3**). This is a very effective method of traction for the correction of scoliosis and kyphosis. In this technique, continuous traction of between 20 and a maximum of 25 kg, depending on body weight, is performed, generally for a period of two to three weeks. To avoid skin complications, the patient is placed in a rotary bed and turned at least twice a day. Complete immobilization of the patient and marked loss of friction on the support are significant drawbacks.

Halo–Gravity Traction in a Wheelchair

(Fig. 2.**4**)

The patient is kept in traction against gravity in a wheelchair. In adults, traction is generally started with about 5 kg, and increased daily by 0.5–1 kg. The upper limit is 10–15 kg in adults, and correspondingly less in children.

This form of traction is particularly suitable for high thoracic curvatures. In the presence of more caudally situated curvatures, the effect is considerably diminished by an increase in the partial weight of the upper part of the body above the curvature. During the night, patients are maintained in traction in a tilted bed.

Halo–Pelvic Traction

The equipment consists of the following parts:

- Cranial halo
- Pelvic ring
- Pelvic pins and anchors
- Threaded rods connecting the cranial halo to the pelvic ring

Adjustment of the Halo–Pelvic Apparatus

To begin with, the cranial halo is applied in the usual way. For application of the pelvic rods, the patient is placed in a semilateral position; the upper half of the pelvis is prepared for surgery and draped. To avoid misplacement, which might involve dangerous complications, a drill guide is supplied with the original instrumentation. It is advisable to use a hand drill. The following points are identified for orientation (Figs. 2.**5**, 2.**6**):

The anterior site, for insertion of the pelvic rod, is at the iliac crest in the region of the iliac tubercle, about 5 cm more proximal and posterior than the anterior superior iliac spine; the latter must never be used as the entry site for the nail, as dangerous complications may ensue. A stab incision is made at this point.

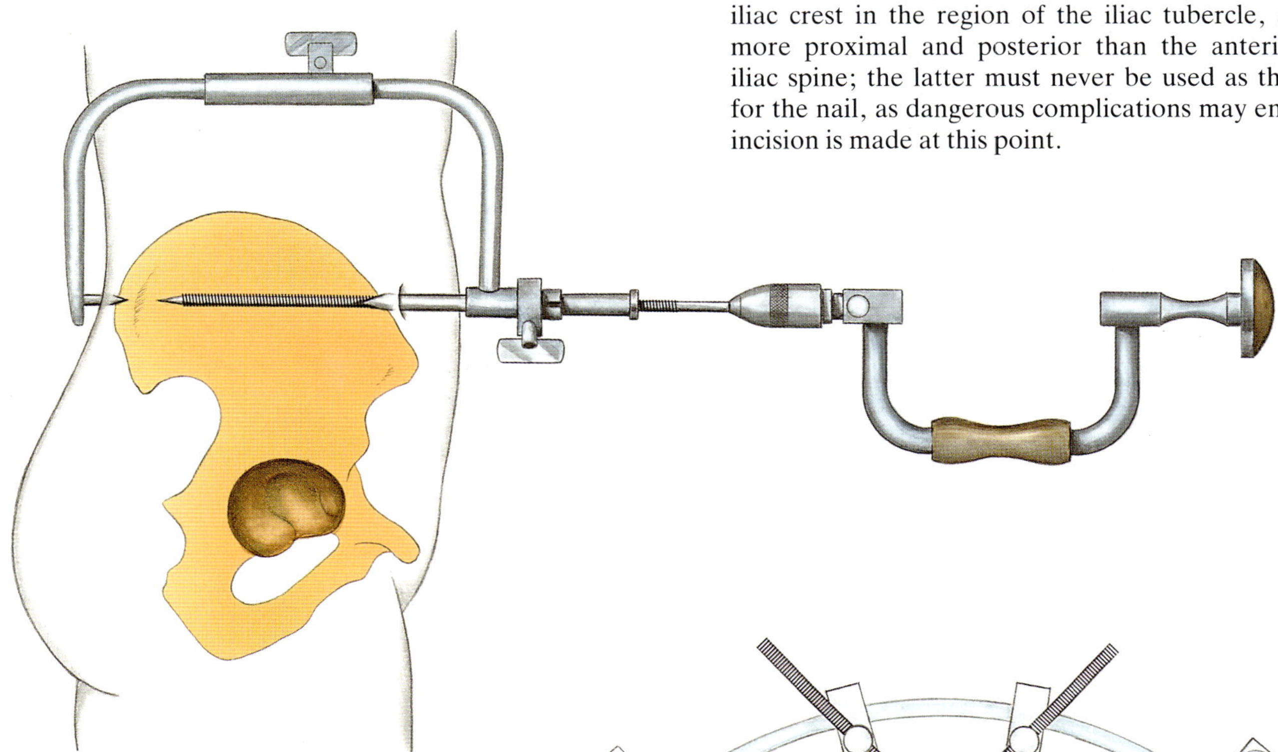

Fig. 2.**5** Insertion of the pelvic rod with the aid of a drill jig.

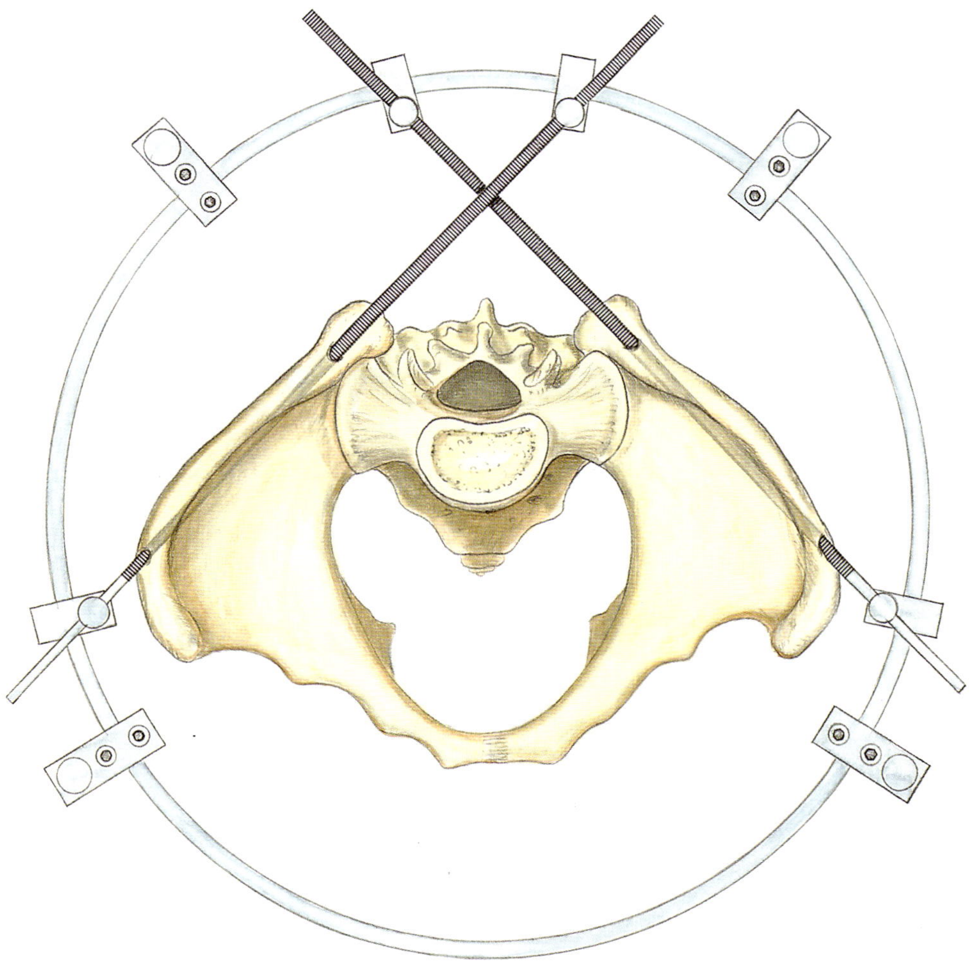

Fig. 2.**6** Correct position of pelvic rods in transverse section.

The exit site is the posterior superior iliac spine on the same side; here, too, a stab incision is made. The tips of the telescopically adjustable drill guide are introduced into the two incisions and anchored in the bone by compression. After this, the drill guide is locked in. While drilling, care should be taken to ensure that the pelvic pin does not slip down the inside of the iliac bone; further drilling would then cause the peritoneum to be wound around the drill, as shown by visible retraction of the abdominal wall. If there is any doubt, it is advisable to make a small incision above the iliac crest and to palpate the iliac fossa with the finger.

Once the pelvic pin has been fixed on one side, the patient is similarly placed in the contralateral position, and the second pin is inserted. The patient is then shifted to the supine position; the pelvic ring is pulled up over the legs and attached to the pelvic pins.

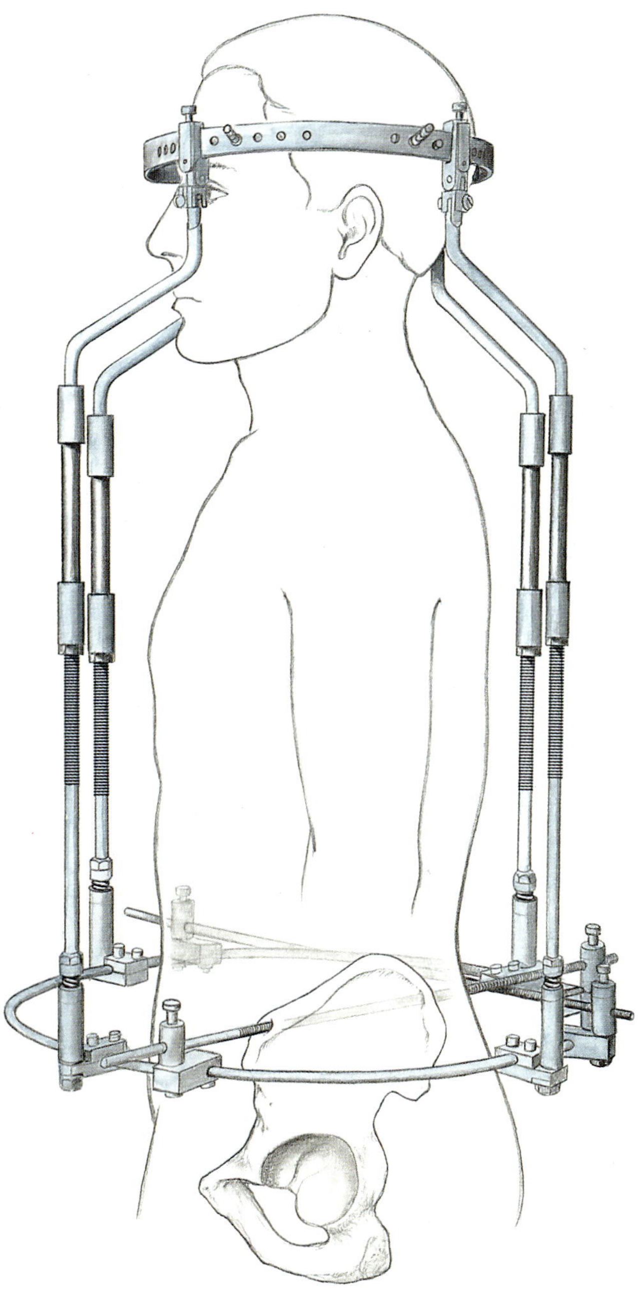

Fig. 2.**7** Halo–pelvic apparatus after assembly.

The rods joining the skull ring to the pelvic part are put in place when the patient has recovered from the anesthesia and is able to sit again (Fig. 2.**7**).

Postoperative Treatment

In order to avert complications, or to detect them at an early stage, the following guidelines should be followed:

- Regular care of screw and pin entry sites
- Regular clinical observation of the patient
- Slow increase in distraction
- Lateral X-rays of the cervical spine
- Daily neurologic assessment with reference to a check list (Table 2.**1**).

In the event of neurologic deficits, the traction should be reduced at once. The chances for remission improve with prompt release of the traction.

Table 2.**1** Checklist for skeletal traction

	Questions	Tests
Spine	– Weakness of legs? – Numbness of legs? – Urinary incontinence?	– Wiggling of toes – Ankle and knee clonus
Cranial nerves (tests VI, IX, X, XII)	– Double images? – Difficulty swallowing? – Difficulty coughing? – Voice alterations? – Weakness of tongue?	– Eye movements (VI) – Palatal reflex (IX) – Vigorous coughing (X) – Ability to speak, nasal voice (IX or X) – Tongue extended to middle position (XII)
Upper extremities	– Difficulty with hand, shoulder or arm movements? – Numbness or weakness of hands?	– Abduction of shoulder joints (C5, C6) – Flexion of forearm (C5, C6) – Test hand pressure (C7–T1) – Sensibility test at finger tips (C6–C8)

Pitfalls and Complications

Perforation by halo screws, brain abscess, pin infection, infection of pelvic pins, secondary degenerative changes in the cervical spine, paralyses of peripheral nerves and cranial nerves; paraplegia.

Further Reading

Bauer R. Die operative Behandlung der Skoliose. Berne: Huber, 1979.

Brinckmann P. Halo-Schwerkraftbehandlung für Skoliosepatienten. In: Hoke M, Bally G, eds. Proceedings of the Symposium 1976;2:369.

Brinckmann P, Krenz J, Polster J. Measurements of the tensile force in the halo–pelvic apparatus and in the halo–Milwaukee brace: internal report. Münster, Germany: Westfälische Wilhelms-Universität, 1974.

Brinckmann P, Krenz J, Polster J. Dynamic halo–gravity traction in scoliosis: internal report. Münster, Germany: Westfälische Wilhelms-Universität, 1974.

Daymond K. Use of halo–femoral traction in spinal surgery. J Bone Jt Surg 1977;59-B:117.

Letts RM, Palakar G, Bobechko WP. Preoperative skeletal traction in scoliosis. J Bone Jt Surg 1975;57-A:616.

O'Brien JP. The halo–pelvic apparatus: a clinical, bioengineering and anatomical study. Acta Orthop Scand 1975;suppl 163.

O'Brien JP. The management of severe spinal deformities with the halo–pelvic apparatus. J Bone Jt Surg 1977;59-B:117.

O'Brien JP, Yau ACMC, Smith TK, Hodgson AR. Halo–pelvic traction. J Bone Jt Surg 1971;53-B:217.

O'Brien JP, Yau ACMC, Hodgson AR. Halo–pelvic traction: a technique for severe spinal deformities. Clin Orthop 1973;92:127.

Perry J, Nickel VL. Total cervical spine fusion for neck paralysis. J Bone Jt Surg 1959;41-A:37.

Ransford AO, Manning CWSF. Complication of halo–pelvic distraction for scoliosis. J Bone Jt Surg 1975;57-B:131.

Wilkins C, MacEwen GD. Cranial nerve injury from halo traction. Clin Orthop 1977;126:106.

Posterior Scoliosis Operations

Harrington Operation

Indications

Principal indication: Thoracic and thoracolumbar scoliosis, with no defect in the posterior vertebral elements.

Secondary indications: Combined scoliosis, lumbar scoliosis (alternatives are anterior procedures such as Dwyer's and ventral derotation spondylodesis).

Approach

See Chapter 1, pp. 64–72.

Operative Technique

Instrumentation

The principal components of the Harrington instrumentation are the following (Figs. 2.**8**, 2.**9**):

Distraction rod: 6 mm diameter; at one end, there are conical sections with a length of 7.5 cm.

Distraction hooks: Thoracic, lumbar, sharp, blunt.

Harrington compression system: This consists of a thick (3/16 inch) and a thin (1/8 inch) threaded rod with hooks and nuts. As a rule, the thinner rod is used in the treatment of kyphoscoliosis. It is flexible, and adjusts to the kyphotic curve.

Modifications:
Moe hook or rod (Fig. 2.**8d**): This is used when lordotic or kyphotic bending of the implanted Harrington rod becomes necessary in the lumbar or thoracolumbar region in order to preserve a physiologic spinal configuration. A square-shaped rod or hook opening is needed to avoid rotation of the rod. This type of hook is also advantageous when the Harrington distraction rod is combined with sublaminar Luque wires (p. 129).

Wisconsin compression system (Fig. 2.**8j**; see also Fig. 2.**31**): This facilitates insertion of the compression rod on the convex side. The posteriorly open compression hooks may be placed first, after which the rod is inserted and secured in the hook with bushings.

Transverse stabilization (DTT, device for transverse traction according to Cotrel): This allows a transverse force to be introduced into the system (Fig. 2.**8k**).

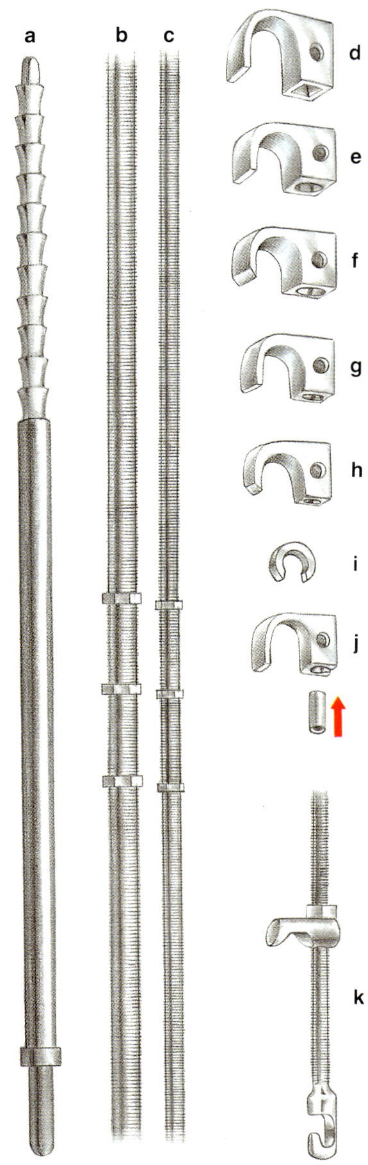

Fig. 2.**8** Harrington instrumentarium, implants.
a Distraction rod.
b Compression rod, 3/16 in.
c Compression rod, 1/8 in.
d Moe hook.
e Blunt thoracic distraction hook.
f Sharp thoracic distraction hook.
g Compression hook for thick threaded rod; also, a caudal end hook for a distraction rod.
h Compression hook for a narrow threaded rod.
i C-ring.
j Open compression hook with shaft insert (Wisconsin system).
k Transverse stabilization (DTT).

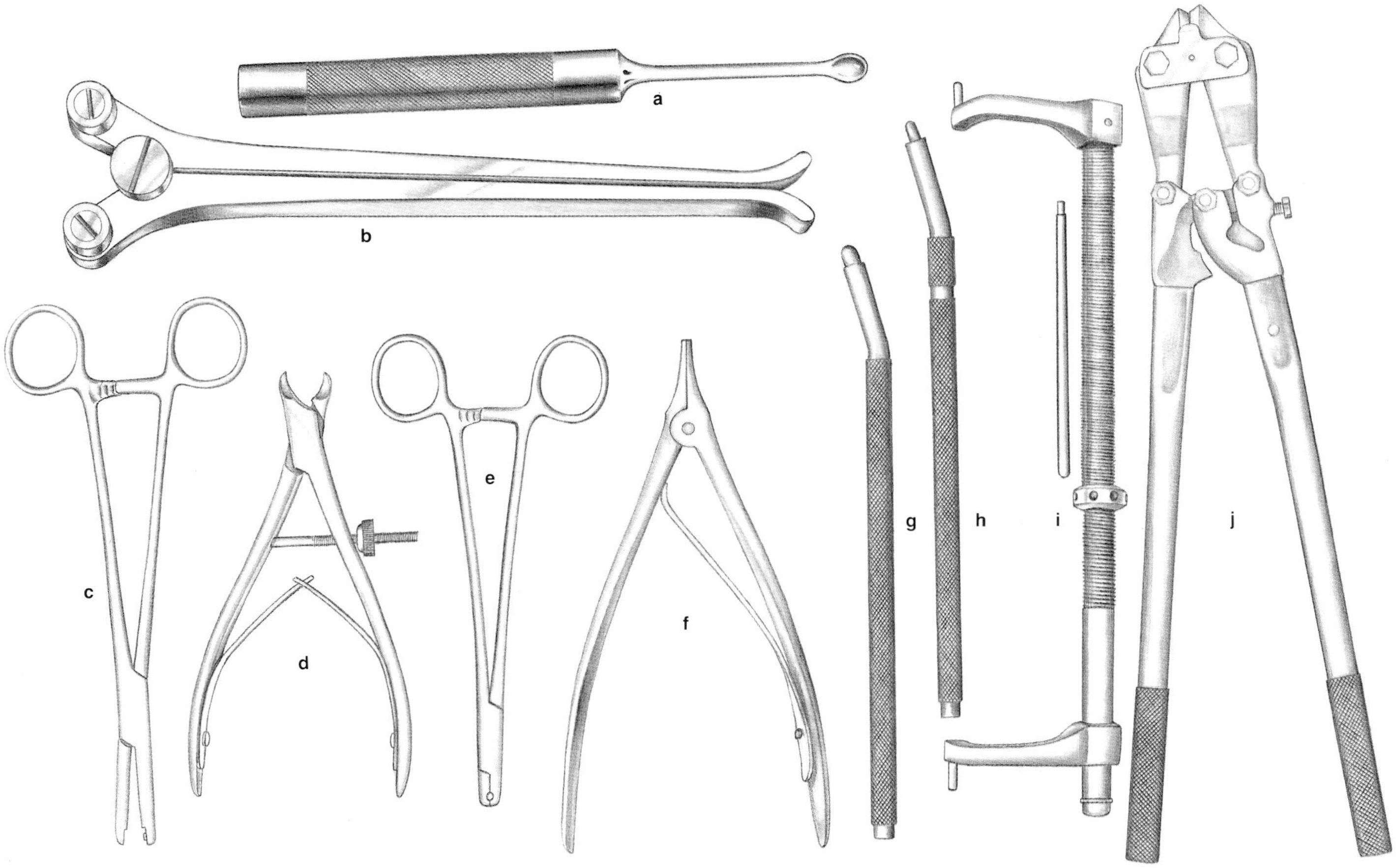

Fig. 2.**9** Harrington instrumentarium.
a Cobb elevator.
b Bending device for the rod.
c Hook holder.
d Compression forceps for the C-ring.
e Holder for the threaded rod.
f Spreading forceps for distraction hook.
g, h Hook inserters.
i Outrigger for distraction.
j Cutting forceps for the rod.

Principles of Correction

- Distraction on the concave side
- Compression on the convex side
- Transverse traction using a DTT.

Hook Position

The following X-ray films are needed to determine hook placement:

- Anteroposterior and lateral films of the entire spine in the standing position
- Bending film in the frontal plane
- Bending films in the sagittal plane if there is a deformity in this plane
- Suspension film

The curvature is measured by the Cobb method from end vertebra to end vertebra. The end vertebra of a structural curve shows the greatest obliquity. Vertebral rotation is determined by the Nash and Moe method. When the pedicles on both sides of the vertebral body are at the same distance, the vertebra is in neutral rotation. The end vertebra is not necessarily identical with the neutral vertebra.

Classification

The four main types of idiopathic scoliosis, according to Ponseti, are:

– Type I: Dorsal scoliosis
– Type II: Lumbar scoliosis
– Type III: Dorsolumbar scoliosis
– Type IV: Combined scoliosis (dorsal and lumbar curve)

These basic types have been subdivided as follows by King et al.:

Type I (Fig. 2.**10**)
S-shaped (13%). The thoracic and the lumbar curve go beyond the midline. The lumbar curve is larger than the thoracic curve. The flexibility index is negative (that is, on the bending film, the percentage of the thoracic correction is greater than that of the lumbar correction).

Definition of the flexibility index: The percentage correction of the thoracic curve as shown on the bending film is subtracted from the percentage correction of the lumbar curvature.

Type II (Fig. 2.**11**)
S-shaped (33%). The thoracic and the lumbar curve pass beyond the midline. The thoracic curve is bigger than the lumbar curve. The flexibility index is 0 or greater (that is, the percentage of lumbar correction on the bending film is greater than that of the thoracic correction).

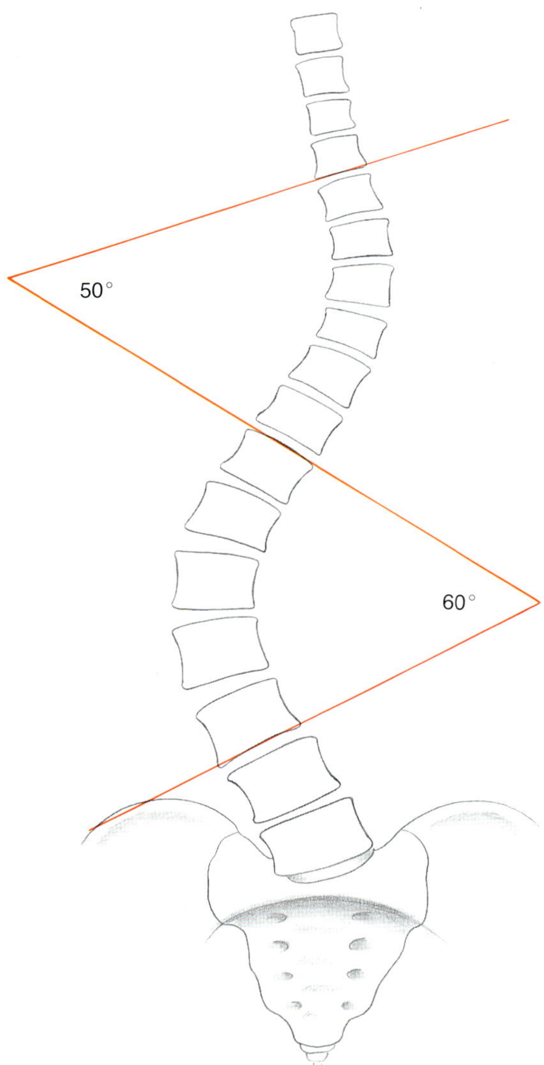

Fig. 2.**10** King classification, Type I.

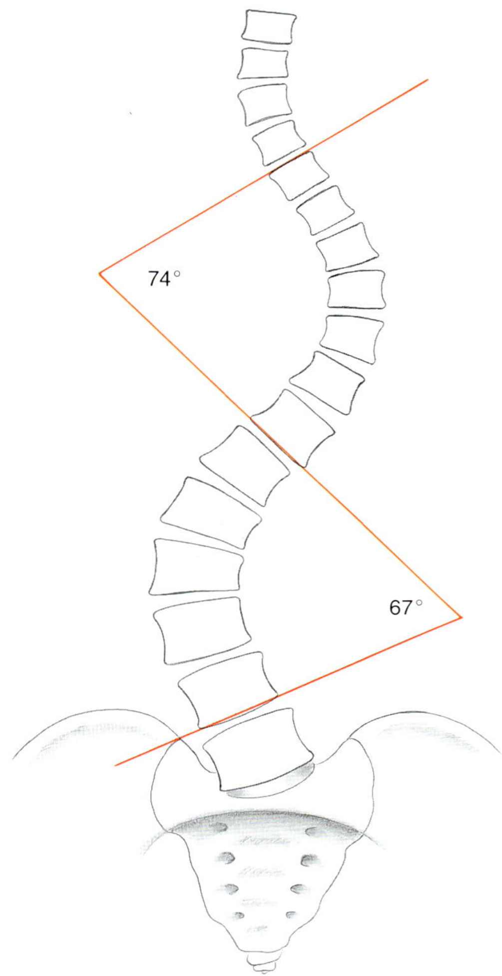

Fig. 2.**11** King classification, Type II.

Type III (Fig. 2.**12**)
Thoracic curve (33%). The lumbar curve does not go beyond the midline.

Type IV (Fig. 2.**13**)
Large thoracic curvature (9%), with L5 centered over the sacrum. L4 inclines into a long thoracic curve.

Type V (Fig. 2.**14**)
Thoracic double curve (11%). T1 inclines in the convexity of the upper curve. Upper curve structural.

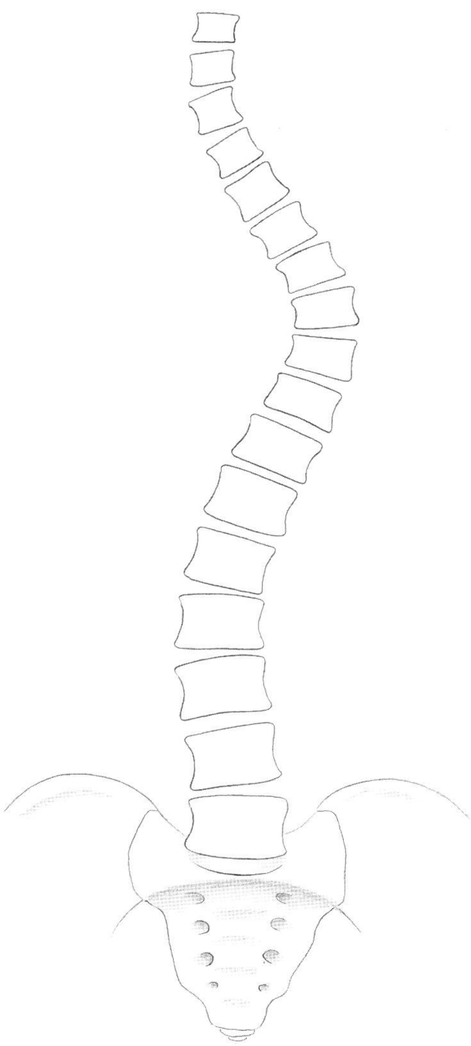

Fig. 2.**12** King classification, Type III.

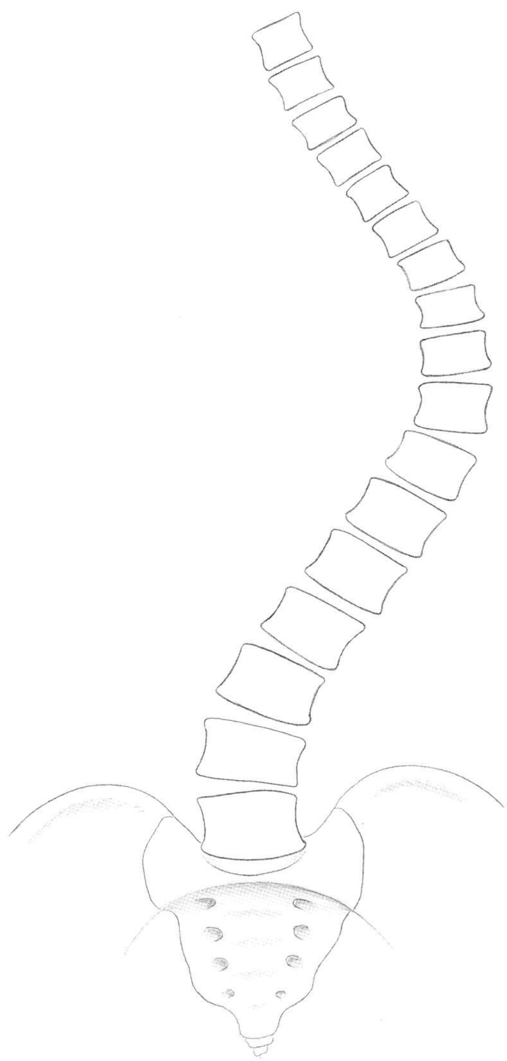

Fig. 2.**13** King classification, Type IV.

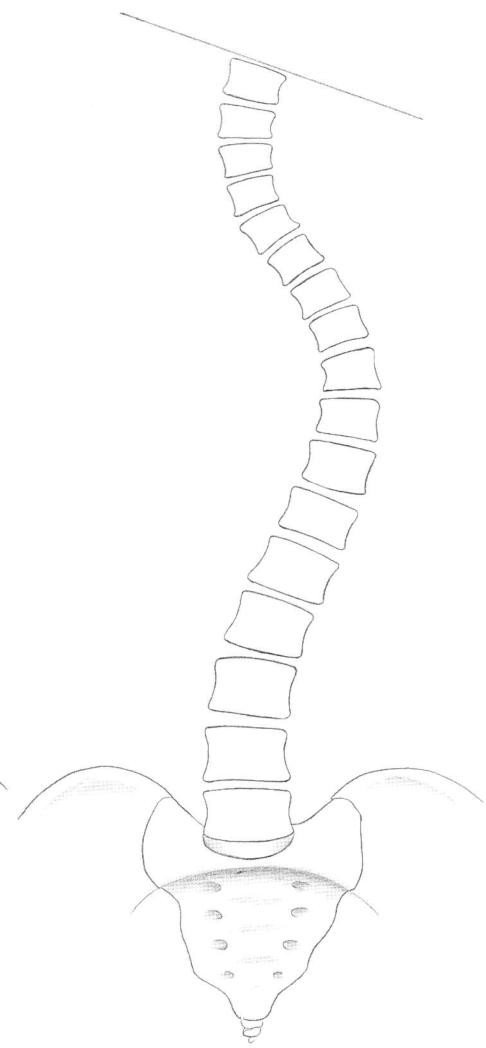

Fig. 2.**14** King classification, Type V.

Fusion Area

Choice of the area of fusion, particularly in thoracic and combined scoliosis, is a controversial subject. Various recommendations for determining the fusion area have been put forward. For thoracic curvature, Harrington recommends extending the fusion from above the curve to two vertebrae below the curve. Fusion from the upper neutrally rotated vertebra to the lower neutrally rotated vertebra has been recommended as well (Goldstein 1930, 1966, 1971, Moe et al. 1978). If the rotation continues distal to the end vertebra, the fusion should extend at least to the first neutrally rotated vertebra. The younger the patient, the greater the advisability of a long fusion. Harrington (1962) pointed out the significance of the so-called *stable zone,* into which the lower end of the fusion should extend. This is defined by two parallel lines running vertically through the lumbosacral joints. The vertebrae lying inside these lines are in the stable zone. According to King et al. (1983), a more precise definition is provided by a single line through the middle of the sacrum and perpendicular to the line joining the iliac crests. If the legs differ in length, the difference has to be eliminated by leg length correction with wood blocks before radiography. The vertebra that is divided into two halves, completely or approximately, by this line is the so-called *stable vertebra* (Fig. 2.**16**). Fusion requirements according to the type of the curve have been explained as follows by King et al.:

Type I (Fig. 2.**15**): Both curves have to be fused. Applying the above criteria (lowermost vertebra in neutral rotation and within the stable zone), a stable outcome with no progression can be achieved. It is possible, as a general rule, to work with two distraction rods, or to use the so-called dollar method in conjunction with a compression instrument in the area of the thoracic spine.

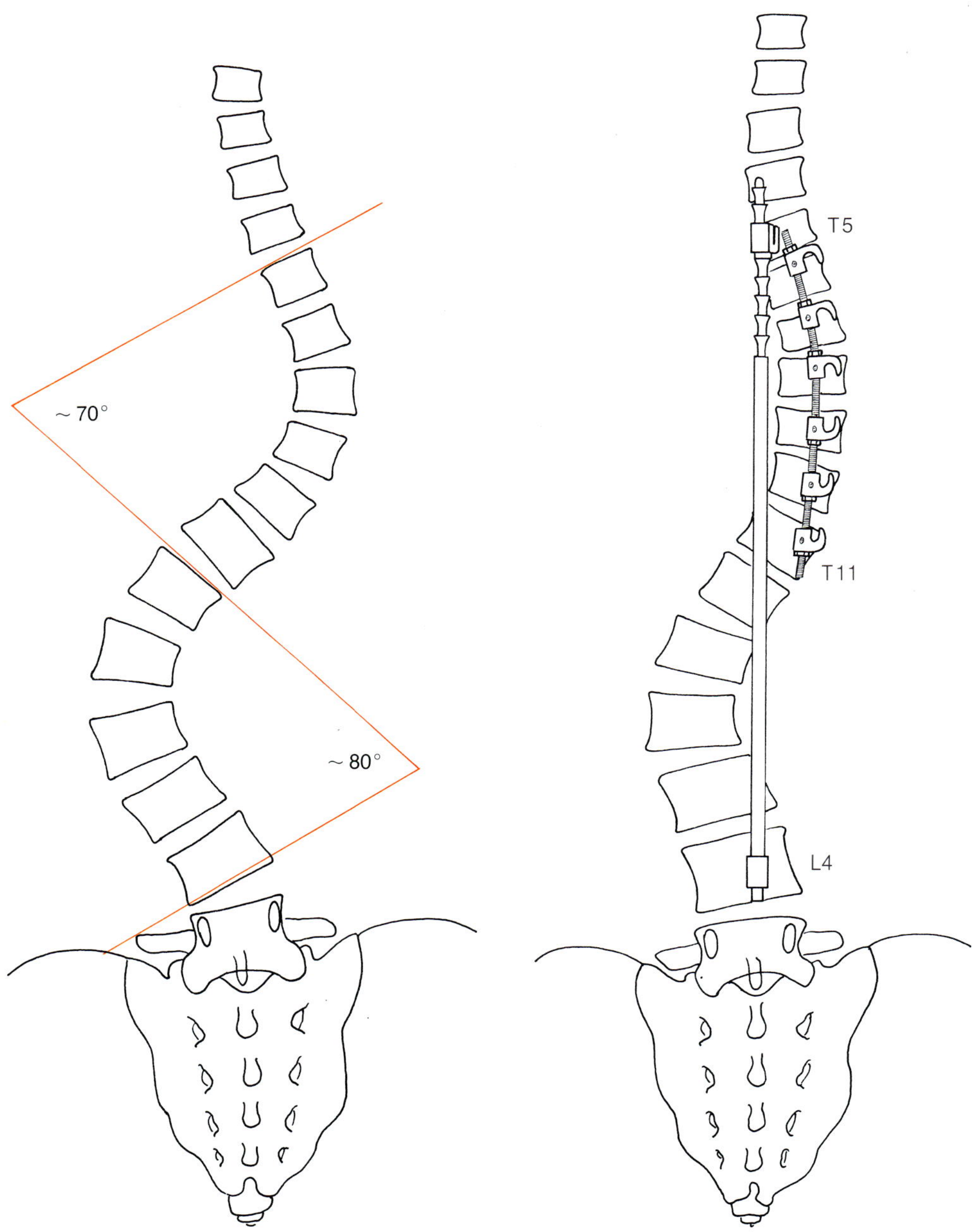

Fig. 2.**15** King Type I curve. Both curves have to be fused. The so-called dollar method is shown here.

Type II: Fusion exclusive of the thoracic curve is adequate. However, vertebral rotation and the stable vertebra are very important for the choice of the caudal vertebra. The neutral vertebra and stable vertebra often are identical. In this case, fusion up to that point is sufficient. If they are not identical, fusion should extend as far as the stable vertebra.

Type III (Fig. 2.**16**): Fusion as far as the neutral vertebra may lead to an increase in the thoracic curvature if the stable vertebra is more distally located. In every case, therefore, fusion as far as the stable vertebra is required.

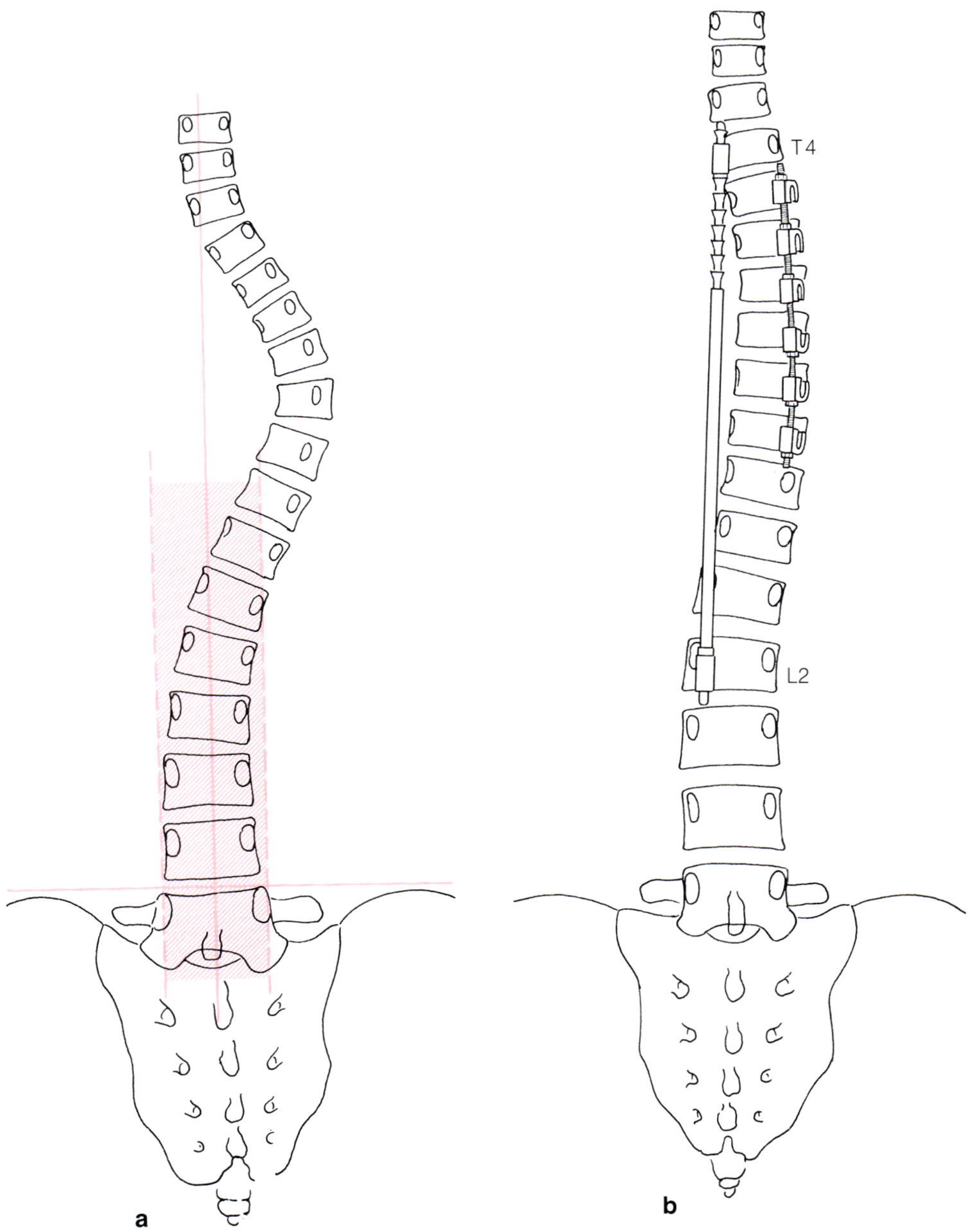

Fig. 2.**16** King Type III thoracic curve.
a Harrington's stable zone (between the vertical lines through the lumbosacral vertebral joints). King's stable vertebra: divided by vertical lines through the middle of the sacrum.
b Correct fusion as far as L2. The vertebra is neutrally rotated within the Harrington stable zone and conforms to the stable vertebra according to the King classification.

Type IV (Fig. 2.**17**): If the fusion is carried only to the neutrally rotated vertebra, a distal prolongation of the curve may result. Fusion to the stable vertebra gives reliable results.

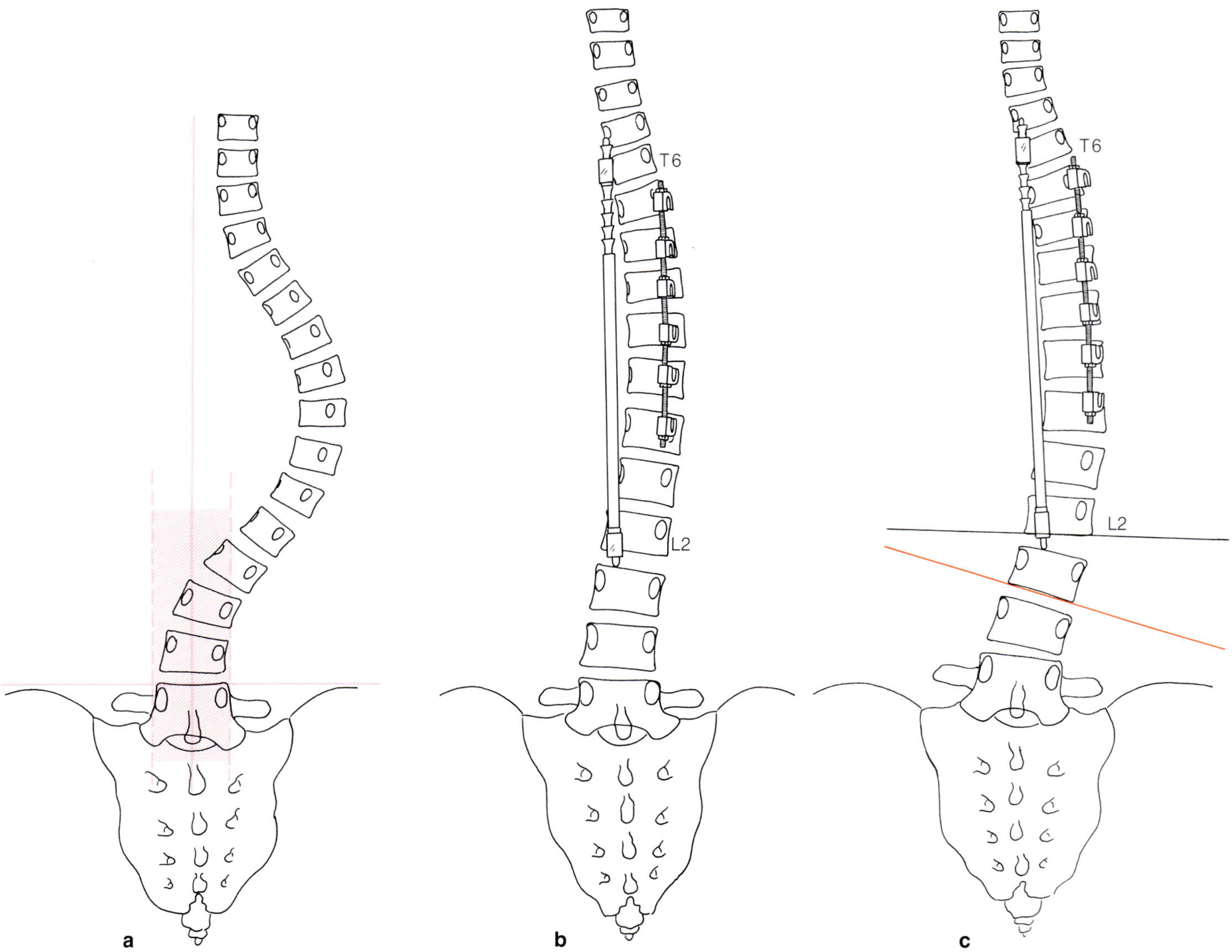

Fig. 2.**17** Long thoracic curve, King Type IV.
a Harrington stable zone (between the vertical lines through the lumbosacral vertebral joints). King's stable vertebra: divided by vertical lines through the middle of the sacrum.
b L2 is neither neutrally rotated nor inside the stable zone. The fusion is too short.
c Despite a good primary correction, distal extension of the curve can be expected.

Type V (Fig. 2.**18**): In this case, a high thoracic curve has to be included in the fusion in order to correct the slant of the shoulder. Distally, the fusion should extend to the stable vertebra. If fusion is carried only as far as the neutrally rotated vertebra and this lies proximal to the stable vertebra, the curve may be moved in a distal direction.

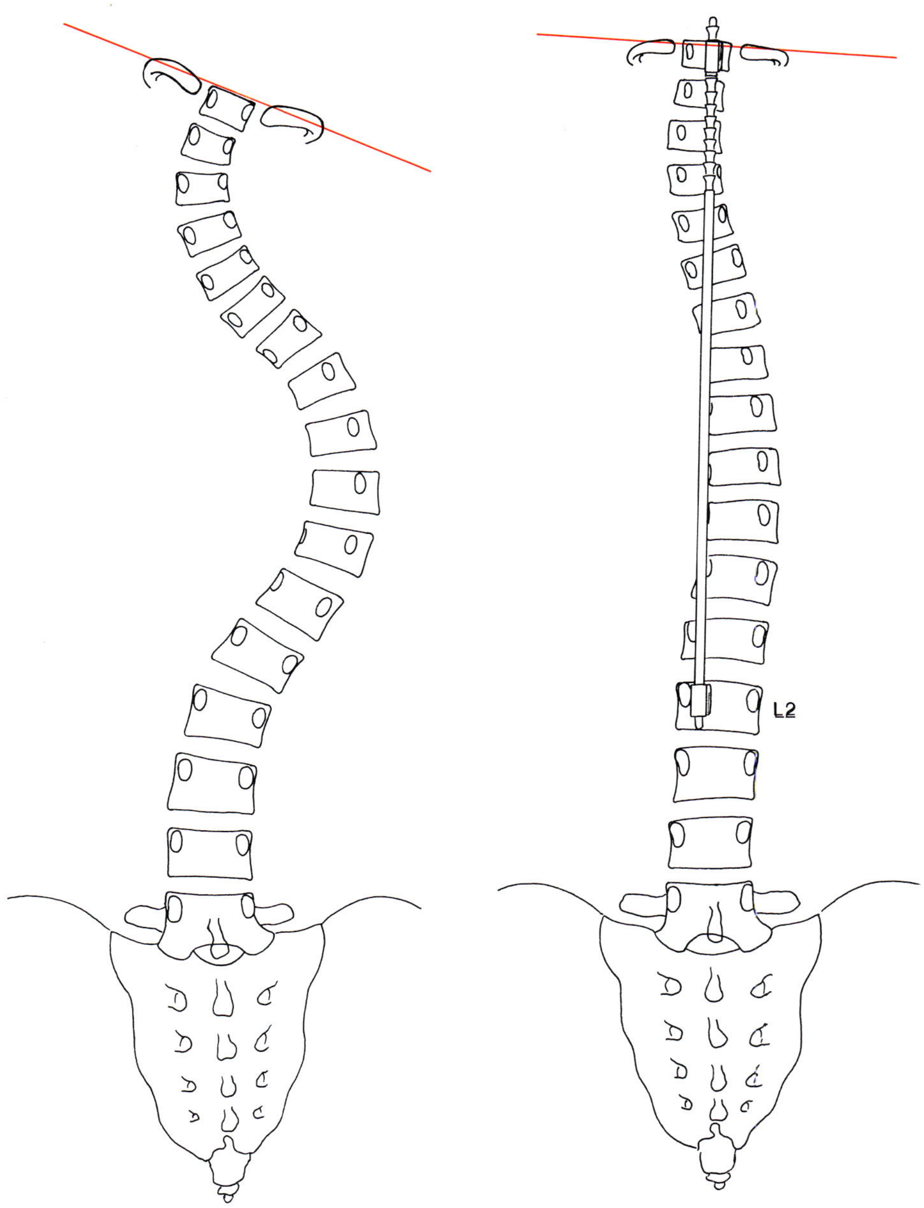

Fig. 2.**18** King Type IV curve. The proximal thoracic curve has to be instrumented to correct the obliquity of the shoulder.

Thoracolumbar curve (Fig. 2.**19**): This is usually left-convex, beginning between T8 and T11, and extending in a distal direction to L3, L4, or L5. Fusion as far as L4 is generally sufficient. Fusion to L5 may be necessary if there is a marked thoracic overhang, or if there are long thoracic curves.

Lumbar scoliosis: This generally extends from T11 to L3 or L4 and is often left-convex. Fusion to the end vertebra is usually sufficient. If the end vertebra lies at the level of L3 or L4, but rotation continues more distally so that the neutral vertebra is at L5, for example, it is generally sufficient to fuse to the end vertebra only.

Note

At the present state of the art, anterior procedures (Dwyer, Zielke) may be preferable for thoracolumbar and lumbar curves. Correction is more efficient, and it may be possible to limit fusion to a shorter distance (pp. 163–185). For combined scoliosis (mainly of King type I), concomitant use of anterior procedures for the caudal curve and of posterior procedures for the thoracic curve is advisable (p. 167).

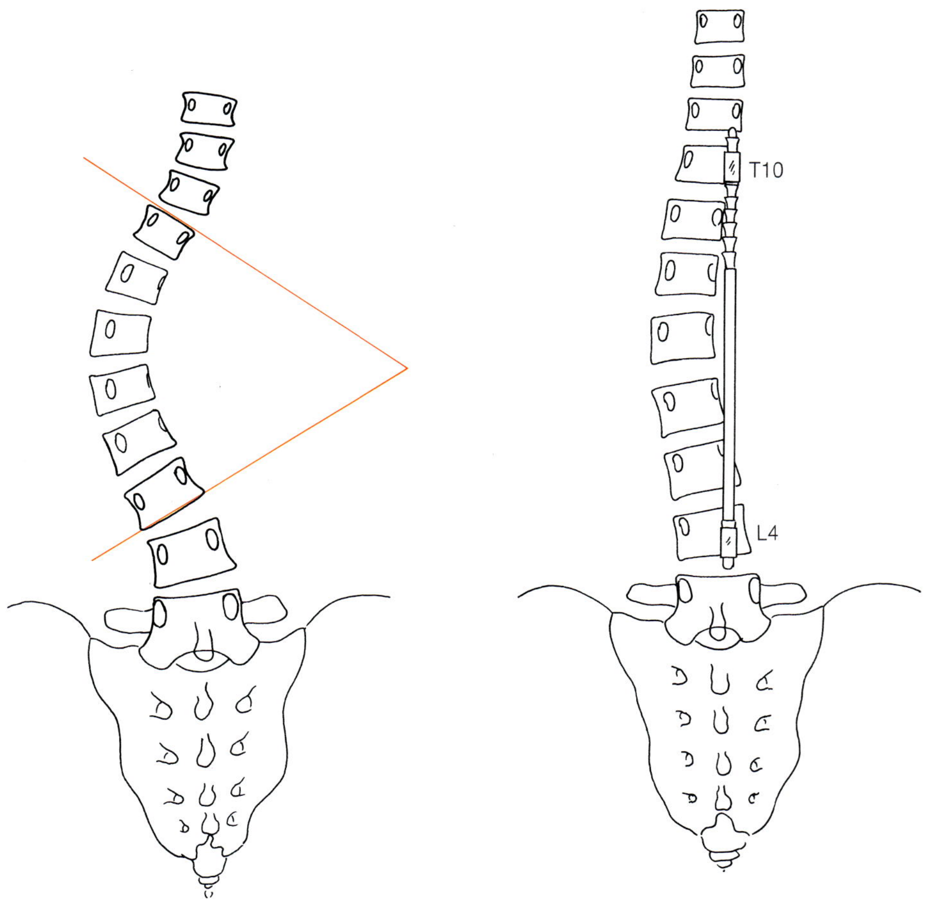

Fig. 2.**19** Thoracolumbar scoliosis; correct fusion as far as L4. Neutrally rotated and within the stable zone.

Instrumentation

Following clear exposure of the area of fusion and interim collection of bone chips from the posterior parts of the iliac crest, the site for the proximal distraction hook is prepared initially, i.e., on the concave side at the upper end of the curve, in accordance with the preoperative plan.

With the chisel, a small piece of bone is removed from the inferior articular process of the selected vertebra (Fig. 2.**20**). The transverse plane of decortication should ascend slightly in a medial direction. This provides a good site for application of the distracting forces and prevents lateral slippage of the hook. A sharp Harrington hook is first inserted into the interarticular portion with a hook holder, until it is felt that the hook has penetrated into the facet joint and is firmly anchored in it. For the instrumentation, this hook is usually replaced by a blunt one (Figs. 2.**21**–2.**23**).

After this, the seat of the caudal distraction hook is prepared. This is also located on the concave side of the curve and is generally in the area of the lumbar spine (Figs. 2.**24**, 2.**25**).

The hook straddles the cranial border of the lamina of the selected vertebra; the internal limb of the hook lies between the dura and the vertebral arch. To allow easy insertion of the hook, it is sometimes necessary to resect the caudal portion of the lamina, or portions of the inferior articular process of the next higher vertebra. The yellow ligament is then transversely incised at the upper margin of the vertebral arch in the region of the half of the vertebra that lies on the concave side and is retracted proximally or partly resected. Any bleeding epidural veins have to be coagulated with the aid of bipolar forceps. Using a bone rongeur, the upper border of the lamina is leveled off; the caudal distraction hook may then be inserted by a small rotary movement with the use of a hook holder and the hook-seating instrument.

After positioning of the two distraction hooks, the so-called outrigger can be applied, and continuous distraction can now begin (Fig. 2.**9i**). This distraction is facilitated by manual pressure on the convex side of the scoliosis, with the outrigger thread merely tracking behind. Use of the outrigger is not mandatory; alternatively, the Harrington distraction rod may be used to begin with. However, the facet joints on the concave side need to be debrided beforehand, and the fusion sites must be prepared in areas that will no longer be accessible after introduction of the Harrington distraction rod. For severe curvatures, the Harrington distraction rod may also be applied primarily, without covering up the operative field. The correction is carried out continuously during the operation. Distraction of the Harrington rod (Fig. 2.**35**) with the spreaders requires sensitivity and experience on the part of the surgeon. There must be no breakage of the hook seat, particularly cranially (neurologic limit: somatosensory evoked potentials and a wake-up test; see p. 96).

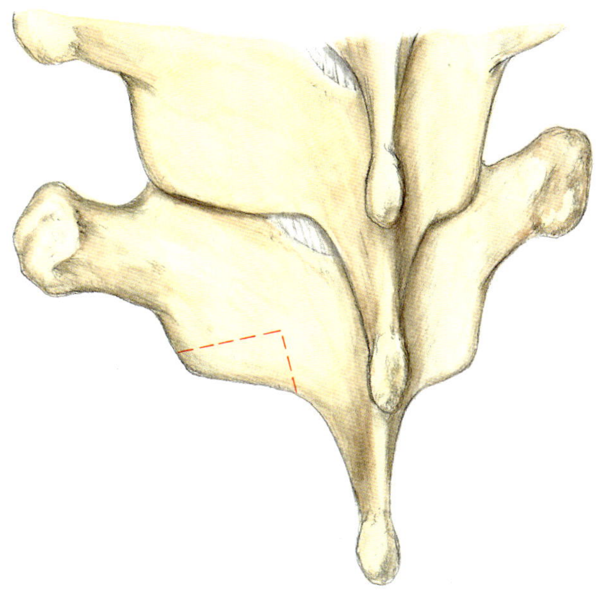

Fig. 2.**20** Dissection for placement of cranial distraction hooks. Choice of chisel plane.

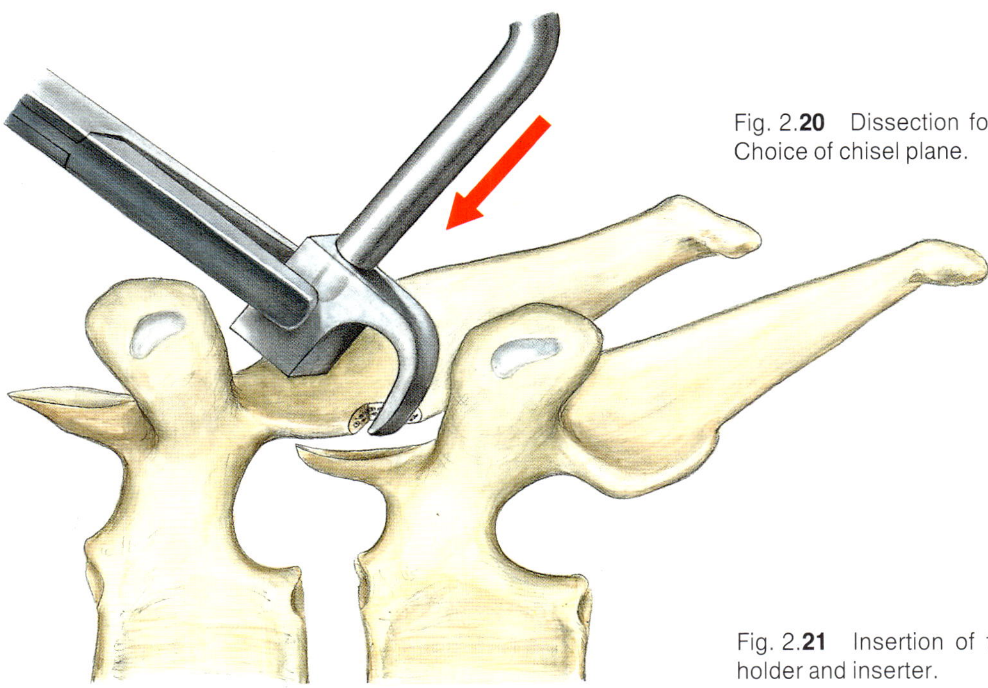

Fig. 2.**21** Insertion of the cranial distraction hook with a hook holder and inserter.

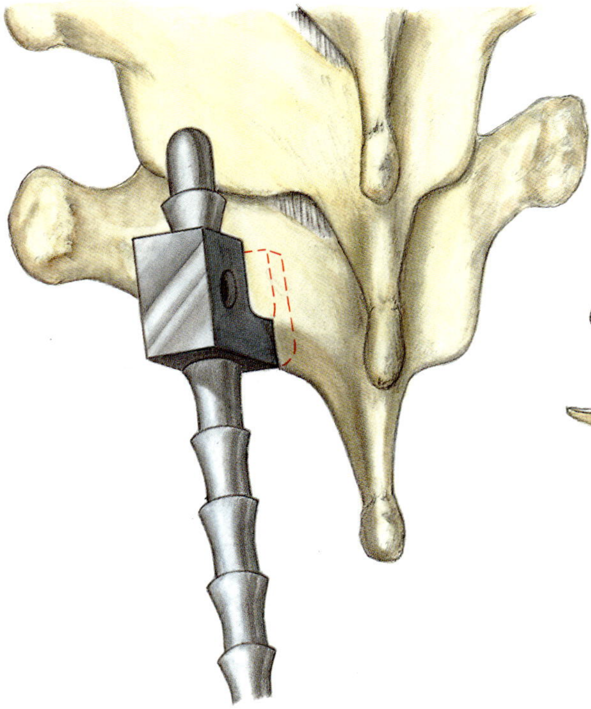

Fig. 2.**22** Distraction hook in place, seen from above.

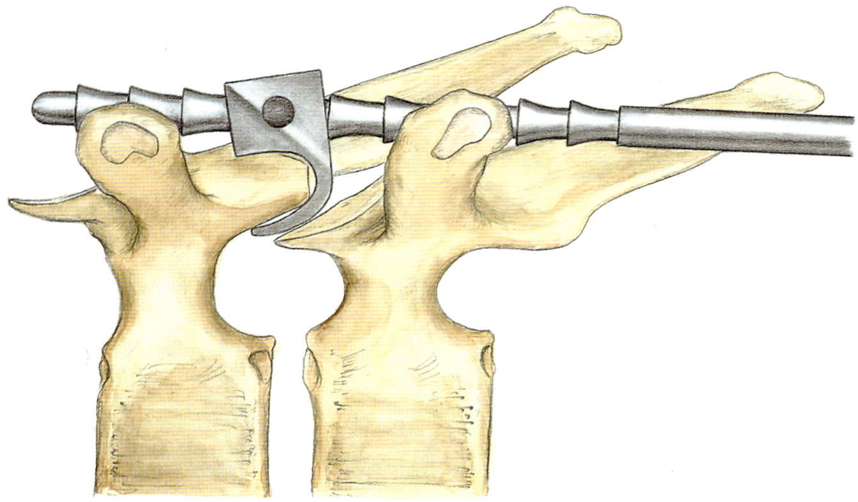

Fig. 2.**23** Distraction hook in the facet joint, seen from the side.

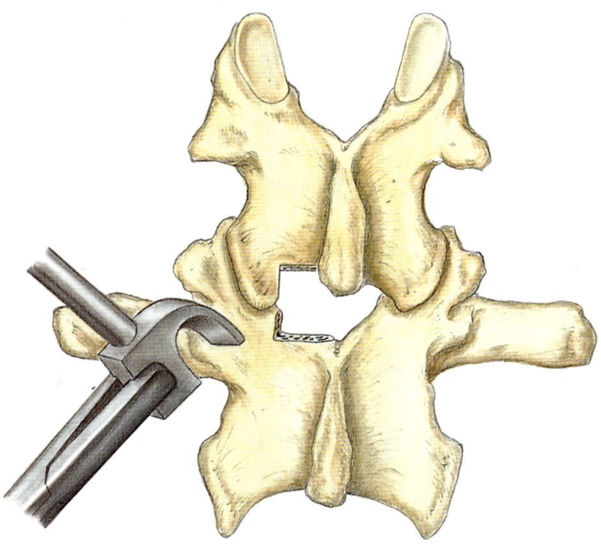

Fig. 2.**24** Dissection for placement of caudal distraction hooks and insertion of a hook.

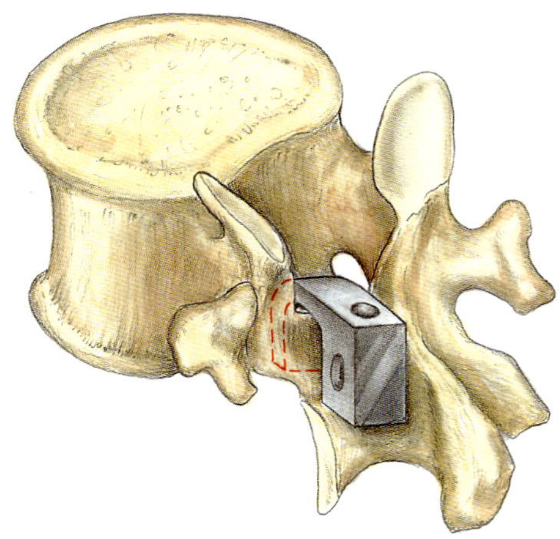

Fig. 2.**25** Caudal distraction hook in place.

Fusion

The first step is resection of the facet joints on the concave side, based on the Moe technique. The resected facet joints in the lumbar spine region that have been partly resected with a gouge or rongeur are covered with cancellous bone chips (Fig. 2.**26**). In the area of the thoracic spine, the facet joints are also resected, and this can provide increased mobility of the spine and thus improved correction. We essentially follow the Hall technique: using a gouge, the inferior articular process of the upper thoracic vertebra is removed. The superior articular process of the nearest caudal thoracic vertebra is debrided with the gouge. The spinous processes are divided in the midline with a blade chisel and cut off at the base with a Liston rongeur. The spinous processes are crushed and used as bone chips. The vertebral arches are also debrided as far as the transverse processes, using the gouges, to obtain a cortical–cancellous graft. The excavation in the region of the resected vertebral joints is bridged with a massive cancellous-bone chip (Figs. 2.**27**, 2.**28**). Subsequently, the facet joints of the convex side are similarly treated.

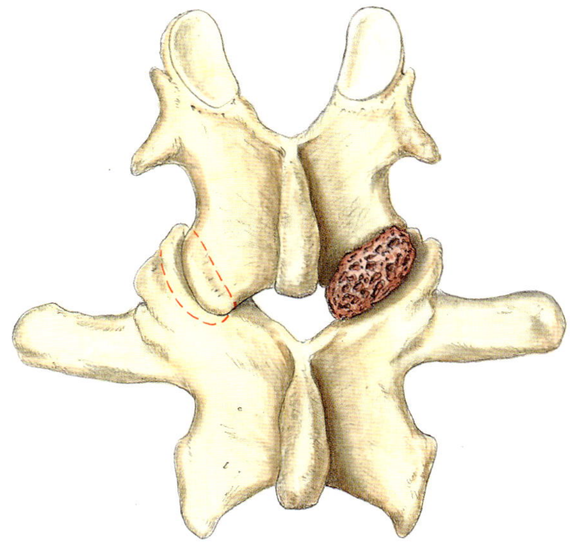

Fig. 2.**26** Debridement and bridging of facet joints in the lumbar spine.

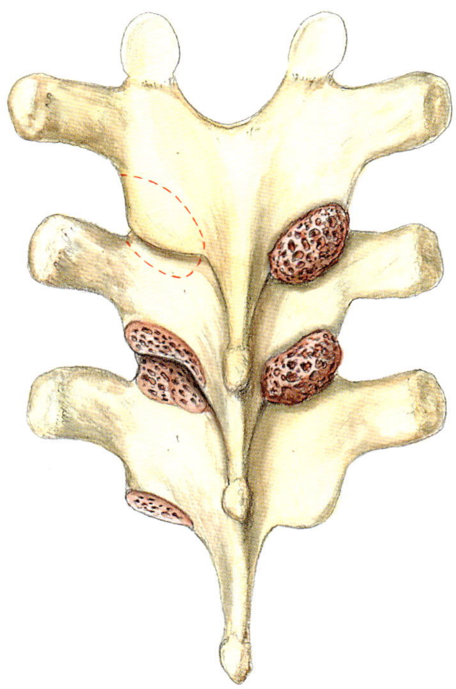

Fig. 2.**27** Debridement and bridging of facet joints in the thoracic spine.

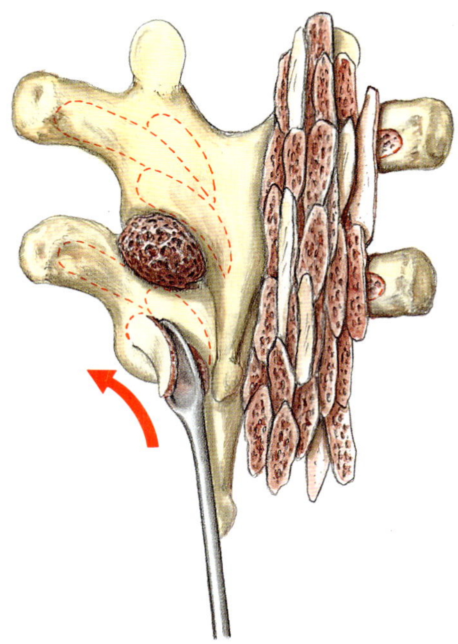

Fig. 2.**28** Debridement of posterior vertebral elements and grafting of corticocancellous chips in the area of the thoracic spine.

After this, the *compression system* is applied (Figs. 2.**29**–2.**34**). Generally, up to six compression hooks are used; these are attached to the bases of the transverse processes on the convex side in the thoracic area. The direction of compression depends on the apex of the curve: proximal to it, the hooks are aligned distally, and distal to it they are aligned proximally. In the area of the thoracolumbar junction (weak transverse processes), the hooks may also be applied to the lamina from the caudal side (Figs. 2.**32**–2.**34**; see also p. 218).

The hook seat is prepared either with a special instrument replicating the shape of the hook, or directly with the clamp-anchored hook. First of all, the hook is rotated around the transverse process in immediate contact with the bone, which generally makes it necessary to overcome soft-tissue resistance (corresponding to transection of the costotransverse ligament, Fig. 2.**29**). The hook is removed again, passed into the depth between the transverse processes without rotation, and then applied to the transverse process. This is necessary, as the individual hooks can no longer be rotated when the compression rod that engages

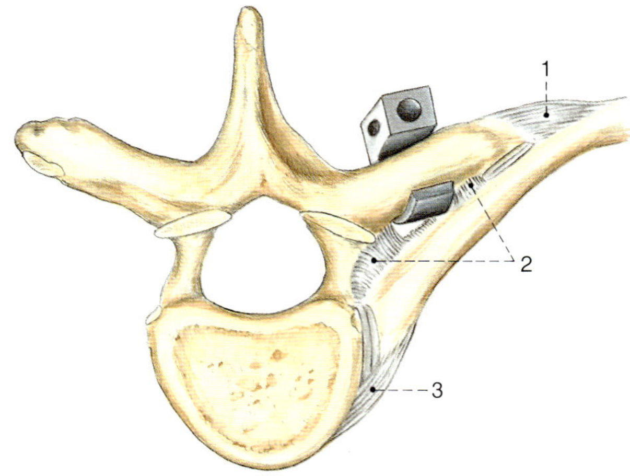

Fig. 2.**29** Cross-section of thoracic vertebra, with a compression hook. Note the division of the costotransverse ligament.

1 Lateral costotransverse ligament
2 Costotransverse ligament
3 Radiate ligament of the head of the rib

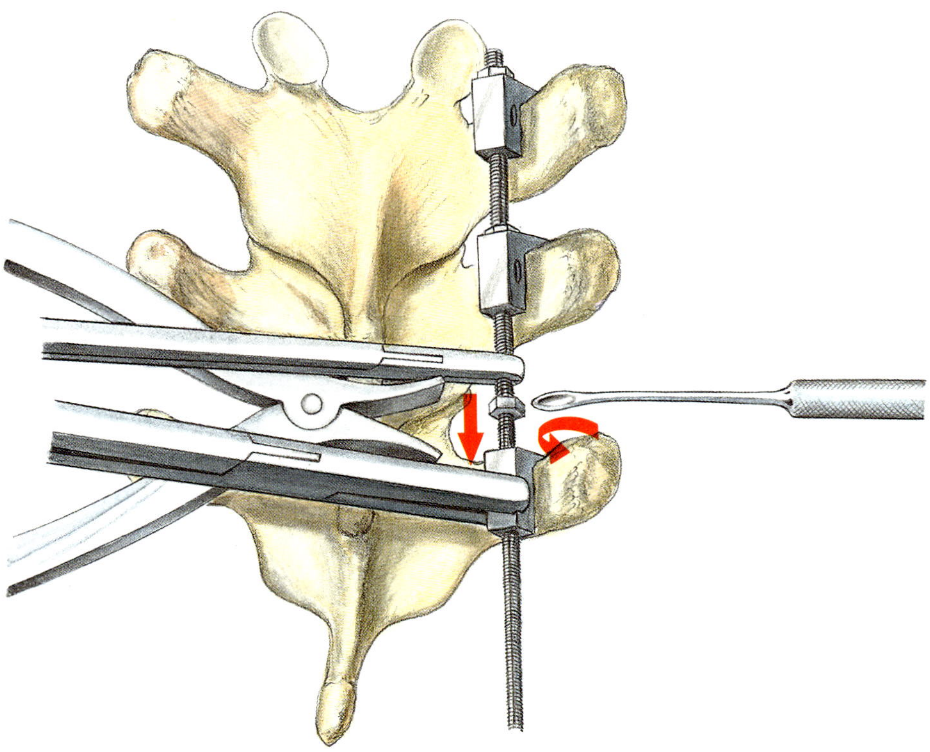

Fig. 2.**30** Harrington compression system, attached to the transverse process of the thoracic spine. Compression is effected by applying spreaders between the rod holder and the hook holder.

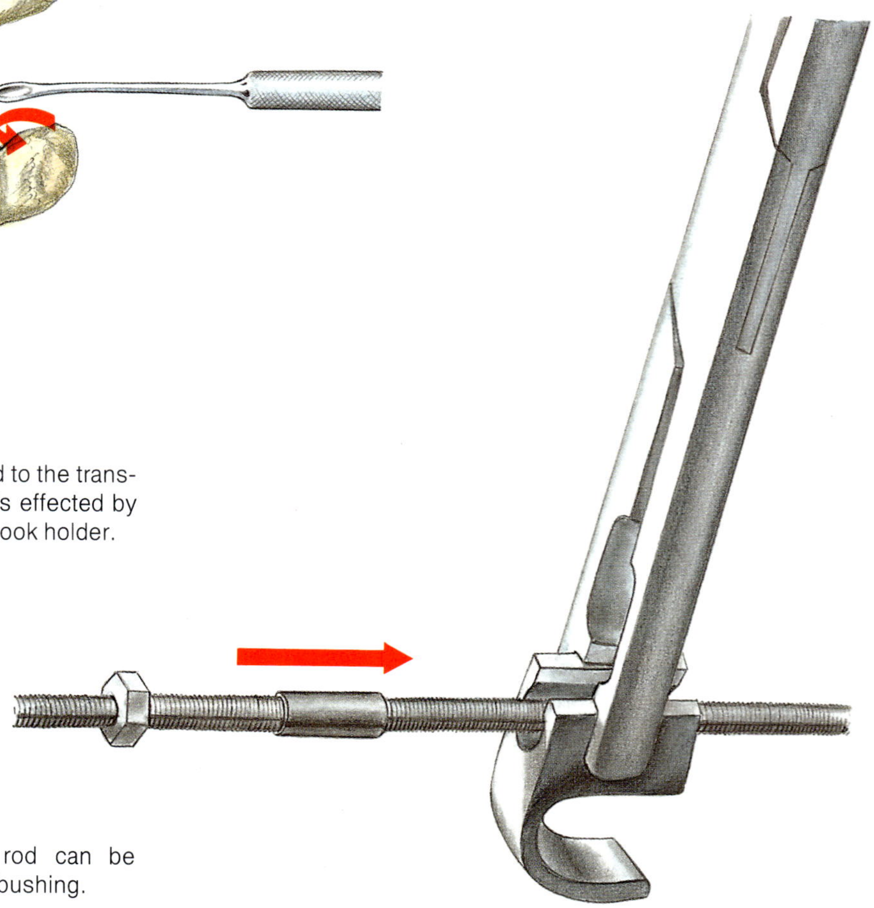

Fig. 2.**31** Wisconsin system. The compression rod can be inserted into the hooks afterward and secured with a bushing.

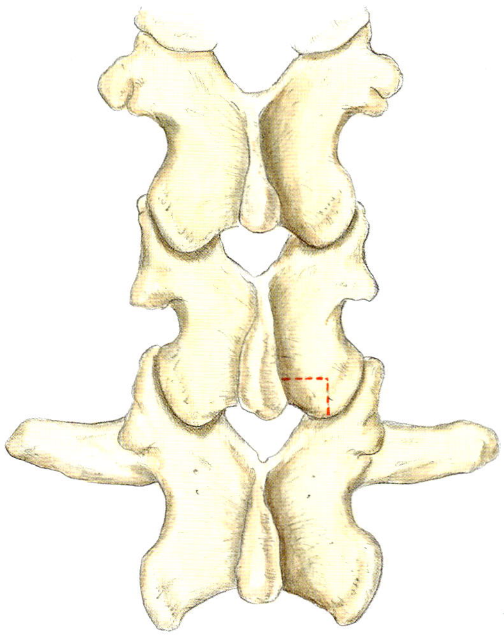

Fig. 2.**32** Dissection for placement of caudal compression hooks in the lumbar spine. Choice of chisel plane.

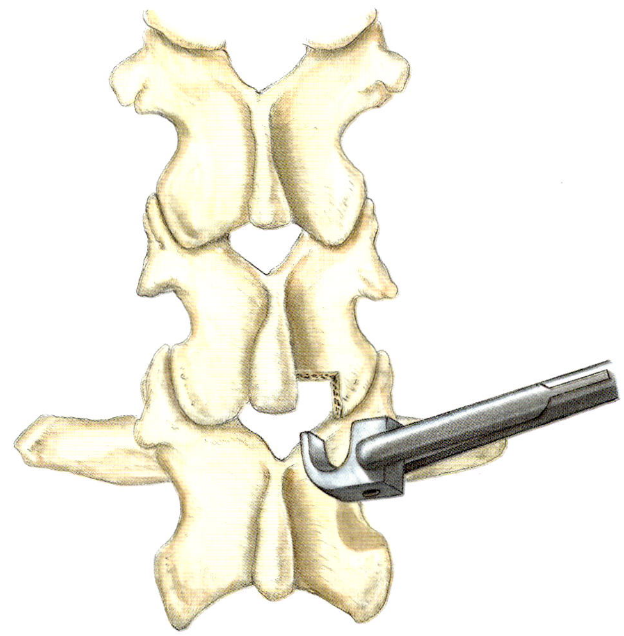

Fig. 2.**33** Insertion of a caudal compression hook.

all the hooks is introduced. Adequate practice is required. Positioning of the compression hooks may present difficulties (Fig. 2.**36**). This can be circumvented by use of the so-called Wisconsin system: there is a slit in the back of the hook through which the threaded rod can be inserted after positioning of the hook. The rod is fixed by means of a bushing that is introduced into the hook (Fig. 2.**31**).

Once all the hooks have been placed, compression is exerted by applying spreaders between the hook holder and the rod holder. The hexagonal nuts are placed afterwards and are finally tightened with a wrench (Fig. 2.**30**).

When the compression instrumentation is put under tension, further corrections can be made with the distraction rod (when an outrigger is used, it may be eventually replaced by the definitive Harrington rod). The distraction should be carried out cautiously and continually.

Finally, the vertebral arches on the convex side as well are debrided in the usual way. However, if a compression system is used, resection should not be carried beyond the transverse process bases, in order not to compromise stability.

For further rigidity—how much extra correction is obtainable is a subject of controversy in the literature—a transverse stabilization according to Cotrel may be performed with the DTT (device for transverse traction). The proximal distraction hook is locked by means of a C-ring, in order to prevent the hook from slipping down the rod postoperatively.

The cancellous bone chips taken from the ilium are now applied in the targeted fusion area; the bone chips collected upon decortication of the vertebral column are now also placed. The cortical–cancellous iliac bone chips are applied at the top. It is important to include the end vertebrae of the fusion site (hook seat) in the fusion (Figs. 2.**35**–2.**38**).

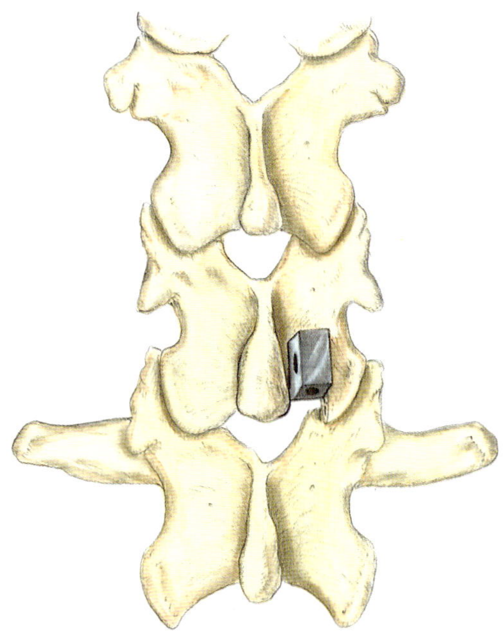

Fig. 2.**34** Caudal compression hook in place.

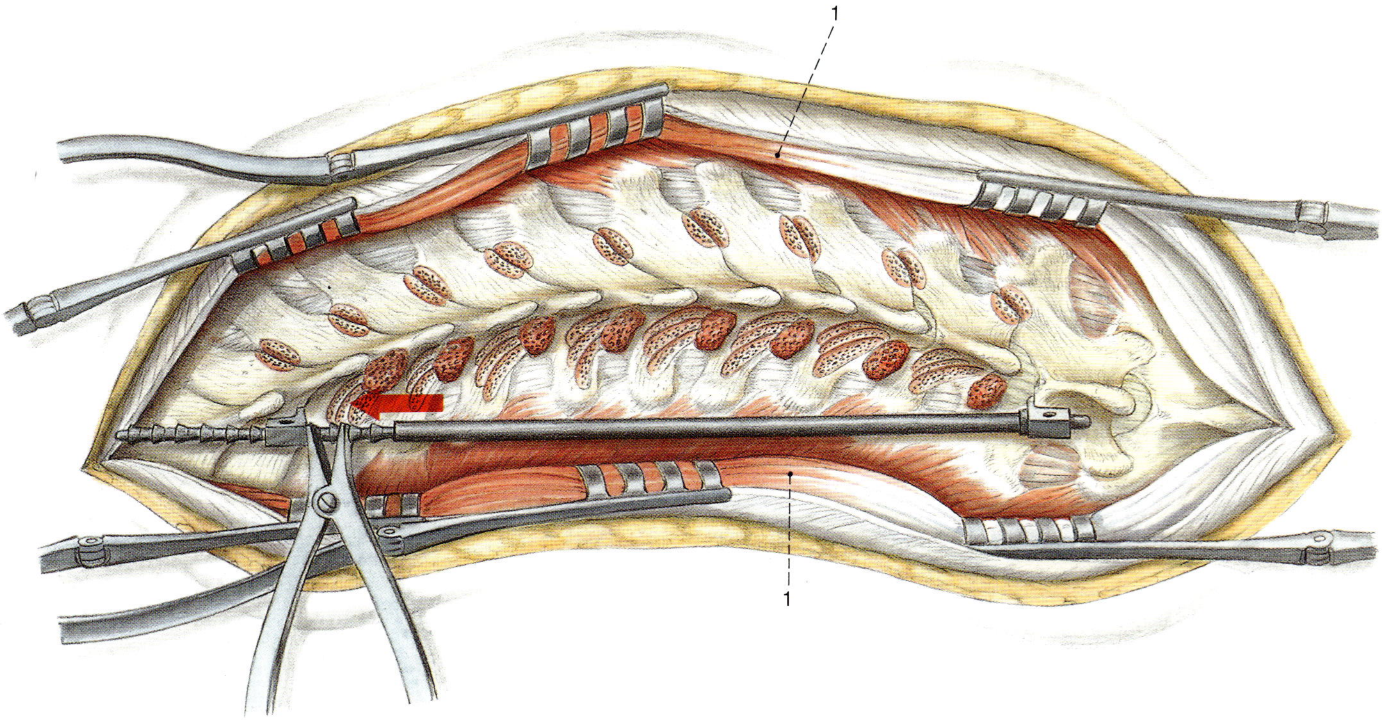

Fig. 2.**35** Operative site. Status after debridement of the facet joints and insertion of the Harrington distraction rod. The distraction is performed with spreaders.

1 Erector muscle of the spine

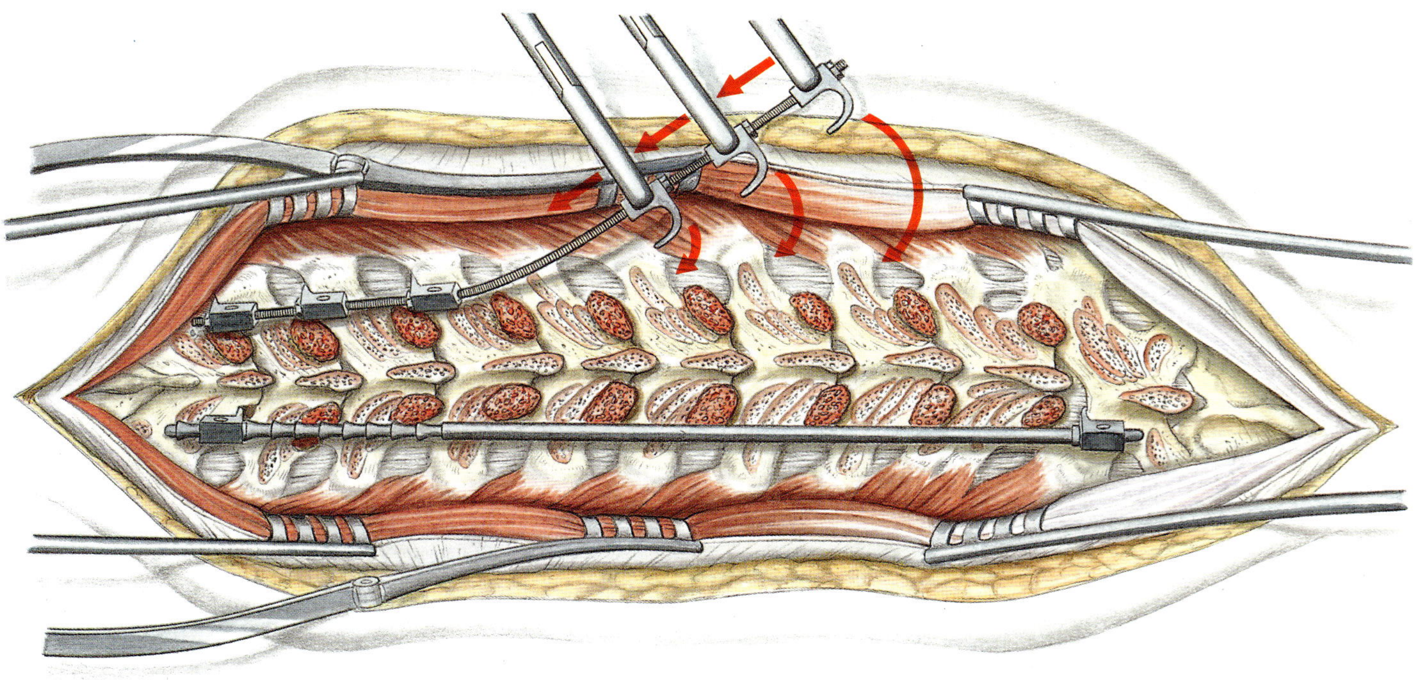

Fig. 2.**36** Operative site. Introduction of a Harrington compression system.

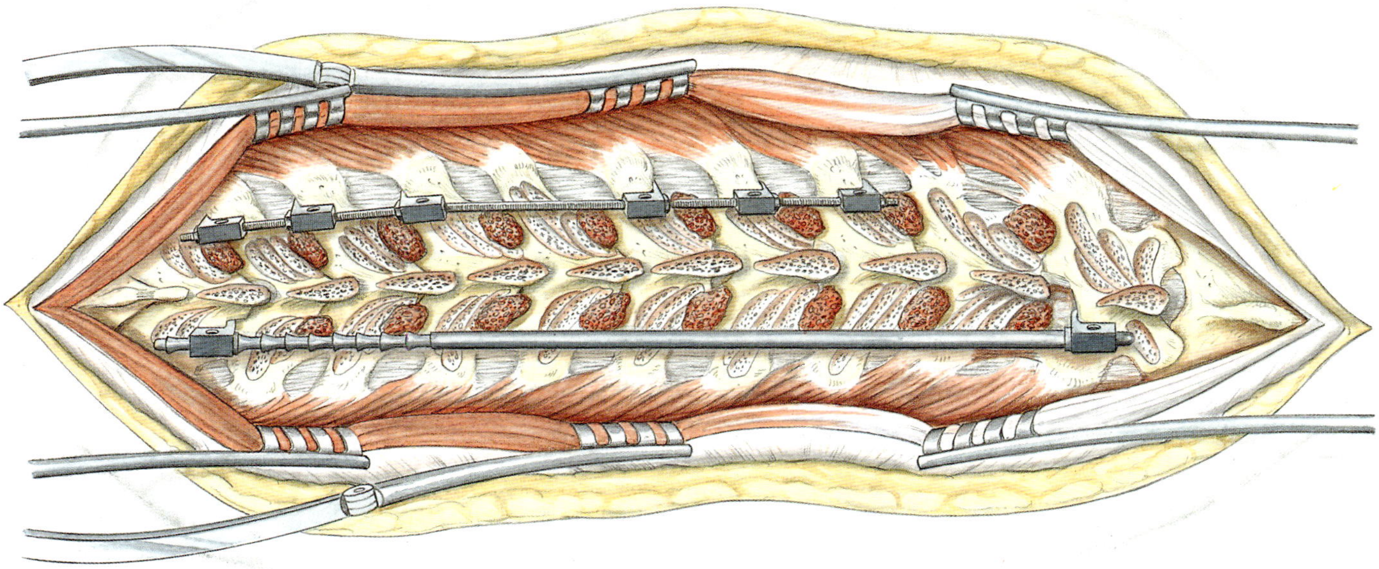

Fig. 2.**37** Status after definitive correction by distraction and compression.

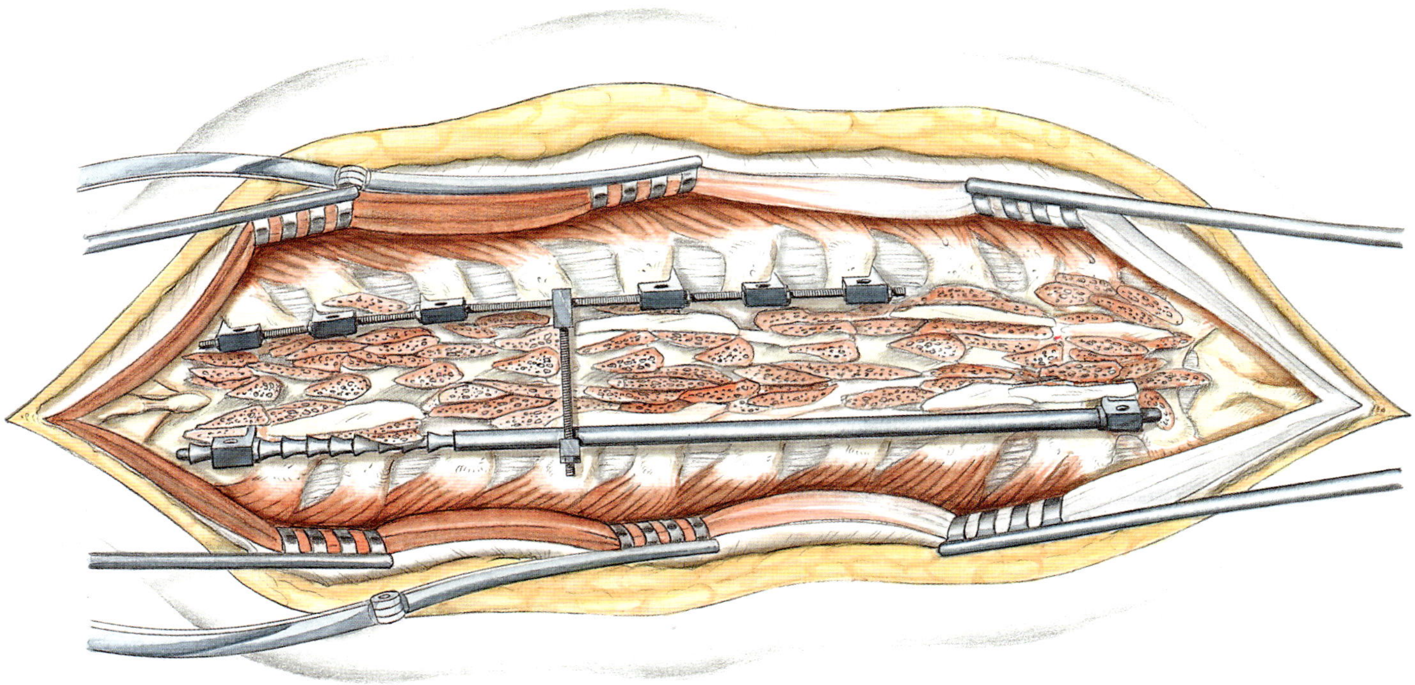

Fig. 2.**38** Status after bone grafting and transverse stabilization with a DTT.

Wound Closure

Wound closure is effected in two layers by suture of the paraspinal musculature and the overlying fascia.

In children and adolescents, the split spinous process apophyses are readily united by sutures. An intracutaneous wire suture is used for skin closure.

Postoperative Treatment

The patient is generally placed in bed without any external fixation. If preoperative correction has been performed by halo traction, it is left in place and continually dismantled within a week after the operation. Immediately after the operation, the patients are taken to the intensive care unit, where all necessary diagnostic and therapeutic measures can be taken. A neurologic assessment is made immediately after the operation, and movement of the extremities is tested, first at 15-minute and later at hourly intervals. For three days, patients are given antibiotics to prevent infection.

The patient's position is shifted in a revolving bed. The sutures are removed between the twelfth and fourteenth postoperative days; after this, the patient is discharged from hospital with a plaster jacket. A spinal orthosis has to be worn for 6–9 months.

Pitfalls and Complications

There is considerable blood loss in the Harrington operation (literature data vary between 300 and 3800 mL). Blood-saving measures and modern blood replacement techniques are therefore of great importance. They comprise prone positioning without pressure, infiltration of the operative site with a 1 : 500,000 norepinephrine solution, subperiosteal dissection, careful hemostasis, operation under controlled hypotension, autotransfusions, and use of a Cell Saver.

The Harrington operation entails an appreciable neurological risk. In order to verify possible neurologic lesions, the so-called wake-up test (Vaucelle et al. 1973) should be applied. About 5–10 minutes after reaching maximal distraction, the patient is allowed to wake up, and is asked to move his feet. If neurologic function is unremarkable, anesthesia is continued and the operation completed. If there is a definitely positive neurological finding, the Harrington instrumentation is removed, and the distraction thus discontinued.

Another means of monitoring spinal cord function is the use of somatosensory evoked potentials.

Numerous complications have been described:

- Cardiovascular complications: cardiac arrest, cor pulmonale with secondary complications, pulmonary embolism, anemia (severe intraoperative hemorrhage, wound hematoma, gastric ulcers, hemothorax).
- Pulmonary complications: adult respiratory distress syndrome, hemothorax, atelectases, pneumonia, pneumothorax.
- Gastrointestinal complications: Gastritis, stress ulcers, ileus.
- Wound infections.
- Neurological complications: spinal cord lesions (complete or incomplete transverse lesions); lesions of cranial and peripheral nerves (observed especially in connection with skeletal traction).

According to a 1975 report of the American Scoliosis Research Society, the neurological risk in a total of 7885 scoliosis operations amounted to 0.72%; on the other hand, in 1987 the Society reported that the standard Harrington operation carried a neurological risk of 0.12% (Edmonson 1975, Lowe 1987).

- Complications related to the instrumentation: hook avulsion, rod fracture, loss of lumbar lordosis, pseudarthrosis.

Alternative Methods

Cotrel–Dubousset technique: used mainly for thoracic and thoracolumbar scoliosis.
Advantage: orthosis-free follow-up.
Luque operation: Used mainly for neuromuscular scoliosis.
Advantage: orthosis-free follow-up.
Dwyer, VDS: Used mainly in lumbar and thoracolumbar scoliosis as well as for defects of the posterior vertebral elements.

Further Reading

Edmonson AS. Morbidity report. American Scoliosis Research Society, 1975.

Goldstein LA. The surgical management of scoliosis. South Med J 1930;23:116.

Goldstein LA. Surgical management of scoliosis. J Bone Jt Surg 1966; 48-A:167.

Goldstein LA. The surgical management of scoliosis. Clin Orthop 1971;77:32.

Hall JE. Harrington instrumentation and spine fusion. Follow-up study in 157 cases. J Bone Jt Surg 1968;50-A:848.

Harrington PR. Treatment of scoliosis: correction and internal fixation by spine instrumentation. J Bone Jt Surg 1962;44-A:591.

King AH, Moe JH, Bradford DS, Winter RB. The selection of fusion levels in thoracic idiopathic scoliosis. J Bone Jt Surg 1983;65-A:1302.

Lowe TG. Morbidity and mortality report. American Scoliosis Research Society, 1987.

MacEwen GD, Bunnell WP, Sriram K. Acute neurological complications in the treatment of scoliosis: a report of the Scoliosis Research Society. J Bone Jt Surg 1975;57-A:404.

Moe JH. Methods of correction and surgical techniques in scoliosis. Orthop Clin N Amer 1972;3:17.

Moe JH, Winter RB, Bradford DS, Lonstein JE. Scoliosis and other spinal deformities. Philadelphia: Saunders, 1978.

Nash CL, Moe JH. A study of vertebral rotation. J Bone Jt Surg 1969; 51-A:223.

Ponseti IV, Friedmann B. Prognosis in idiopathic scoliosis. J Bone Jt Surg 1950;32-A:381.

Vauzelle C, Stagnara P, Jouvinroux P. Functional monitoring of spinal cord activity during spinal surgery. J Bone Jt Surg 1973;55-A:441.

Scoliosis Operations in Children

The main indication is congenital scoliosis, for which surgical criteria different from those for idiopathic scoliosis need to be applied. The fundamental problem is a difference in growth potential between the concave and the convex side of the curvature (Fig. 2.**39**). The magnitude of the difference determines the prognosis of the curvature. One-sided segmentation failures cause the most severe progressions (Fig. 2.**39f**), but failures of formation—particularly several hemivertebrae lying in the contour of the same curve—can lead to a marked increase in curvature. The worst progression is likely to be caused by a combination of the above malformations.

When a severe curvature is already present in adolescence, the possibilities for correction are not the same as with idiopathic scoliosis. The treatment of congenital scoliosis, therefore, differs significantly from that of idiopathic scoliosis, in which corrections of 50–60 percent and more are obtainable, even after the arrest of growth. By contrast, congenital scoliosis is very difficult to correct after the completion of growth; the percentage attained generally does not exceed 10–20 percent. The neurological risk, too, is relatively high when distraction correction is employed.

It should be mentioned that diastematomyelia and a tethered cord have to be ruled out prior to any operation for congenital spinal alterations.

The goal of surgical treatment of congenital scoliosis is the prevention of progression of the deformity.

Occasionally, surgical measures also have to be taken in earlier childhood in the presence of infantile idiopathic scoliosis with malignant progression.

Generally, the following options are available:

- Posterior fusion in situ
- Posterior fusion with instrumentation
- Epiphysiodesis on the convex side, with posterior vertebral fusion on the convex side
- Subcutaneous Harrington instrumentation
- Hemivertebra resection

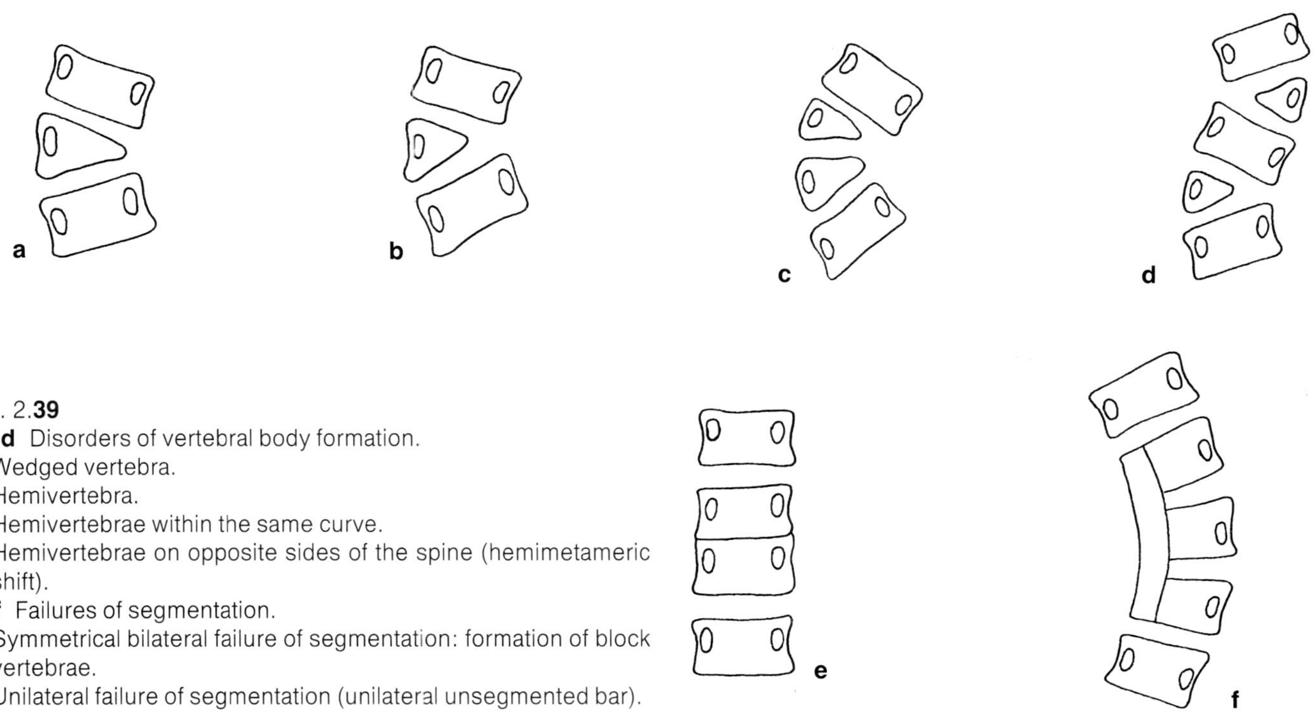

Fig. 2.**39**
a–d Disorders of vertebral body formation.
a Wedged vertebra.
b Hemivertebra.
c Hemivertebrae within the same curve.
d Hemivertebrae on opposite sides of the spine (hemimetameric shift).
e, f Failures of segmentation.
e Symmetrical bilateral failure of segmentation: formation of block vertebrae.
f Unilateral failure of segmentation (unilateral unsegmented bar).

Posterior Fusion in Situ

Indication

In unilateral segmentation disorders (unsegmented bar), early bilateral vertebral fusion (Fig. 2.**40**) is recommended. As a rule, posterior fusion is sufficient, since it has been found that the risk of thoracic lordosis due to posterior fusion exists only in children who had thoracic lordosis to begin with. In these situations, posterior fusion should be combined with anterior transthoracic fusion.

The operation should be performed as early as possible (from the sixth month of life onward), provided there is no severe deformity present so far (Cobb angle less than 50 degrees). The best results are obtained in patients in whom the fusion is carried out before they reach the age of three.

Extent of fusion: Normally, one segment cranial and one caudal to the segmentation failure is added. However, the fusion will not encompass the entire curvature. Application of a corrective cast is required postoperatively. Long-term monitoring of the patient is needed, since the curvature may progress, on the one hand, and the curve may increase, on the other. In some circumstances, refusion with extension of the fusion length may become necessary. An exploration has to be carried out 4–6 months after the first operation, since this is the only way to detect a possible pseudarthrosis. Additional bone grafting has to be carried out.

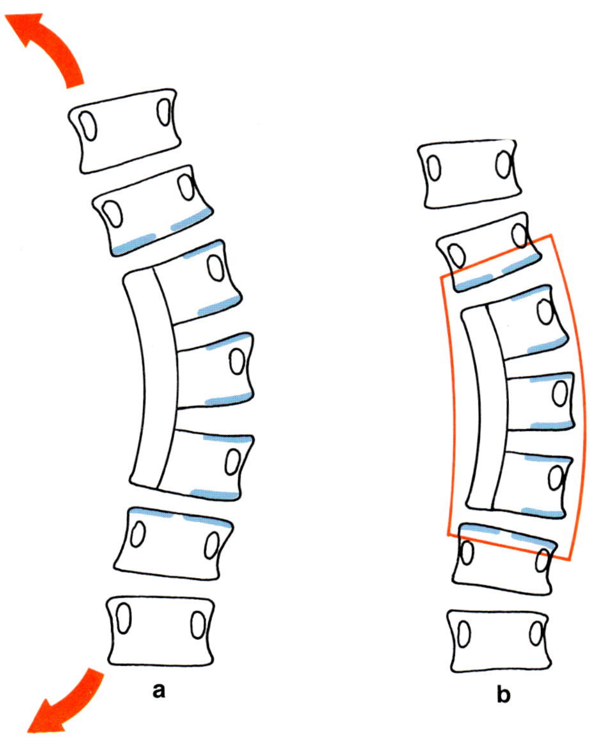

Fig. 2.**40**
a Unilateral failure of segmentation.
b Treatment by bilateral posterior vertebral fusion in early childhood. Note that vertebral fusion exclusively on the convex side is not effective, since there is no growth potential on the concave side.

Operative Technique

See Harrington Operation, Fusion, on p. 91.

In the case of congenital malformations, a radiograph may have to be obtained intraoperatively to identify the correct level. The fusion has to be performed with great precision, and has to include all the vertebral elements, including the transverse processes. It may be possible to extend the fusion to one more segment on the convex side than on the concave side, in order to induce a spontaneous correction. There is no evidence, however, that this is a successful method.

Collection of Chips

Bone chips may be obtained mostly when debriding the posterior vertebral elements; they are used to bridge over the facet joints. In young children, it may be necessary to have access to bank bone or hydroxyapatite. Starting at three years of age, the iliac crest can be used for harvesting of bone graft.

Postoperative Treatment

A plaster jacket is applied in the corrected position, followed by a spinal orthosis.

Pitfalls and Complications

Pseudarthrosis; elongation of the curvature.

Posterior Fusion with Instrumentation

Indication

It was originally thought that internal fixation should not be performed in congenital scoliosis, due to the high neurological risk; more recent experience, however, shows that implants may also be applied with congenital spinal deformities. The neurologic risk remains. The advantage of the added instrumentation lies in the possibility of greater correction, a higher fusion rate, and the reduced significance of postoperative immobilization. With adequate instrumentation (e.g., Cotrel–Dubousset, pp. 131–146), only a spinal orthosis may be needed postoperatively, or external support may be dispensed with altogether. The instrumentation may be carried out in adolescent patients with bones of satisfactory quality. The operative technique and the fusion length are generally the same as in idiopathic scoliosis (pp. 84–88). Preoperative evaluation of dysraphic disorders is of utmost importance. Somatosensory evoked potentials should be monitored for the operation; the Stagnara wake-up test is mandatory.

Convex-Side Epiphysiodesis with Posterior Convex-Side Spinal Fusion

Owing to the drawbacks of extensive spinal fusion in early childhood, there has been growing clinical interest in the principle of surgical growth control in scoliosis. Still, the operation has not fulfilled the original expectations. However, in congenital as well as in malignant scoliosis, progressive idiopathic scoliosis epiphysiodesis may be justified. Fusion on the convex side is indicated only for curvatures that have a specific growth potential on the concave side (such as several hemivertebrae lying in the contour of the same curve; malignant, progressive infantile scoliosis). To avoid consecutive kyphosis, an anterior convex-sided epiphysiodesis has to be combined with a posterior convex-sided fusion (Fig. 2.**41**). In the presence of kyphosis, this procedure is contraindicated.

Indications

Epiphysiodesis should be performed only in the presence of documented or definitely anticipated progression, and at an early age (generally under age six), as well as for curvatures that are not very pronounced (less than 50–60 degrees).

Operative Technique

See under Epiphysiodesis, pp. 160–162.

Following epiphysiodesis, the patient is repositioned. Under the same anesthesia, a posterior vertebral approach is made in the area of the curve convexity. A spinal fusion is performed on the convex side that includes the same number of vertebrae as the anterior treatment.

Postoperative Treatment

A body cast is applied in the reduced position for six months, and this is followed by orthotic therapy, which may have to be continued for several years.

The convex-sided epiphysiodesis may be combined with a subcutaneous Harrington implant.

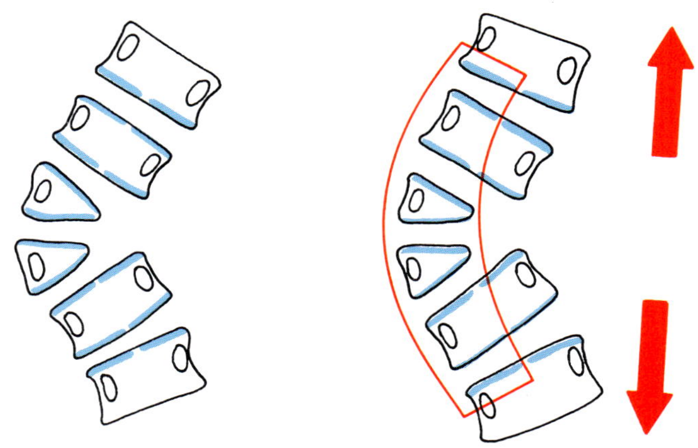

a b

Fig. 2.**41**

a Congenital scoliosis with two hemivertebrae on the convex side.

b Treatment by convex epiphysiodesis with posterior spinal fusion on the convex side; some spontaneous correction is possible. There is a growth potential on the concave side.

Subcutaneous Harrington Instrumentation

Indications

Malignant, progressive idiopathic scoliosis in early childhood, for correction and growth control without fusion, or at least, without concave-sided fusion. Depending on the severity of the deformity in the frontal and the sagittal plane, this operation is combined with an anterior convex-sided epiphysiodesis, and posterior spinal fusion on the convex side (Fig. 2.**42**).

This technique offers the advantage of efficient intraoperative correction without the need for fusion of the entire curvature in early childhood.

Operative Technique

(Fig. 2.**43**)

A so-called children's Harrington instrumentation is used, with appropriately small implants. With the patient in prone position, the cranial end vertebra is exposed from a short longitudinal incision, and the Harrington hook is placed in the usual way. A short longitudinal incision is then made over the caudal end vertebra, and here, too, the hook is applied to the lamina in the usual manner. A suitable instrument is then used to produce a subcutaneous channel between the two hooks, and the threaded Harrington rod is inserted. The correction is made with the help of a nut, causing distraction (Fig. 2.**44**).

Special Note
Care should be taken to make sure that an excess rod length is available proximally to begin with. At intervals of six months, the proximal hook may then be exposed and retightened by a small operation.

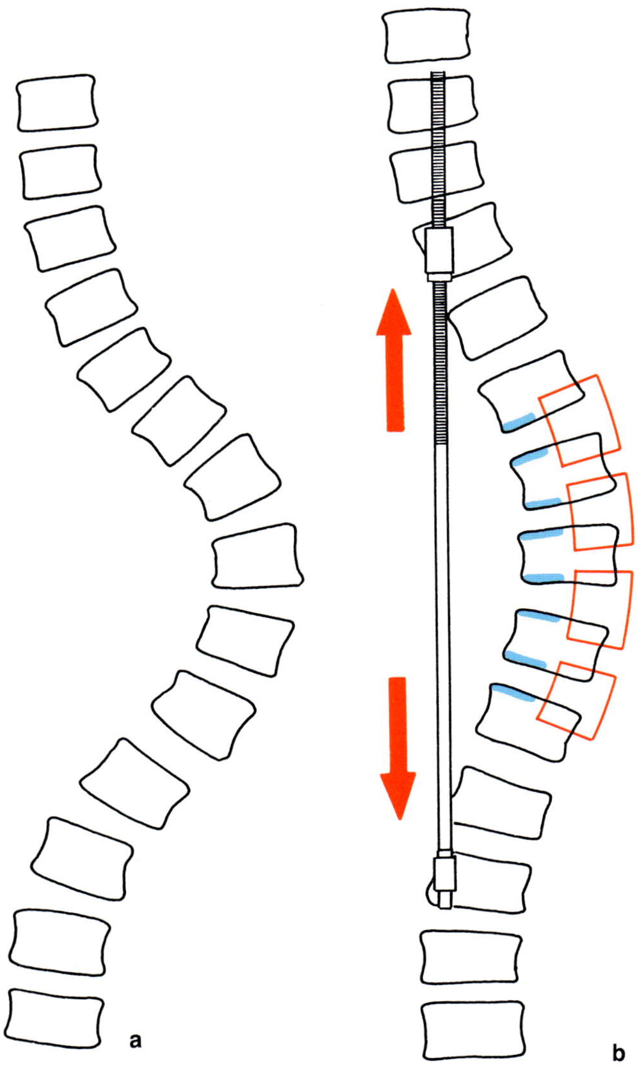

Fig. 2.**42**
a Infantile malignant progressive idiopathic scoliosis.
b Treatment by subcutaneous Harrington distraction combined with posterior and/or anterior spinal fusion on the convex side. The advantage is effective correction with no need to fuse the entire curve in early childhood. Further corrections can be effected by retightening the distraction rod.

Hemivertebra Resection

Indication

The indication for hemivertebra resection remains a controversial issue. The presence of a hemivertebra is not in itself an indication for its removal. Hemivertebra excision is sometimes recommended for demonstrated progression; on the other hand, less invasive measures may yield the desired result. An example of the latter is the combination of a convex-sided anterior epiphysiodesis with posterior fusion on the convex side and postoperative treatment with a molded body cast.

Generally speaking, wedge or hemivertebra excisions should be reserved for severe progressive deformities that lead to spinal decompensation or pelvic obliquity, or both. This is the case with a hemivertebra at the lumbosacral junction, for example.

Operative Technique

See under Hemivertebra Resection, p. 151.

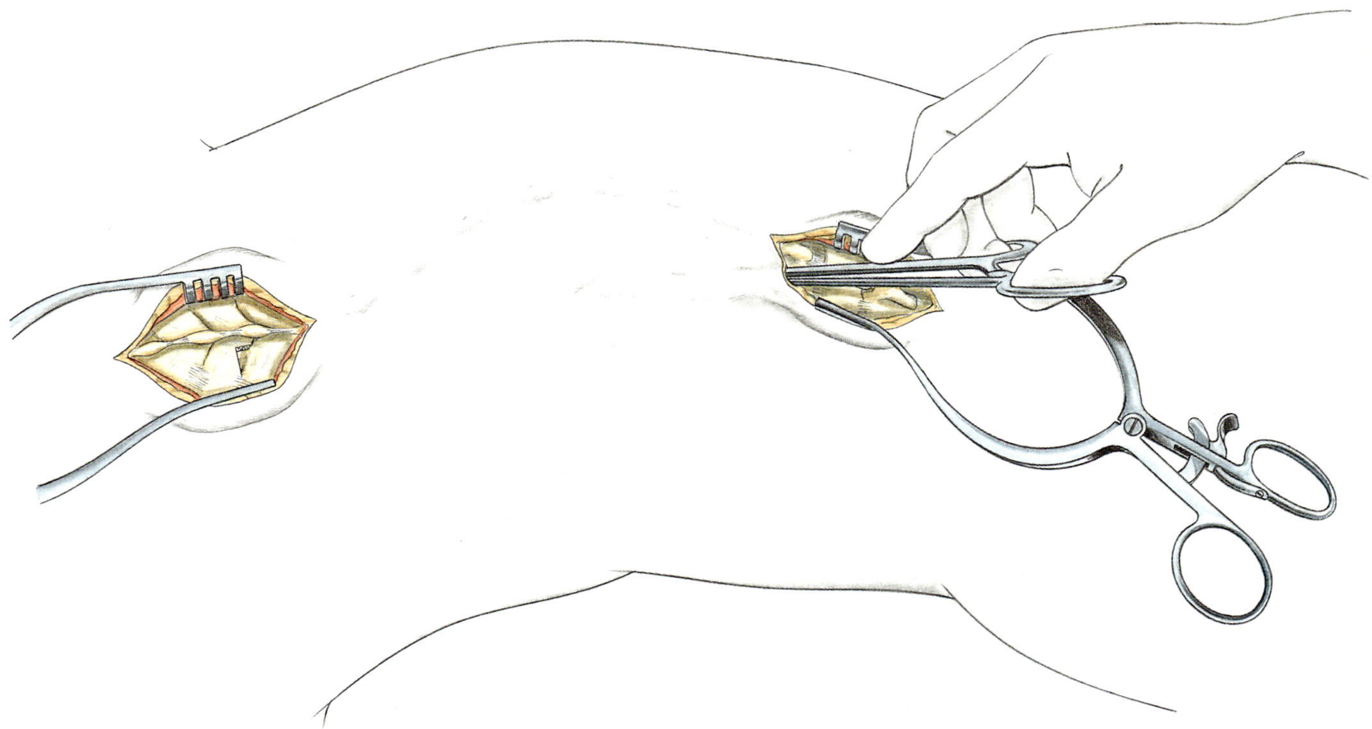

Fig. 2.**43** Subcutaneous Harrington instrumentation. Starting out from short skin incisions, the hook seat at the cranial and caudal end vertebrae is prepared; a tunnel is then made subcutaneously between the two incisions with a curved clamp.

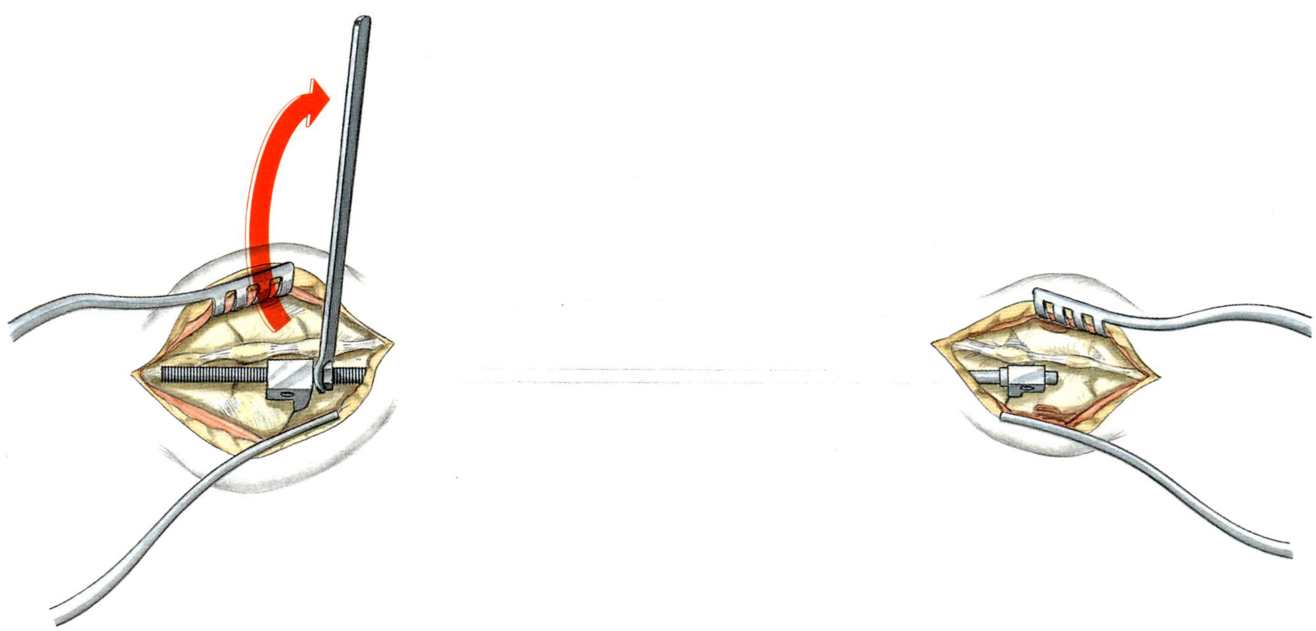

Fig. 2.**44** The Harrington distraction rod is inserted subcutaneously. Correction is effected by manual pressure on the apex of the scoliosis and tightening of the nut on the threaded rod.

Further Reading

Andrew T, Piggott H. Growth arrest for progressive scoliosis: combined anterior and posterior fusion of the convexity. J Bone Jt Surg 1985;B-67:193.

Bauer R. Die operative Behandlung der Skoliose. Berne: Huber, 1979.

Blake NS, Lynch AS, Dowling FE. Spinal cord abnormalities in congenital scoliosis. Ann Radiol 1986;29:377.

Bradford DS. Partial epiphyseal arrest and supplemental fixation for progressive correction of congenital spinal deformity. J Bone Jt Surg 1982;A-64:610.

Bradford DS. Die angeborene Skoliose. Orthopäde 1989;18:87.

Gillespie R, Faithfull DK, Roth A, Hall JE. Intraspinal anomalis in congenital scoliosis. Clin Orthop 1973;93:103.

Götze HG. Indikation, Technik und Ergebnisse der ventralen Spondyloepiphysiodese. In: Zielke K, ed. Skoliose und Kyphose. Stuttgart: Hippokrates, 1978.

Hall JE, Herndon WA, Levine CR. Surgical treatment of congenital scoliosis with or without Harrington instrumentation. J Bone Jt Surg 1981;A-63:608.

Morscher E. Experiences with the transthoracic, hemilateral epiphysiodesis in the treatment of scoliosis. In: Chapchal G, ed. Operative treatment of scoliosis. Stuttgart: Thieme, 1973.

Roaf F. The treatment of progressive scoliosis by unilateral growth arrest. J Bone Jt Surg 1963b;45-B:637.

Roaf R. The late results of unilateral growth arrest of the spine for scoliosis. Acta Orthop Scand 1963a;33:393.

Winter RB. Diastematomyelia and spina bifida in scoliosis. In: Keim HA, ed. First annual postgraduate course on the management and care of the scoliosis patient. New York:1969:67.

Winter RB. Congenital scoliosis: postgraduate course on the management and care of the scoliosis patient. New York:1970:27.

Winter RB. The effect of early fusion on spine growth. In: Zorab PA, ed. Scoliosis and growth. Edinburgh: Churchill Livingstone, 1971:98.

Winter RB. Congenital scoliosis. Clin Orthop 1973a;93:75.

Winter RB. Congenital spine deformity. Israel J Med Sci 1973b;9:719.

Winter RB. Scoliosis and other spinal deformities. Acta Orthop Scand 1975;46:400.

Winter RB, Moe JH, Eilers VA. Congenital scoliosis study of 234 patients treated and untreated. J Bone Jt Surg 1981;50-A:1.

Winter RB. Congenital deformities of the spine. Stuttgart: Thieme, 1983.

Winter RB. Congenital spine deformity. In: Bradford DS, Lonstein JE, Ogilvie JW, Winter RB, eds. Scoliosis and other spinal deformities. Philadelphia: Saunders, 1987.

Winter RB, Moe JH, Lonstein JE. Posterior spinal arthrodesis for congenital scoliosis: a analysis of the cases of two hundred and ninety patients, five to nineteen years old. J Bone Jt Surg 1984;A-55:1188.

Fig. 2.**45** Severe adult scoliosis.
a Preoperative situation.
b Correction can possibly be performed after a mobilizing osteotomy and halo traction.
c Stabilization with two Harrington distraction rods.

Operations for Scoliosis in the Adult

Two groups of patients may be distinguished:

- Patients who have previously undergone a fusion operation and whose curvature has decidedly worsened;
- Patients with severe scoliosis without previous surgery. Also in this group of patients, correction of the scoliosis may be complicated by the following factors: spontaneous ankylosis of the facet joints, synostosis of transverse processes and ribs, a pronounced kyphotic component, cor pulmonale, and a restrictive pulmonary disorder.

Indications

- Severe spinal pain, particularly in the lumbar region
- Cardiorespiratory problems
- Neurologic complications
- Severe deformities, for cosmetic purposes (especially in younger women)
- Marked progression after completion of growth

Operative Technique

Harrington Instrumentation

One-Stage Operation

When the curvature is relatively mobile or there has been satisfactory preoperative correction, the operation is performed in a single session. For severe curvatures, it may be necessary to insert two distraction rods on the concave side (Fig. 2.**45**). In the presence of synostoses, or if preoperative correction has not produced the desired result, two sessions should be planned.

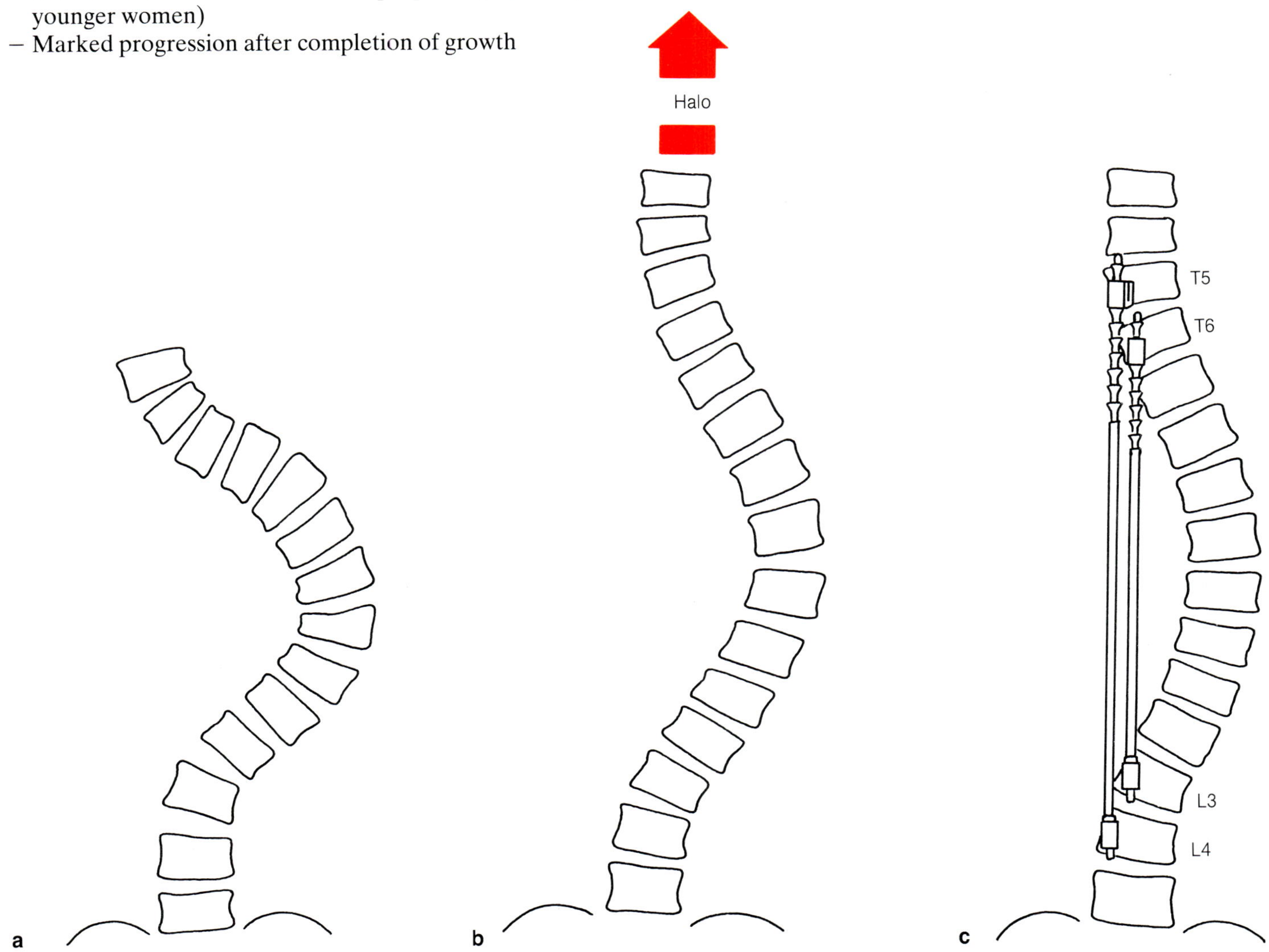

Multistage Procedure

First session: Osteotomy of the spine, release measures, and possibly rib resection on the concave side and provisional introduction of the Harrington distraction rod. The rib resection is occasionally required so that the Harrington distraction rod—particularly when there is a strong kyphotic component—need not be bent at all, or at least not appreciably. Sharper bending of the Harrington rod entails a long-term risk of metal fatigue, besides the chance that the lamina in the region of the proximal hook will break under a nonaxial load.

After the first operation, progressive correction is achieved by halo traction.

Second session: The provisionally inserted distraction rod is replaced by a definitive rod of adequate length. Severe curvatures may require the use of a second, shorter distraction rod (Fig. 2.**45**). The usual posterior spinal fusion follows. In segmental osteotomies, care should be taken that the bone chips being placed do not press on the dura.

Note
Instead of the Harrington rod, other implant systems, such as Cotrel–Dubousset, for example, can obviously be used as well (p. 143).

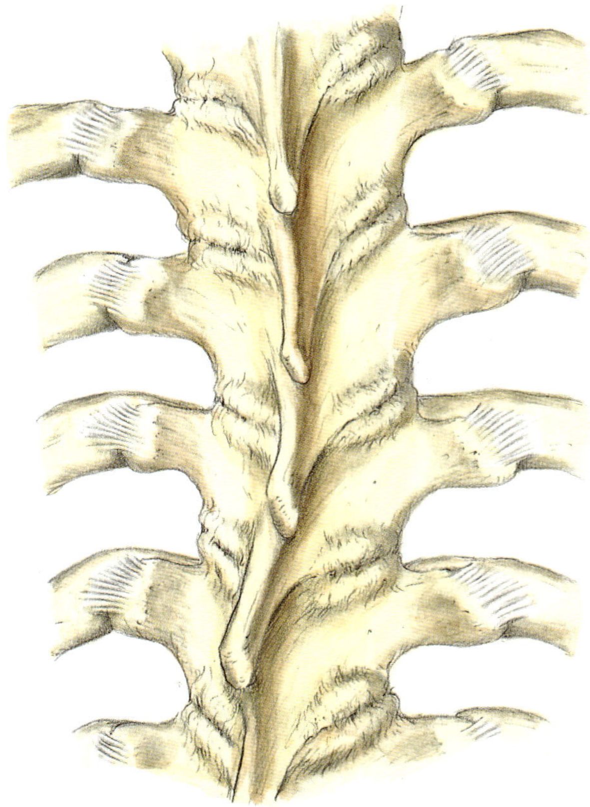

Fig. 2.**46** Spontaneous ankylosis of facet joints.

Mobilizing Spinal Osteotomy

A spontaneously synostosed or surgically fused spine has to be mobilized by multiple osteotomies before corrective measures are initiated. A number of procedures involving slight technical differences may be mentioned:

Osteotomy of Facet Joints (Without Prior Operation)

(Figs. 2.**46**–2.**49**)

Following posterior exposure of the spine, the ankylotic masses in the region of the facet joints are bilaterally removed with a hollow chisel. A spreader is then placed between two contiguous transverse processes, in order to verify whether the debrided motor segment already has mobility. If mobility is not adequate, the articular processes have to be removed with a bone rongeur after a sparing laminotomy, until the foramen is completely free. Good spinal mobility can thus be obtained, unless there is fusion in the vertebral body region, which of course has to be ruled out preoperatively. In the event that mobility still is not adequate—possibly due to fusion in the area of the costotransverse joints—a costotransversectomy may have to be carried out at the apex of the scoliotic curve, on the concave side, with resection of a rib portion approximately 2 cm long. Additionally, a soft-tissue release can be performed, with separation of the contracted muscle groups, especially on the concave side of the curve.

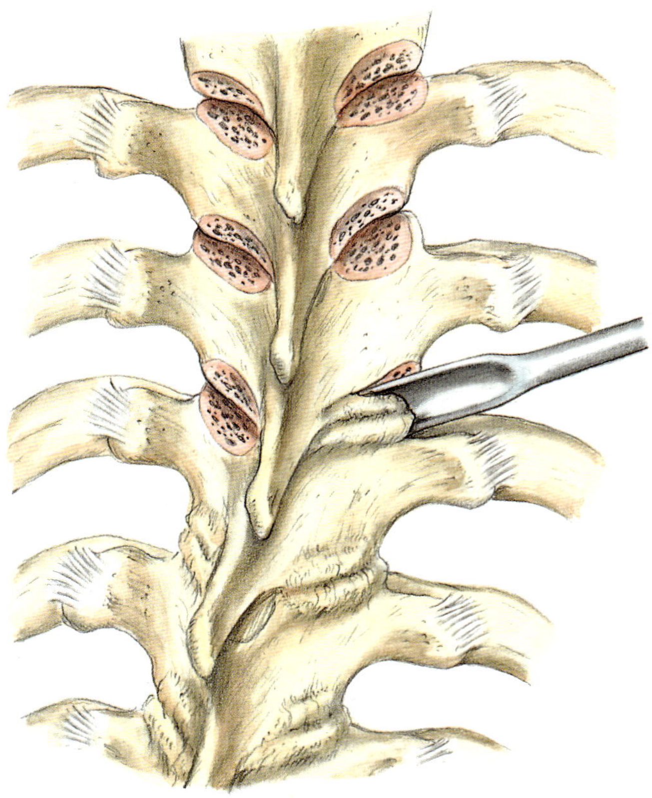

Fig. 2.**47** Resection of the ankylotic mass or the articular processes with a hollow chisel.

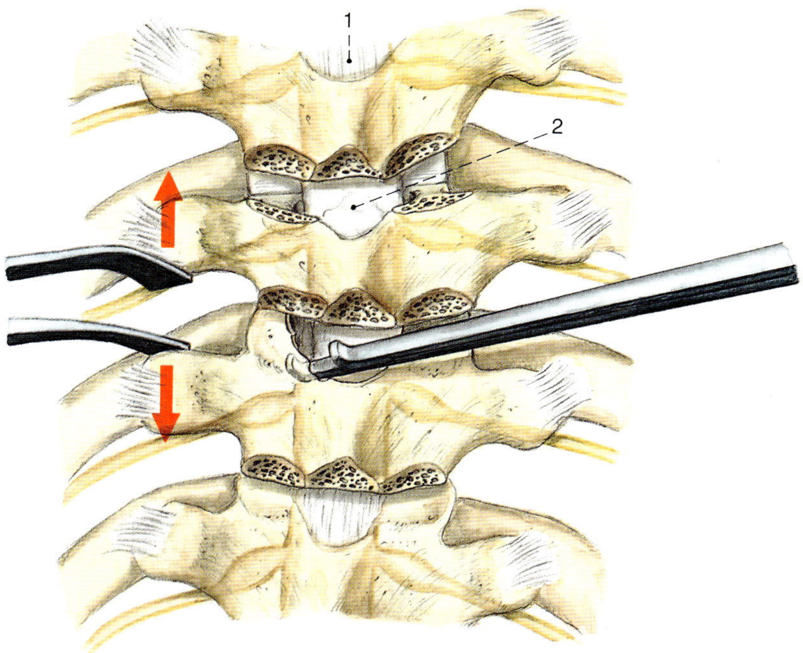

Fig. 2.**48** Resection of the ligamentum flavum and articular processes with a bone punch.

1 Ligamentum flavum
2 Dura mater of spinal cord

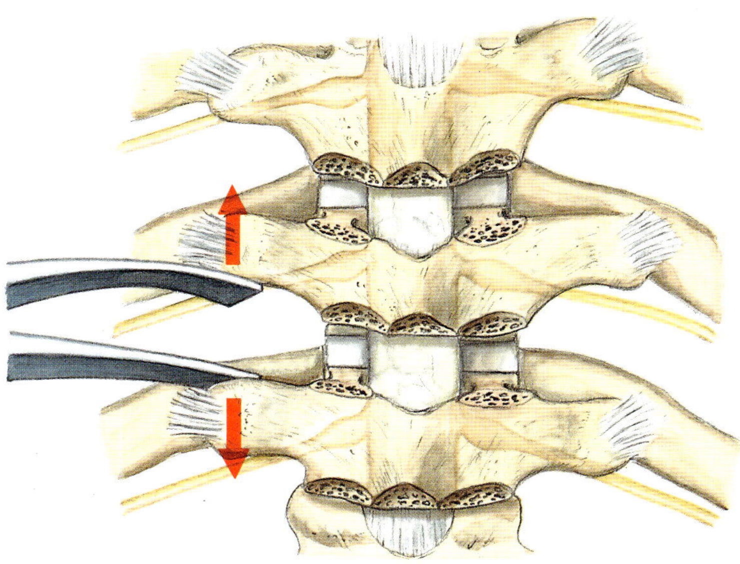

Fig. 2.**49** Testing mobility with an osteotomy spreader.

Posterior Spinal Osteotomy (Status After Fusion)

(Figs. 2.**50**–2.**55**)

A somewhat modified technique has to be used when there has been posterior spinal fusion. The number of osteotomies required is determined, and the level of osteotomy chosen preoperatively on the basis of radiographs. The osteotomy is performed at the site showing the greatest curvature between two comparatively straight segments of the fusion mass. As a rule, osteotomies are needed at several levels.

First of all, the fusion mass is exposed by a posterior approach. Following level identification, to select the desired segment, the osteotomy level is determined intraoperatively by localization of the intervertebral foramina (between the transverse processes). These may have to be palpated with a dissector. Using a gouge, transverse grooves are then produced between the transverse processes in the area of the fusion mass; these grooves will eventually extend as far as the cortical portion of the lamina or the ligamentum flavum.

After this, the yellow ligament, emerging at the center of the groove, is resected. The ankylosed joints are thinned out further with the gouge; the remnants are bilaterally removed with the bone rongeur until segmental mobility can be verified with the aid of a spreader.

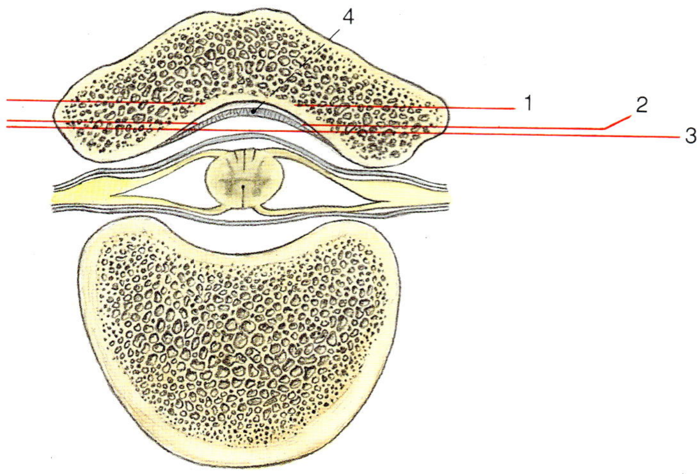

Fig. 2.**50** Status after spinal fusion, cross-section. Numbers 1 to 3 mark the dissection steps taken for a posterior mobilizing osteotomy. The posterior cortical layer (1) or remnants of the yellow ligament (2) are the first to be visualized at the center. Status after central opening of the vertebral canal (3).

4 Ligamentum flavum

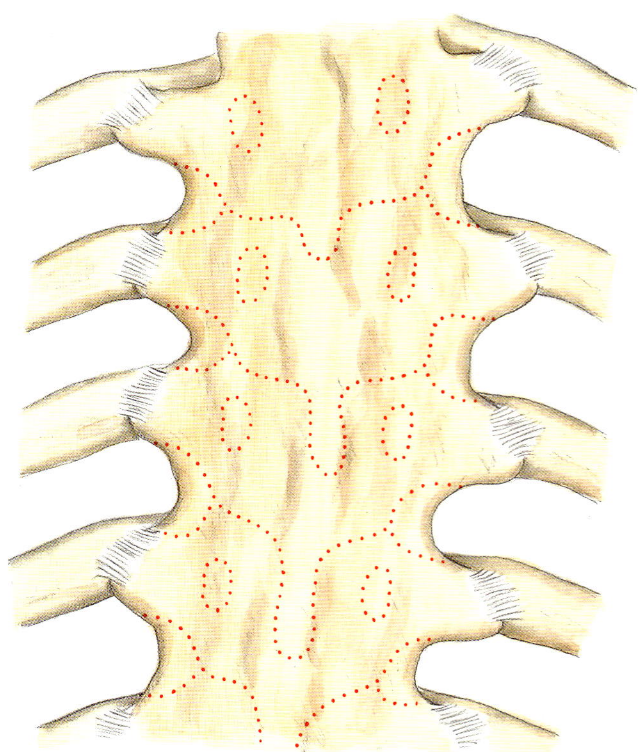

Fig. 2.**51** Position of posterior vertebral elements and pedicles inside the fusion mass (dotted lines).

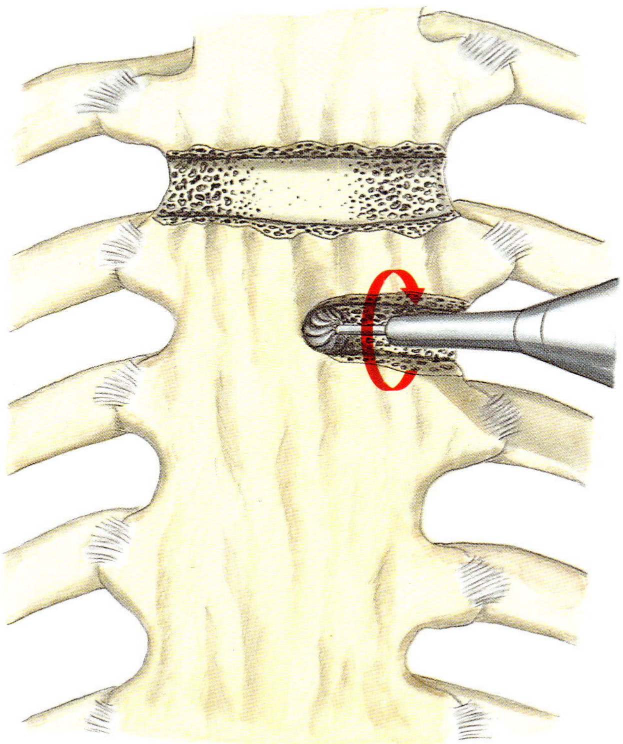

Fig. 2.**52** At the level of the foramina (between the transverse processes), a transverse groove is made with the spherical cutter.

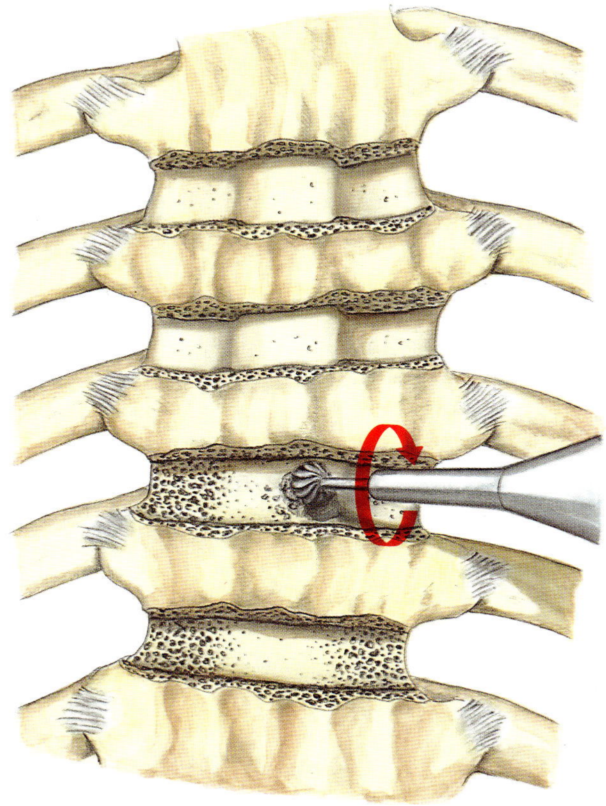

Fig. 2.**53** The internal cortical substance of the lamina is visualized at the center.

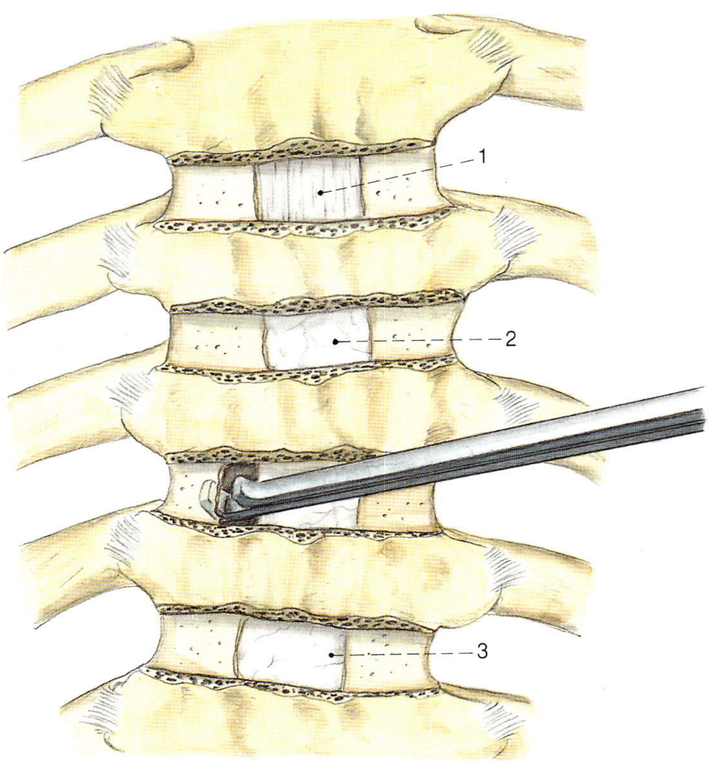

Fig. 2.**54** The ligamentum flavum is visualized. After its resection, the articular processes are removed with a bone punch.

1 Ligamentum flavum
2, 3 Dura mater of spinal cord

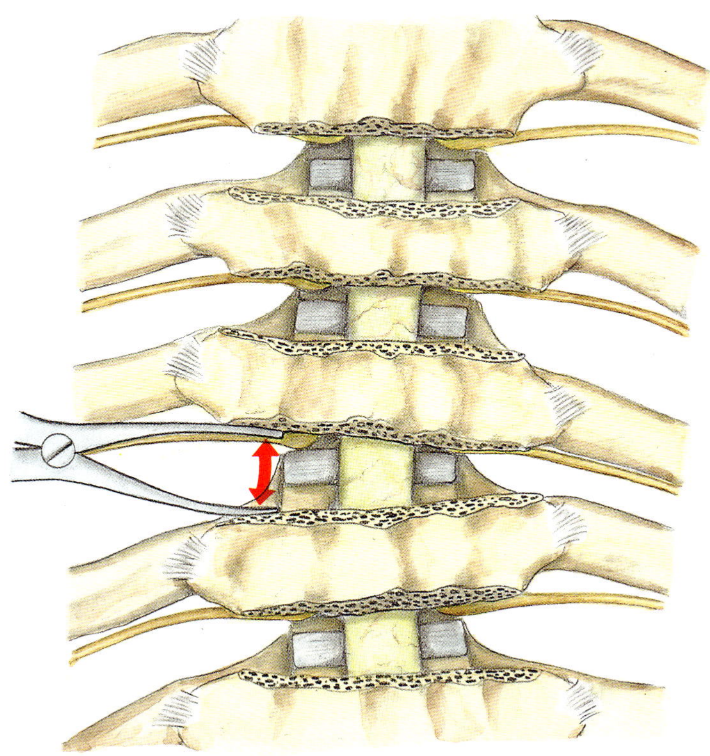

Fig. 2.**55** Segmental mobility is tested with the osteotomy spreader.

Rib Resection on the Concave Side

(Figs. 2.**56**–2.**58**)

For a typical exposure of the posterior vertebral elements, the ribs on the concave side lying in the area of the kyphotic apex are exposed close to the spine. In the region of the connecting line between the cranial and the caudal Harrington rods, a rib section 2–4 cm wide is resected, at the site where the Harrington rod is to be placed later on. In this area, the ribs are exposed subperiosteally. The dissection is quite difficult, for in cases of severe kyphoscoliosis some ribs may present a triangular profile and lie in very close proximity to one another. Pleural injuries must be avoided as far as possible. A provisional Harrington distraction rod may then be inserted into the resultant groove, intrathoracically but extrapleurally, and mild distraction can be initiated.

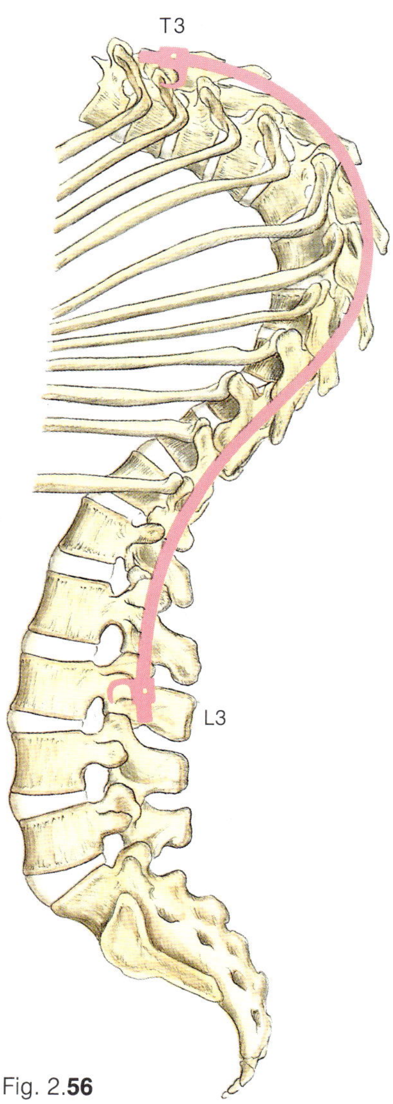

Fig. 2.**56**

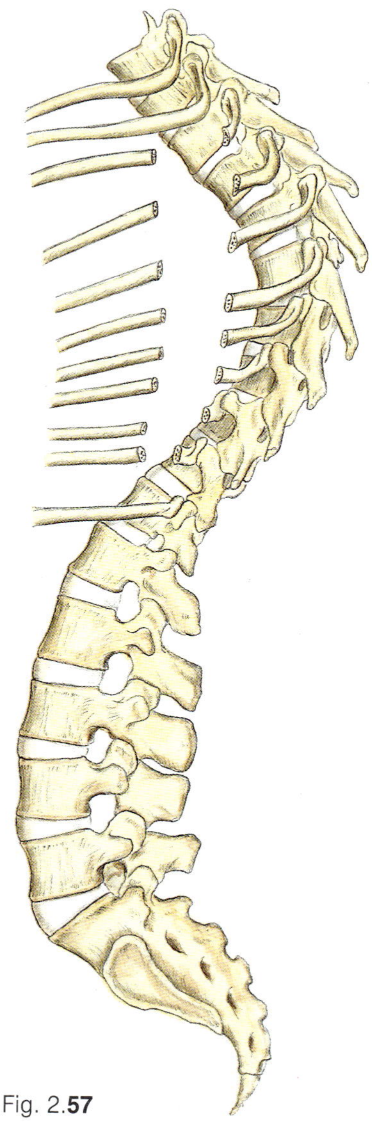

Fig. 2.**57**

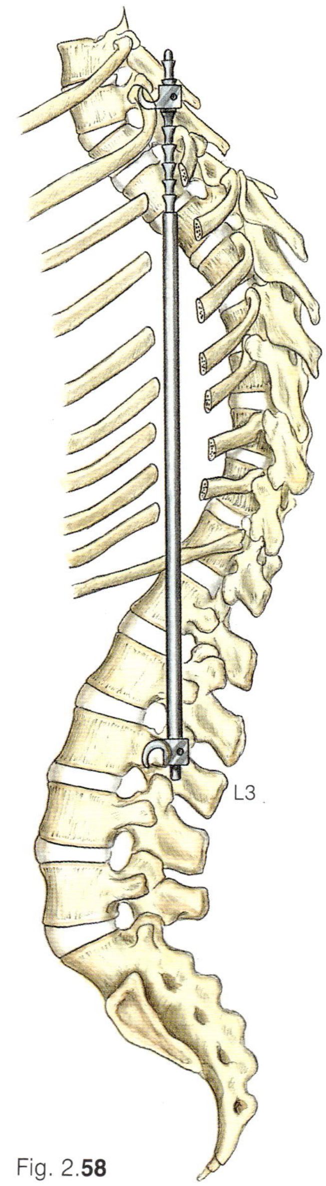

Fig. 2.**58**

Fig. 2.**56** In the presence of a severe kyphotic component, the Harrington rod has to be bent sharply consequently, distraction is hardly possible, and posterior avulsion of the proximal hook is possible.

Fig. 2.**57** Status after rib resection on the concave side, which allows the Harrington distraction rod to be inserted without appreciable bending.

Fig. 2.**58** Intrathoracic but extrapleural position of the Harrington distraction rod.

Resection of Rib Hump on the Convex Side

Indication

The indication can be established by tangential radiography and particularly by computed tomography. The operation is indicated only if the corresponding ribs clearly protrude beyond the vertebra. If the vertebral body lies directly behind the rib as a result of the severe torsion, no cosmetically satisfactory results can be obtained (Fig. 2.**59**).

Resection of the rib hump can be performed in the course of a posterior spinal fusion. However, if the cosmetic result is unsatisfactory (no derotation!), it may also be carried out during a second session.

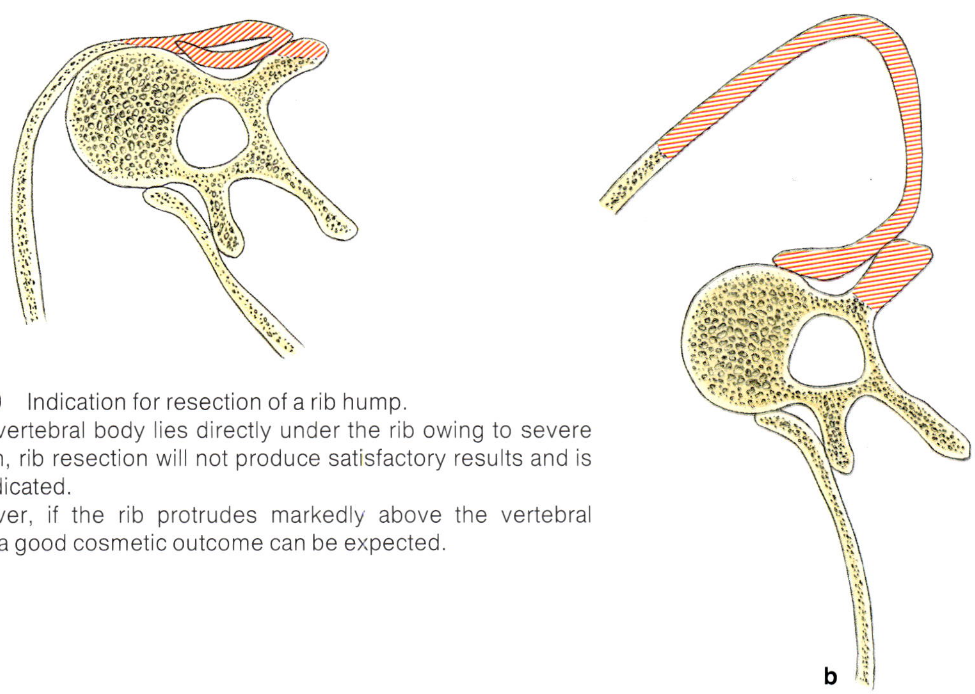

a

b

Fig. 2.**59** Indication for resection of a rib hump.
a If the vertebral body lies directly under the rib owing to severe torsion, rib resection will not produce satisfactory results and is not indicated.
b However, if the rib protrudes markedly above the vertebral body, a good cosmetic outcome can be expected.

Operative Technique

(Figs. 2.**60**–2.**64**)

As a rule, a midline incision is used. The trapezius muscle and the latissimus dorsi muscle are divided paravertebrally in a longitudinal direction, as is the subjacent greater rhomboid muscle. Following broad exposure of the rib hump by lateral retraction of the chest wall musculature, the most prominent ribs are exposed subperiosteally. Extreme care should be taken in dissecting the severely deformed ribs, to avoid pleural injuries. The ribs are then undermined, divided peripherally, and raised. After this, the costotransverse ligaments are transected with a sharp elevator or a knife, and the head of the rib is cautiously displaced. If the transverse processes protrude posteriorly as a result of the severe torsion, these, too, are ablated; the extensors of the back are merely retracted medially.

At the end of the operation, the pleura is inspected to detect possible injuries. If there are injuries, a thoracic drain has to be placed; otherwise, Redon drainage is adequate. The chest wall musculature is then reinserted, and the wound closed in layers.

Pitfalls and Complications

The rib resection may be complicated by a hemopneumothorax. This complication can be caused intraoperatively by direct injury to the pleura. Hemothorax can also occur postoperatively, however, if an extensive wound hematoma penetrates the pleural cavity.

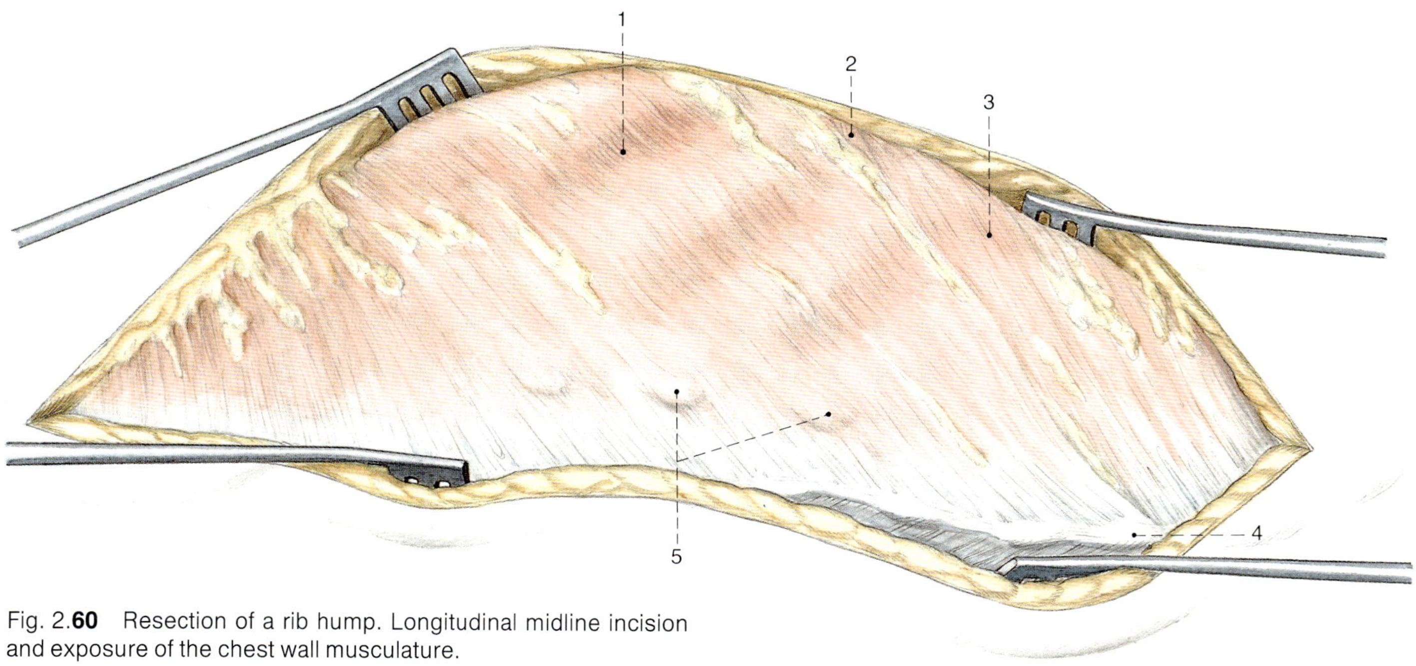

Fig. 2.**60** Resection of a rib hump. Longitudinal midline incision and exposure of the chest wall musculature.

1 Trapezius muscle
2 Greater rhomboid muscle
3 Latissimus dorsi muscle
4 Spinous process of thoracic vertebra
5 Transverse processes of thoracic vertebrae

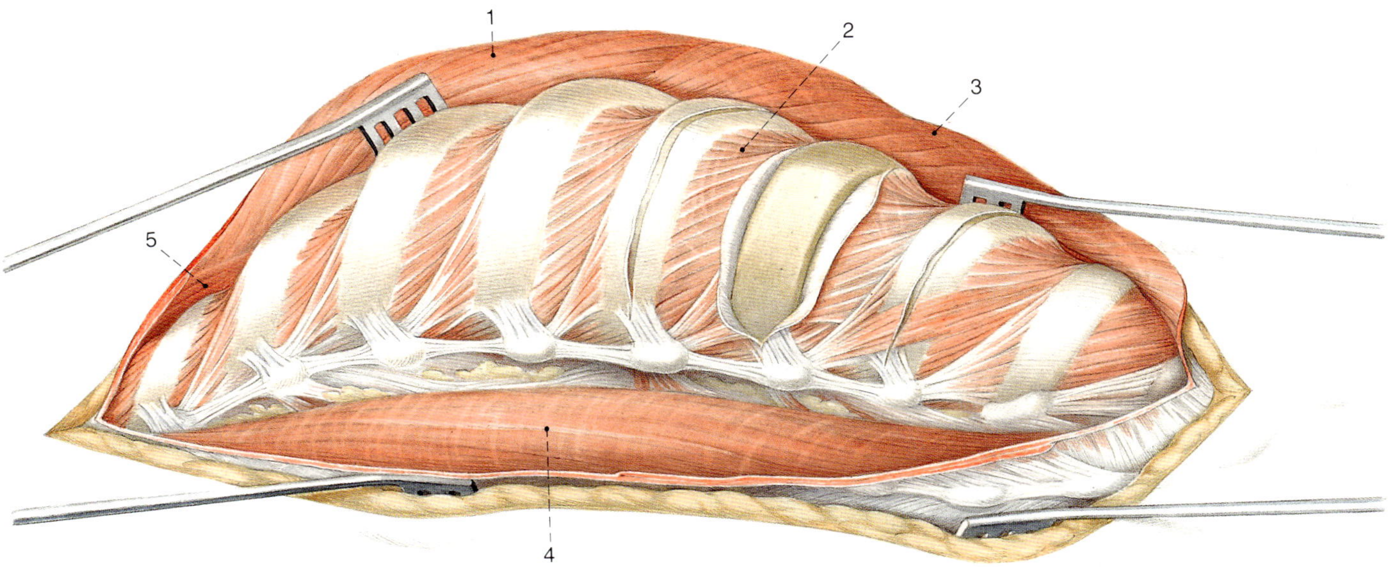

Fig. 2.**61** The chest wall musculature has been liberated laterally; the rib hump is visualized. The rib periosteum is incised.

1 Trapezius muscle
2 External intercostal muscle
3 Latissimus dorsi muscle
4 Erector muscle of the spine
5 Lesser rhomboid muscle

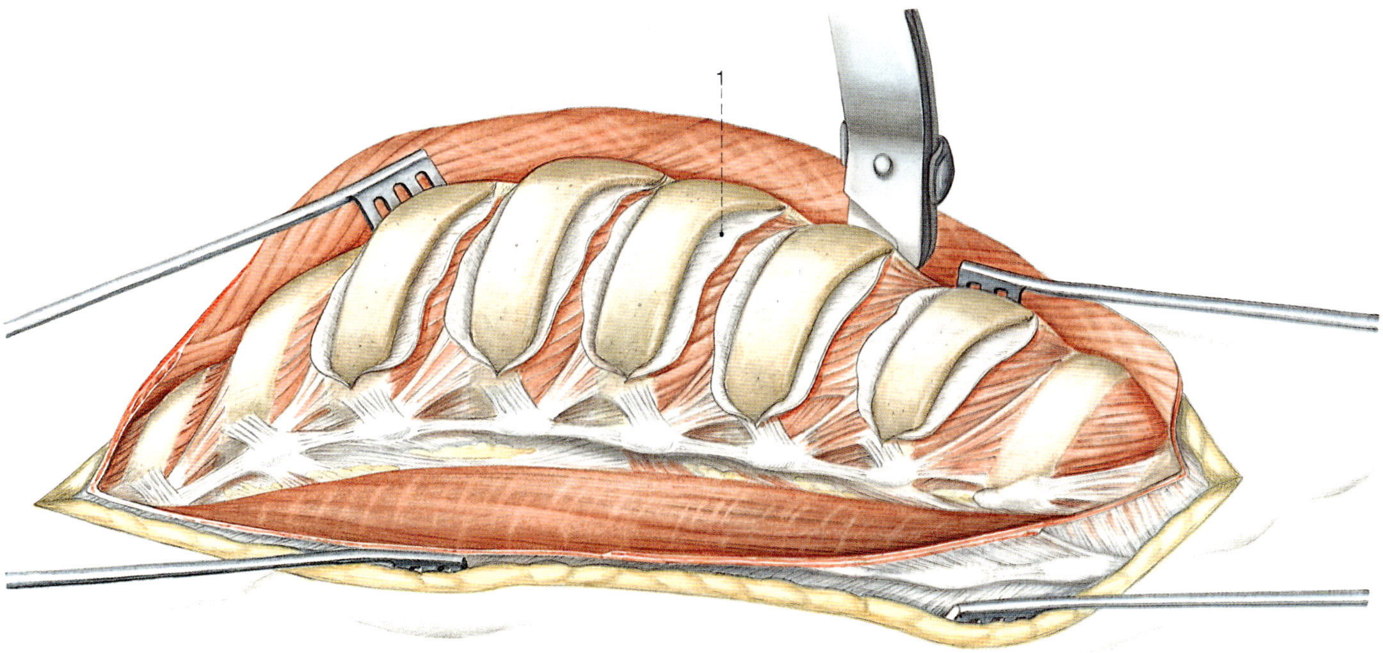

Fig. 2.**62** Peripheral division of the rib with rib shears.

1 Periosteum

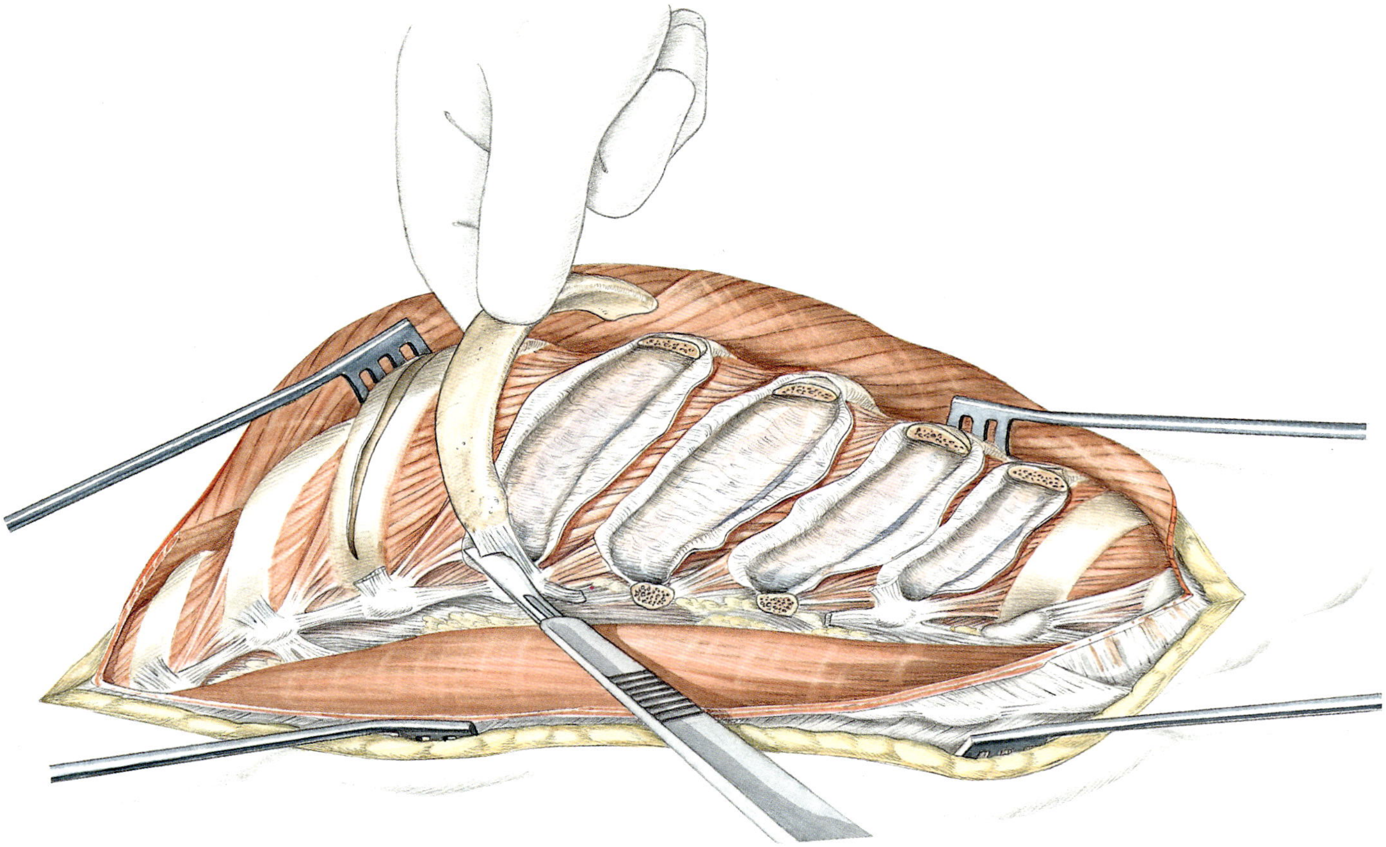

Fig. 2.**63** Elevation of the separated rib and transection of the costotranverse ligament.

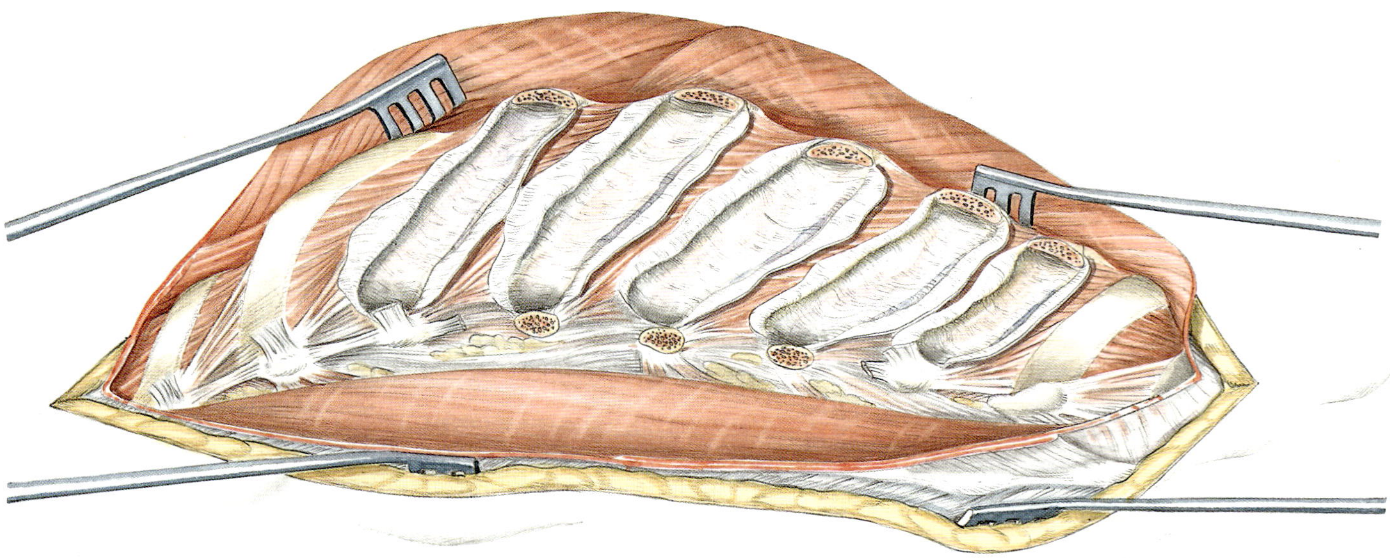

Fig. 2.**64** Status after resection of the prominent ribs and posteriorly protruding transverse processes.

Further Reading

Aaro S, Dahlborn M. The effect of Harrington instrumentation on the longitudinal axis rotation of the apical vertebra and on the spinal and rib-cage deformity in idiopathic scoliosis studied by computer tomography. Spine 1982;7:456.

Aaro S, Ohlen G. The effect of Harrington instrumentation on the sagittal configuration and mobility of the spine in scoliosis. Spine 1983;8:570.

Fauchet MR. Traitement chirurgical des scolioses. Rev Lyon Méd 1968;17:415.

Goldstein LA. Concave rib resection and ligament release for correction of idiopathic thoracic scoliosis. In: Symposium on the Spine. St. Louis: Mosby, 1969:254.

Houghton GR. Cosmetic surgery for scoliosis. In: Dickson R, Bradford D, eds. Management of spinal deformities. London: Butterworth, 1984:237.

Kostuik JP. Treatment of rigid spinal deformities in adult kyphoscoliosis. 11th Annual Meeting of the American Scoliosis Research Society, Ottawa, Canada, 1976.

Kostuik JP, Israel J, Hall JE. Scoliosis surgery in adults. Clin Orthop 1973;93:225.

Manning CW, Prime FJ, Zorab PA. Partial costectomy as a cosmetic operation in scoliosis. J Bone Jt Surg 1973;55-B:521.

Pellin B, Zielke K. Scolioses sévères de l'adulte et du grand adolescent. Rev Chir Orthop 1974;60:623.

Piggott H. Posterior rib resection in scoliosis. J Bone Jt Surg 1971;53-B:663.

Stagnara P. Utilization of Harrington's device in the treatment of adult kyphoscoliosis above 100°. In: Chapchal G, ed. Operative treatment of scoliosis. Stuttgart: Thieme, 1973.

Stagnara P, Fleury D, Rauchet R, Mazoyer L, Biot B, Vauzelle C, Jouvinroux P. Scolioses majeures de l'adulte supérieures à 100°. Rev Chir Orthop 1975;61:101.

Steel HH. Rib resection and spine fusion in correction of convex deformity in scoliosis. J Bone Jt Surg 1983;65-A:920.

Thulbourne T, Gillespie R. The rib hump in idiopathic scoliosis: measurement analysis and response to treatment. J Bone Jt Surg 1976;58-B:64.

Zielke K, Pellin B. Ergebnisse operativer Skoliosen- und Kyphoskoliosen-Behandlung beim Adoleszenten über 18 Jahre und beim Erwachsenen. Z Orthop 1975;113:157.

Luque Operation

SSI, Segmental Spinal Instrumentation.

Indications

According to a survey by the A.S.R.S. (American Scoliosis Research Society, 1987), the Luque operation is associated with four times as high a neurologic risk as the Harrington operation. This operative technique should therefore be reserved primarily for neuromuscular scoliosis.

Note
The Luque instrumentarium can generally be used in scoliosis, kyphosis, fractures, tumors, and degenerative spinal alterations.

Approach

See Chapter 1, pp. 64–69.

Operative Technique

Instrumentarium

The principal components of the Luque instrumentarium (Fig. 2.**65**) are as follows:

Implants:

– Straight rods, L-rods 3/16 in. (4.8 mm)
– Straight rods, L-rods 1/4 in. (6.4 mm)
– Prebent wire loops, coil wire (1.0 mm, 1.2 mm)

Instruments:

– Bending press
– Bending device
– Wire-grasping forceps
– Jet twister

Principles of Correction

Essentially, transverse forces are applied, chiefly in the apical area of the curvature. There also is a certain potential for derotation in the transverse plane, provided the concave-sided wires are first tightened.

Fusion Length

In cases of compensated scoliosis, fusion should be carried out at least from neutral vertebra to neutral vertebra. Generally speaking, the guidelines for Harrington instrumentation also apply here. The last caudal vertebra included in the fusion should lie within Harrington's stable zone, or should be divided by King's line (stable vertebra).

However, in keeping with the indication for SSI, the special etiology of the scoliosis (neuromuscular scoliosis) and the contour of the spine in the sagittal plane have to be taken into consideration in choosing the fusion length. Long, decompensated curves may require fusion from the upper thoracic spine to the pelvis (for special fusion techniques including the pelvis, see p. 126).

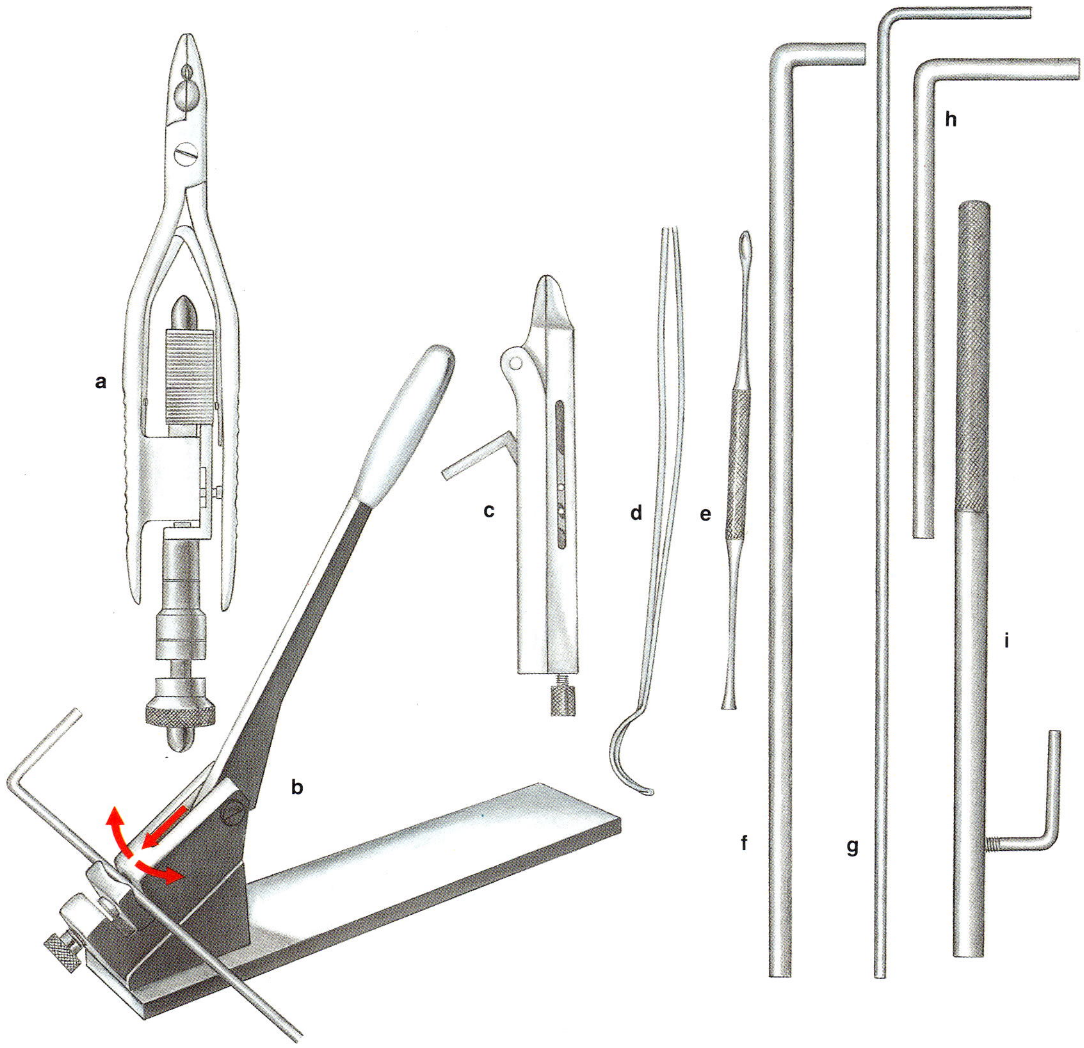

Fig. 2.**65** Luque operation; implants and instruments.
a Jet twister (wire-tensioning device).
b Bending press (for arcuate curvature).
c Wire-grasping forceps.
d Wire.
e Dissector.
f Long Luque rod, $^1/_4$ in.
g Long Luque rod, $^3/_{16}$ in.
h Short Luque rod, $^1/_4$ in.
i Bending device (for angular curvature).

Pre-Bending of the Luque Rod

The difficulty is that the Luque rod has to be pre-bent approximately to the extent of the desired correction. There are various means of arriving at a useful approximate value. In accordance with the operative technique, it is not so much the scoliotic curvature as the alignment of the series of spinous processes that needs to be considered. The Cobb angle is of little help in this evaluation. There are three possibilities:

- *Bending film:* If the bending film shows a nearly vertical contour of the series of spinous processes, complete correction of the posterior vertebral elements can generally be achieved. However, this is not equivalent to full correction of the scoliosis in terms of the Cobb angle.
- *Traction film:* If the spinous processes do not show a good alignment on the bending films, a film is obtained under traction combined with lateral pressure. A line is drawn from the spinous process of the superior end vertebra to the inferior end vertebra of the curve, and the rectangular distance between this line and the spinous process of the apical vertebra is measured. The Luque rod is then bent to a degree slightly smaller than this lateral deviation (Fig. 2.**66**).
- It often proves sufficient to make an estimate after exposure of the spine. The attainable correction is estimated through manual pressure on the apex of the scoliosis. The degree to which the Luque rod is bent then falls somewhat short of the maximally obtained intraoperative correction. As indicated by Luque, neurological considerations dictate that the intraoperative correction should not exceed 10 degrees compared with the maximal correction attained preoperatively, and this regardless of the method by which the preoperative correction was carried out.

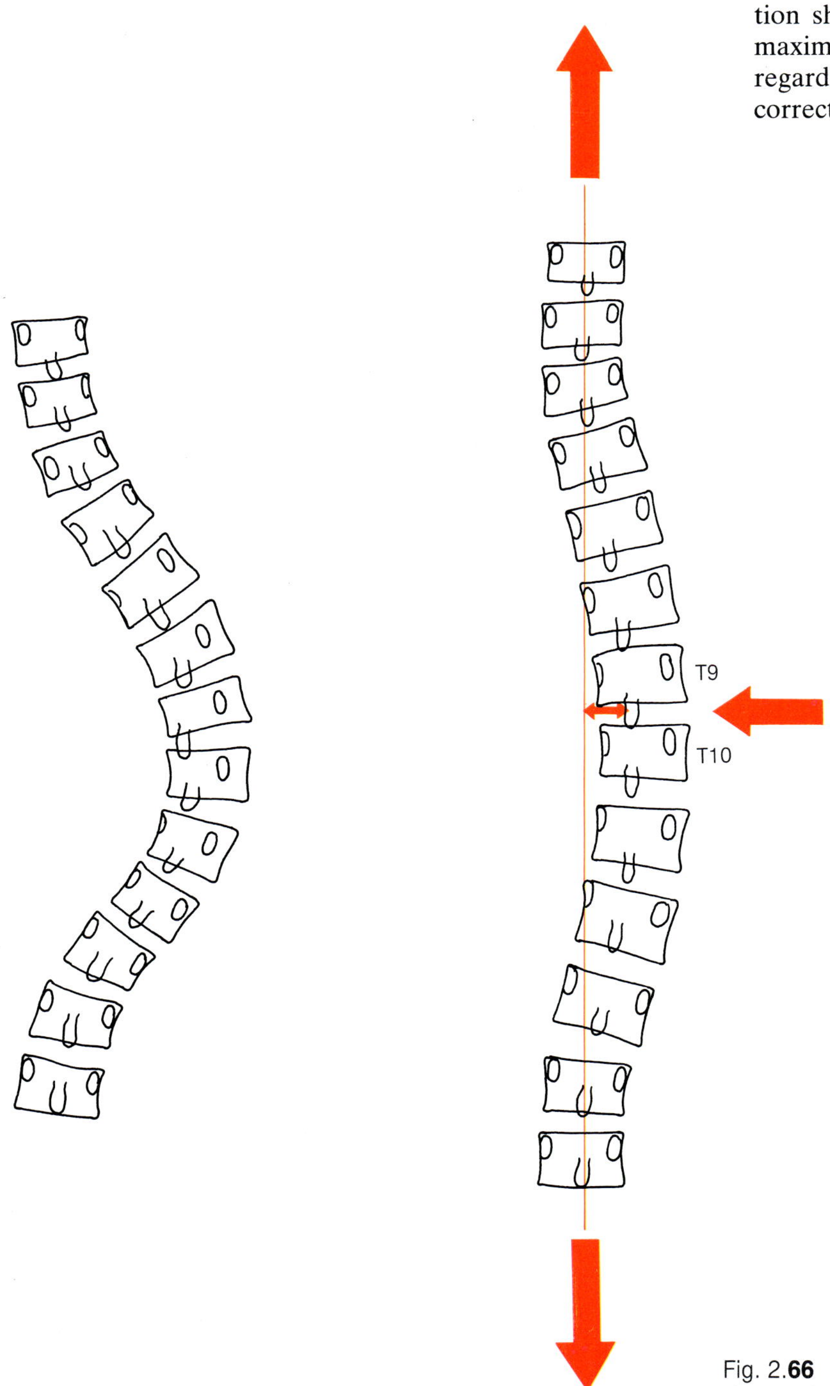

Fig. 2.**66** Measuring the bend of a Luque rod. The correction film shows the distance between the vertical line and the spinous process of the apical vertebra.

A point of special importance is that the rod should be shaped in the sagittal plane in accordance with the physiological spinal curvatures, thus showing a thoracic kyphosis or lumbar lordosis. It is important to bend the rod so that kyphosis and lordosis lie in the same rod plane, with the short limb of the L-rod serving as the reference plane. The three-dimensional bending of the rod brings strong rotary forces to bear on the rod when the wires are tightened. These forces can be absorbed only through strong fixation of the short limb to the lamina with two double wires. Otherwise the rod will be twisted, and the primarily specified physiological curves in the sagittal plane (thoracic kyphosis and lumbar lordosis) will no longer lie in the right plane. In order to secure the rotation further, it is advantageous for the free end of the second rod to lie posterior to the short limb of the L-rod. This transfers the rotary forces via several segments of the second rod (Fig. 2.**67**).

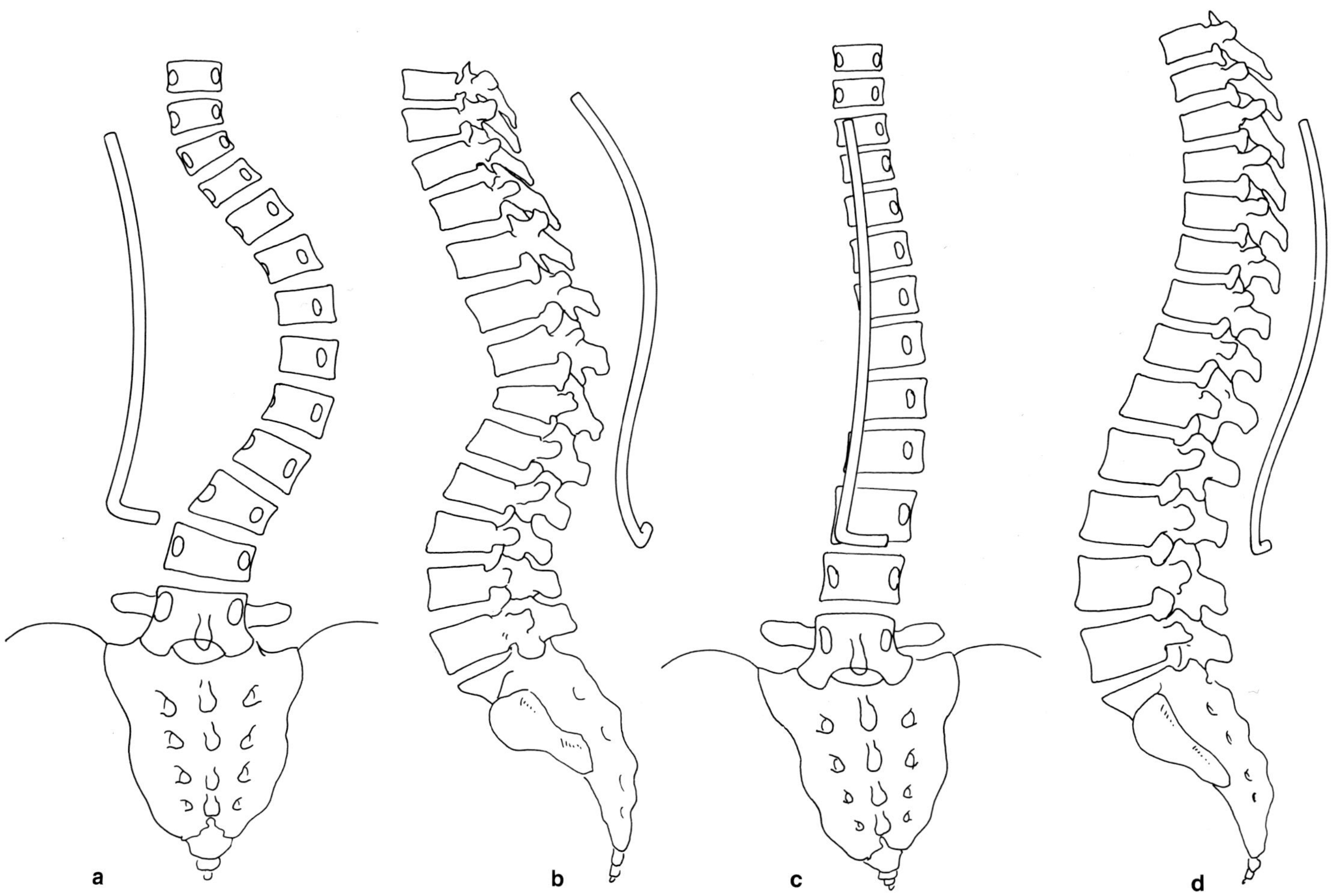

Fig. 2.**67**

a The Luque rod is bent in the frontal plane, following the anticipated correction of the curve.

b In the sagittal plane, the Luque rod is pre-bent following the desired thoracic kyphosis and lumbar lordosis (three-dimensional alignment).

c, d The spinal deformity is corrected in both the frontal and the sagittal planes.

Insertion of Sublaminar Wires

After exposure of the posterior vertebral elements in the proposed area of fusion and debridement of the facet joints (Harrington operation, p. 91), the yellow ligament has to be exposed at all fusion levels. In the area of the thoracic spine, pituitary forceps have to be used to remove distally aligned parts of the spinous processes. The rongeur is deeply inserted until contact is made with the yellow ligament. The ligamentum flavum is carefully stripped in the midline from the upper border of the lamina of the caudal vertebra, using a knife; it is separated from the epidural tissue with a dissector, and its central portion is resected with a Hajek punch (Figs. 2.**68**–2.**70**).

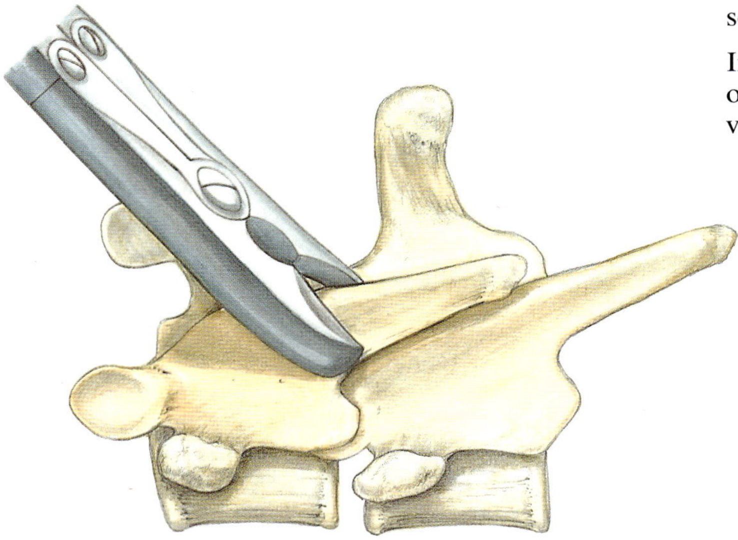

Fig. 2.**68** Resection of spinous processes in the thoracic spine that bridge the ligamentum flavum.

The doubled and semicircularly pre-bent wires are then passed through below the lamina with a circular movement, going from caudal to cranial, with very close attention being paid to ensure that the wires do not penetrate into the depth. As soon as the tip of the wire emerges at the cranial border of the lamina, it is fixed by an assistant using wire holders and is then pulled through under tension, using traction in a posterior direction, until the two wire ends are of equal length (Figs. 2.**71**, 2.**72**). The "eye" of the wire loop is now clipped off, so that two individual wires are obtained. It is important that the wires should be kept steadily under posterior traction. One wire is then passed to the right side of the lamina, and the other wire to the left side. While still being pulled posteriorly, the wires are now bent around the lamina (Fig. 2.**73**). During subsequent manipulations, this will prevent inadvertent intrusion of the wire into the vertebral canal and resultant neurological sequelae.

In this manner all the wires are placed in the proposed area of fusion, two double wires being used at each of the end vertebrae.

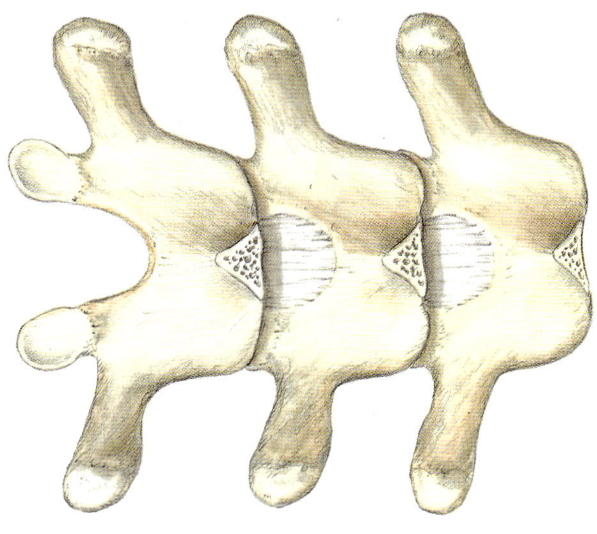

Fig. 2.**69** The ligamentum flavum is exposed.

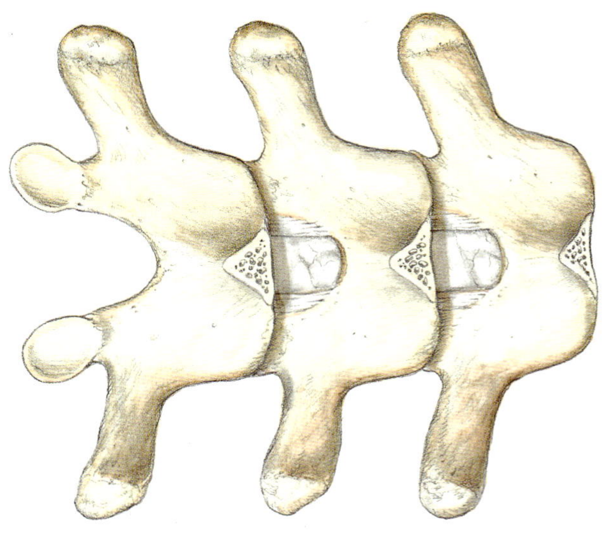

Fig. 2.**70** Status after resection of the ligamentum flavum.

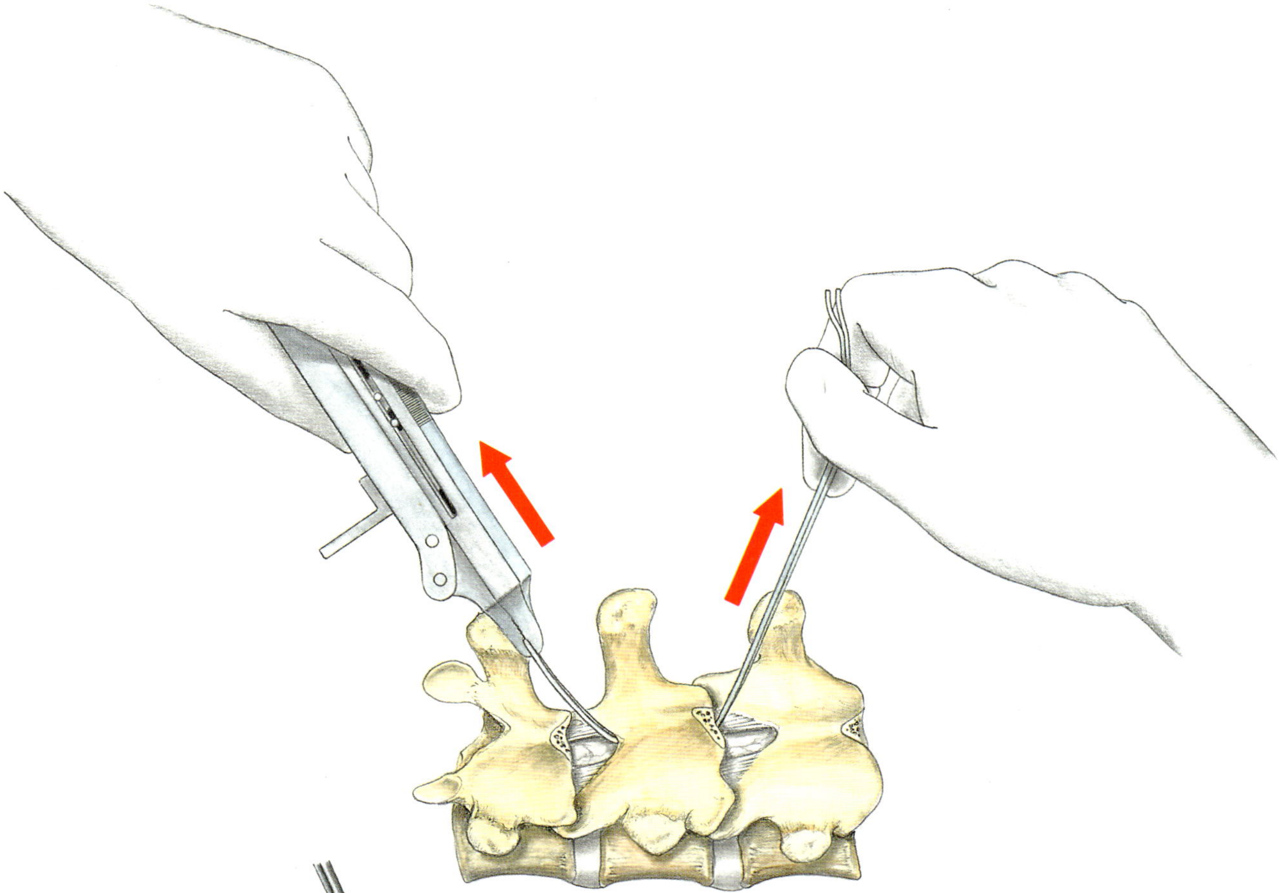

Fig. 2.**71** The Luque wire is pulled through from caudal to cranial while being kept under constant tension.

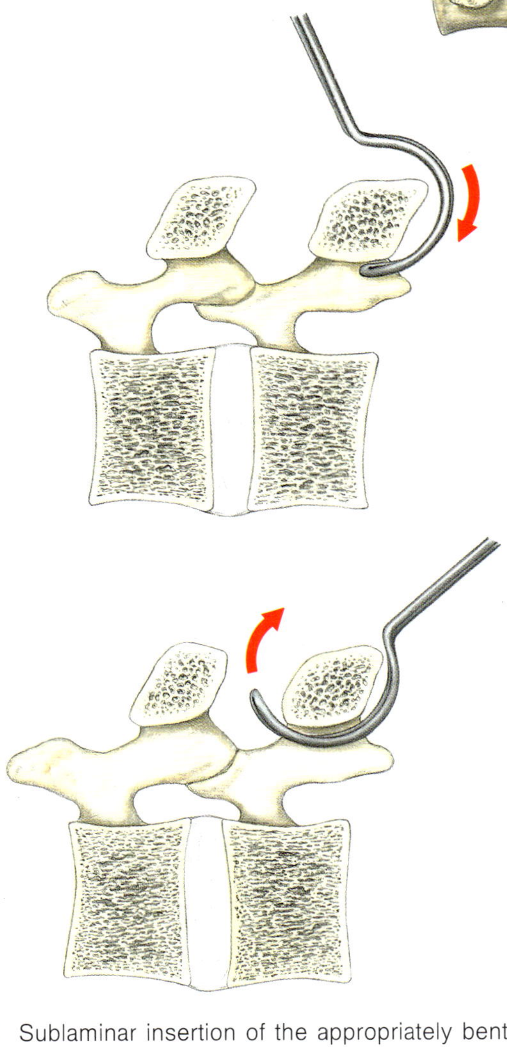

Fig. 2.**72** Sublaminar insertion of the appropriately bent Luque wire.

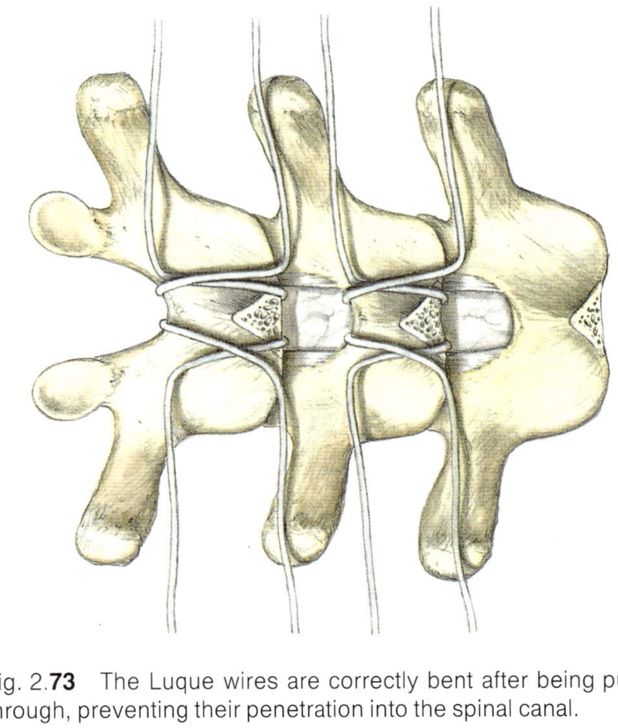

Fig. 2.**73** The Luque wires are correctly bent after being pulled through, preventing their penetration into the spinal canal.

Correction Technique

There are essentially two possible methods of correction: the convex-side L-rod technique and the concave technique. The type used depends on which rod is implanted first.

The convex technique is recommended, above all, for cases of thoracic scoliosis in which the physiologic thoracic kyphosis is to be maintained. For lumbar curvatures, on the other hand, the concave technique is advantageous, and it is also indicated for lordoscoliosis in the thoracic region.

Convex Technique (example: thoracic scoliosis)

To begin with, the convex-sided rod is introduced. The transverse limb of the L-rod is first placed on the neutral vertebra, or one segment above it, in a narrow excavation of the lamina when all the wires have been positioned in the fusion area. Using double wires, the transverse part of the rod is first fixed over the lamina in such a way as to ensure rotational stability. Then the wires of the next three to four vertebrae are tightened. After this, the convex-sided rod is advanced toward the spine with continuous pulling on the wires from cranial to caudal (Fig. 2.**74**). Prior to final fixation of the convex-sided rod, the concave-sided rod is attached to the caudal end of the fusion by its short transverse limb (Fig. 2.**75**) in a groove at the lower margin

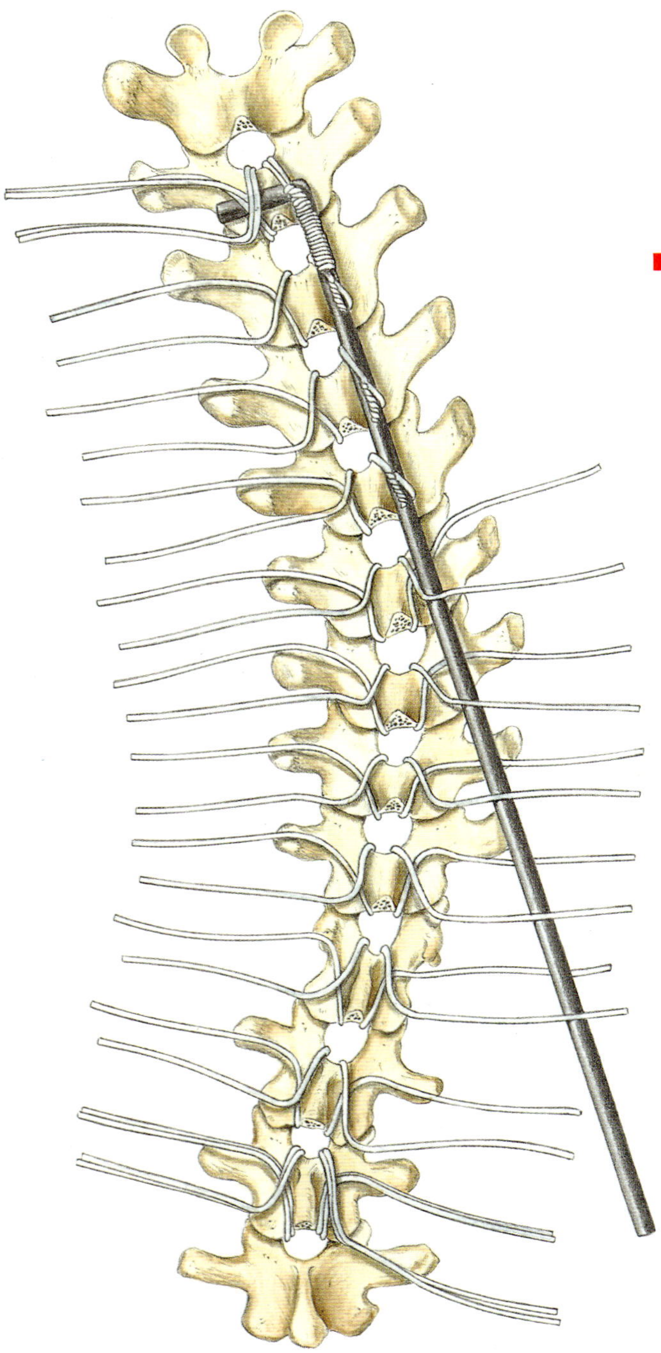

Fig. 2.**74** Operative technique for the convex side. Fixation of the L-rod and tightening of the wire from cranial to caudal.

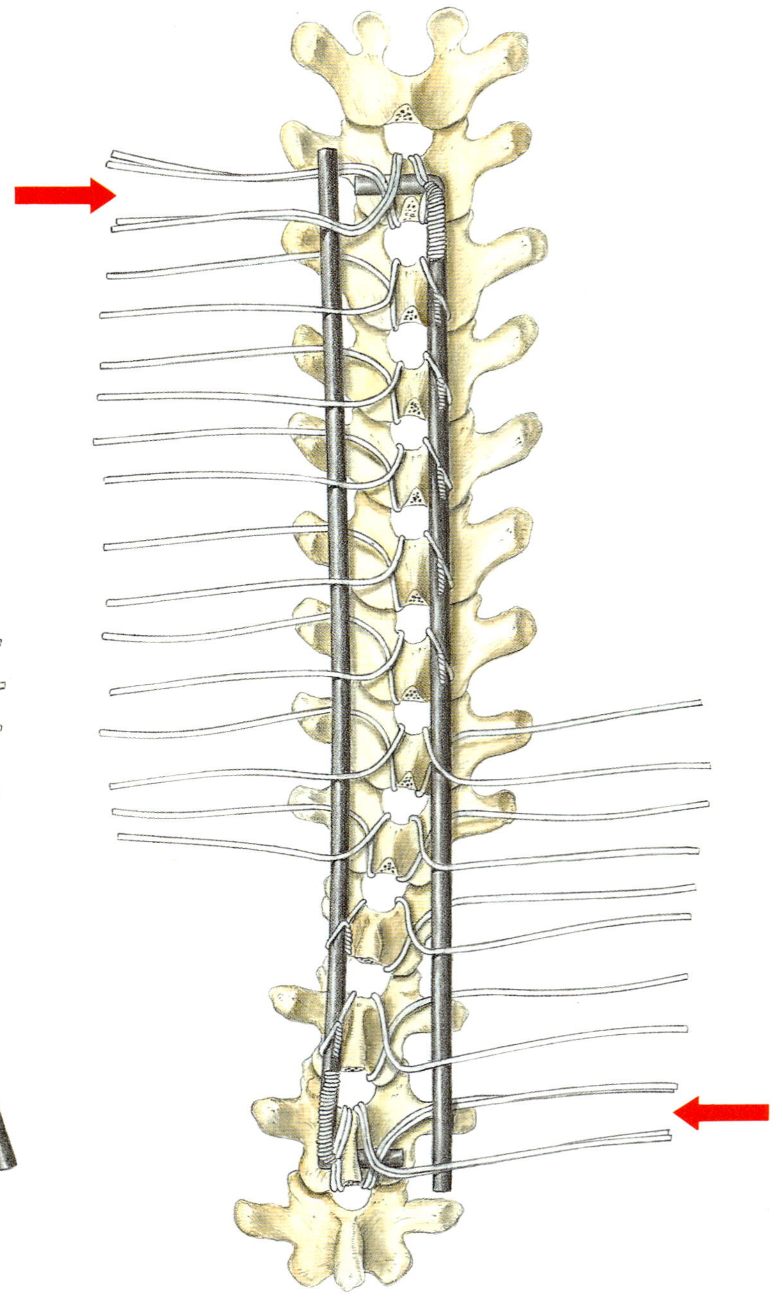

Fig. 2.**75** Operative technique for the convex side. Insertion of the L-rod for the concave side and fixation from caudal to cranial.

of the spinous process or in a hole at the base of the spinous process. The transverse limb is once again fixed by a double cerclage, after which the next three or four segments are tightened on the concave side from caudal to cranial. Both rods are now placed in parallel positions in such a way that the straight end of one rod will come to rest *on top of* the short L-limb. Finally, all the wires are tightened once more; they are then shortened to a length of about 1 cm and bent in the direction of the midline (Fig. 2.**76**).

Special Note
It is important to use two double wires, each at both end vertebrae of the fusion. According to Allen, it is advisable to secure the cranial decussation of the two rods by a double wire, which—in contrast to the usual rule—runs over the lamina from cranial lateral to caudal medial. The wires otherwise travel over the rod from cranial medial to caudal lateral (Fig. 2.**76**, inset).

For maximum stability of the fixation, it is important that the rods should be firmly apposed to the lamina at the base of the spinous process. The correction should not only be effected by tightening of the wires, but should also be supported by traction or by manual lateral pressure on the apex of the scoliosis.

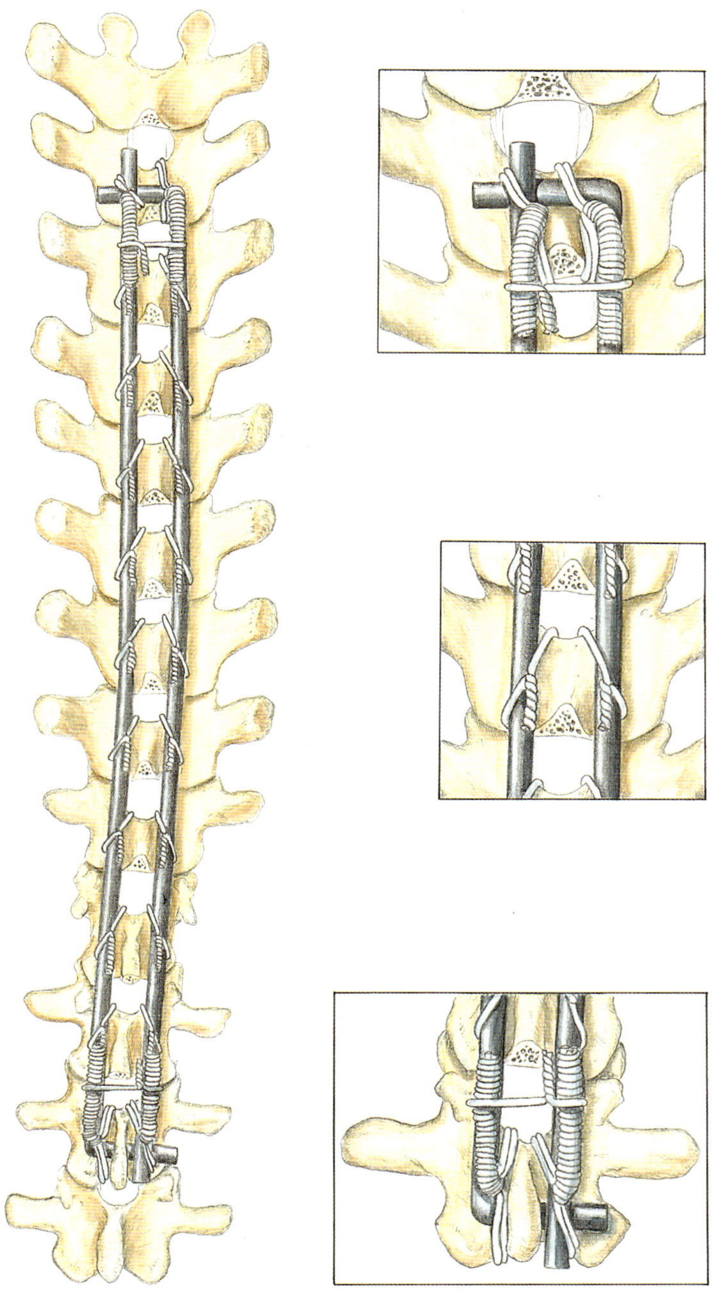

Fig. 2.**76** Luque operation. Status after completion of the final correction. The three insets show the correct wiring.

The convex technique is shown in Figures 2.**71**–2.**81** in a case of thoracic scoliosis.

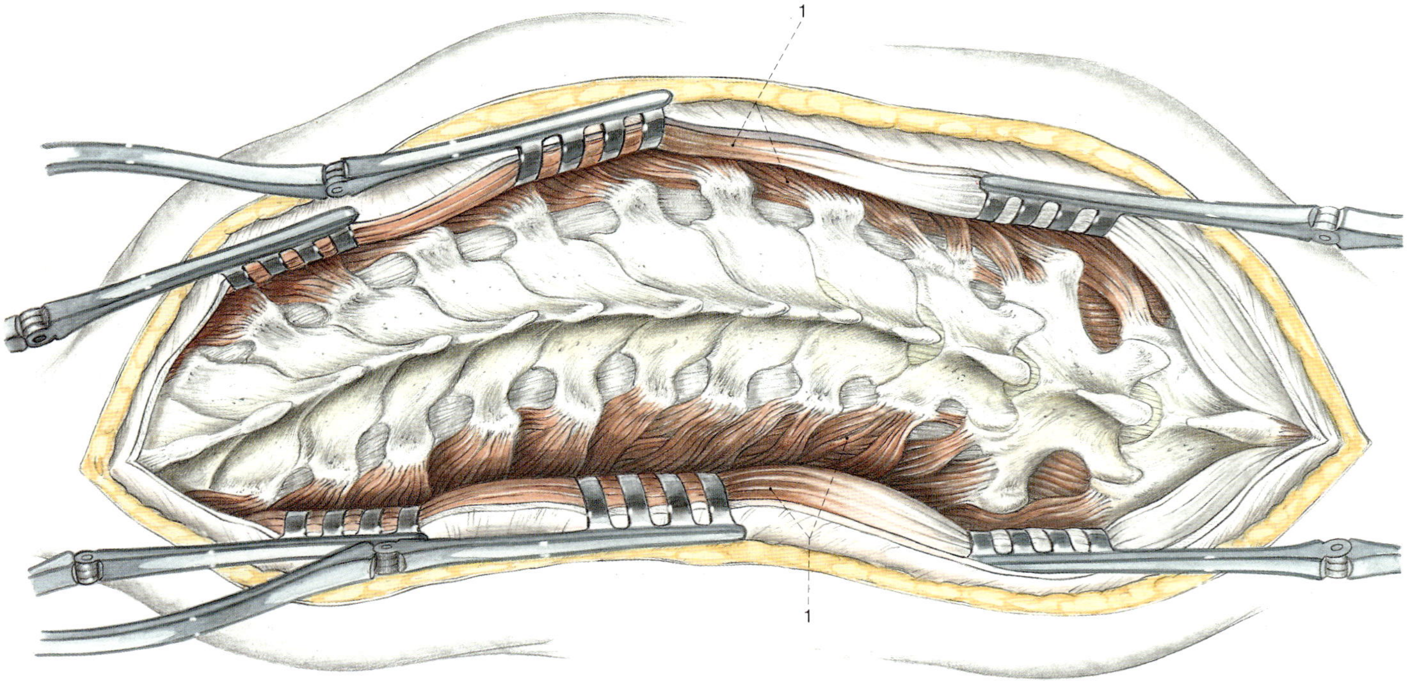

Fig. 2.**77** Exposure of the posterior vertebral elements of a right-convex thoracic scoliosis.

1 Erector muscle of the spine

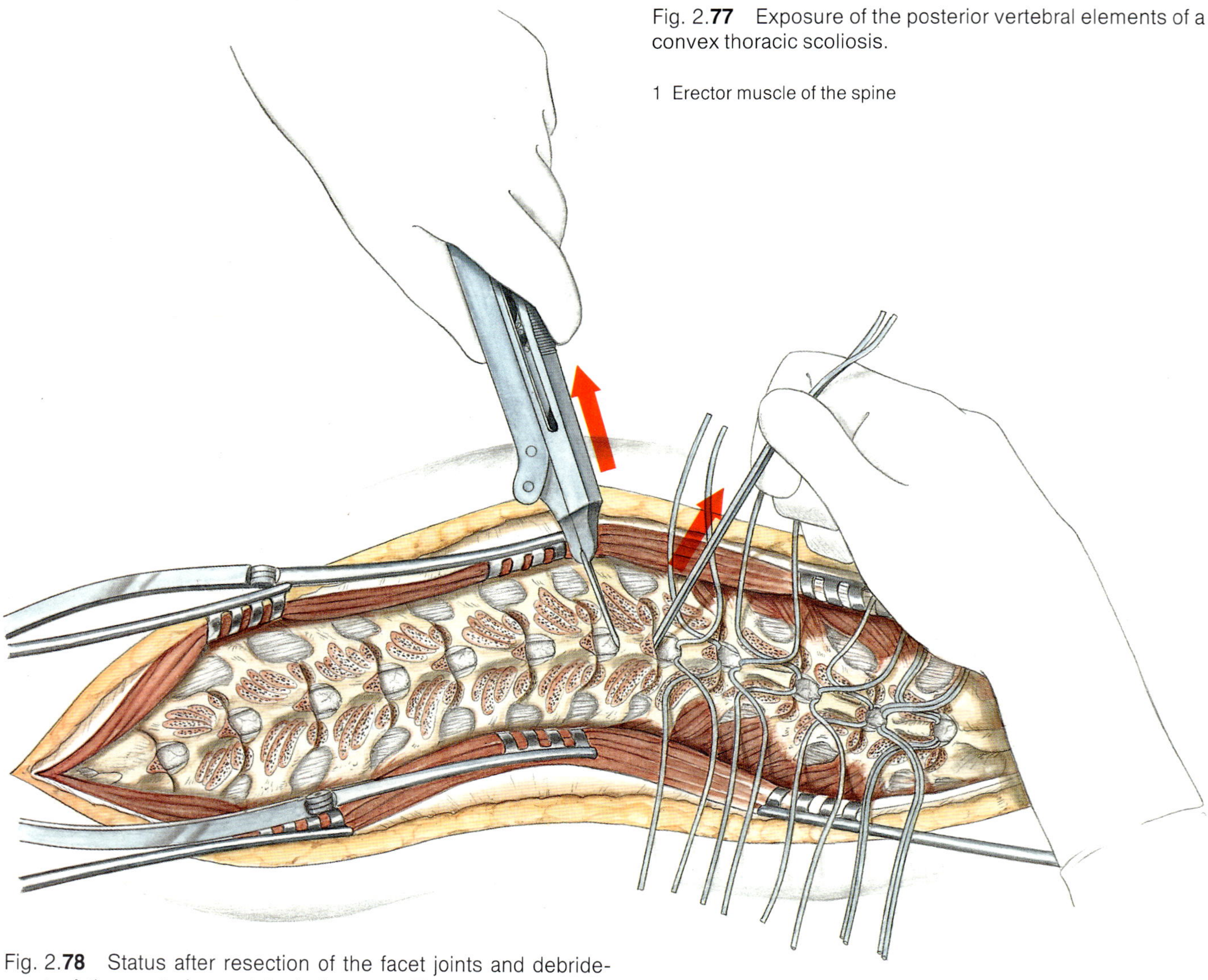

Fig. 2.**78** Status after resection of the facet joints and debridement of the posterior vertebral elements. The Luque wires are pulled through from caudal to cranial and are appropriately bent over the vertebral arches.

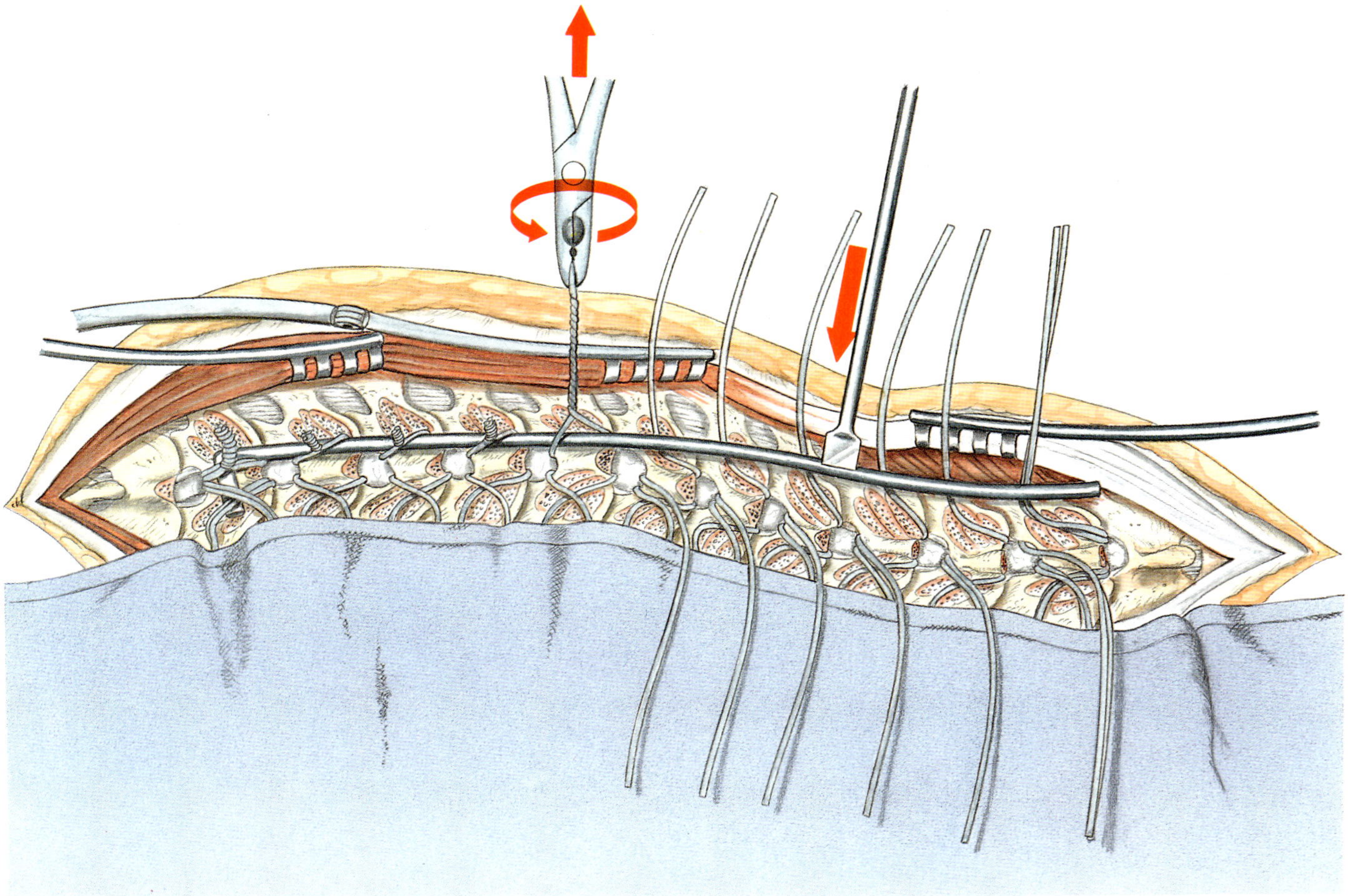

Fig. 2.**79** Operative technique for the convex side. The rod for the convex side is inserted and is fixed from cranial to caudal. The concave-side Luque wires are covered with a drape so that they will not be mistaken for convex-side wires.

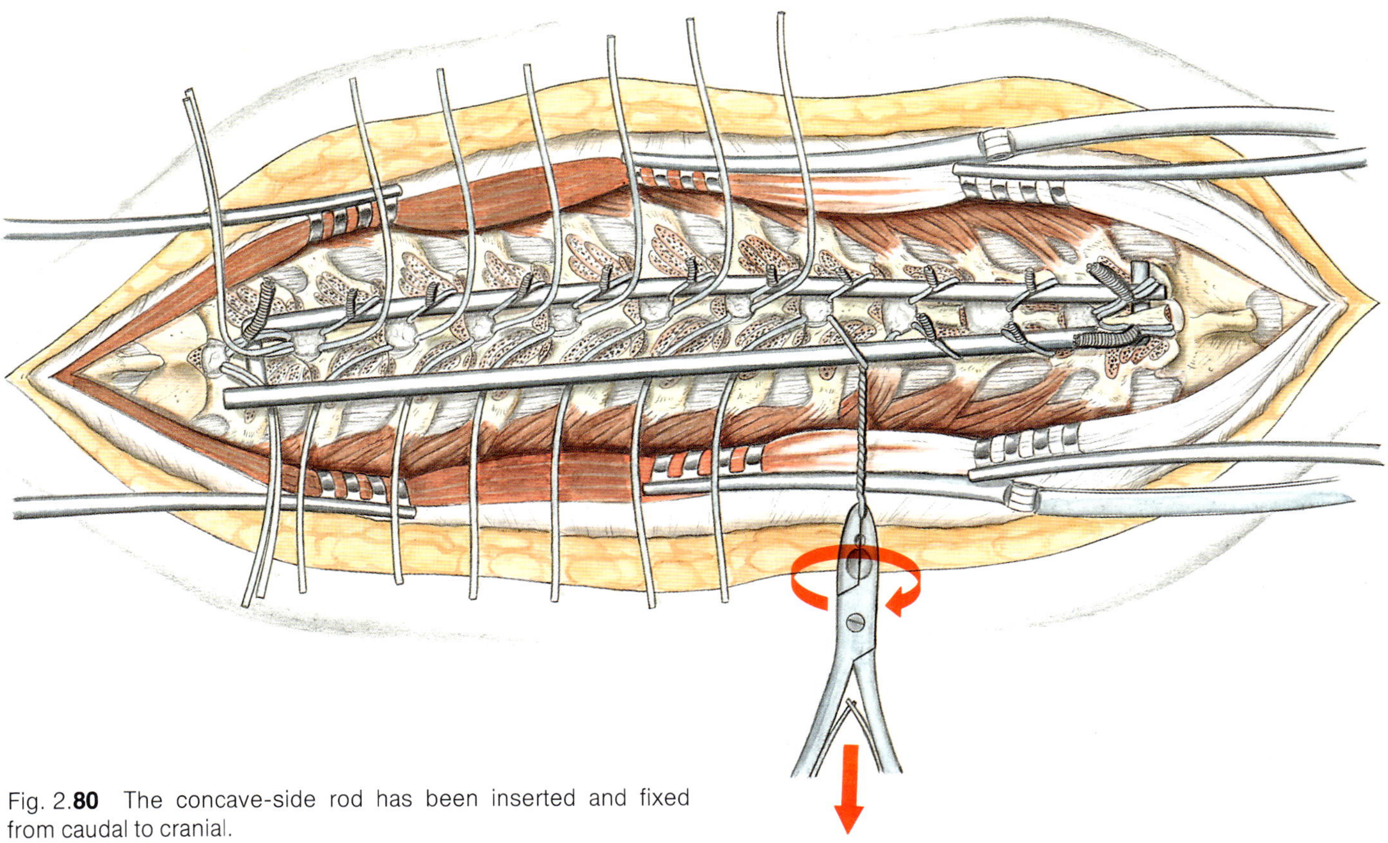

Fig. 2.**80** The concave-side rod has been inserted and fixed from caudal to cranial.

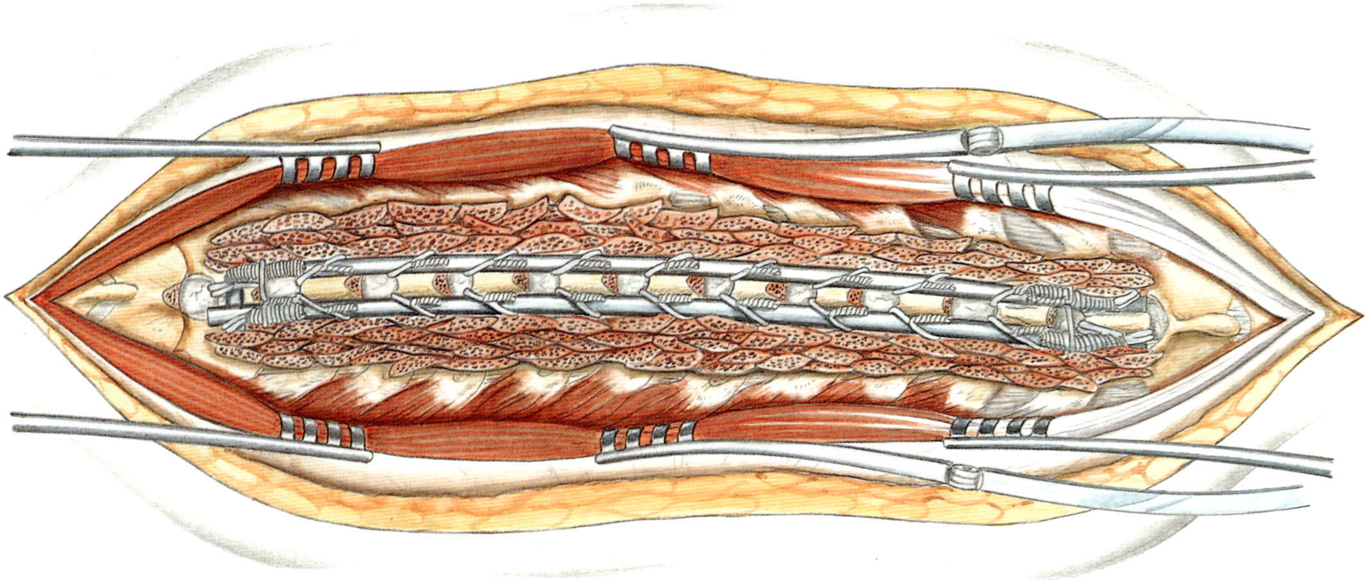

Fig. 2.**81** Status after fixation of both Luque rods and introduction of bone chips into the fusion area. Firm enclosure of the two end vertebrae is important.

Concave Technique (example: lumbar scoliosis)

The short transverse limb of the Luque rod is fixed over the lamina of the caudal end vertebra of the proposed fusion. As a rule, it is inserted through a hole at the base of the spinous process; the double wire on the concave side is drawn tight. If greater lordosis was specified for the Luque rod, strong torsional forces are produced. In this case, it is necessary to fix the short limb of the L-rod temporarily on the convex side as well. After this, the correction is performed: manual pressure is exerted from the convex side of the scoliotic curve. On the concave side, the wire is tightened, first on the apical vertebra and then on adjacent vertebrae (Fig. 2.**82**). The rod on the convex side is now fixed, from cranial to caudal (Fig. 2.**83**), with the short limb coming to rest below the long limb of the concave-sided rod. The wires in the area of the concave-sided rod are subsequently tightened more and more. If the rod at the apex of the scoliosis is still not in apposition to the lamina, the convex-sided rod is alternatively fixed further from cranial to caudal. After complete fixation of the rod on the convex side, the concave-sided rod will have loosened up somewhat, so that the wires have to be retightened. In the concave technique, too, the short ends of the L-rod lie below the long limb, just as in the convex technique. Again, the wire ends are clipped off at a length of about 1 cm and bent toward the inside (Fig. 2.**84**).

Wound Closure

The wound is closed in two layers by suturing the musculature and the overlying fascia. In children and adolescents, the split spinous process apophyses are readily united by sutures.

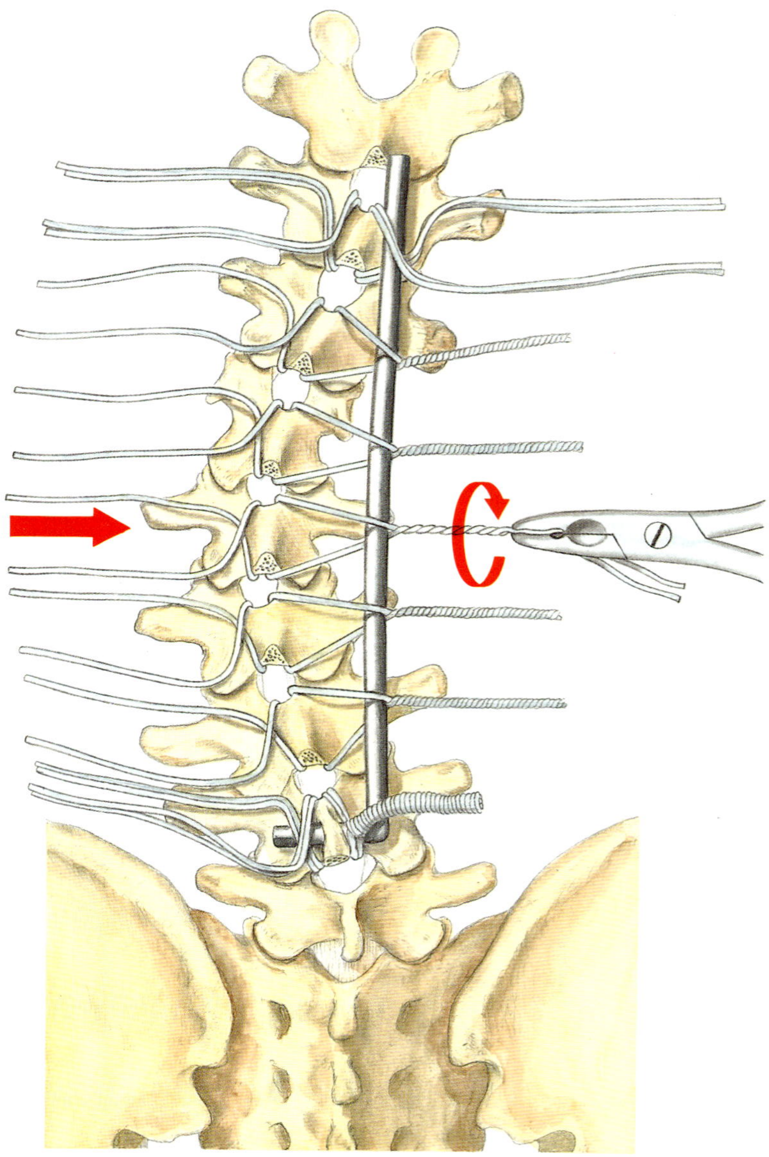

Fig. 2.**82** Operative technique for the concave side. The concave-side L-rod is inserted and tightened first.

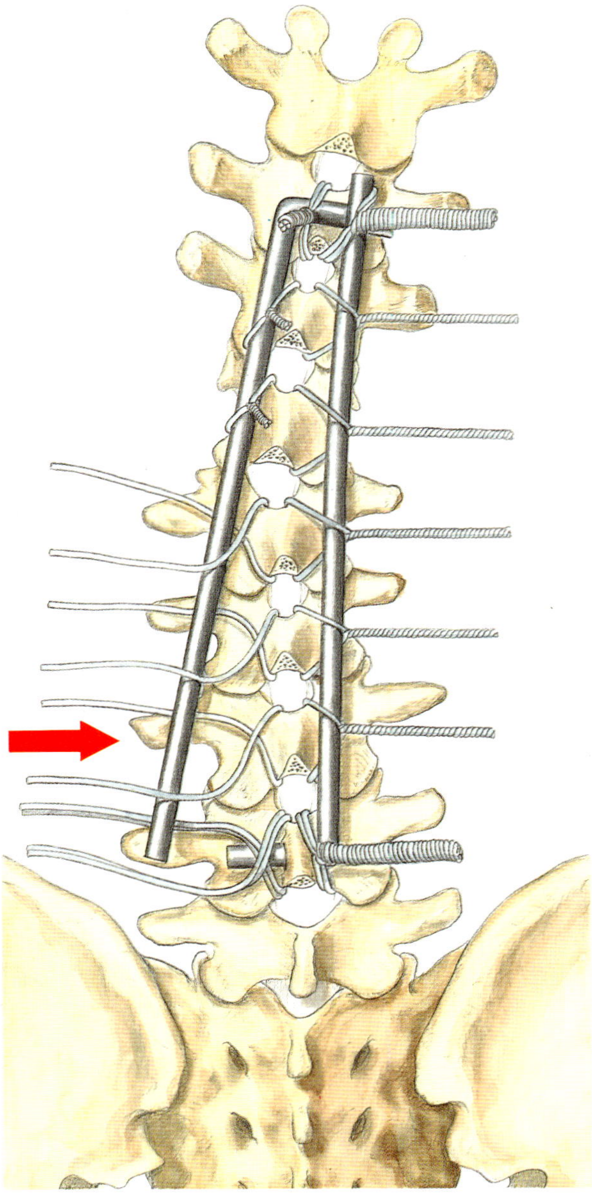

Fig. 2.**83** Insertion of convex-side rod and fixation from cranial to caudal.

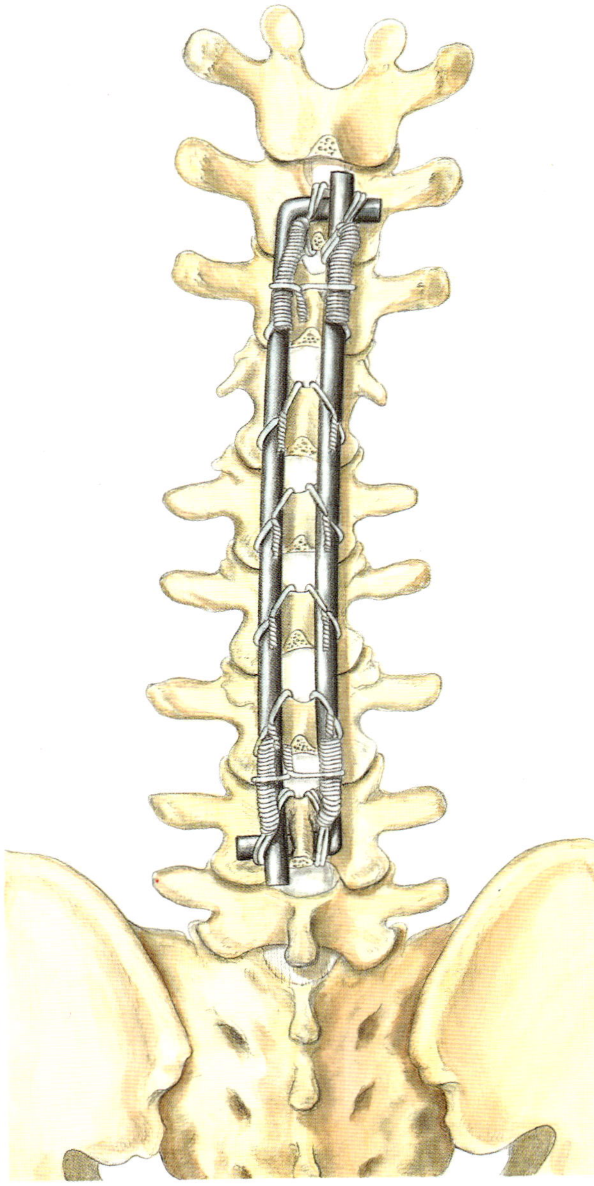

Fig. 2.**84** Status after correction of scoliosis and fixation of both Luque rods. Note that the long limb of the L-rod always overlies the short tranverse limb.

Postoperative Treatment

The patient is placed in bed without any external supports. Immediately after the operation, the patients are transferred to the intensive care unit, where the necessary diagnostic and therapeutic measures are taken. About a week after the operation, the patients are mobilized without external supports.

Pitfalls and Complications

The specific risk in this operation is neurologic complications. According to a report of the American Scoliosis Research Society (1987), sublaminar instrumentation is four times as risky as the Harrington instrumentation; the neurologic risk in the Luque operation is reported to be 1.77%.

Alternative Methods

Possible alternatives are, first of all, the Cotrel–Dubousset instrumentation and, for thoracolumbar and lumbar scoliosis, anterior procedures, such as Dwyer's and VDS.

Lumbosacral Fixation

The segmental spinal instrumentation according to Luque permits orthosis-free postoperative mobilization. Whereas in the case of idiopathic scoliosis, for example, the omission of a postoperative support is not of critical importance when compared with the neurological risk of the Luque operation, orthosis-free postoperative mobilization affords a tremendous advantage, particularly in neuromuscular scoliosis or in paralytic scoliosis involving various skin problems. In this group of patients, it is often necessary to also stabilize the pelvis, or to correct pelvic obliquity. Various modifications of the Luque technique offer the possibility of stable pelvic fixation.

Luque originally described a pelvic fixation technique in which the Luque rod over S1 is angulated by 90 degrees. The transverse limb is then passed through a drill hole in the posterior segments of the iliac bone (Fig. 2.**85**).

The Galveston techniques, proposed by Allen and Ferguson (1982), is worth recommending.

Indications

- Markedly decompensated neuromuscular scoliosis
- Pelvic obliquity

Galveston Technique

(Figs. 2.**86**–2.**91**)

See the Luque operation (p. 122); in addition to this, surgical exposure of the lumbosacral junction is carried out. The Luque rod is fixed in the ilium immediately above the greater ischiadic foramen. Here the bone is very strong, and provides good stabilization. For safety reasons, it is advisable to strip the gluteal musculature from the ilium in the median line of the back, so that the greater ischiadic foramen can be palpated with the finger from the outside for orientation as to the drilling direction. Approximately at the level of S1, a drill of a width equivalent to the thickness of the Luque rod is introduced into the ilium from the posterior superior iliac spine, in such a way that the drilling is done directly above the greater ischiadic foramen inside the two cortical tables of the ilium.

Bending the Luque rod appropriately for the Galveston technique is difficult. The following suggestions may help in the procedure. Neuromusculatur scoliosis often requires fusion from the upper thoracic spine down to the pelvis. As a rule, therefore, a long L-rod has to be used. The short transverse limb is positioned cranially. It is advisable to first produce a rectangular bend with the bending device 8–12 cm from the caudal end of the rod. About 2–3 cm (equal to half the sacral width) to the side of this rectangular bend, a second curvature of 50–75 degree (open laterally) is made, conforming to the inclination of a Steinmann nail temporarily inserted into the drill hole in the ilium. The caudal end, which is now free, should have a length of at most 8 cm in the adult, and should be appropriately shorter in children (average 5–6 cm). The bending device is then used to produce the lumbar lordosis; this automatically causes the distal limb to go toward the right direction. More cranially, the physiological thoracic kyphosis is produced. The segmental fixation with wires follows the customary procedure. The transverse limb is fixed over the lamina of S1 with two double wires. For this purpose, it is advisable to make a drill hole between S1 and S2. The short transverse limb at the cranial end of the rod can serve as an orientation aid in the frontal plane, and should be clipped off only after the rod has been completely bent.

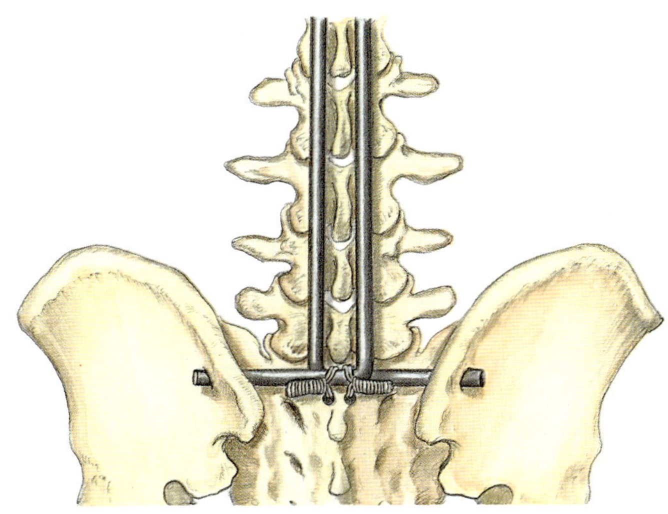

Fig. 2.**85** Pelvic fixation with the Luque technique. Note the drill hole in S1 for double-wire fixation of the Luque rods. Disadvantage: No lumbosacral stability in the sagittal plane.

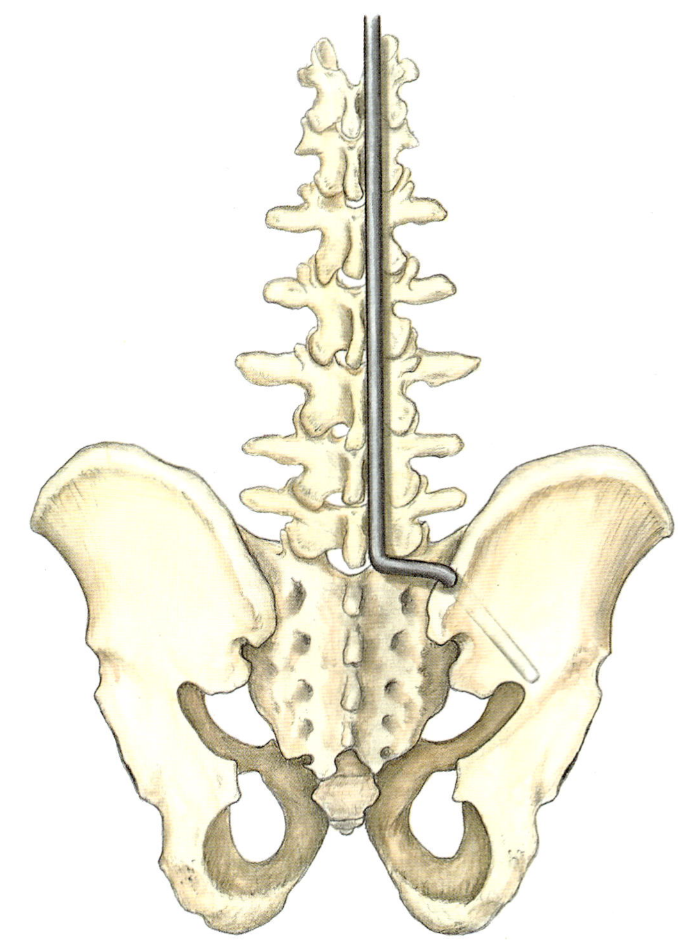

Fig. 2.**86** Pelvic fixation with the Galveston technique.

Special Note

In neuromuscular diseases, in particular, the alae of the ilium are not aligned laterally at the usual angle, but lie very close to the sagittal plane. If correction of a lumbar kyphosis is required, fixation of the Luque rod in the ilium offers very little resistance to any posterior slippage (Fig. 3.**29**). An alternative that can be recommended is pelvic fixation with the Dunn technique (p. 209). Another option for lumbosacral fixation is to use the Cotrel–Dubousset system in combination with sacral screws.

Pelvic Obliquity

There is another special indication for the Galveston technique, in pelvic obliquity, particularly in neuromuscular scoliosis. In incomplete obliquity, especially, the fusion frequently has to be extended as far as the sacrum. For the distinction between complete and incomplete obliquity, reference can be made to the Dwyer instrumentation (p. 68). As a rule, a two-stage procedure is required.

1. Anterior mobilization, intervertebral disk resection, and preparation for spinal fusion in the area of the lumbar curvature

In the case of curves that can be readily corrected after anterior release, an anterior systemic corrective operation (Dwyer or Zielke instrumentation) may be suitable. If, however, effective correction of the curvature is not possible by the anterior approach (posterior adhesions of facet joints, soft-tissue contractions, etc.), instrumentation is not applicable, since it may present an obstacle to possible correction in a second, posterior operation. See pp. 173 and 181, respectively, for the operative technique. The intervertebral disks are resected by the anterior approach; the upper plates are debrided, and bone graft material is introduced intervertebrally in preparation for fusion.

2. Posterior Operation

The posterior operation usually consists of extensive muscle release by the posterior approach on the concave side, followed by Luque instrumentation using the Galveston technique. For correction of the pelvic obliquity, the long limb of the L-rods has to be perpendicular to the line of the transverse iliac crest.

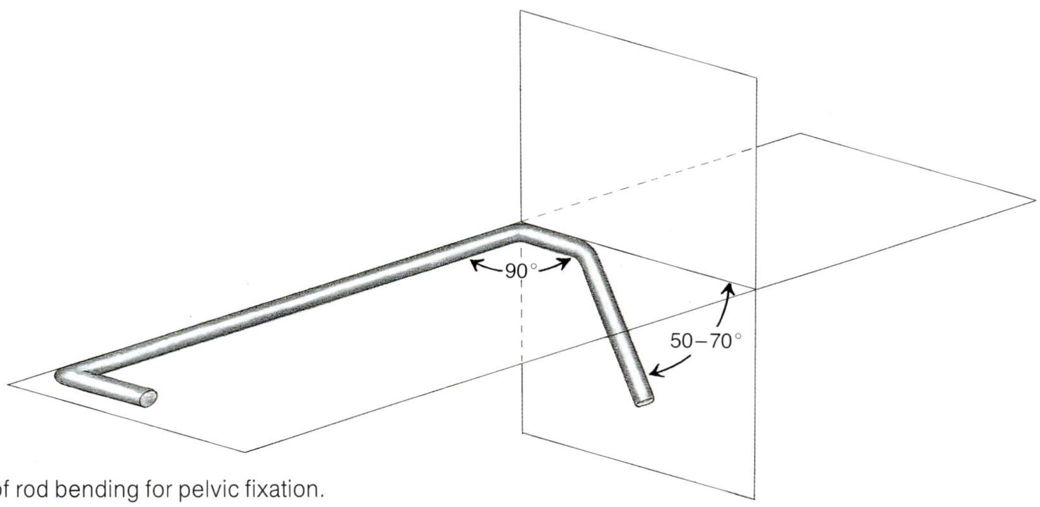

Fig. 2.**87** Planes of rod bending for pelvic fixation.

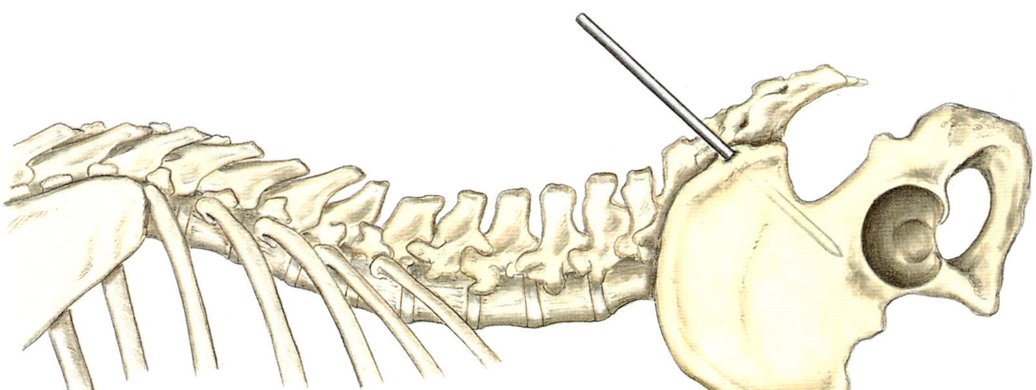

Fig. 2.**88** Pelvic fixation. The drill hole runs from the posterior iliac spine in the direction of the greater ischiadic foramen. The direction of the drill channel for bending of the Luque rod is marked by temporary insertion of a Steinmann pin.

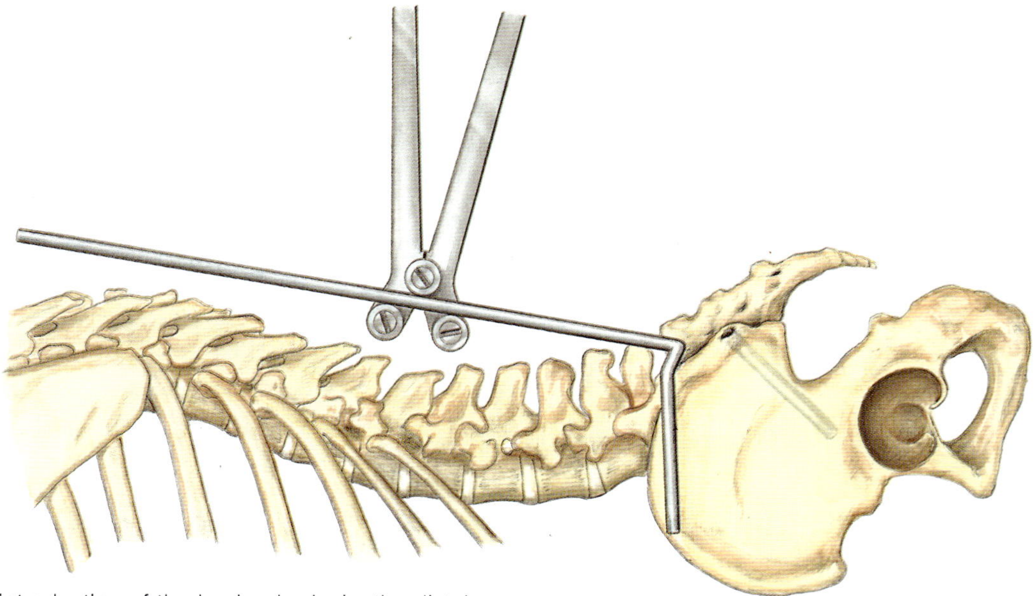

Fig. 2.**89** Through introduction of the lumbar lordosis, the distal limb of the rod is caused to move in the direction of the drill hole.

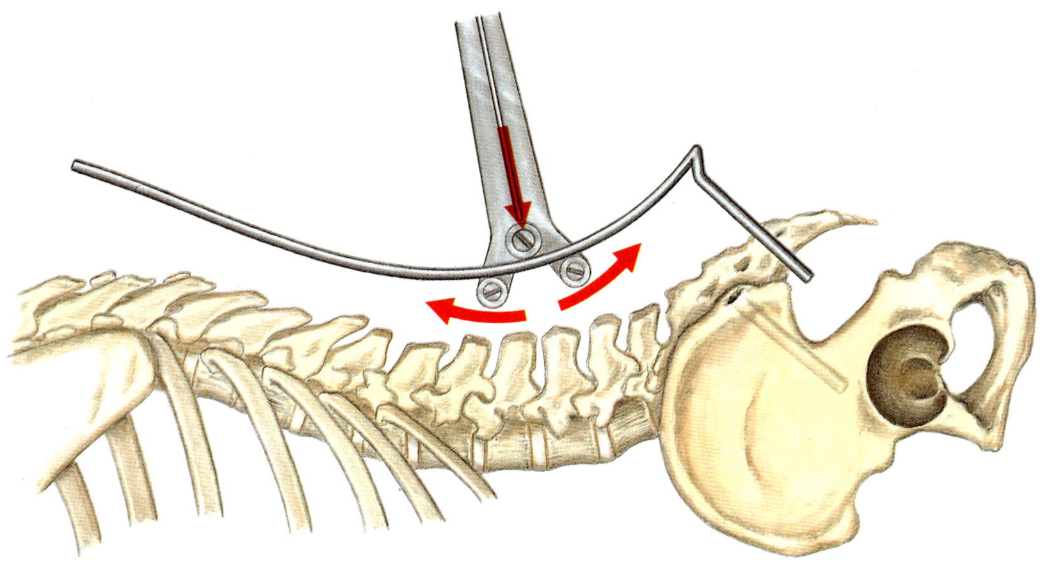

Fig. 2.**90** Final bending of the Luque rod.

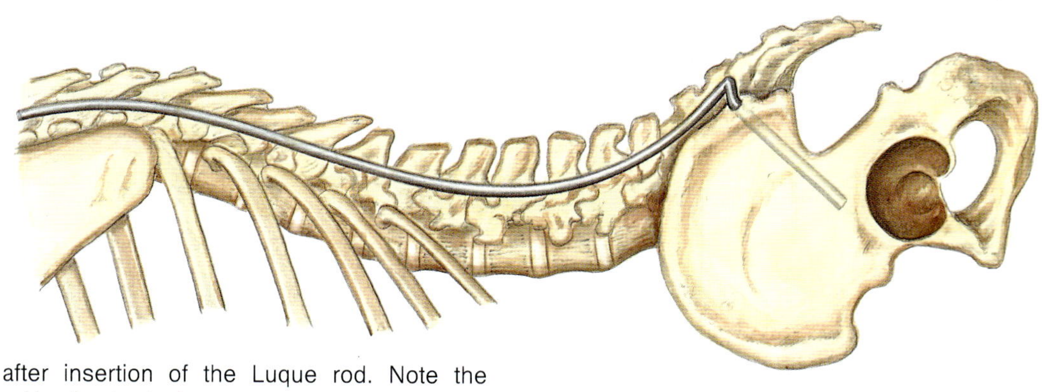

Fig. 2.**91** Status after insertion of the Luque rod. Note the thoracic kyphosis and lumbar lordosis.

Harrington Operation Combined with Sublaminar Luque Wires

Indication

The operation is indicated in patients with a higher risk of pseudarthrosis (e.g., adult scoliosis, thoracolumbar and lumbar curves, status after a preliminary operation). There is also a limited possibility of modifying the spinal curvature in the sagittal plane. The resultant rotational component has to be absorbed by means of a square-ended rod and a square-ended hook (Moe). The possibilities for treating torsion are therefore limited.

Operative Technique

See Harrington operation (pp. 89–95) and Luque operation (p. 118; Figs. 2.**92**, 2.**93**).

The advantages of this system include more stable fixation than with the Harrington system alone; further simple instrumentation and use of less metal in the canal than in the original Luque system with the double-rod techniques; and more room for bone-chip fusion on the convex side. However, there is a limited potential for correction in the sagittal plane.

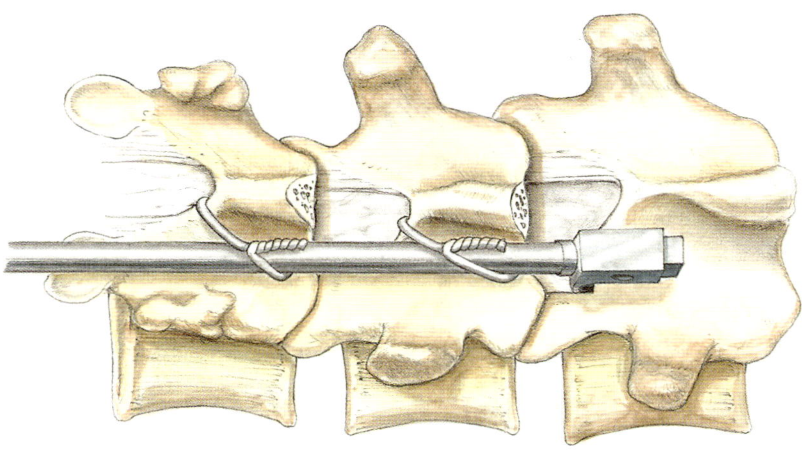

Fig. 2.**92** Combination of Harrington instrumentation with sublaminar wires. The rotational forces are absorbed by rectangular hooks (Moe).

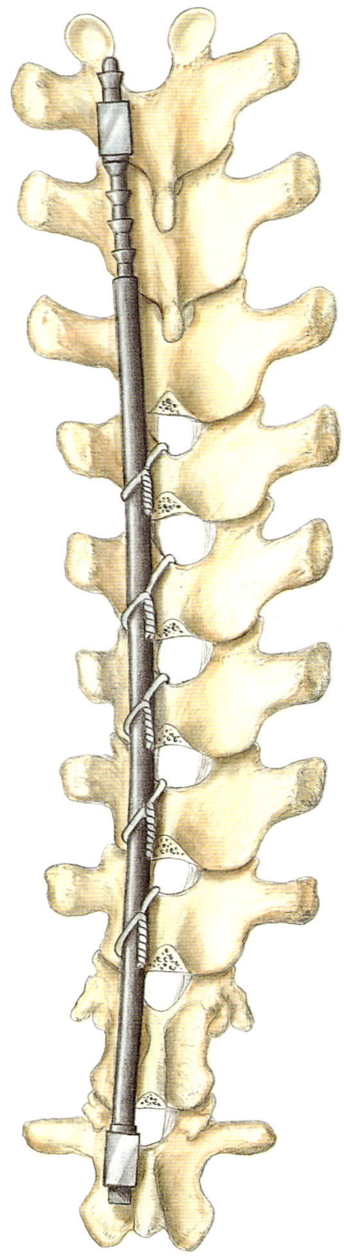

Fig. 2.**93** Harrington instrumentation with sublaminar wires. Example of instrumentation of thoracic scoliosis.

Further Reading

Allen BL, Ferguson RL. The operative treatment of myelomeningocele spinal deformity. Orthop Clin N Am 1979;10:845.

Allen BL, Ferguson RL. L-rod instrumentation for scoliosis in cerebral palsy. J Pediatr Orthop 1982;2:87.

Bernard TN, Johnston CE, Roberts JM, Burke SW. Late complications due to wire breakage in segmental spinal instrumentation. J Bone Jt Surg 1983;65-A:1339.

Bradford DS, Lonstein JE, Moe JH, Ogilvie JW, Winter RB. Scoliosis and other spinal deformities. Philadelphia: Saunders, 1987.

Dubousset J, Guillaumat M, Cotrel Y. Correction and fusion to the sacrum of pelvic obliquity with CD instrumentation in children and adults. 21st Annual Meeting of the American Scoliosis Research Society, 1986.

Luque ER. The correction of postural curves of the spine. Spine 1982;7:270.

Luque ER. Segmental spinal instrumentation (SSI) bei neuromuskulären Skoliosen. Orthopäde 1989;18:28.

Wenger DR, Carollo JJ, Wilkerson JA. Biomechanics of scoliosis correction by segmental spinal instrumentation. Spine 1982;7:260.

Cotrel–Dubousset Instrumentation

Indications

Principal indication: thoracic lordoscoliosis with no defect of the posterior vertebral elements.

Secondary indications: combined scoliosis, thoracolumbar and lumbar scoliosis (alternatives include anterior procedures such as Dwyer's and VDS, q.v.).

Note
The Cotrel–Dubousset instrumentation is generally applicable in scoliosis, kyphosis, fractures, tumors, and degenerative spinal conditions.

Approach

See Chapter 1, pp. 64–69.

Operative Technique

Instrumentarium

The following are the principal components of the Cotrel–Dubousset instrumentarium (Figs. 2.**94**, 2.**95**):

Cotrel rod: this has a diamond-rough surface and can be bent as required using bending forceps or a plate bender.

As a rule, one rod is used on the concave and one on the convex side. The rods are fixed to the vertebrae with hooks.

Hooks:

- Pedicular hook: open, closed.
- Laminar hook, thoracic: open, closed.
- The anterior surface of the body of the hook is slanted so that the hook, when inserted into the sublaminar space, tends to slip off posteriorly and will therefore not penetrate deeper into the spinal canal.
- Laminar hook, lumbar: open and closed.
- Transverse hook.
- C-ring: this serves to prevent longitudinal dislocation of the hook on the rod during the derotation phase.

Various implants: vertebral screws for transpedicular fixation. Various hook modifications are possible, but cannot be discussed here.

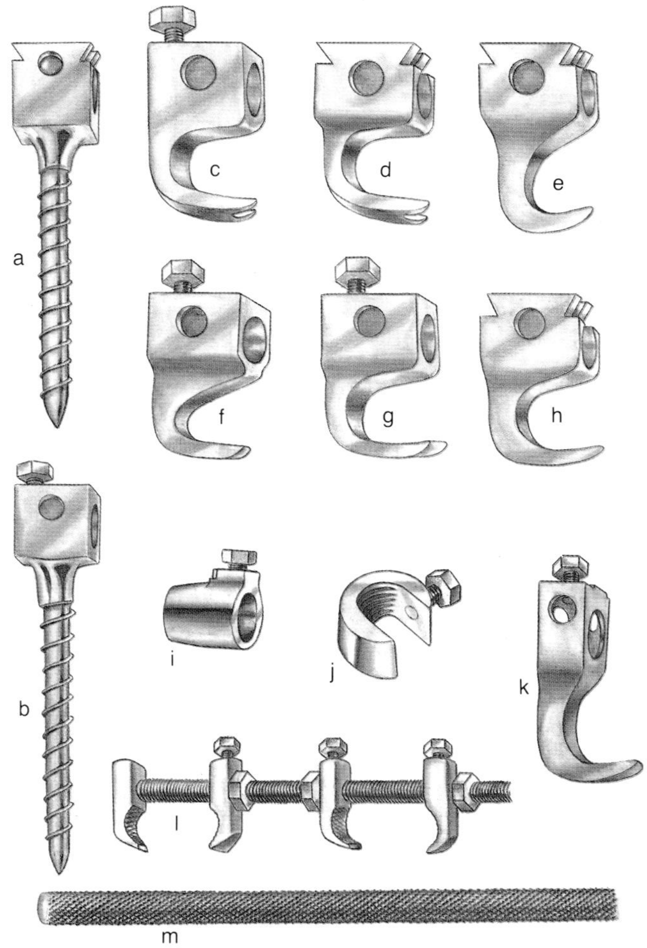

Fig. 2.**94** Cotrel–Dubousset implants.
a pedicular screw. Open.
b pedicular screw. Closed.
c pedicular hook. Closed.
d pedicular hook. Open.
e Open thoracic laminar hook.
f Closed thoracic laminar hook.
g Closed lumbar laminar hook.
h Open lumbar laminar hook.
i Hook blocker.
j C-ring.
k Transverse hook.
l DTT (device for transverse traction).
m Cotrel rod.

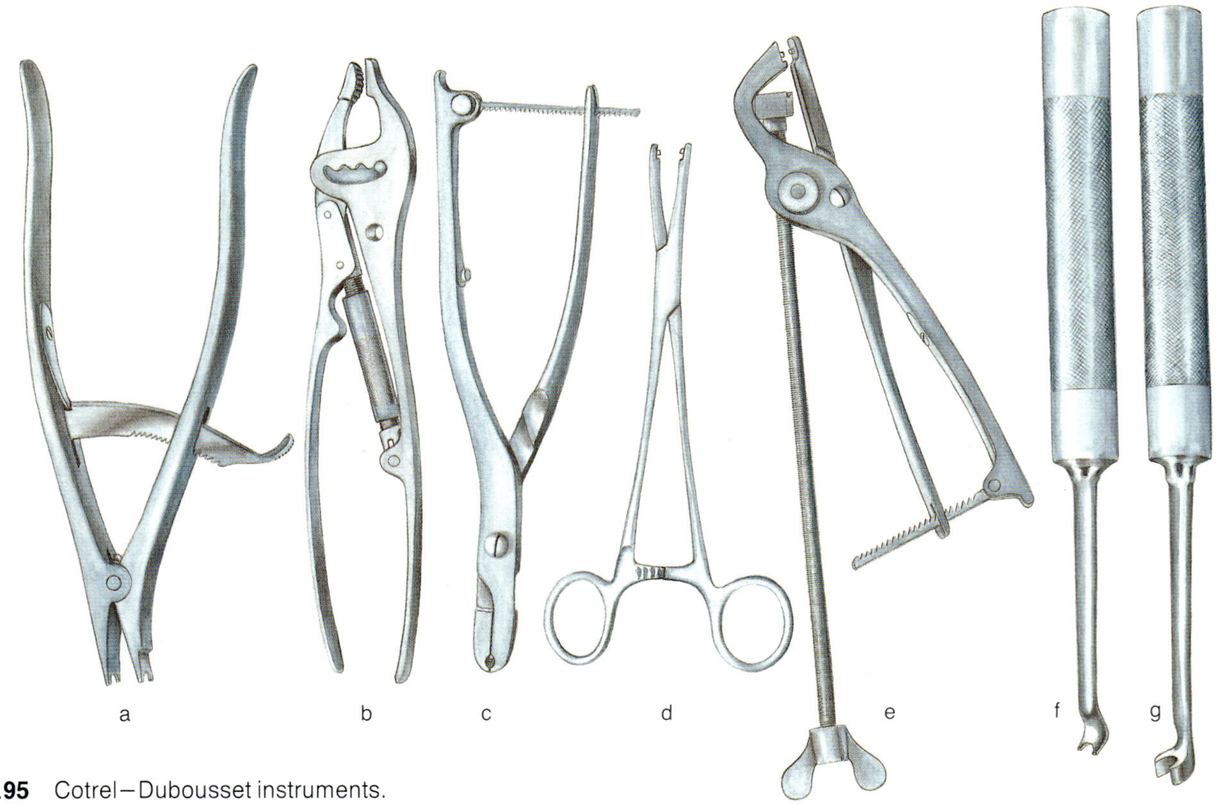

Fig. 2.**95** Cotrel–Dubousset instruments.
a Spreading forceps.
b Rod rotator.
c Grasping forceps.
d Hook holder.
e Curved hook holder with an attachment for insertion of the Cotrel rod into an open hook (cf. Fig. 2.**97**).
f Pedicle elevator.
g Hook inserter.

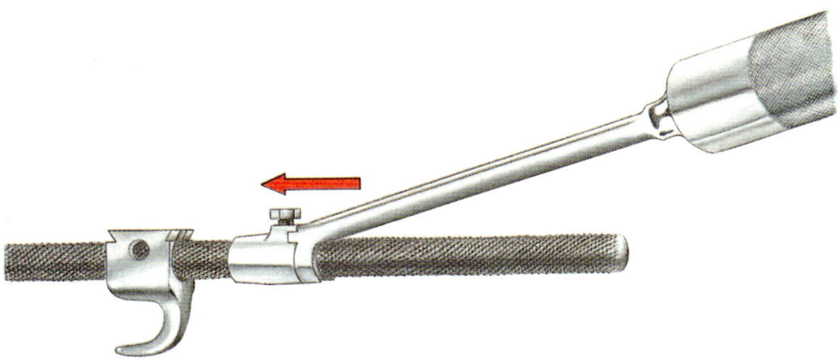

Fig. 2.**96** The Cotrel rod is locked into an open hook by introducing the hook cleat using guiding instrument.

Fixation of hook on rod: closed hooks are fixed with screws, and open hooks by means of a clamplike hook cleat that is introduced into the hook (Fig. 2.**96**).

Bent hook holder with attachment for insertion of the rod: the hook holder is fitted with a threaded rod serving as impactor. By rotating the threaded rod clockwise, the Cotrel rod is inserted into the open hook (Fig. 2.**97**/1), and fixation is then effected by driving in the hook blocker (Fig. 2.**97**/2). This instrument is particularly helpful when introducing the Cotrel rod into the intermediate hooks. The distance between the rod and the hook opening should not exceed 1 cm; the rod will otherwise have to be re-bent.

Rod rotator (Fig. 2.**95 b**): this is essentially a grasping forceps, with which the derotation can be carried out (see also Figs. 2.**101 a**, 2.**110**).

Distraction or compression procedure (Fig. 2.**98**). A clamp is fixed behind the hook, and a spreader is applied between them for distraction; after this, the hook is secured to the rod with a screw.

Transverse stabilization (DTT, Figs. 2.**94 l**, 2.**112**, 2.**113**). When both the concave-sided and the convex-sided rod have been inserted and the final correction has been achieved, the DTT (device for transverse traction) is applied as well. This can be used to approximate, distract, or merely fix the longitudinal rods. The DTT additionally allows rotational stabilization of the longitudinal rods in any position and enhances the stability of the construction.

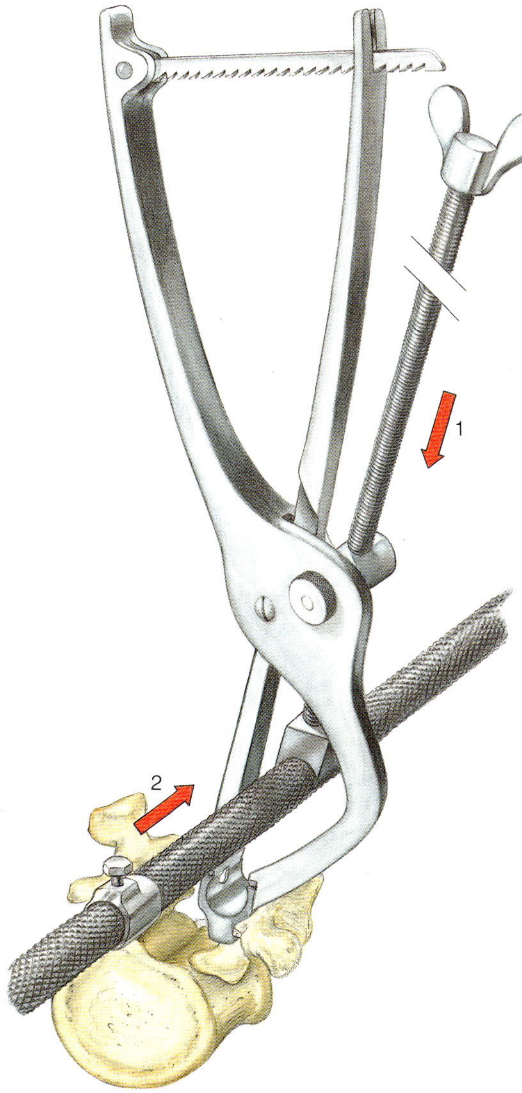

Fig. 2.**97** Curved hook holder with attachment. By turning the threaded rod clockwise (1), the Cotrel rod is inserted into the open hook. As soon as the rod is in the depth of the hook opening, it is locked by driving in the hook cleat (2) (cf. Fig. 2.**96**).

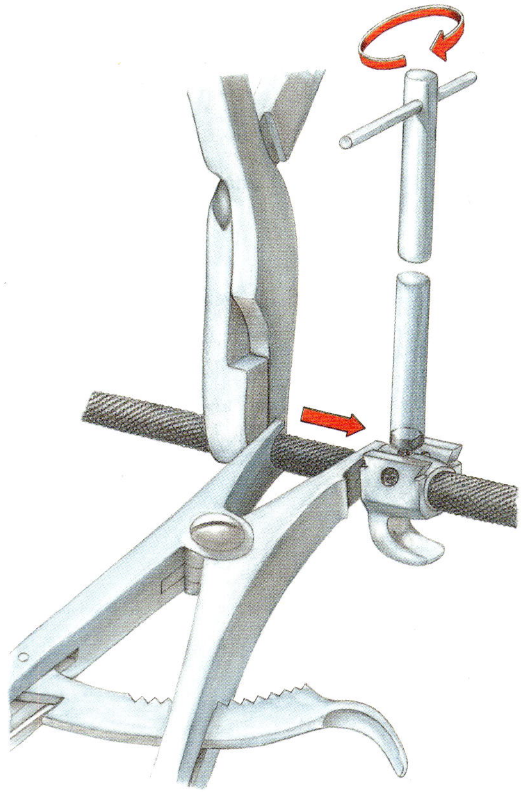

Fig. 2.**98** Carrying out distraction or compression. Behind the hook, a grasping forceps serving as an abutment is mounted on the Cotrel rod. Distraction between the two is now effected with spreaders. During the distraction, the hook screw has to be open. The screw is then tightened to maintain the correction.

Principles of Correction

The scoliotic (possibly also kyphotic) curvature is corrected by various forces:

- Distraction on the concave side.
- Compression on the convex side.
- Transverse traction and derotation at the apex of the curve.
- Wide intervertebral spaces are compressed.
- Narrow intervertebral spaces are distracted (applies to the frontal and sagittal planes).
- Lordosis (lordoscoliosis) is distracted.
- Kyphosis is compressed.

The correction is carried out with the aid of rods, which are attached to the so-called strategic vertebrae with various hooks. As a rule, two rods are used: one on the concave side of the curve, and another on the convex side. The rods have to be bent individually. The extent of bending required depends on the location, the magnitude, and the rigidity of the spinal curvature in the frontal and sagittal planes. When bending the rod, the utmost attention should be paid to postoperative restoration of physiological curvatures in the sagittal plane (i.e., thoracic kyphosis and lumbar lordosis). With mobile curves, rotation of the bent rod around the longitudinal axis leads to a three-dimensional correction of the instrumented vertebrae.

Hook Position

(on the "strategic" vertebrae)

The following radiographs are needed to determine the hook position:

- Standing anteroposterior and lateral film of the entire spine.
- Bending films in the frontal plane.
- Bending films in the sagittal plane (flexion and extension) when deformity is present in this plane.
- Suspension film.

On the basis of these radiographs, the following strategic vertebrae need to be identified:

- End vertebra, upper and lower.
- The last vertebra, cranially and caudally, included in the fusion. In simple curvatures, this may be identical with the neutral vertebra. However, if there are deformities on another level—in the sagittal plane, for example—the scoliotic curve may have to be instrumented beyond the neutral vertebra. Positioning of the lower-end vertebra is important, especially for curves that end in the area of the lumbar spine. Positioning of the hook is defined as shown in Figure 2.**99**: the bending films must show an opening of the segment that is distal to the proposed fusion in both planes.
- Neutral vertebra, upper and lower.
- Apical vertebra.
- Intermediate vertebra, upper and lower. The intermediate vertebrae are located at the cranial and caudal ends of the rigid zone at the apex of the curvature (segments that open least on the bending films).

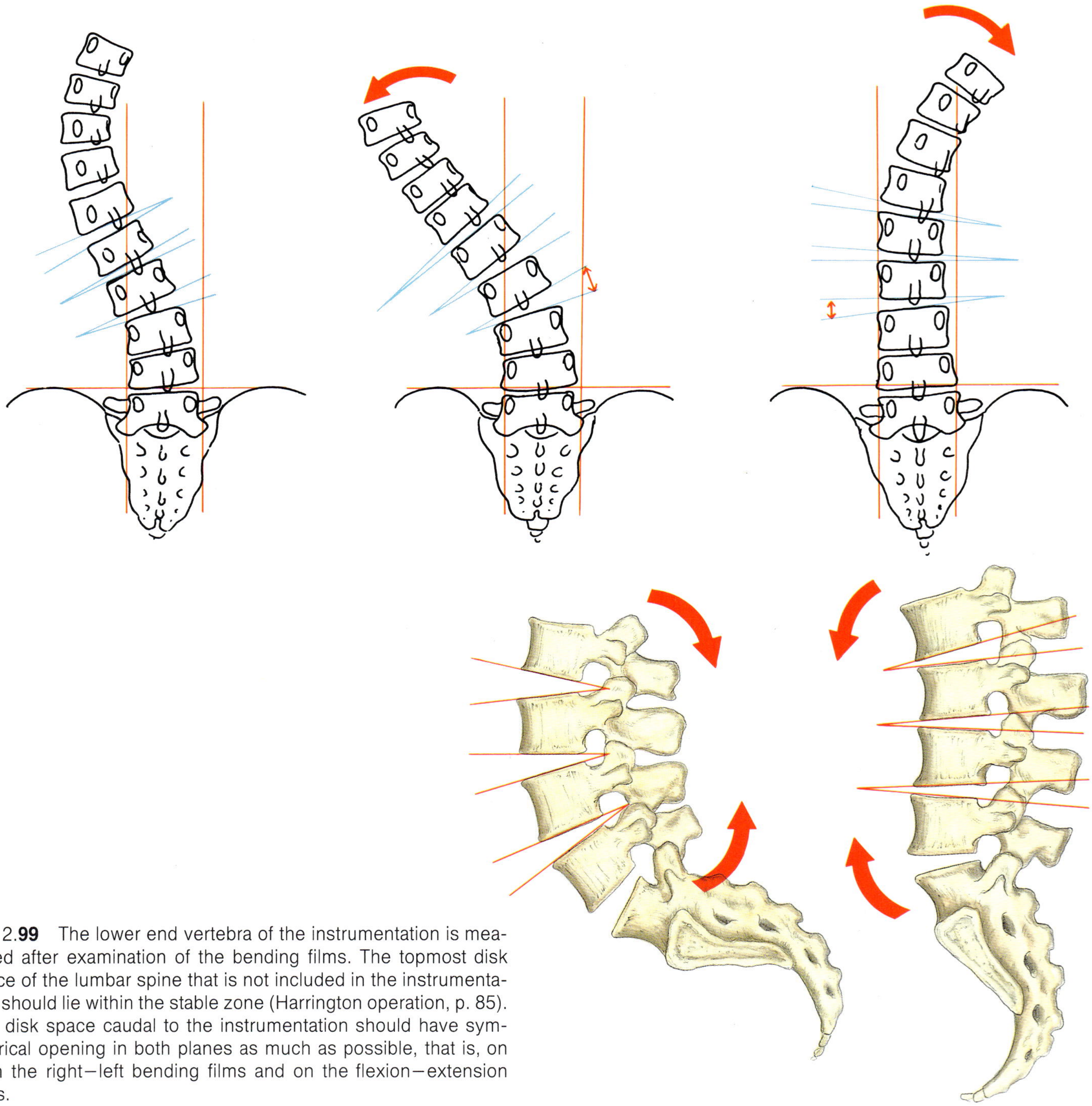

Fig. 2.**99** The lower end vertebra of the instrumentation is measured after examination of the bending films. The topmost disk space of the lumbar spine that is not included in the instrumentation should lie within the stable zone (Harrington operation, p. 85). The disk space caudal to the instrumentation should have symmetrical opening in both planes as much as possible, that is, on both the right–left bending films and on the flexion–extension films.

After review of the radiographs in both planes, a working diagram with the appropriate hook positions is drawn and placed on the suspension film.

Mobile Thoracic Lordoscoliosis

(End vertebrae are also neutral vertebrae)

An example of the instrumentation and the principles of correction is given in Figure 2.**100**.

The end vertebrae (neutral vertebrae) are fitted with closed hooks, and the other strategic vertebrae with open hooks. On the convex side, the pedicular hook is combined with a transverse hook, forming a clamp (Fig. 2.**106**). On the concave side, the hooks are aligned by applying distraction (the intervertebral spaces are opened), and on the convex side by applying compression (the intervertebral spaces are closed).

Following the theory (end vertebrae are neutral vertebrae), hooks are applied to the intermediate vertebrae and the apical vertebrae as well as the end vertebrae.

Principle of three-dimensional correction by derotation in mobile lordoscoliosis (Figs. 2.**101a**, **b**). The Cotrel rod on the concave side is bent in accordance with the scoliotic curvature and, above all, following the desired postoperative thoracic kyphosis; in the lower portion, lumbar lordosis is already initiated in the region of L1. Before derotation, the concave rod appears curved in the frontal plane but straight in the sagittal plane (Fig. 2.**101a**). After correction by derotation, the concave rod appears straight in the frontal plane and bent in the sagittal plane according to the physiologic thoracic kyphosis. At L1, the lumbar lordosis has been initiated.

If the lordotic component of the scoliosis is fixed (bending films in the sagittal plane), an anterior polysegmental mobilization (see p. 147 for the operative technique) is advisable prior to the posterior Cotrel–Dubousset instrumentation.

Another correction is then performed by distraction on the concave side, followed by compression on the convex side in the order of numbers 1 to 5 in Figure 2.**101b**.

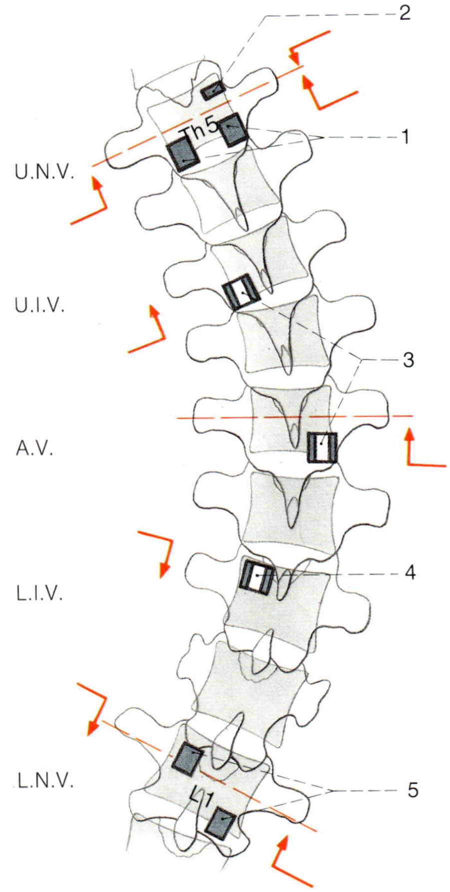

Fig. 2.**100** Working diagram for the positioning of hooks, using a mobile thoracic lordoscoliosis as example (end vertebrae are neutral vertebrae).

U.N.V.	Upper neutral vertebra
U.I.V.	Upper intermediate vertebra
A.V.	Apical vertebra
L.I.V.	Lower intermediate vertebra
L.N.V.	Lower neutral vertebra

1 Closed pedicular hook
2 Transverse hook
3 Open pedicular hook
4 Open thoracic laminar hook
5 Closed lumbar laminar hook. The hook direction is identified by arrows.

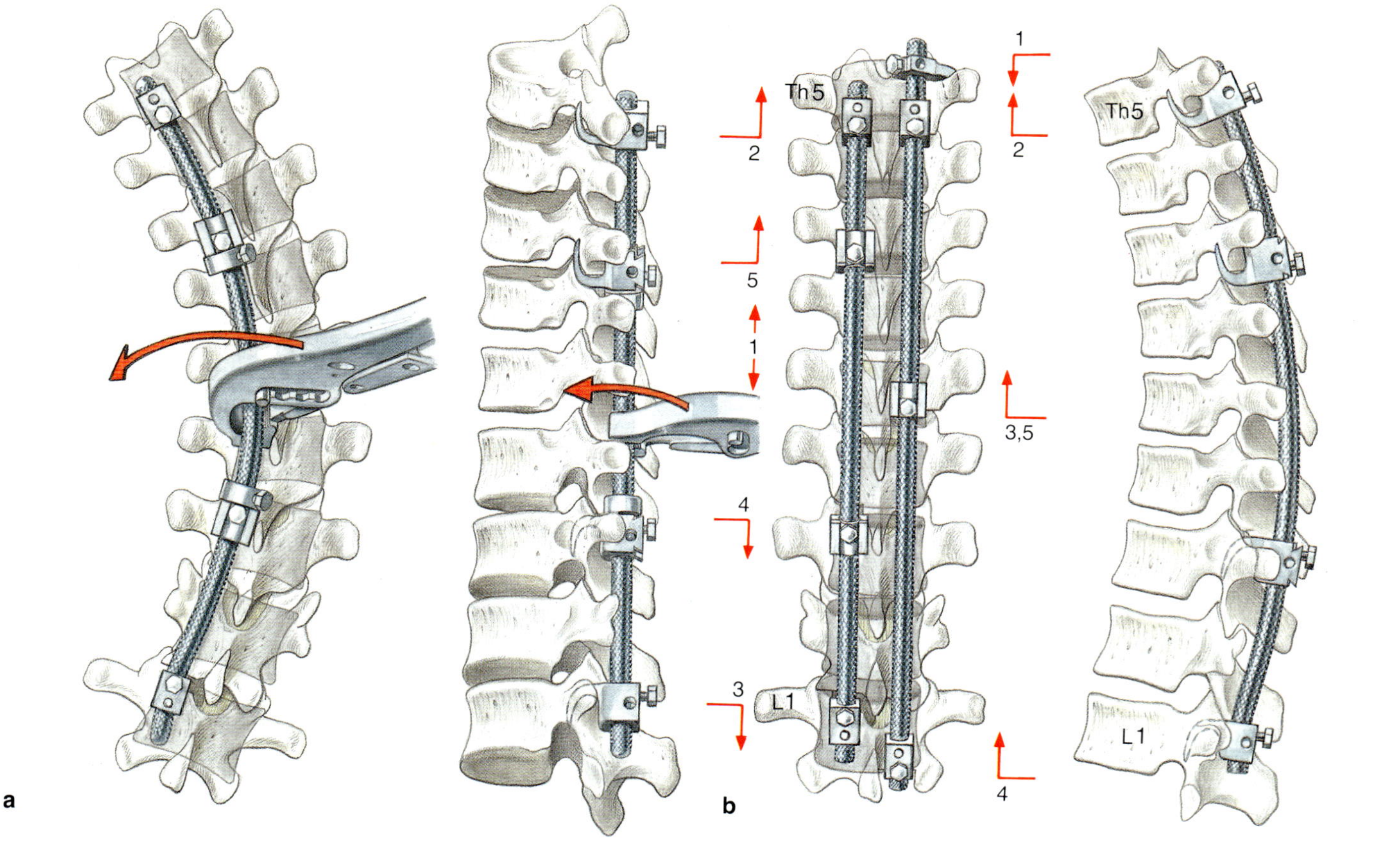

Fig. 2.**101** Mobile thoracic lordoscoliosis. Projection of the Cotrel rod in the frontal and sagittal planes *before* and *after* correction by derotation.

a Hook position corresponding to Fig. 2.**100**. The intermediate hooks are blocked by C-rings. The rod rotator is used to initiate the derotation (arrow).

b Status after correction of scoliosis by derotation. After derotation, the scoliosis is corrected by distraction in the area of the concave-side rod, in the order of 1 to 5. After this, the convex-side rod is introduced and corrected by compression, again in the order of 1 to 5.

Technique of Hook Fixation

Pedicular hooks (Figs. 2.**102**–2.**104**). The facet joint is partly opened. First, a square osteotomy of the inferior articular process is carried out 4 mm caudal to the line joining the inferior transverse process border. Perpendicularly to it, a longitudinal groove is produced at the boundary between the articular process and the lamina (transition point between convex and concave vertebral contours) and parallel to the spinous process.

A pedicle elevator is now inserted into the facet joint, parallel to the spinous process. The elastic resistance of the joint capsule is overcome until the pedicle's hard resistance is felt at the point of entry into the lamina. By raising or *lateral* translation of the tip of the instrument, the stability of the seat can be tested (beware of medial translation, which would risk neurologic complications). The pedicular hook is then driven in with a hammer, using a hook holder and the inserter. The spikes of the hook must be anchored in bone to the posterior part of the pedicle and must have good contact with the bone at the caudal articular process.

Thoracic laminar hook (Fig. 2.**105**). Small spreaders are placed between the spinous processes of two adjacent thoracic vertebrae. The ligamentum flavum is then resected near the midline, and medial portions of the caudal articular process of the lamina of the next higher vertebra are removed with a bone punch. The cranial border of the caudal vertebral arch is merely leveled off. The thoracic laminar hook is then inserted, and the spreader is removed.

Lumbar laminar hook. This is applied to the lamina from cranial or caudal, as required (compression or distraction) following retraction of the ligamentum flavum and narrow laminotomy with a punch (Harrington operation, p. 90).

Transverse hook (Fig. 2.**106**). A special instrument (the transverse-process elevator) is entered between the rib and the transverse process, dividing portions of the costotransverse ligament. Dissection close to the transverse process is indicated, since there may otherwise be bleeding from the posterior intercostal artery. The combination of pedicular and transverse hooks provides for a very stable fixation at the cranial end of the curvature.

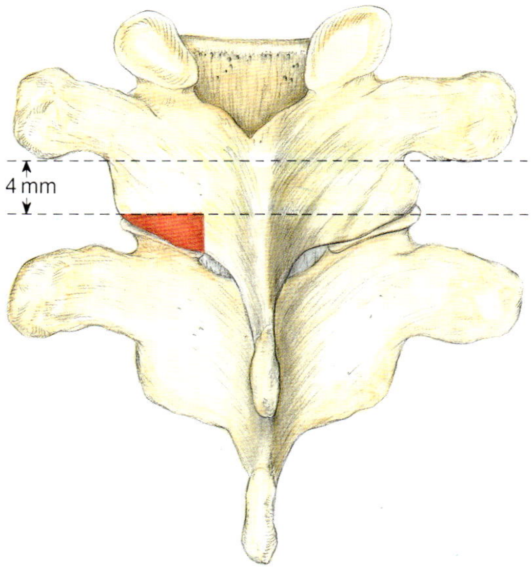

Fig. 2.**102** Fixation of the pedicular hook. The inferior articular process is partially resected by two perpendicular osteotomies.

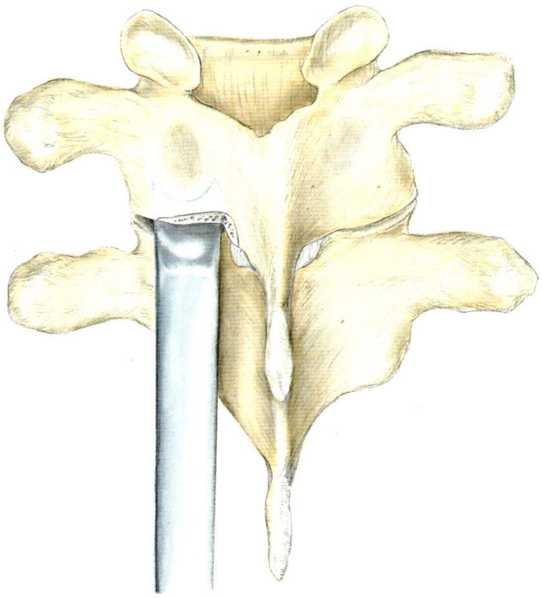

Fig. 2.**103** Fixation of the pedicular hook. After partial resection of the inferior articular process corresponding to Fig. 2.**102**, the pedicle elevator is inserted (Fig. 2.**95 f**).

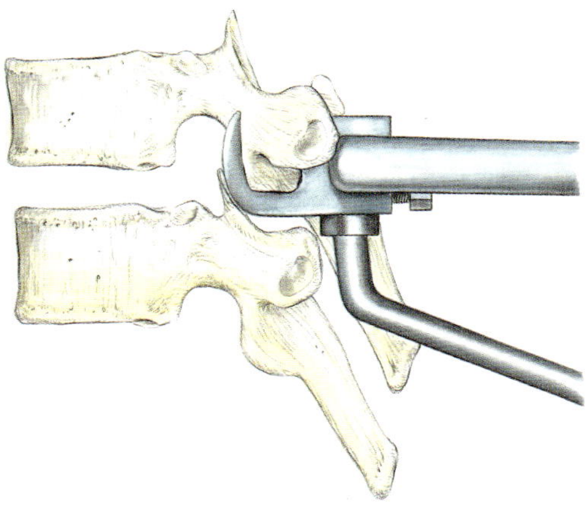

Fig. 2.**104** Fixation of the pedicular hook. After appropriate dissection, the pedicular hook is driven in with the hook inserter with the aid of the hook holder.

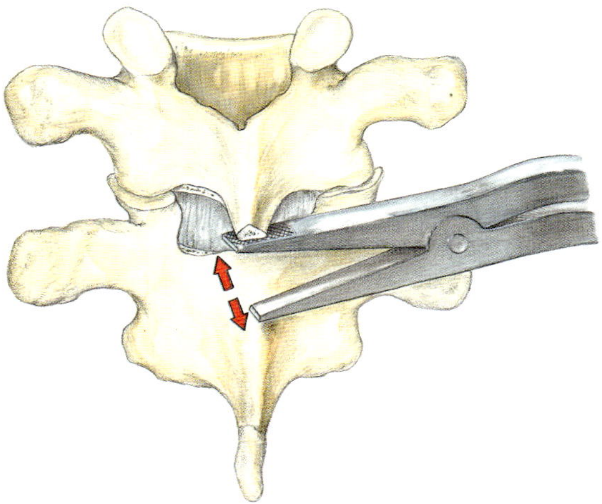

Fig. 2.**105** Fixation of the thoracic laminar hook.

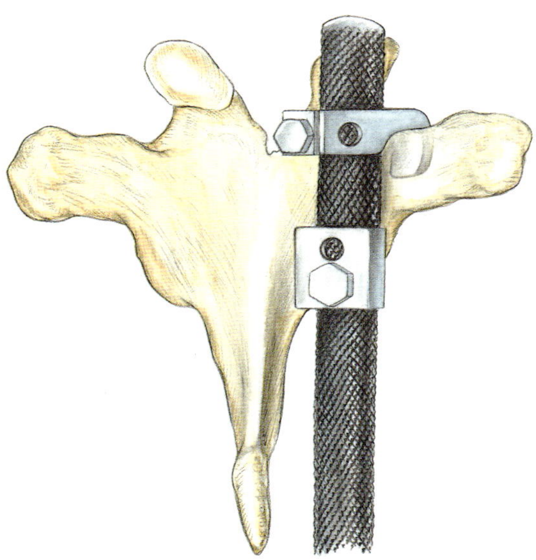

Fig. 2.**106** Preparation of a claw grip on the convex side of the cranial end vertebra by combination of pedicular and transverse hooks.

Bending of the Rod

After careful exposure of the spine (Fig. 2.**107**) and implantation of the hooks (Fig. 2.**108**), a flexible rod is manually bent according to the hook positions. It serves as a template for the bending of the implant. The rod should be continuously bent in numerous small steps, using the bending device and avoiding any sharp kinking. The utmost importance should be attached to producing a physiological curvature in the sagittal plane postoperatively (Fig. 2.**101**). To avoid bending of the rod in the wrong plane, a C-ring is temporarily attached to one end of the rod as a rotation marker.

Decortication

When all the hooks have been implanted and the concave rod has been appropriately bent, a typical decortication of the posterior vertebral elements (spinous process, lamina, transverse process) is performed (Harrington operation, pp. 80–96). The decortication is essentially carried out at sites that are no longer accessible after the instrumentation. This prevents hemorrhages. The spinous processes are left intact to ensure a normal posterior configuration. In vertebrae not fitted with hooks, the facet joints are debrided. The previously harvested cancellous bone chips are then packed at the sites that are no longer accessible after insertion of the concave rod. The facet joints on the convex side (watch the hook position!) are also debrided.

Insertion of the Concave Rod
(Fig. 2.**109**)

The rod is fitted with two oppositely-placed cleats for the open intermediate hooks. The rod is then seized with the rod holder and is first inserted through the cranial hook with rotary movements. This is made easier if the convexity of the rod is first directed anteriorly. After this, the rod is turned according to the spinal curvature, introduced into the intermediate hooks fitted with hook holders and advanced into the inferior end-vertebra hook. Insertion into the lower intermediate hook, in particular, may be difficult. In this case, use can be made of the special hook clamp with an impactor (Fig. 2.**97**).

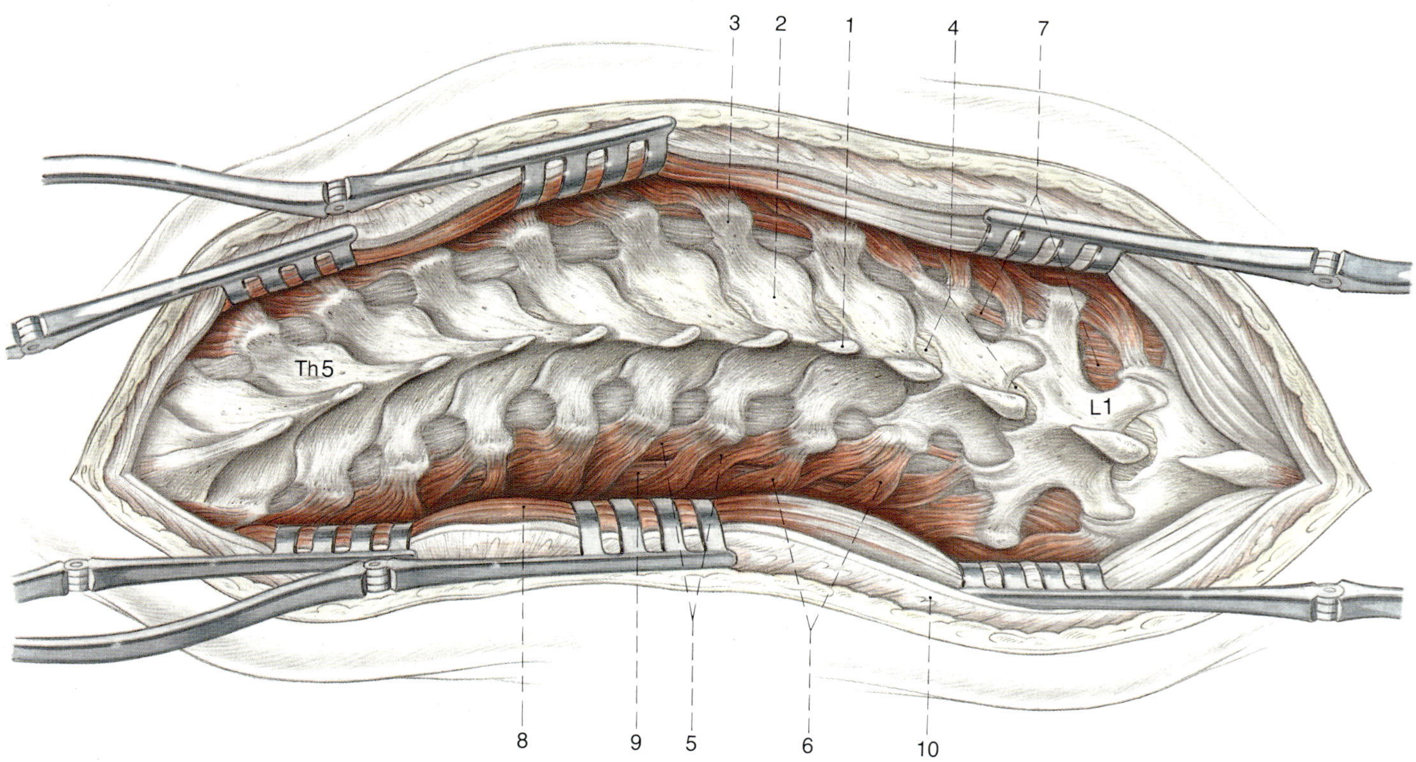

Fig. 2.**107** Exposure of the posterior vertebral elements of a right-convex thoracic lordoscoliosis. Owing to vertebral torsion, the spinous processes at the apex of the curve deviate toward the concave side.

1 Spinous process
2 Lamina of vertebral arch
3 Transverse process
4 Ligamenta flava
5 Rotator muscle
6 Multifidus muscles
7 Intertransverse muscles
8 Longissimus muscle
9 Spinal muscle
10 Thoracolumbar fascia

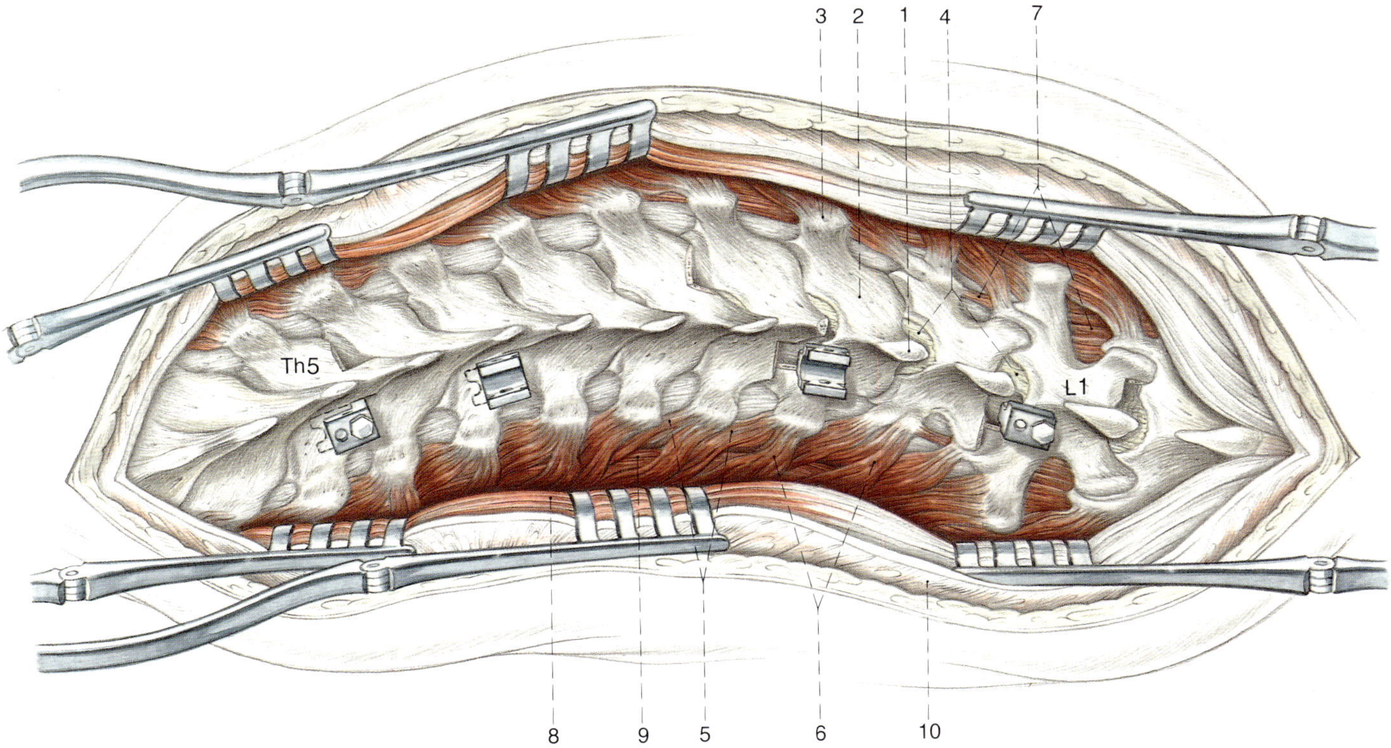

Fig. 2.**108** Dissection of hook placement corresponding to the working diagram (Fig. 2.**100**). The hooks for the concave side have been placed.

1 Spinous process
2 Lamina of the vertebral arch
3 Transverse process
4 Ligamenta flava
5 Rotator muscles
6 Multifidus muscles
7 Intertransverse muscles
8 Longissimus muscle
9 Spinal muscle
10 Thoracolumbar fascia

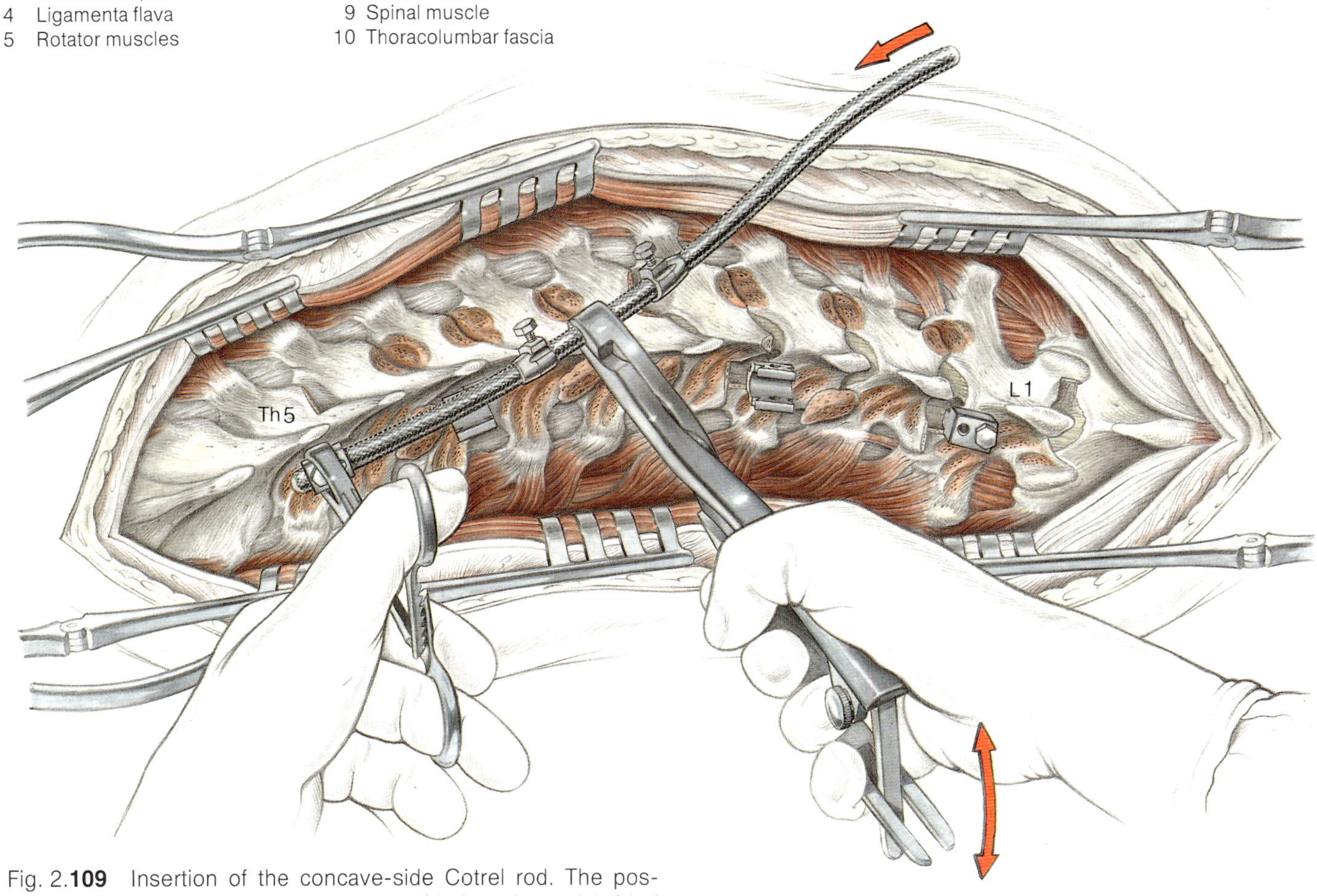

Fig. 2.**109** Insertion of the concave-side Cotrel rod. The posterior vertebral elements on the concave side have been debrided and the facet joints resected on both sides.

Correction by Derotation

First, the intermediate hooks are blocked with C-rings (Fig. 2.**110**). The screws of the C-rings should first be seated on the convex side, since they will otherwise be inaccessible after derotation. Using the rod rotator, the derotation is then carried out, with slow, cautious movements. (Note: derotation produces elongation and may therefore loosen the hook seat. The hooks then have to be driven in once again before derotation can continue.) The rotation should amount to 90 degrees, if possible. After completion of the derotation, the implanted rod appears straight in the frontal plane (Fig. 2.**111**). On the other hand, appropriate bending of the rod should produce a physiological kyphosis in the sagittal plane. The hooks are then provisionally fixed with the aid of the screws, and the C-rings are removed. Another correction is obtained by distraction of the hooks in the order shown in Figure 2.**101b**. The intermediate hooks are distracted first. After distraction of the end hooks, the intermediate hooks have to be readjusted.

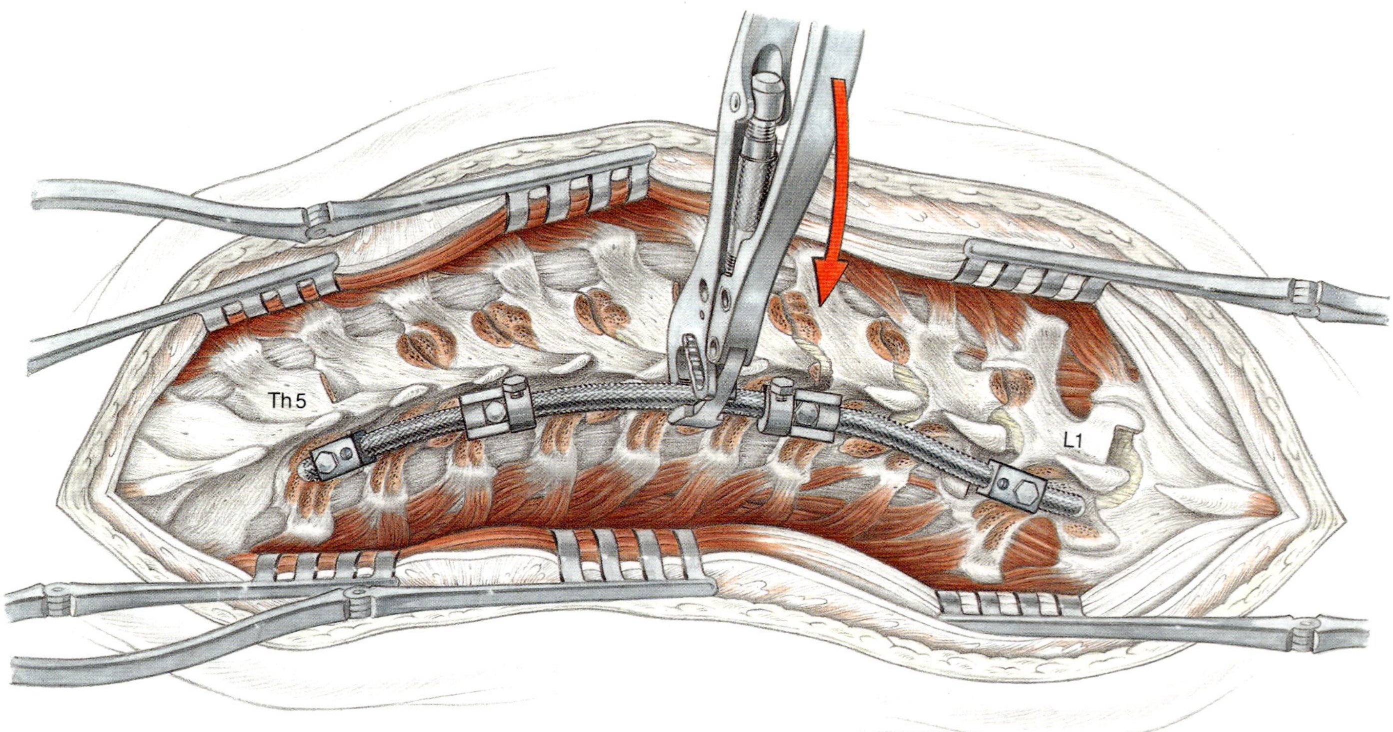

Fig. 2.**110** Correction of thoracic lordoscoliosis by derotation.

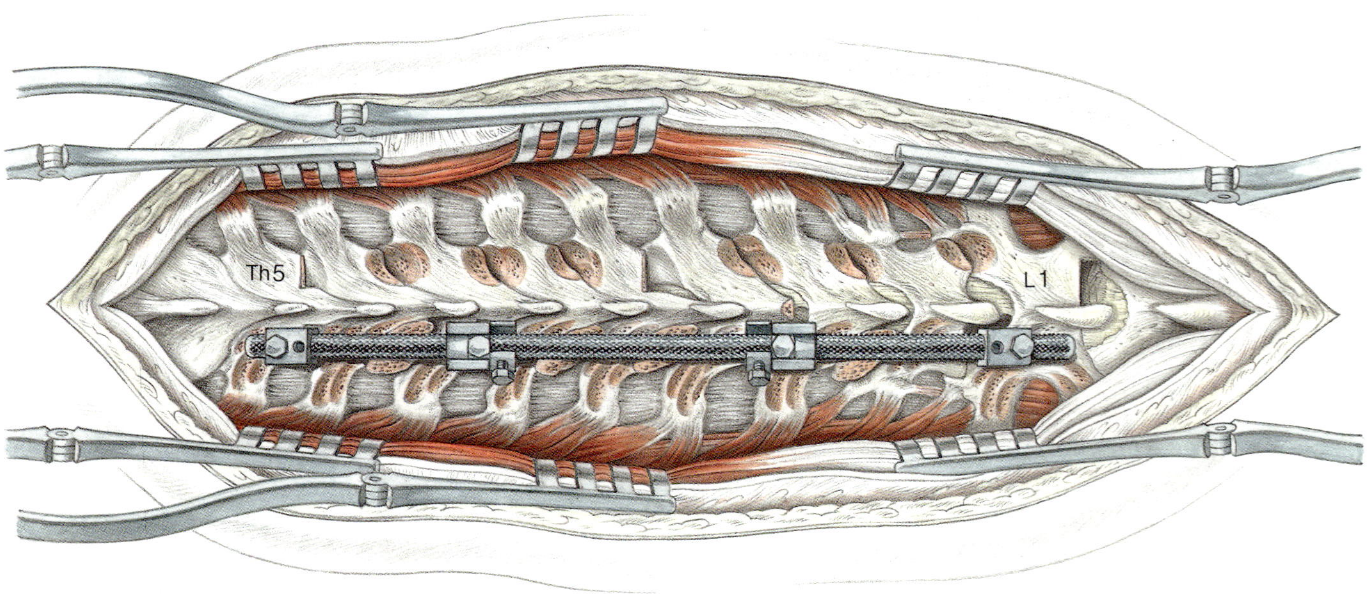

Fig. 2.**111** After derotation, the scoliosis curvature has been transformed into a physiological thoracic kyphosis. Seen from the top, the appropriately bent Cotrel rod now appears straight (cf. Fig. 2.**101**). The rod position is fixed by provisional tightening of the hook screws. Another correction is then performed by distraction as in Fig. 2.**101**. The distraction is carried out as shown in Fig. 2.**98**.

Introduction of the Convex Rod

(Fig. 2.**112**)

The rod on the convex side is bent appreciably less than the one on the concave side and contributes to the derotation by exerting pressure on the posterior vertebral elements. A typical decortication of the posterior vertebral elements is now carried out on the convex side. The convex-sided hooks are inserted. The Cotrel rod is once again inserted, first through the proximal hooks, then into the open pedicular hook at the apical vertebra, and finally into the lumbar laminar hook with appropriate displacement.

The correction on the convex side is effected by compression, following the sequence shown in Figure 2.**101 b**. First, the transverse hooks and pedicular hooks are approximated at the cranial end vertebra by means of special compression forceps, so that the end vertebra is fixed in a stable grip (Fig. 2.**106**). The pedicular hook at the apical vertebra is then placed under compression, followed by the laminar hook at the inferior end vertebra.

Note

If the convex-sided laminar hook at the inferior end vertebra is not well seated, the complication of a hook dislocation may develop in the postoperative phase. If there is any doubt as to its stability, a kind of claw grip can also be set up at the lower end of the instrumentation by implanting a caudally-aligned laminar hook in the next higher vertebra.

Since compression of the caudal laminar hook leads to loosening of the hook at the apical vertebra, this has to be corrected by compression at the end. During the process of compression (Fig. 2.**98**), the hook screws should be opened and subsequently fixed once again.

Once the final correction has been accomplished, the hook screws are maximally tightened and finally stripped. Decortication is continued in the areas not covered by implants. As large an amount of additional bone graft as possible is then applied at the proposed fusion site.

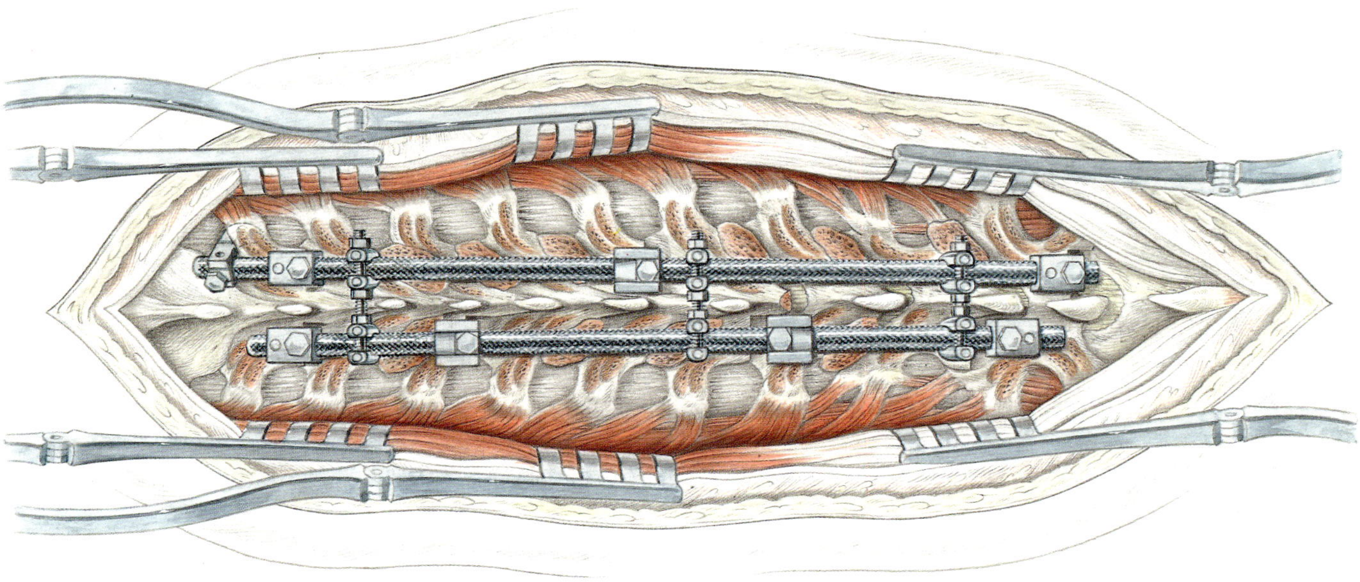

Fig. 2.**112** Status after fixation of both Cotrel rods and the DTTs. With thoracic lordoscoliosis, the spinous processes are not resected, so that a better cosmetic appearance can be obtained for the back.

Introduction of the DTT

The concave and convex-sided Cotrel rods are linked by the DTT system, creating a stable frame construction. At least two DTTs are applied, one as closely as possible below the hooks at the superior end vertebra, and a second one as closely as possible above the hooks at the inferior end vertebra. For longer instrumentation systems, several DTTs are used (about one DTT per 15 cm; Fig. 2.**113**). It is advisable to record somatosensory evoked potentials while carrying out the operation. After completion of the correction a Vauzelle–Stagnara wake-up test should be performed.

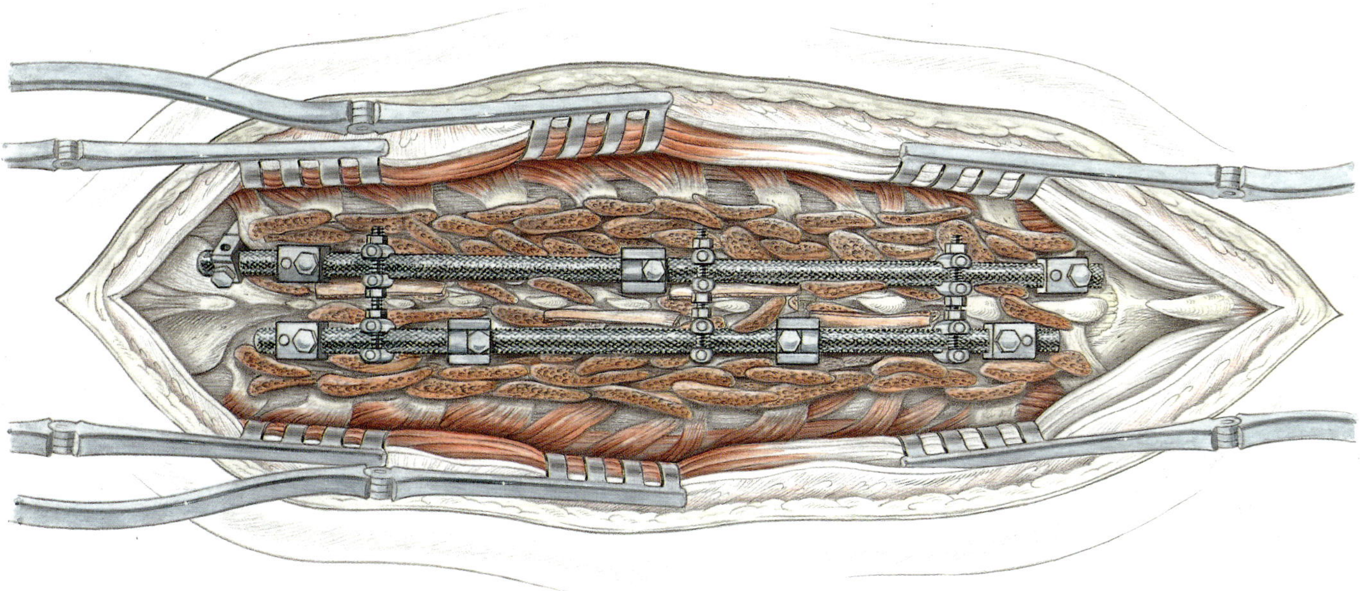

Fig. 2.**113** Status after implantation of bone chips in the area of fusion. Firm inclusion of the two end vertebrae in the fusion is important.

Rigid Thoracic or Thoracolumbar Scoliosis

(Fig. 2.**114**)

Correction by derotation alone is not possible. In this situation, correction is achieved by using two distraction rods on the concave side, with substantially the same hook positioning.

To begin with, a short rod (about 6–8 cm) is placed in the intermediate hooks, and then a long rod is fixed in the hooks of the end vertebrae. Distraction is now applied in the area of both rods, after which two DTTs are introduced to approximate the two rods. This maneuver not only corrects the scoliosis, but also determines the extent of the kyphosis or lordosis. Bending the long rod and rotating it into the appropriate plane increases the distance between the two rods and consequently enhances the extent of the possible correction. The convex rod is inserted in the usual way and placed under compression (mobile thoracic lordo-scoliosis, p. 141).

Multistage procedure. With very severe curves, notably in adult patients, the operation may have to be carried out in several stages. In the first session, a mobilizing osteotomy is performed in the usual way in the apical zone of the curvature, with excision of the facet joints (mobilizing osteotomy, p. 104).

After this, the intermediate hooks are inserted. In some circumstances, a short distraction rod can be introduced even now. After a traction phase of 2–3 weeks, the instrumentation is then completed as described above.

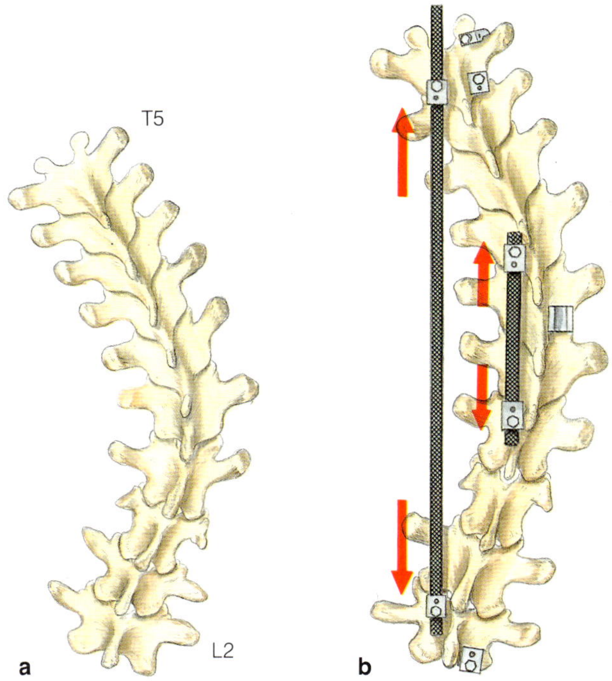

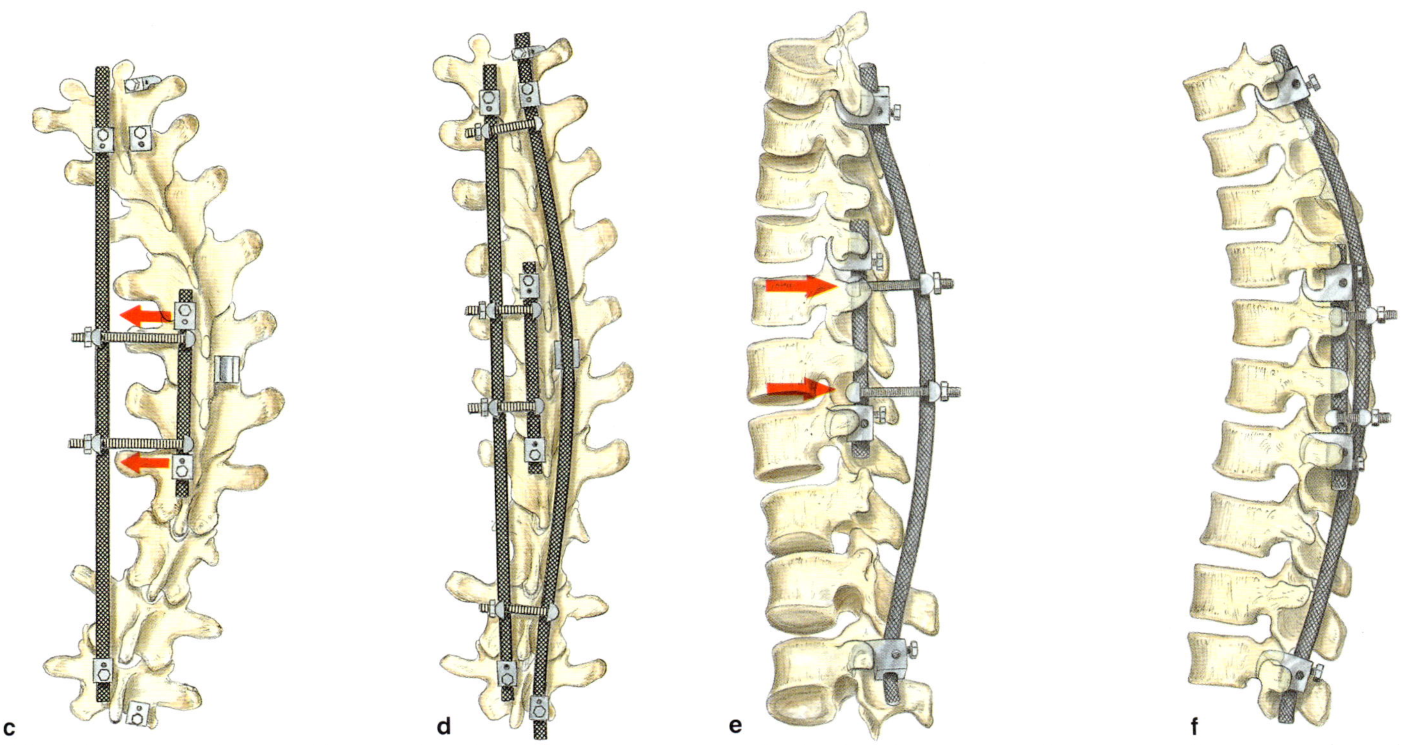

Fig. 2.**114** Correction of a rigid thoracic scoliosis.
a Initial status.
b Insertion of two rods.
c Approximation of the long distraction rod by the short one, using a DTT.
d Final status after insertion of the convex-side compression rod.
e, f Modification of lordosis, depending on the bending of the long distraction rod.

Mobile Double Curve

(Fig. 2.**115**)

Since the hooks on the CD rod can be fixed in any direction and position, it is possible, in principle, to exert both compression and distraction on the same rod. The scoliosis is instrumented with hooks in accordance with the criteria set forth above. The initially inserted rod is first bent into an S-shape in conformity with the scoliosis. As a result of a 90-degree derotation, the rod appears straight in the frontal plane. In the sagittal plane, a physiological thoracic kyphosis and lumbar lordosis are produced.

Rigid Double Curve

A rigid double curve can, in principle, be corrected with the CD instrumentation by the distraction method. The curves need to be individually instrumented using four rods, which are eventually linked. In this case, however, a two-stage procedure is recommended:

1. Correction of caudal curvature using VDS by the anterior approach.
2. Correction of cranial curvature with CD instrumentation by the posterior approach, the caudal curve being included in the fusion for reasons of stability (Fig. 2.**146**).

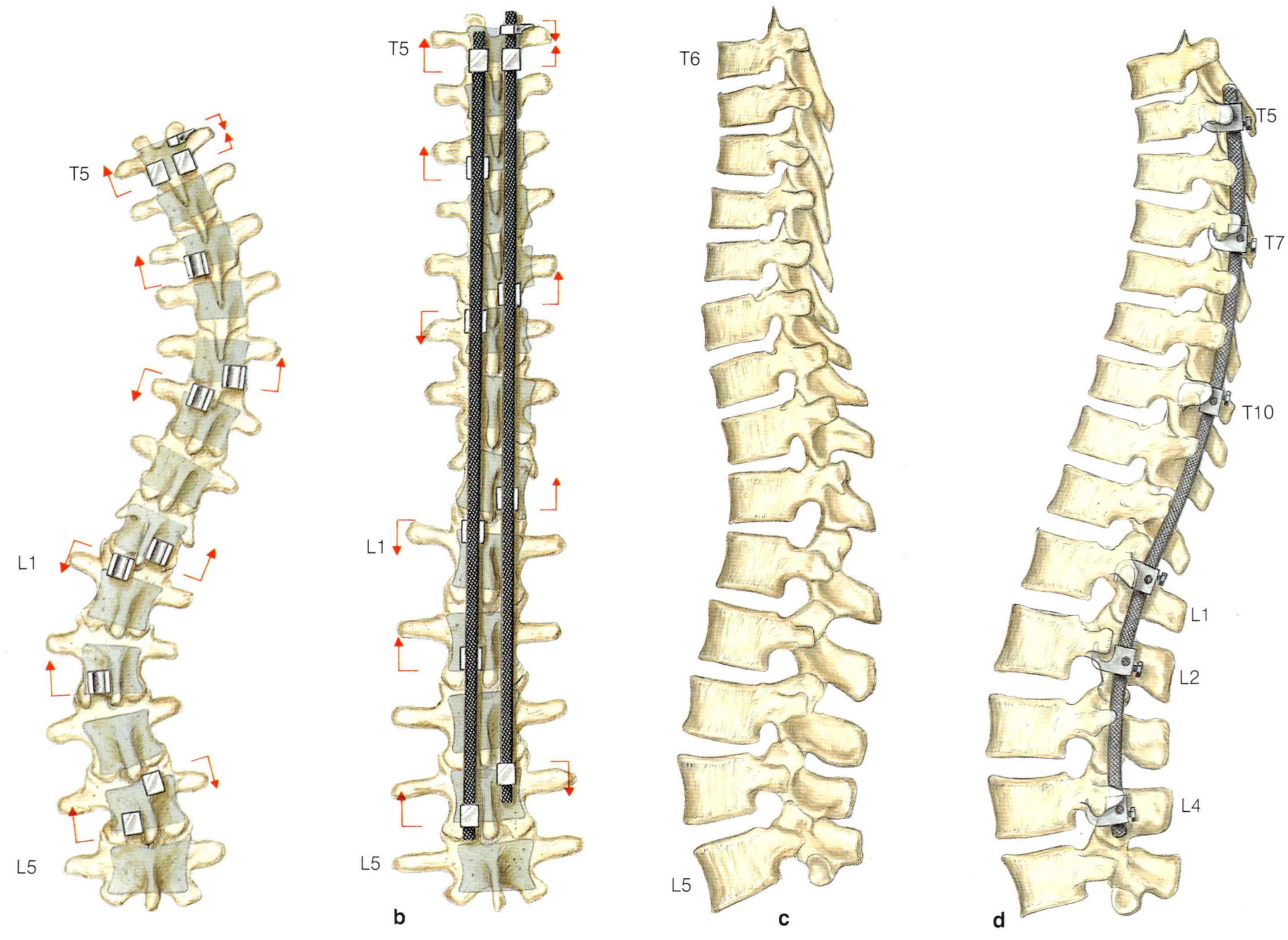

Fig. 2.**115** Mobile double curve.
a Initial status.
b Status after correction in the frontal plane. The rods appear straight in this plane.
c, d Thoracic kyphosis and lumbar lordosis are restored by rotating the S-shaped rod.

Lumbar Kyphoscoliosis

(Fig. 2.**116**)

In many cases, there are two apical vertebrae (L2 and L3) that exhibit a marked kyphotic component. In this situation, the facet joints should be resected bilaterally. The two apical vertebrae are instrumented for compression, to assist lordosis by shortening of the dorsal elements.

In this situation, the rod on the convex side is introduced, and an initial compression is effected in the apical region. The rod is then rotated to the convex side, which at the same time leads to correction of the scoliosis and kyphosis. The concave rod is placed under a distraction load. In the area of the apical vertebrae, hooks as well as pedicular screws can be used on the convex side.

Wound Closure

The wound is closed in two layers by suturing the musculature of the back and the overlying fascia. In children and adolescents, the divided spinous process apophyses are readily united by sutures.

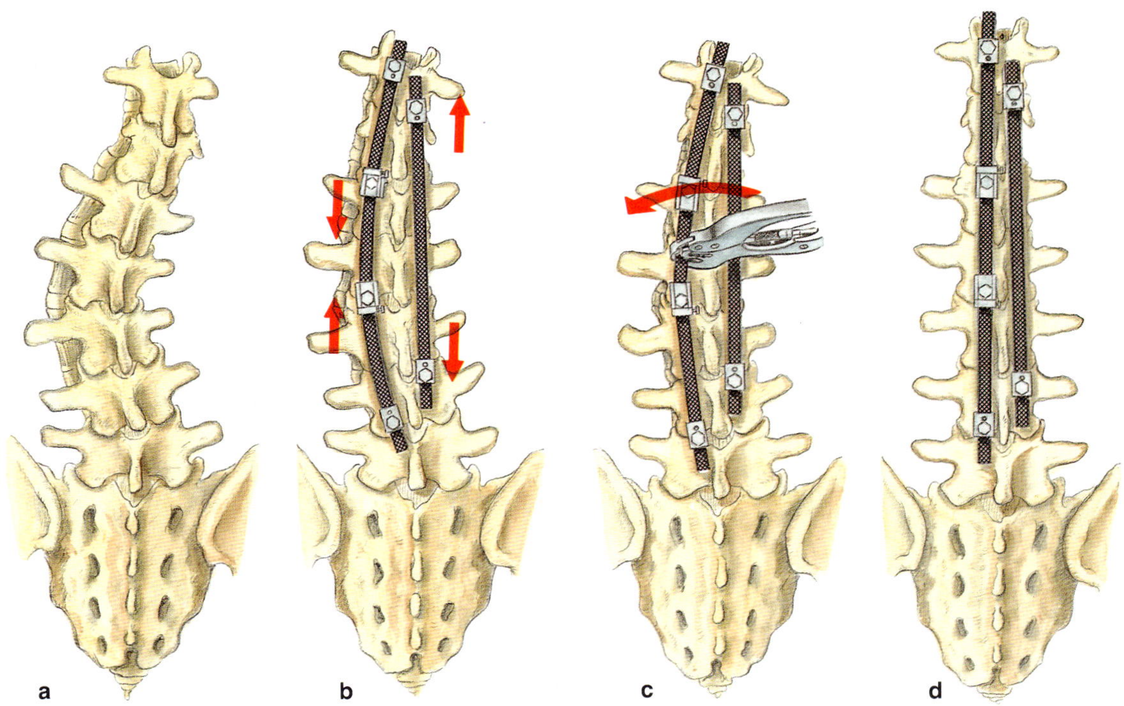

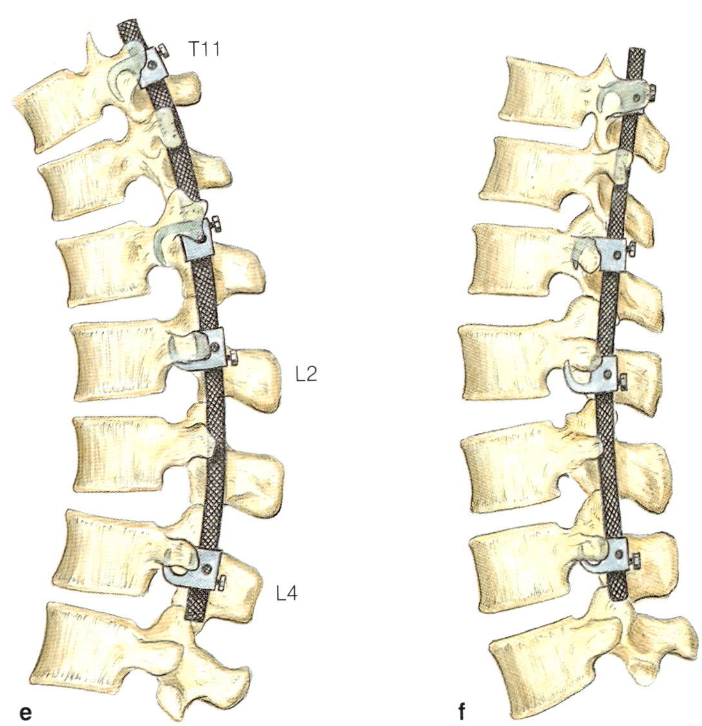

Fig. 2.**116** Lumbar kyphoscoliosis.
a Initial status.
b Distraction on the concave side, compression on the convex side.
c Correction of scoliosis and kyphosis by rotating the rod toward the convex side.
d Final status after correction in the frontal plane.
e, f Correction of the kyphotic deformity in the sagittal plane.

Postoperative Treatment

The patient is generally positioned in bed without any external fixation. Immediately after the operation, patients are taken to the intensive care unit, where the necessary diagnostic and therapeutic measures are carried out. Neurologic monitoring is initiated immediately after the operation; movement of the extremities is assessed at 15-minute intervals at first, and at hourly intervals later on. The patient is mobilized 3–7 days after the operation and is discharged after removal of the sutures.

As a rule, postoperative management does not require the wearing of a brace; physical activity should be restricted until ossification of the fusion is complete (about nine months after the operation). Prescription of a spinal orthosis should be considered for unreliable or uncooperative patients.

Pitfalls and Complications

The specific risk in the operation lies in neurological complications (Report of the American Scoliosis Research Society, 1987):

- Spinal cord lesions (0.6%)
- Peripheral lesions
- Hyperesthesia.

With the Cotrel–Dubousset operative technique, the total neurological risk amounts to 1.47%.

The most common causes of neurologic complications are radicular lesions due to improper use of the pedicular elevator, or wrong fixation of the pedicular hook; direct spinal-cord contusion; medial displacement of hooks during derotation; faulty positioning of hooks (e.g., fixation of a hook at the kyphotic apex; distraction in the area of kyphosis, etc.).

Alternative Methods

Harrington, Luque, Dwyer and VDS operations (the latter methods may be considered especially for thoracolumbar and lumbar scolioses).

Further Reading

Bauer R, Mostegl A, Hingsammer R. Cotrel–Dubousset (CD) instrumentation for the correction of spinal curvature. Arch Orthop Traum Surg 1988;107:364.

Cotrel Y, Dubousset J. Nouvelle technique d'ostéosynthèse rachidienne segmentaire par voie postérieure. Rev Chir Orthop 1984a;70:489.

Cotrel Y, Dubousset J. New segmental posterior instrumentation of the spine. 19th Annual Meeting of the American Scoliosis Research Society, Orlando, Florida, September 1984b.

Dubousset J, Graf H, Miladi L, Cotrel Y. Spinal and thoracic derotation with CD instrumentation. 20th Annual Meeting of the American Scoliosis Research Society, San Diego, California, September 1985.

Dubousset J, Cotrel Y. Die CD-Instrumentation in der Behandlung von Wirbelsäulendeformitäten. Orthopäde 1989;18:118.

Anterior Scoliosis Operations

Mobilizing Anterior Osteotomy

Indications

Severe kyphosis or kyphoscoliosis of varied etiology, with marked structural alterations or synostoses in the region of the vertebrae.

Approach

It is necessary to plan an anterior approach to the spine dependent on the location of the deformity. As a rule, a thoracotomy or thoracophrenolumbotomy is required.

See Chapter 1, p. 13, and p. 24, ff.

Choice of side of approach. In simple kyphosis, the anatomical conditions determine the choice between a right-sided thoracotomy and a left-sided thoracophrenolumbotomy. In scoliosis or kyphoscoliosis, the approach is made from the side of the convexity.

Operative Technique

Conventional anterior mobilizing osteotomy for structural alterations has to be distinguished technically from those performed in cases of congenital deformities (such as an anterior unsegmented bar, for example).

The parietal pleura is divided longitudinally over the corresponding vertebrae, and the segmental vessels are ligated and transected in the usual way. The dissection may prove relatively difficult in some circumstances, since the segmental vessels are crowded into a narrow space in patients with severe kyphosis. The intervertebral disks in the target area are now exposed over their entire circumference. The intervertebral disks at the apex of the curve are resected; vertebral synostoses are osteotomized (Figs. 2.**117**–2.**120**).

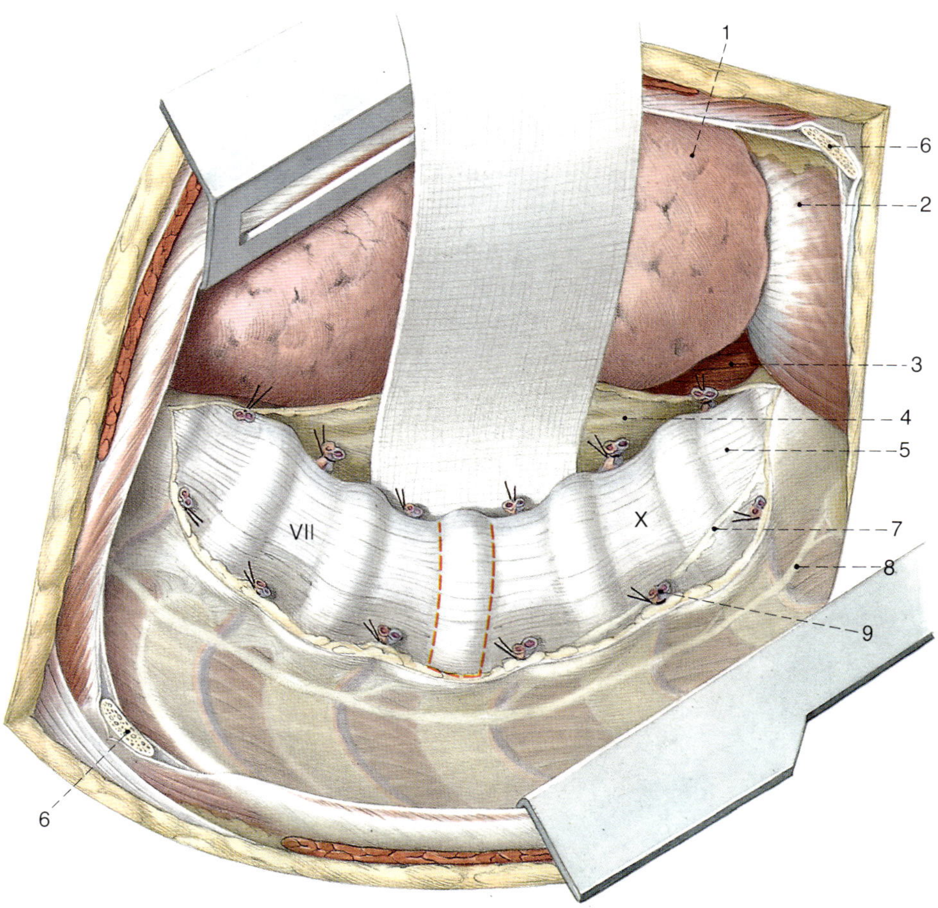

Fig. 2.**117** Status after right-sided thoracotomy. The intervertebral disks are first excised at the apex of the deformity (dashed line).

1 Right lung
2 Thoracic diaphragm
3 Esophagus
4 Parietal pleura
5 Anterior longitudinal ligament
6 6th rib
7 Greater splanchnic nerve
8 Sympathetic trunk
9 Intercostal vessels
VII–X Thoracic vertebrae

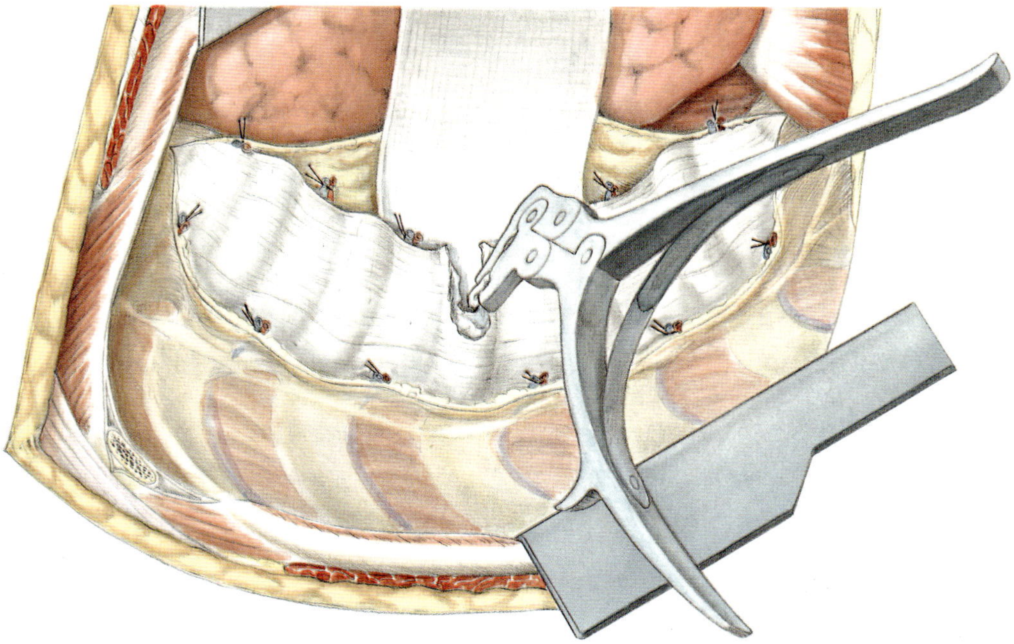

Fig. 2.**118** Removal of intervertebral disks with pituitary forceps as far as the posterior longitudinal ligament.

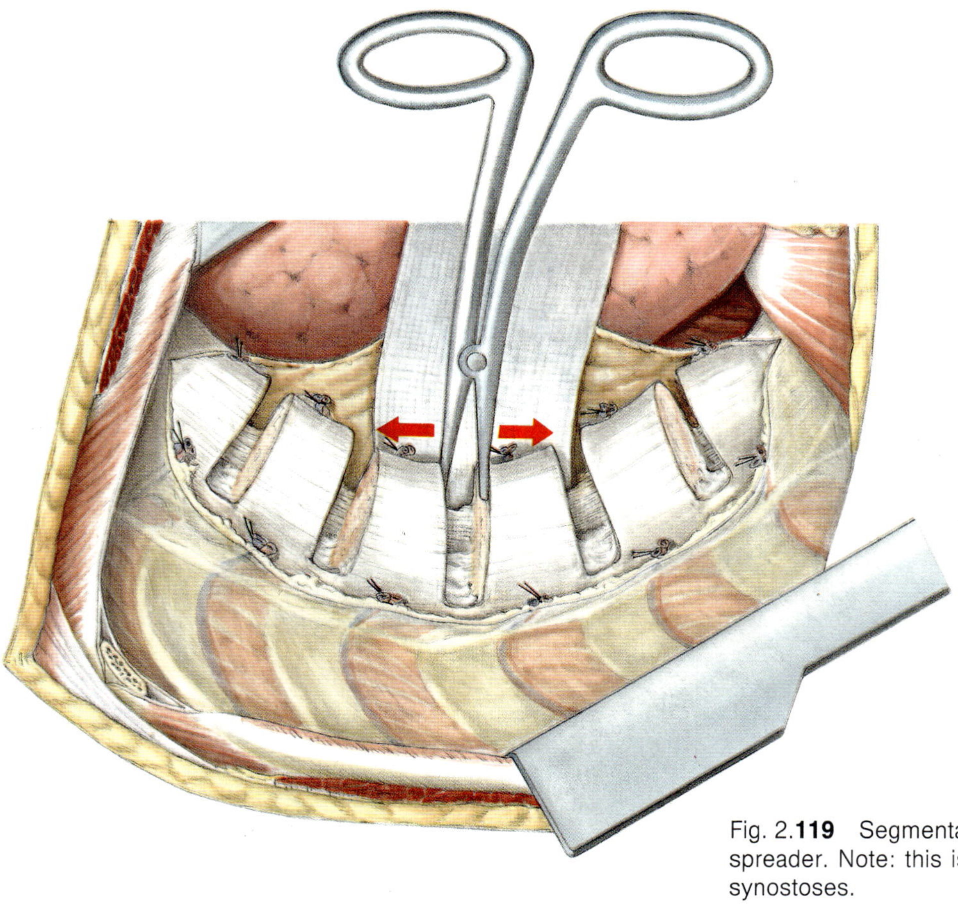

Fig. 2.**119** Segmental mobility is tested with the osteotomy spreader. Note: this is not possible in the presence of posterior synostoses.

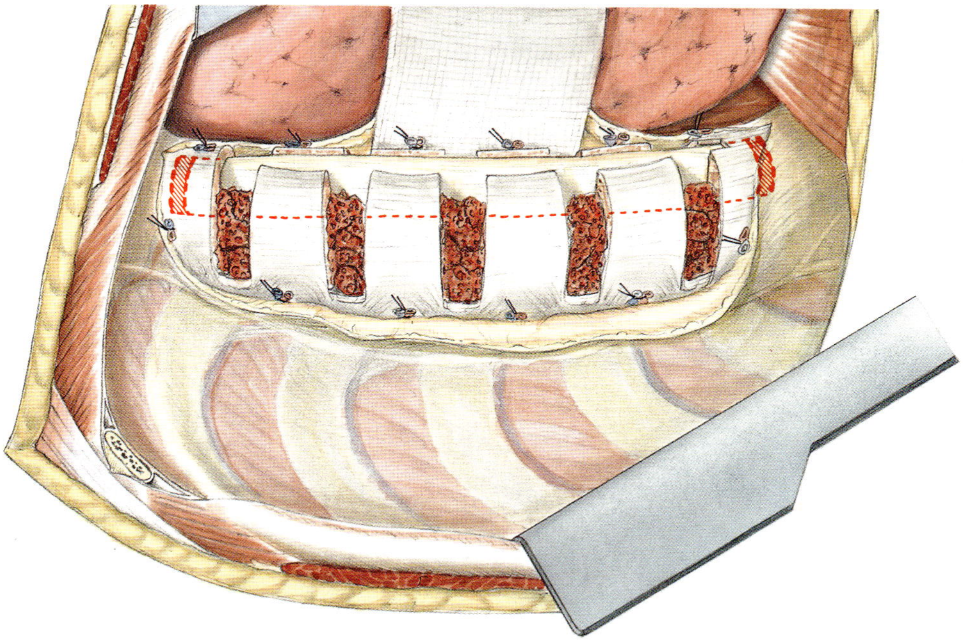

Fig. 2.**120** For preparation of spinal fusion, bone chips are inserted into the intervertebral disk spaces. Alternatively, a sliding graft can be placed in an anterior groove; this will not interfere with further correction.

Special Features of Osteotomy for Anterior Segmentation Failures

(Figs. 2.**121**–2.**122**)

Osteotomy should be performed only if a bony bridge exists anteriorly and intervertebral disk tissue remains at the corresponding levels posteriorly. The osteotomy is always carried out in the direction of the intervertebral disk tissue. After ablation of the anterior bone tissue, the remaining intervertebral disks are removed as far as the posterior longitudinal ligament. In order to achieve an effective correction, it is advisable to resect at least one normal intervertebral disk each, cranial and caudal to the kyphotic area.

The degree of mobility achieved can be tested segmentally by applying a laminar spreader; this is valid only in the absence of any posterior synostoses.

To avoid the need for another intervention after the completed correction, the anterior fusion can be prepared in such a way as not to obstruct any further correction:

- Bone chips are loosely packed into the intervertebral spaces.
- A sliding bone graft is inserted (Fig. 2.**120**).
- A bone graft is introduced into a cavity at the end vertebra, or into a groove in the apical vertebrae (rib, corticocancellous tibial chips, fibula).

In the presence of a concomitant posterior fusion or synostosis, an osteotomy of the posterior vertebral elements at the appropriate levels has to be performed in a second operation.

These mobilizing osteotomies, possibly both anterior and posterior, are followed by an external correction using halo traction (p. 74). Once the desired correction has been accomplished, a posterior spinal fusion is carried out (using the Harrington, Luque or Cotrel–Dubousset techniques, for example).

Wound Closure

See under thoracotomy or thoracophrenolumbotomy, pp. 22, 35.

Pitfalls and Complications

Complications of thoracic surgery, such as pneumothorax, hemothorax, and lung atelectases, may occur. It should be pointed out that mobilizing osteotomies are associated with a high neurologic risk, particularly in patients with congenital deformities.

Further Reading

See p. 155.

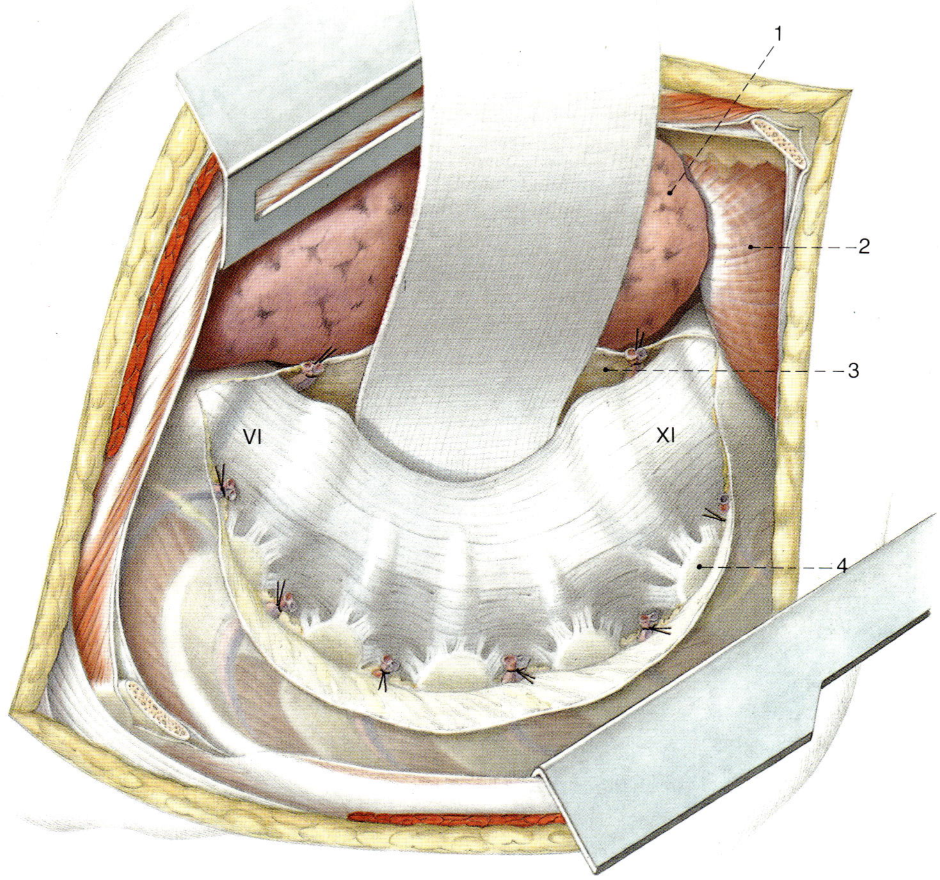

1 Right lung
2 Thoracic diaphragm
3 Parietal pleura
4 Radiate ligament of head of rib
VI–XI Thoracic vertebrae

Fig. 2.**121** Mobilizing osteotomy in anterior failure of segmentation; right-sided thoracotomy. The posterior intervertebral disk remnants are visible at the apex of the kyphosis.

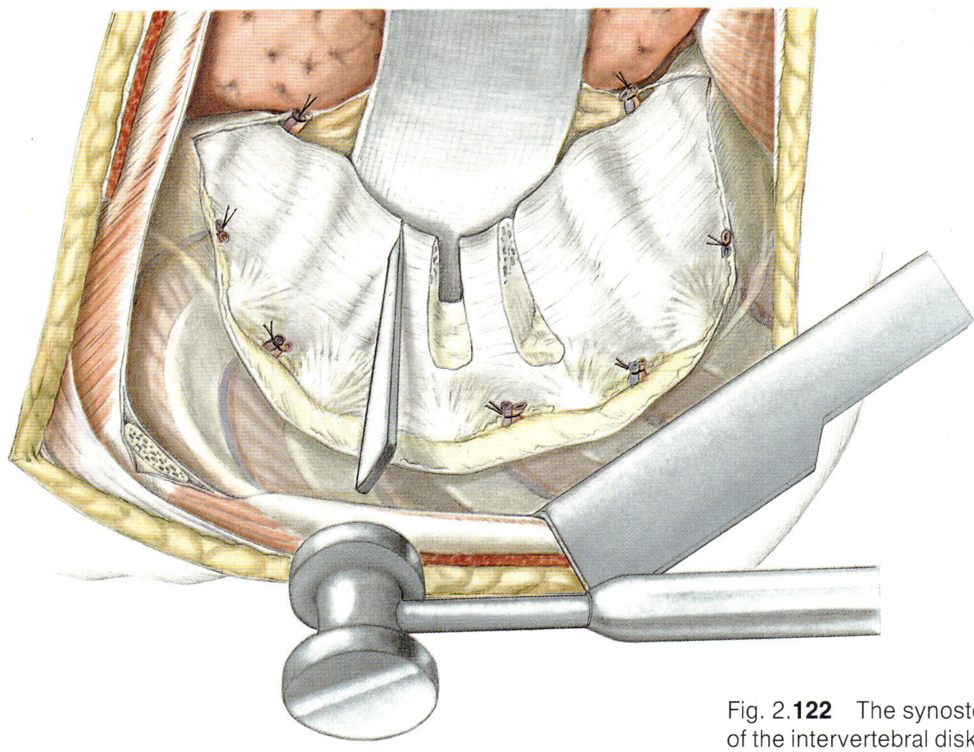

Fig. 2.**122** The synostosis is transected with a chisel at the level of the intervertebral disks.

Resection of Hemivertebrae, Wedge Resection

Indication

Congenital scoliosis with marked progression and spinal decompensation (see also Scoliosis Operations in Children, p. 97).

Approach

This depends on the location of the hemivertebra:

- Thoracic region: thoracotomy (Chapter 1, pp. 13–23).
- Thoracolumbar junction: transthoracic, retroperitoneal approach according to Hodgson (Chapter 1, pp. 24–36).
- Lumbar spine: retroperitoneal approach (Chapter 1, pp. 42–45).
- Lumbosacral: possibly transperitoneal approach (Chapter 1, pp. 52–55).

The operation is completed in a second session from the posterior aspect by removing the corresponding posterior vertebral elements. Here the approach is made via a midline incision. Its length depends on the scope of the posterior fusion and possible spinal instrumentation.

Operative Technique

(Figs. 2.**123**–2.**128**)

Resection of Hemivertebra

With a thoracic hemivertebra, the rib corresponding to the hemivertebra is resected in the course of a thoracotomy.

From this rib, access to the hemivertebra is achieved. The approach has to be made from the convexity of the hemivertebra. A chest spreader is introduced, the parietal pleura is longitudinally divided, and the segmental vessels are ligated, after which the hemivertebra is identified. To begin with, the cranially and caudally situated intervertebral disks are completely removed in the usual way, with the aid of bone rongeurs; only the posterior and medial portions of the annulus fibrosus are left in place. The anterior portion of the hemivertebra is then resected with bone rongeurs, curets, or a gouge. Finally, the posterior cortex of the hemivertebra is removed with a bone punch.

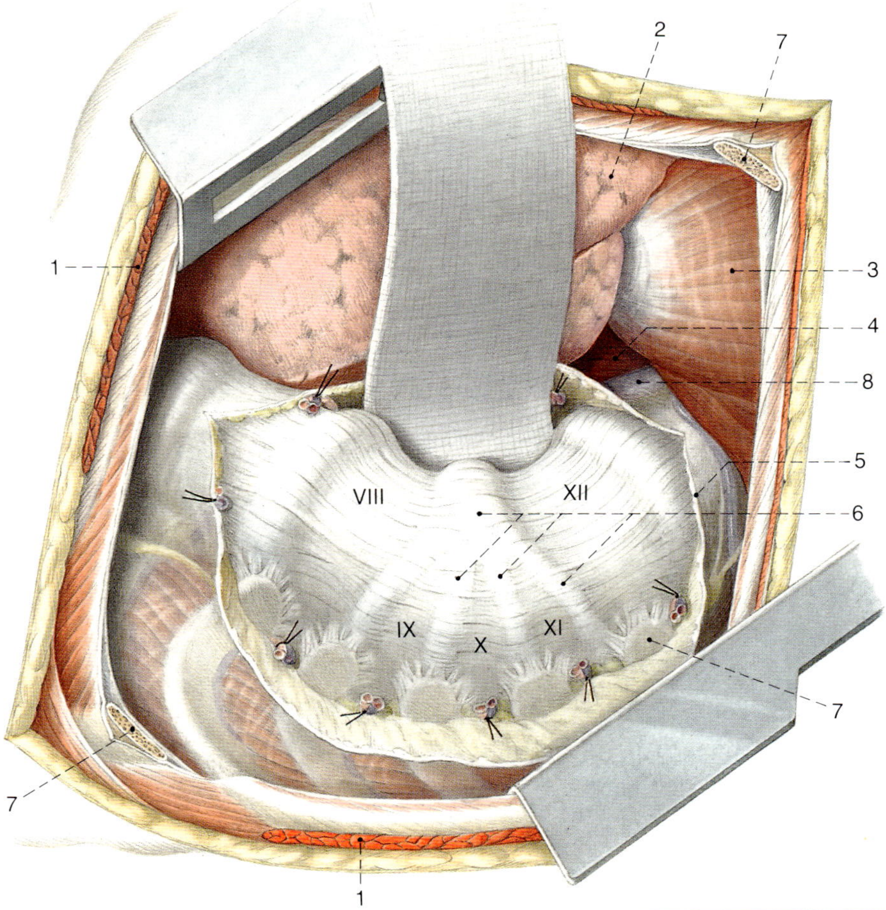

Fig. 2.**123** Wedge resection. Status after right-sided thoracotomy and opening of the parietal pleura. Three hemivertebrae lying within the same curve can be seen.

1 External oblique muscle of the abdomen
2 Right lung
3 Thoracic diaphragm
4 Esophagus
5 Parietal pleura
6 Intervertebral disks
7 Radiate ligament of the head of the rib
8 Azygos vein
VIII–XII Thoracic vertebrae

Together with the vertebral body, the posterior parts of the annulus of the adjacent intervertebral disks are removed. This may lead to massive bleeding from the epidural veins that is difficult to stop. The base of the pedicle is then removed as far in the posterior direction as possible, in order to facilitate posterior removal of the corresponding vertebral parts in a second session. Annulus fibrosus tissue at the apex of the scoliosis (confluence of the two intervertebral disks) can be left in place. This may serve as a stabilizer or as a hinge joint in the subsequent closure of the excision site that is carried out from the posterior side.

Posterior procedure. In a second session, the posterior elements of the hemivertebra are resected via a midline incision.

Hemivertebra resection should always be combined with spinal fusion; mere resection of a hemivertebra without added fusion will not produce the desired result. The extent to which the spine needs to be exposed therefore depends on the length of the proposed posterior vertebral fusion, or on whether or not the fusion is performed with instrumentation (e.g., Harrington). First of all, the posterior portion of the hemivertebra is identified, possibly with the aid of radiography. Then the lamina, the articular processes, the transverse process, and finally the remaining pedicle, are removed from the posterior side.

If the child's age allows it, a compression system can be applied on the convex side (Harrington, Cotrel–Dubousset); the space is slowly closed. If no instrumentation is used, or the child is too young, only a posterior bone fusion is performed with postoperative treatment in a plaster cast.

Hemivertebra resection can generally be carried out in either one or two stages. Most authors recommend the two-stage procedure.

Wedge Resection

Proposed correction of severe congenital deformities (Cobb angle considerably larger than 50 degrees, combination of concave segmentation failure and multiple convex hemivertebrae) requires a wedge resection. The operation is technically performed according to the principles of hemivertebra excision, but several hemivertebrae or a broad-based bone wedge are removed. After the anterior resection, the corresponding posterior vertebral elements are resected in a second session. The correction can be effected with various implant systems from the posterior side. The concave side is stabilized with a distraction rod. On the convex side, the correction is carried out using a compression system (Harrington or Cotrel–Dubousset instrumentation).

Wound Closure

See under Thoracotomy or Thoracolumbophrenotomy, pp. 22, 35.

Pitfalls and Complications

The potential complications are those of thoracic surgery generally, such as pneumothorax, hemothorax, and lung atelectases. Hemivertebra or wedge resection is associated with a high neurologic risk.

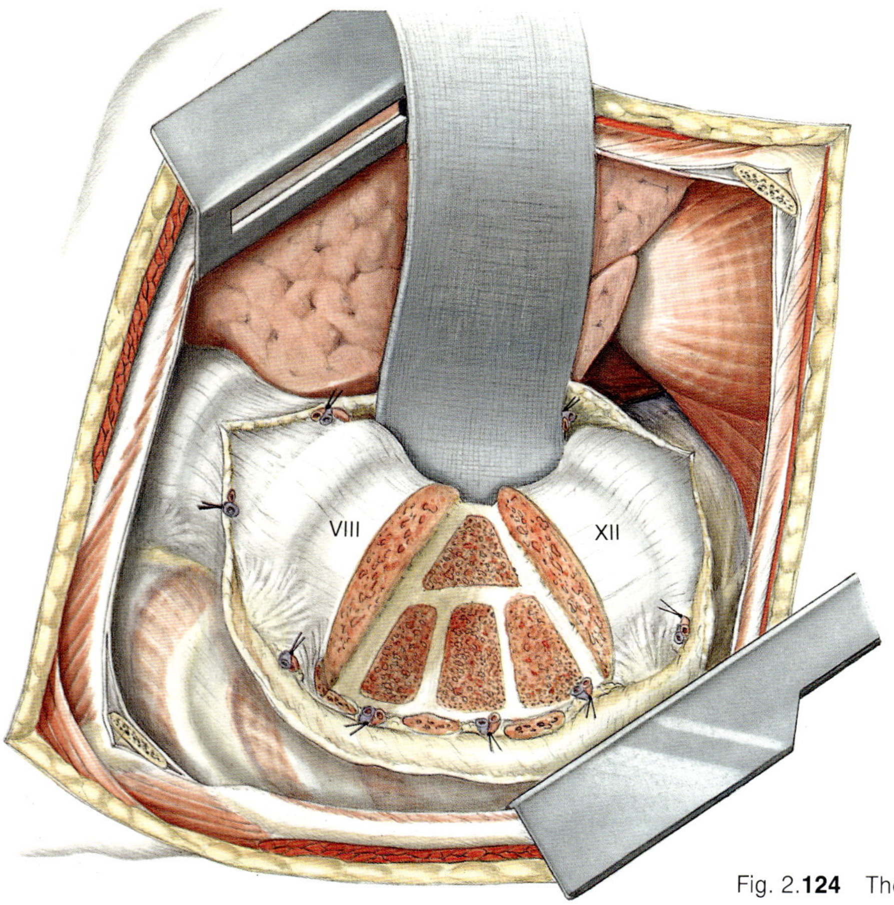

Fig. 2.**124** The hemivertebrae have been partially resected.

Fig. 2.**125** Status after complete resection of the hemivertebrae. The dura is freely exposed; the resection planes of the pedicles and ribs are visible.

1 Spinal dura mater
2 Right pedicle of the vertebral arch
3 11th rib
4 Left pedicle of the vertebral arch
5 Spinal ganglion

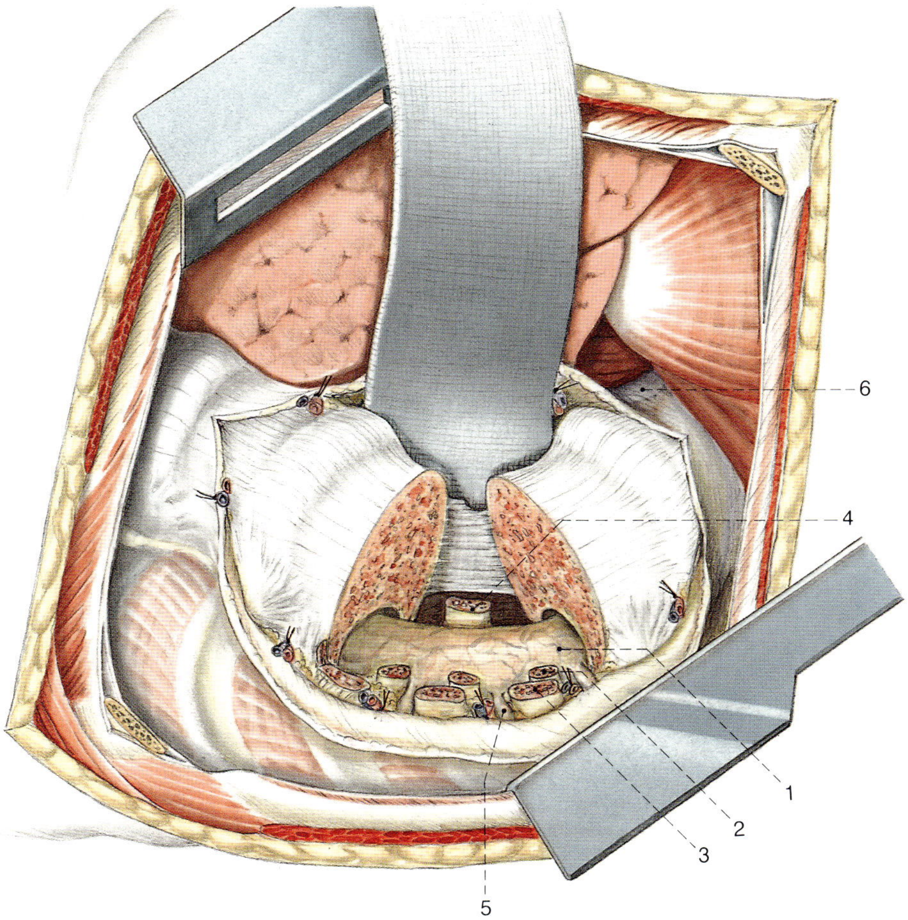

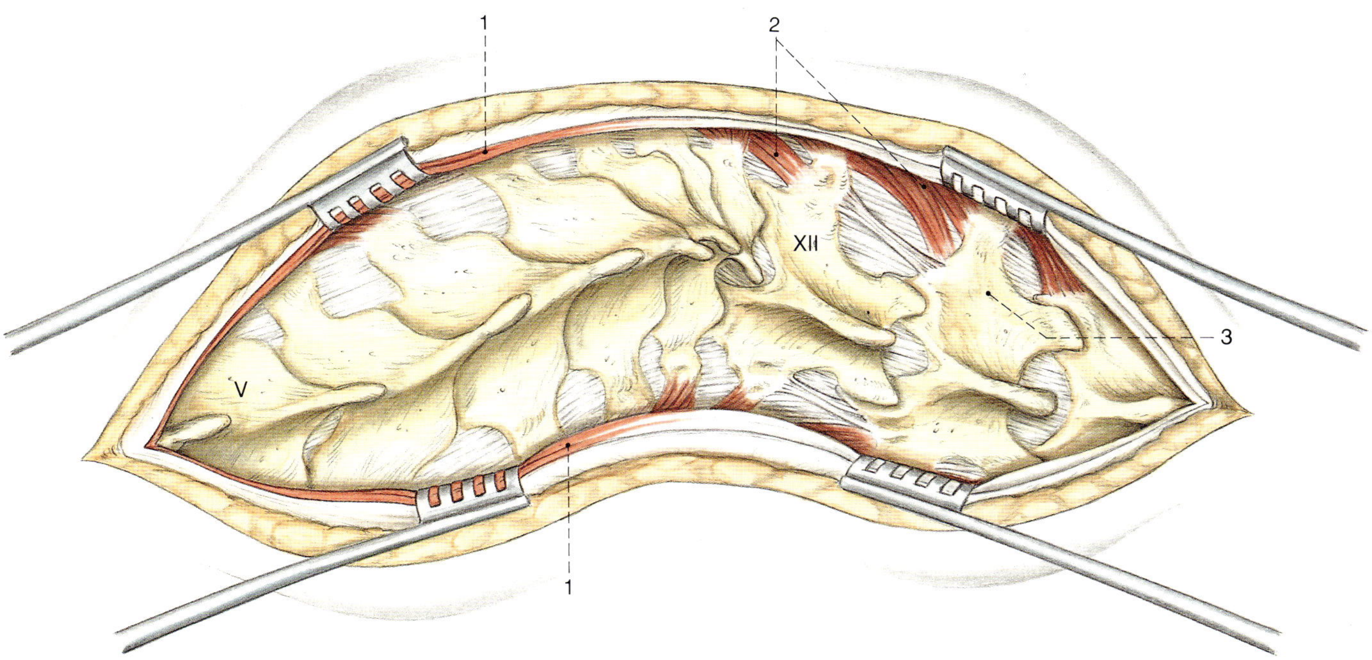

Fig. 2.**126** Wedge resection, posterior operation. Status after exposure of the spine.

1 Erector muscle of the spine
2 Rotator muscles
3 Lamina of the lumbar vertebral arch
V–XII Thoracic vertebrae

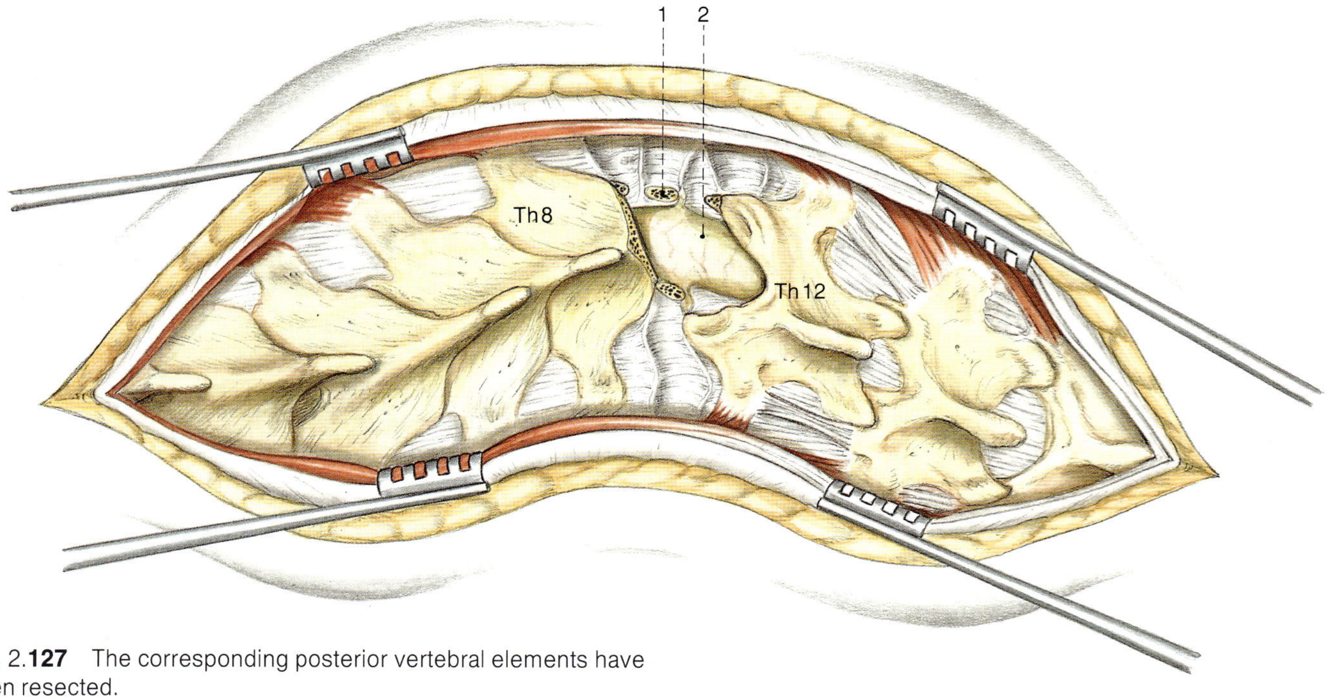

Fig. 2.**127** The corresponding posterior vertebral elements have been resected.

1 Pedicle of the vertebral arch
2 Spinal dura mater

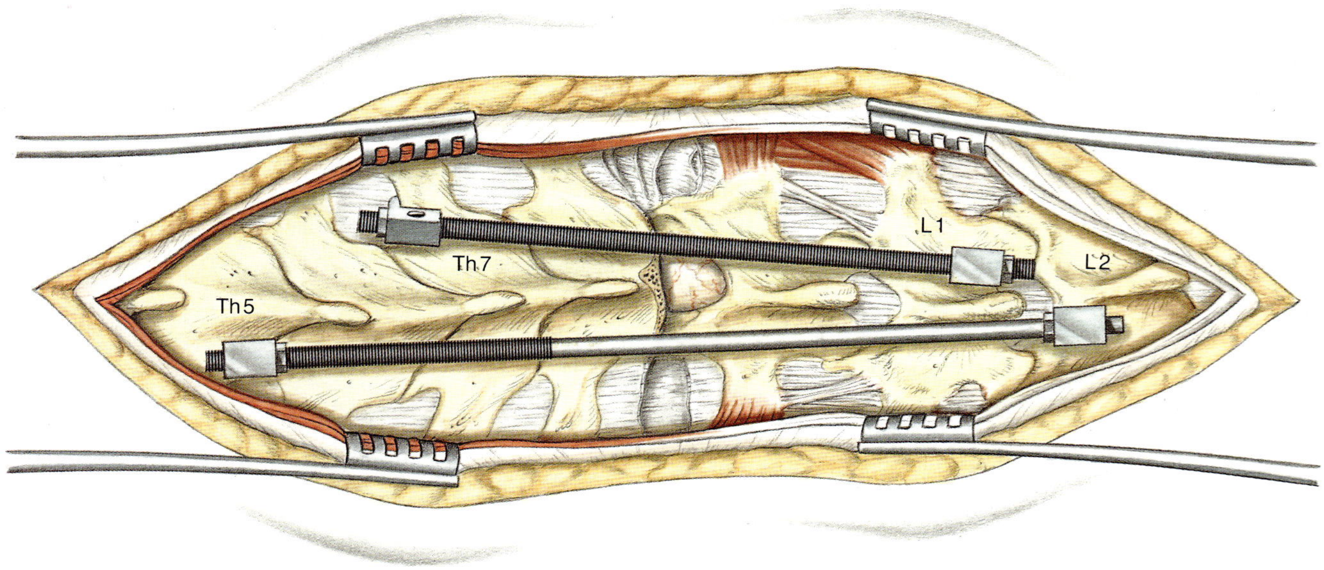

Fig. 2.**128** Correction and stabilization with the Harrington instrumentarium. A distraction rod on the concave side and a compression system on the convex side, with closure of the wedge resection. Posterior spinal fusion should follow.

Further Reading

Bauer R. Die operative Behandlung der Skoliose. Berne: Huber, 1979.

Bradford DS. Partial epiphyseal arrest and supplement fixation for progressive correction of congenital spine deformity. J Bone Jt Surg 1982;64-A:610.

Compere El. Excision of hemivertebrae for correction of congenital scoliosis. J Bone Jt Surg 1932;14:555.

Deburge A, Briard JL. Cervical hemivertebra excision. J Bone Jt Surg 1981;A-63:13350.

Hall JE. Congenital scoliosis. In: Bradford DS, Hensinger RM, eds. Pediatric spine. Stuttgart: Thieme, 1985.

Hall JE, Herndon WA, Levine CR. Surgical treatment of congenital scoliosis with or without Harrington instrumentation. J Bone Jt Surg 1981;63-A:608.

Hodgson AR, Yau ACMC. Anterior surgical approaches to the spinal column. In: Apley AG, ed. Recent advances in orthopedics. London: Churchill, 1969.

Langenskiold A. Correction of congenital scoliosis by excision of one-half of a cleft vertebra. Acta Orthop Scand 1967;38:291.

Leatherman KD. Resection of vertebral bodies. J Bone Jt Surg 1969;51-A:206.

Leatherman KD. The management of rigid spinal curves. Clin Orthop 1973;92:215.

Leatherman KD, Dickson A. Spinal deformity in myelodysplasia–surgical treatment. 11th Annual Meeting of the American Scoliosis Research Society, Ottawa, Canada, 1976.

Moe JH, Winter RB, Bradford DS, Lonstein JE. Scoliosis and other spinal deformities. Philadelphia: Saunders, 1978.

Onimus M, Michel CR. Problèmes posés par la résection des hémivertèbres lombosacrées. Chir Pédiatr 1978;19:119.

Simmons EH. Observations on the technique and indications for wedge resection of the spine. J Bone Jt Surg 1968;50-A:847.

Slabaugh P, Winter R, Lonstein J, Moe J. Lumbosacral hemivertebra. Spine 1980;5:234.

Wils P. Resection of dorsal vertebrae in congenital scoliosis. J Bone Jt Surg 1951;33-A:151.

Winter RB. Congenital scoliosis. Clin Orthop 1973;93:75.

Winter RB. Congenital kyphoscoliosis with paralysis following hemivertebra excision. Clin Orthop 1976;119:116–125.

Complete Vertebrectomy

Indications

- Correction of severe, rigid idiopathic scoliosis, generally in adults when other methods of correction (Harrington operation in adults, p. 103) are no longer effective.
- Spinal tumors.

Approach

The anterior parts of the vertebra are usually removed by thoracotomy on the convex side, and the posterior parts via a conventional posterior approach to the spine. See Chapter 1, pp. 13, 64.

Operative Technique

(Figs. 2.**129**–2.**137**)

Profound, detailed anatomical knowledge is required for the resection of vertebrae. The following circumstances need to be taken into account (Figs. 2.**129**–2.**131**):

In the area from T2 to T10, the rib heads are articularly joined to the corresponding vertebra, as well as to the caudal portions of the next higher vertebra and to the intervertebral disk. The pedicle arises in the upper third of the respective vertebral body; the corresponding segmental nerve leaves the vertebral canal in the intervertebral foramen immediately inferior to the pedicle. The corresponding segmental nerve then courses laterally, lies anterior to the external intercostal muscles, and approaches the inferior surface of the corresponding rib about 4 cm to the side of the vertebral body. The segmental vessels (artery and vein) travel across the midsection of the vertebral body and then join the nerve. Complete resection of the vertebral body requires removal of the rib head. After exposure of the dura in the superior portion of the vertebral body, therefore, the base of the pedicle and, overlapping laterally and in a cranial direction, the site of the rib resection, are identified.

Posterior site. Following resection of the vertebral joint, the superior boundary of the next lower pedicle is encountered. The intervertebral disk is located in the depth and lateral to the spinal cord. The corresponding segmental nerve lies fairly close, below the lamina and directly inferior to the next higher pedicle.

The operation is performed in two sessions. In the first, the vertebral bodies at the apex are resected by way of a convex-sided thoracotomy. In the second session, the corresponding posterior vertebral elements are removed via a posterior approach. In the same session, the scoliosis is corrected, and stabilization is effected with a Luque or Cotrel–Dubousset implant.

Starting from a thoracotomy on the convex side, the vertebral bodies situated at the apex of the scoliotic curvature are exposed; in typical fashion, the parietal pleura is divided and the segmental vessels are ligated. Depending on the severity of the deformity, two or three vertebral bodies are completely resected. First of all, a covering of periosteum, vertebral cortex, and the annulus fibrosus of the intervertebral disks is lifted off, with a medial peduncle being left in place. The remainder of the bone is then completely removed with a rongeur as far as the posterior longitudinal ligament. While properly protecting the spinal cord, the pedicles are resected as far posteriorly as possible, using the rongeur or a pituitary forceps. The cancellous bone harvested on resection of the vertebral body is then loosely packed on the posterior longitudinal ligament. The cortical shell is reattached with approximation sutures, a thoracic drain is inserted, and the wound is closed in layers.

Posterior procedure. About two weeks after the first session, the corresponding posterior vertebral elements at the apex of the kyphoscoliosis are resected; these are the spinous process, vertebral arches, transverse processes, and the remaining pedicles. For effective correction, the ribs on the convex side should be removed at the same time by a rib hump resection (p. 110); in addition, concave-sided rib segments 3–4 cm long in the apical region of the curve have to be resected. After this, correction of the scoliosis and fixation by the Luque system are carried out in the same session.

Wound Closure

See Chapter 1, p. 22.

Pitfalls and Complications

- Complications of thoracic surgery in connection with the anterior procedure.
- Complications of Luque instrumentation.
- Neurologic complications: radicular lesions, spinal cord lesions.

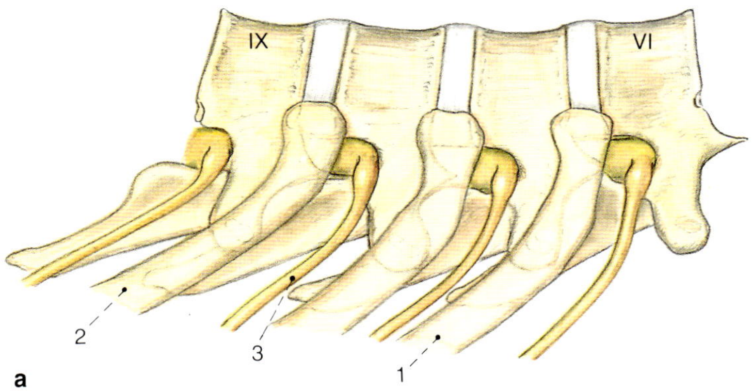

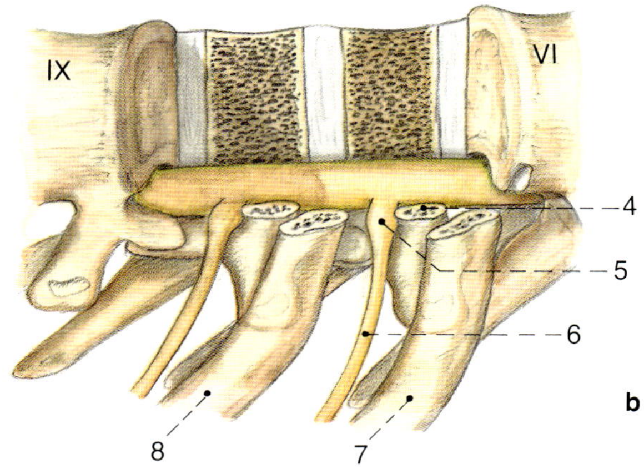

Fig. 2.**129 a** Anatomical site of the thoracic spine. **b** Status after resection of two vertebral bodies. Note the relations between the vertebral body, the corresponding rib, the intervertebral disk, the pedicle, and the segmental nerve.

1 7th rib
2 9th rib
3 Spinal nerve
4 Pedicle of the vertebral arch
5 Spinal ganglion
6 Spinal nerve
7 8th rib
8 9th rib
VI–IX Thoracic vertebrae

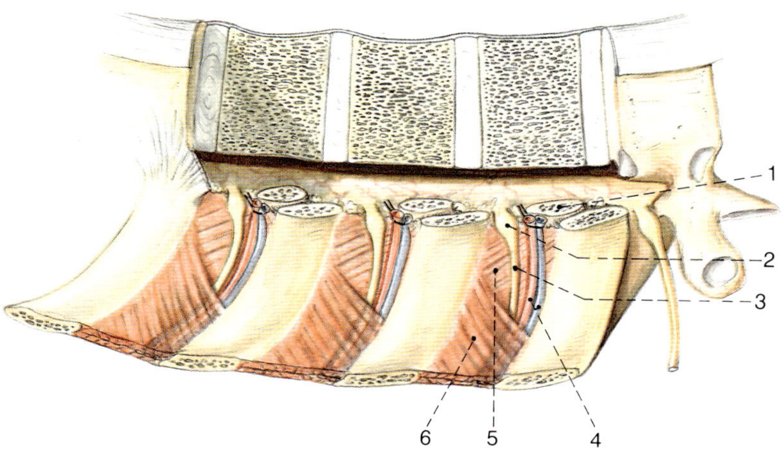

Fig. 2.**130** Status after resection of three vertebral bodies in the thoracic spine. Note the position of the pedicles, of the ribs after resection of the rib head, and of the segmental neurovascular bundle.

1 Pedicle of the vertebral arch
2 Spinal ganglion
3 Spinal nerve
4 Intercostal vessels
5 External intercostal muscle
6 Internal intercostal muscle

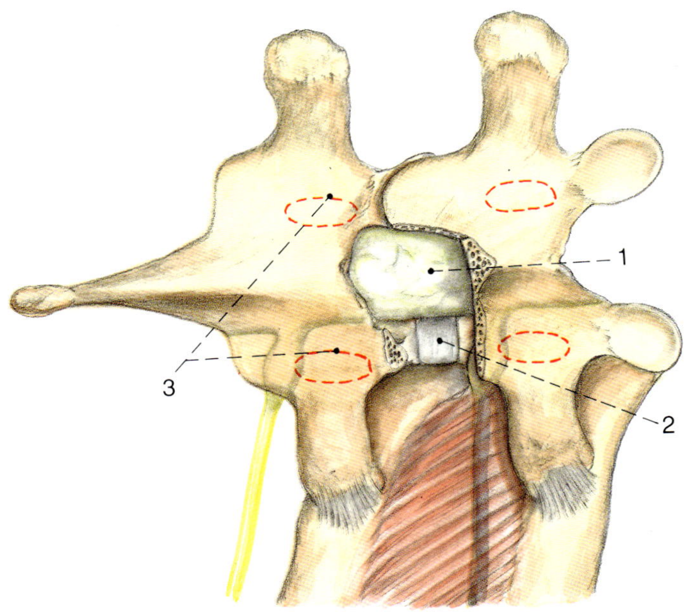

Fig. 2.**131** Anatomical site. Status after resection of the facet joint. Note the position of the pedicle, the intervertebral disk, and the segmental nerve.

1 Spinal dura mater
2 Intervertebral disk
3 Projection of pedicles of the vertebral arch

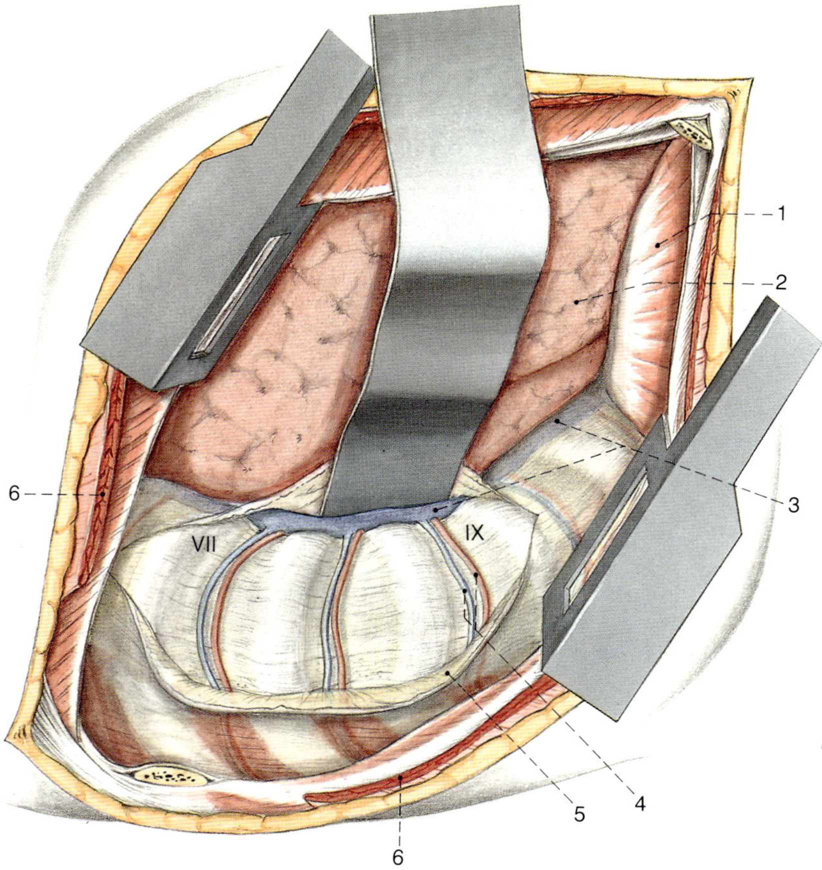

Fig. 2.**132** Complete vertebrectomy. Right-sided thoracotomy; the apical vertebrae are visualized.

1 Thoracic diaphragm
2 Right lung
3 Azygos vein
4 Intercostal vessels
5 Parietal pleura
6 External oblique muscle of the abdomen
VII–IX Thoracic vertebrae

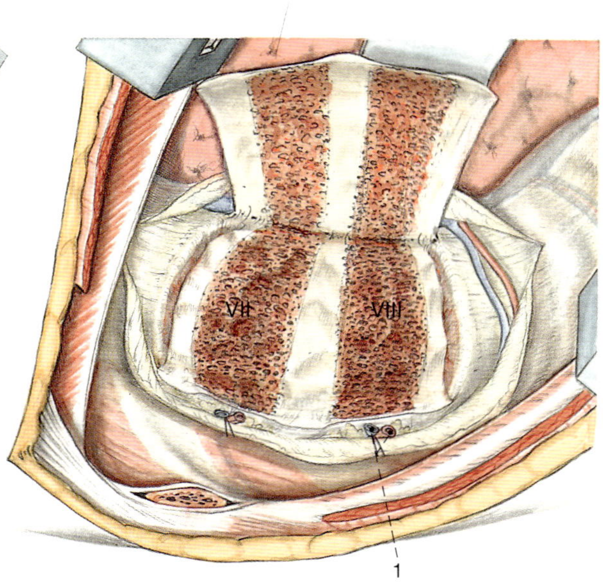

Fig. 2.**133** Elevation of a cortical shell based on the concave side in the area of the apical vertebrae.

1 Intercostal vessels

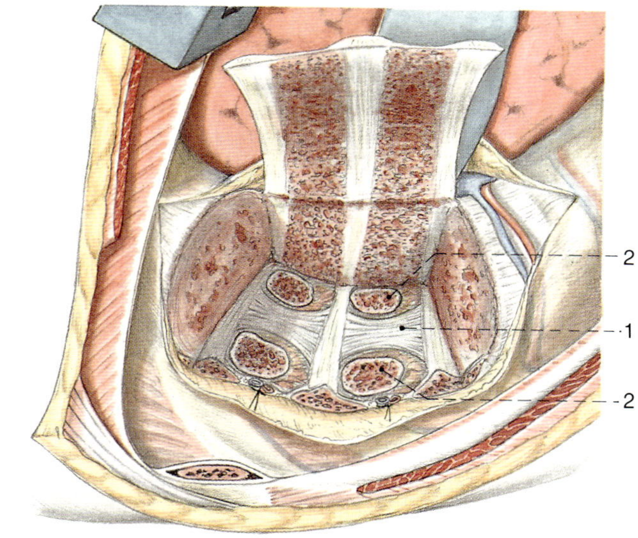

Fig. 2.**134** Status after resection of two vertebral bodies. The pedicles and rib resection surfaces are visible in the depth.

1 Posterior longitudinal ligament
2 Pedicle of the vertebral arch

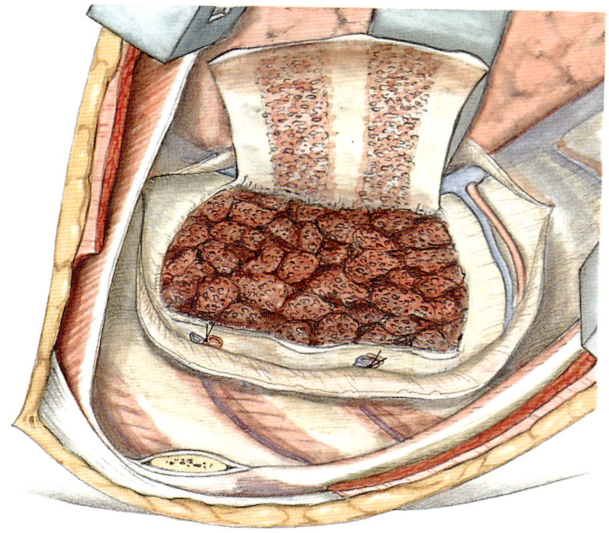

Fig. 2.**135** The cavity is bridged with loosely implanted cancellous tissue, and the bony cover is reattached with approximation sutures.

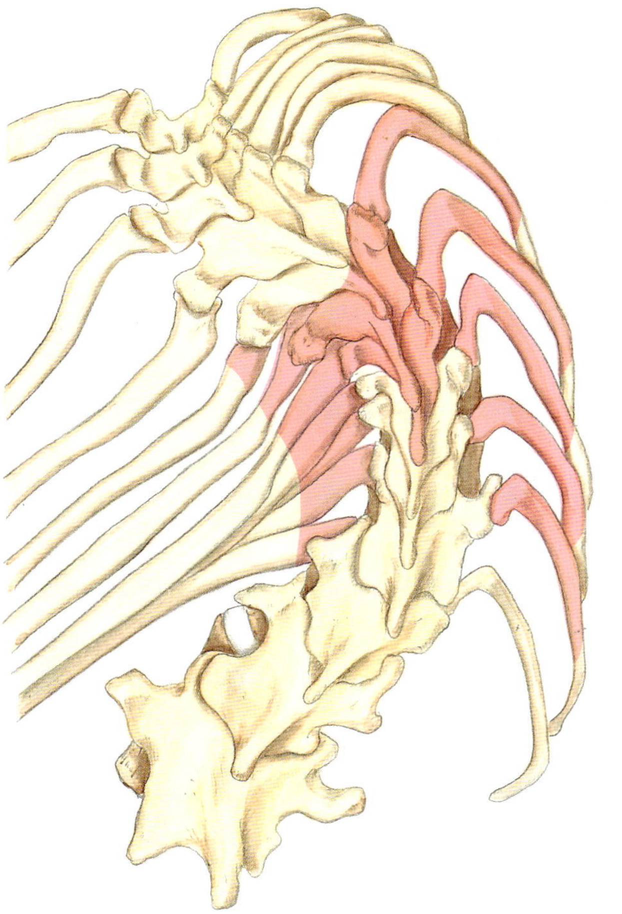

Fig. 2.**136** Bony elements that need to be resected from the posterior side in a second session.

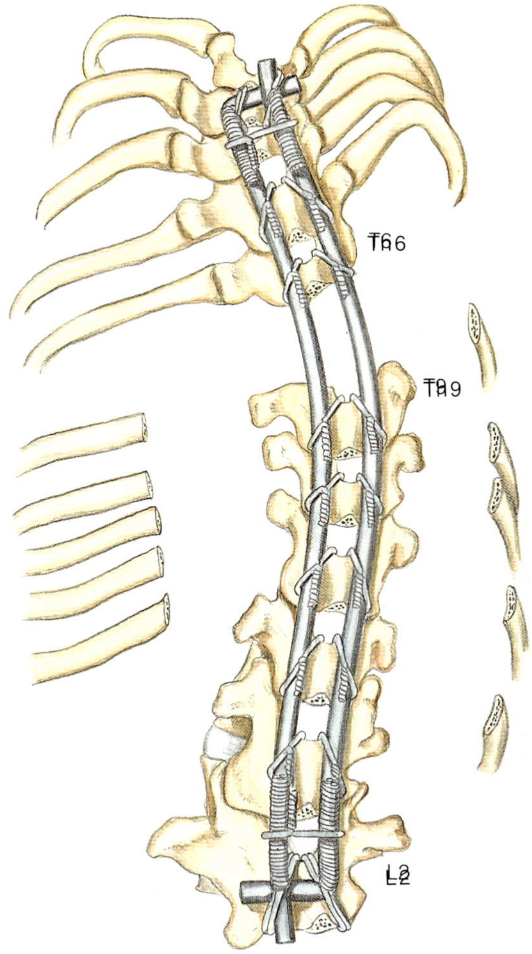

Fig. 2.**137** Status after complete vertebrectomy. Correction of scoliosis and stabilization using the Luque instrumentarium.

Further Reading

Bradford DS. Vertebral column resection. 19th Annual Meeting of the American Scoliosis Research Society, 1984.

Bradford DS. Vertebral column resection. Orthop Trans 1987;11:502.

Epiphysiodesis

Indications

Control of growth in the treatment of certain forms of congenital scoliosis, as well as of malignant, progressive infantile (idiopathic) scoliosis. The curve should not substantially exceed a Cobb angle of 50 degrees and should be short. A severe kyphotic component is a contraindication.

There is controversy in the literature about the indication for epiphysiodesis. The method has generally fallen short of expectations. More stable results can possibly be obtained in combination with posterior fusion on the convex side, or a subcutaneous Harrington instrumentation performed two weeks later (Scoliosis Operations in Children, p. 97).

Approach

Depending on the level of the lesion, thoracotomy or thoracophrenolumbotomy on the convex side of the curve. See Chapter 1, pp. 13–23 and pp. 24–36.

Operative Technique

(Figs. 2.**138**–2.**140**)

Following thoracotomy on the convex side and rib resection (graft material) at the appropriate level (generally two segments above the apex of the scoliosis), the parietal pleura is divided parallel to the intervertebral disks in the area of the scoliotic apex; as a rule, a maximum of four to five segments are fused. With this approach, it is not necessary to ligate segmental vessels. A portion of the convex-sided intervertebral disks is excised with a knife. The adjacent upper plates are removed with a curet; this curettage, however, is carried no further than the middle of the vertebral body. The resulting gap is filled loosely with the bone chips harvested from the resected rib. The parietal pleura is sutured.

Wound Closure

See Chapter 1, p. 22.

Postoperative Treatment

A combination with subcutaneous Harrington instrumentation can be carried out two weeks postoperatively (p. 100); otherwise, removal of the sutures is followed by application of a body cast or a spinal orthosis.

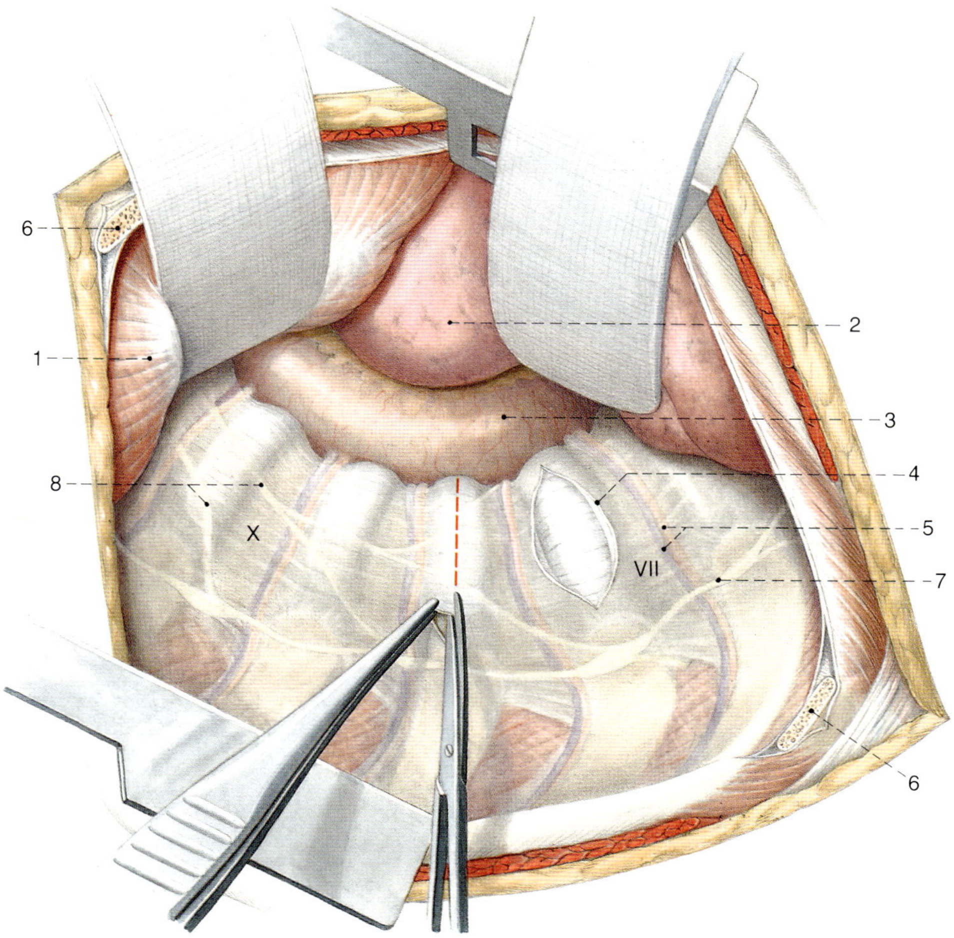

Fig. 2.**138** Status after left-sided thoracotomy. The parietal pleura is transected over the intervertebral disks in the apical region of the scoliosis; the ligation of segmental vessels can therefore be omitted.

1 Thoracic diaphragm
2 Left lung
3 Thoracic aorta
4 Parietal pleura
5 Intercostal vessels
6 6th rib
7 Sympathetic trunk
8 Greater and lesser splanchnic nerves
VII–X Thoracic vertebrae

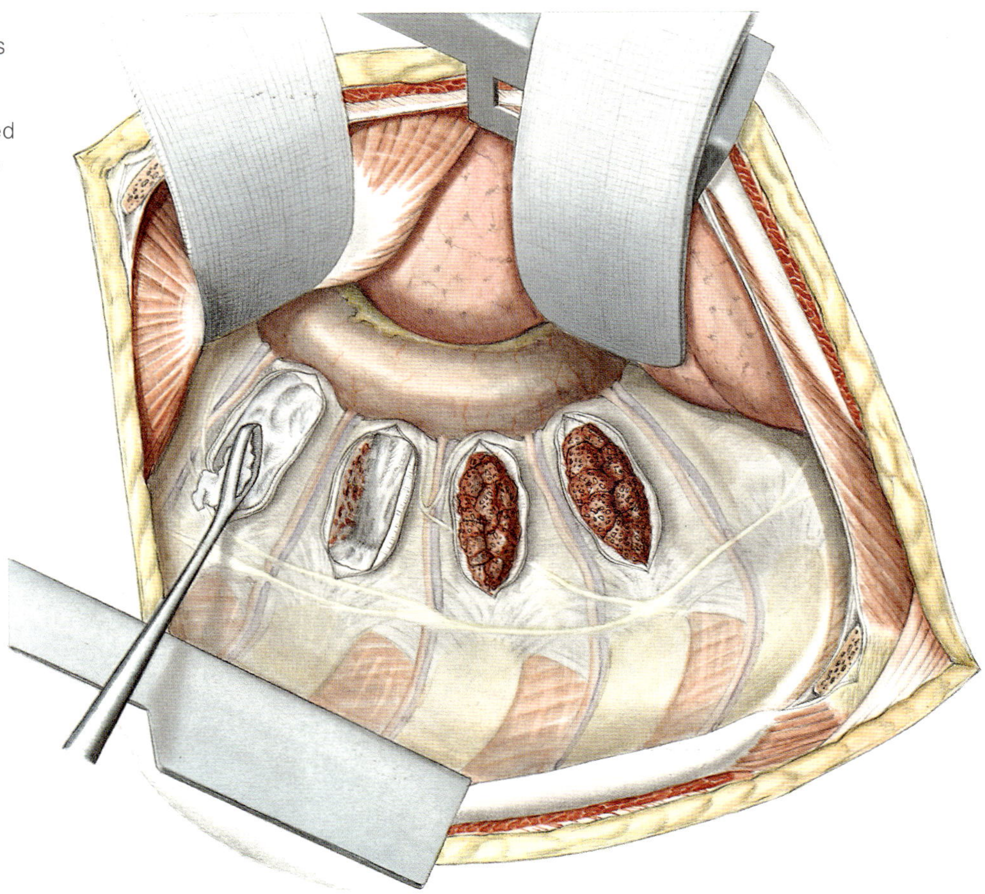

Fig. 2.**139** The intervertebral disk halves on the convex side are removed; the corresponding parts of the upper plates are removed with a curet. The defect is packed with autologous bone graft material (ribs).

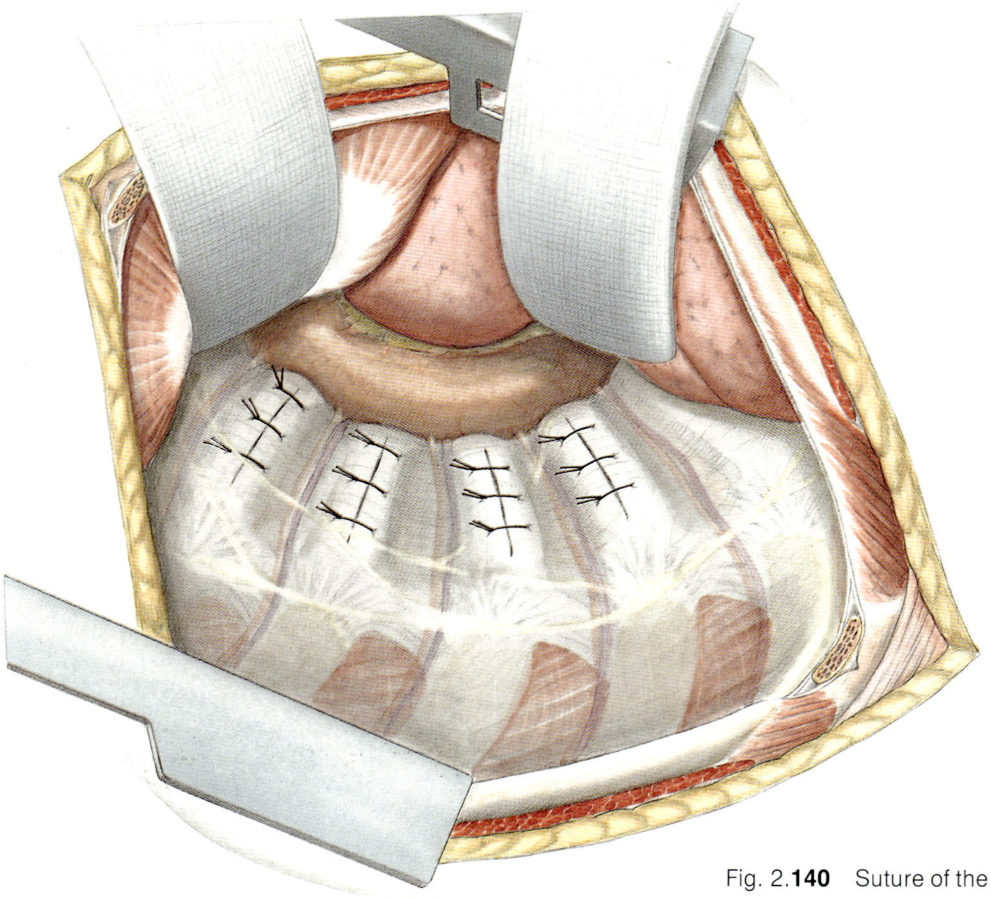

Fig. 2.**140** Suture of the parietal pleura.

Further Reading

Andrew T, Piggott H. Growth arrest for progressive scoliosis. J Bone Jt Surg 1985;67-B:193.

Bradford DS. Partial epiphyseal arrest and supplemental fixation for progressive correction of congenital spinal deformity. J Bone Jt Surg 1982;64-A:610.

Bradford DS. Die angeborene Skoliose. Orthopäde 1989;18:87.

Götze HG. Indikation, Technik und Ergebnisse der ventralen Spondyloepiphysiodese. In: Zielke K, ed. Skoliose und Kyphose. Stuttgart: Hippokrates, 1978.

Morscher E. Experiences with the transthoracic, hemilateral epiphysiodesis in the treatment of scoliosis. In: Chapchal G, ed. Operative Treatment of Scoliosis. Stuttgart: Thieme, 1973.

Roaf R. The last results of unilateral growth arrest of the spine for scoliosis. Acta Orthop Scan 1963;33:393.

The Dwyer Operation

Indications

Principal indication. Thoracolumbar and lumbar curvatures. In combined scoliosis, the lumbar curve is corrected by the anterior approach, and the cranial curve by the posterior approach (Harrington, Luque, Cotrel–Dubousset); decompensation of the spine would otherwise result (p. 166).

Etiologic indication. Defect of posterior vertebral elements (e.g., meningomyelocele).

Secondary indication. Possibly thoracic lordoscoliosis.

Contraindications. Kyphosis and kyphoscoliosis (the operation has a kyphotic effect).

Approach

The approach chosen depends on the extent and the location of the scoliotic curvature. See Chapter 1, pp. 24–36.

Operative Technique

Instrumentarium

The following are the main parts of the Dwyer instrumentarium (Figs. 2.**141**, 2.**142**):

Implants. Clamps of various sizes that are placed on the vertebral body on the convex side, following the original technique.

Screws. The screwheads are fitted with holes for receiving the Dwyer cable.

Titanium cable.

Instruments. Cable-tensioning device; device for crimping the screwheads to the cable.

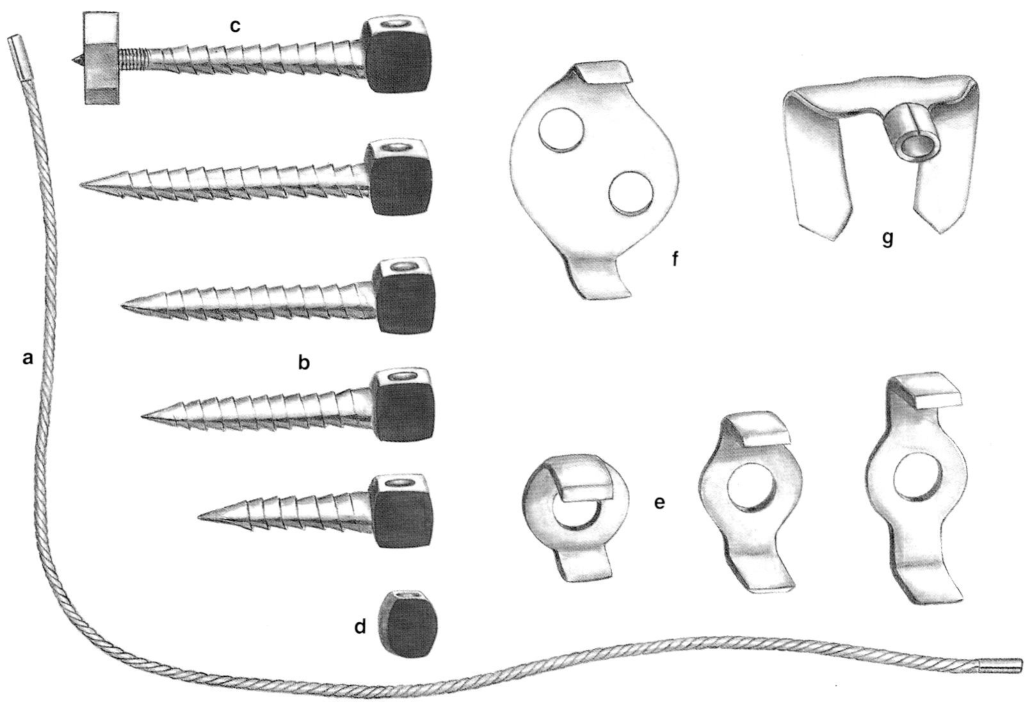

Fig. 2.**141** Dwyer instrumentarium.
a Dwyer cable.
b Dwyer screws.
c Hall screw with lock nut (for porous vertebral bodies).
d Crimp head for anchoring the cable.
e Dwyer clamps.
f Hall two-hole clamp.
g Sacral anchor (Hall).

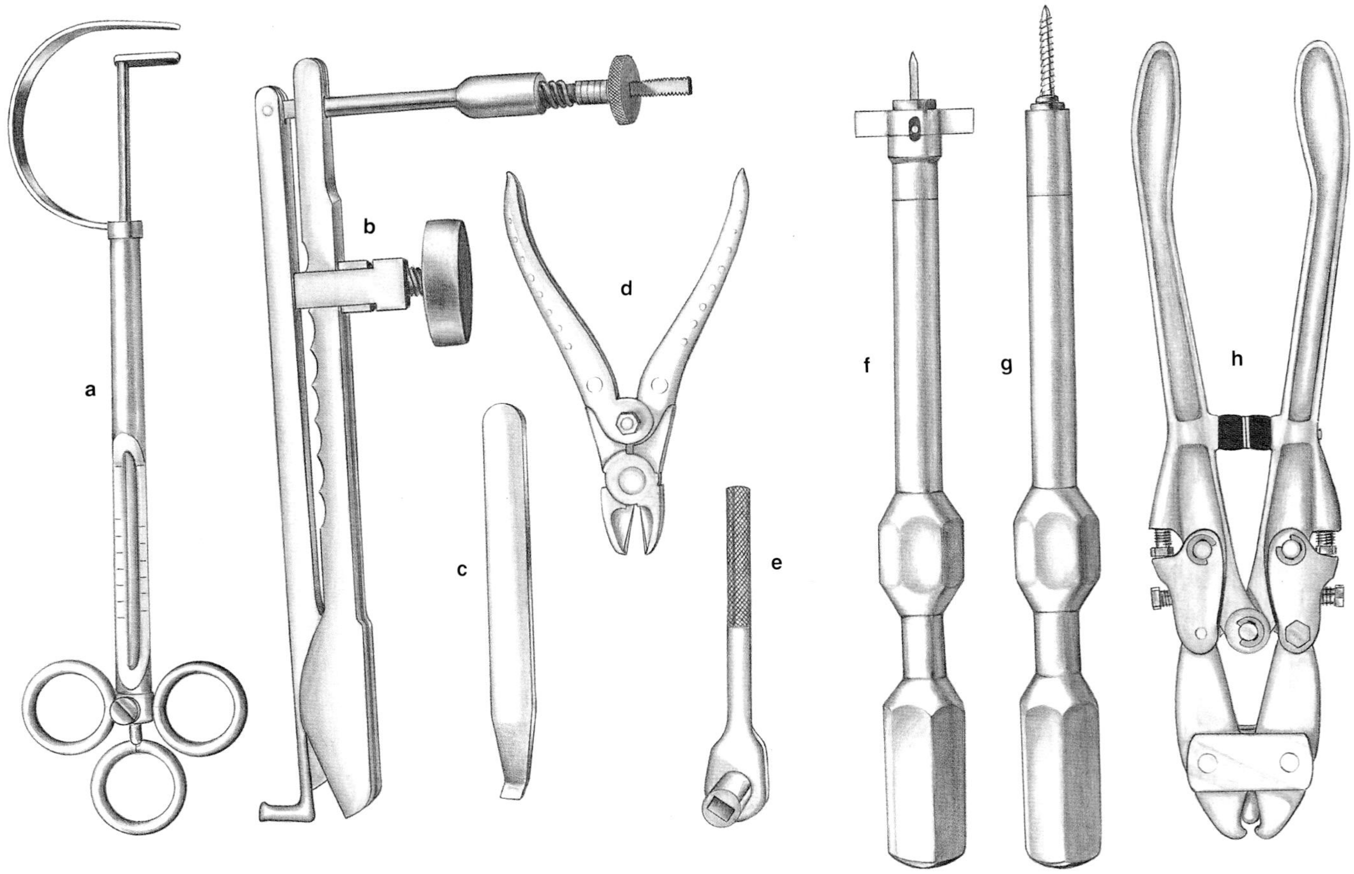

Fig. 2.**142** Dwyer instrumentarium.
a Instrument for measuring screw length.
b Cable-tensioning device.
c Starter for clamp seating.
d Cable-clipping forceps.
e Wrench.
f Clamp applier.
g Screwdriver.
h Screwhead crimper.

Principles of Correction

The scoliotic curvature is corrected by shortening and compressing the convex side with vertebral body screws and the titanium cable (Fig. 2.**143**). The compression is achieved continuously from cranial to caudal.

Fusion Area

Note
Essentially, this also applies to the Zielke derotation spondylodesis.

Evaluation of the fusion area requires the following radiographs:

- Standing anteroposterior and lateral films of the entire spine.
- Bending films in the frontal plane.
- Bending films in the sagittal plane (flexion and extension), if there is a deformity in this plane.
- Suspension film.

According to Dwyer, the fusion should generally be performed from one neutral vertebra to the other. Tensioning of the cable and the correction are carried out from cranial to caudal; continuous retightening (in contrast to the Zielke technique) is not possible. The topmost screw is therefore subjected to a strong tension force. It may be advisable in some circumstances to include in the fusion an additional vertebra cranially, with no correction being performed in this segment. This screw then serves to prevent cut-out of the next screw.

The lowest vertebra included in the fusion should lie in the stable zone according to Harrington (p. 85). The intervertebral disk lying caudal to the fusion should show an opening in both directions on the bending films.

Since the final objective of the operation is restoration of a compensated spine, the utmost attention should be paid to possibly adjoining cranial and caudal curves when selecting the area of fusion. Simple curves without structural reverse curves therefore represent an ideal indication for surgery.

Fig. 2.**143** Dwyer operation–principle of correction. After removal of intervertebral disks, the convex side is shortened by compression with screws and cable.

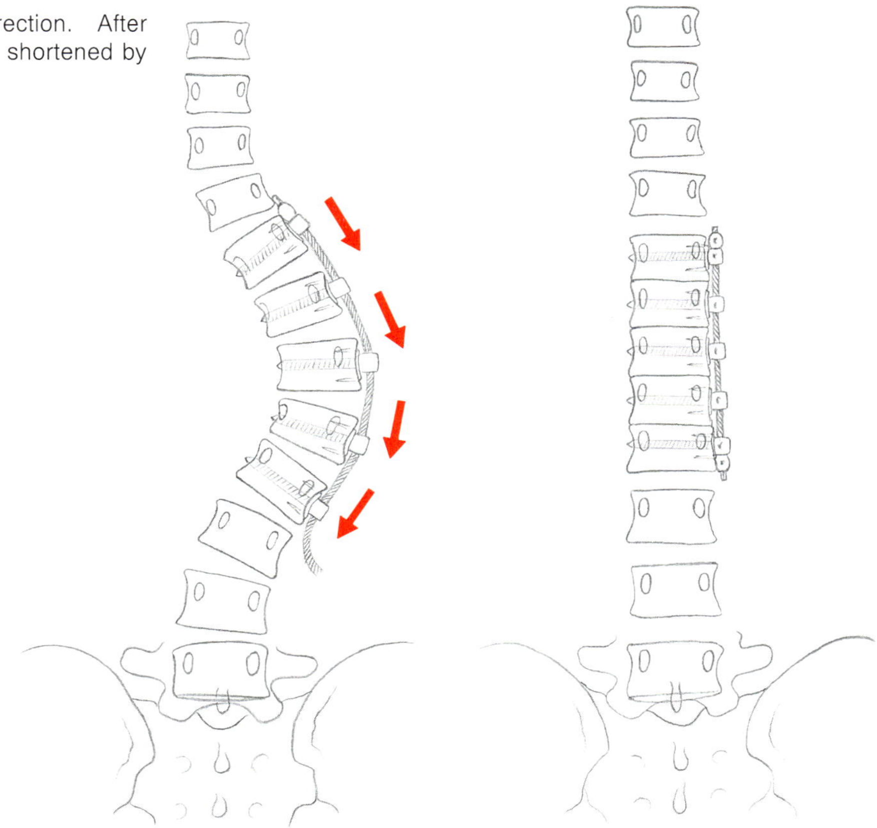

In such a situation, it is even possible to achieve a complete correction of the scoliotic curvature without risking spinal decompensation.

If structural curvatures cranial or caudal to the proposed fusion zones, or both, are present, there is a danger that this technique will lead to a decompensation of the spine as a result of the highly effective correction of the scoliosis.

If there is merely a relatively mobile compensatory curvature cranial to the proposed fusion zone, fusion of the principal lumbar or thoracolumbar curve may be sufficient, since spontaneous correction of the proximal curve may ensue, which will possibly go beyond the straightening obtained on the bending films (Fig. 2.**144**).

With rigid thoracic curves, decompensation results. Corrective measures from the posterior approach should be taken in a second session (e.g., Harrington, Luque, or Cotrel–Dubousset instrumentation). If this is not done, the spine is initially decompensated. If the fusion is relatively short proximally, tilting at the upper end of the fusion may produce compensation.

With the proper length of fusion, however, the compensation is effected by gaping of the intervertebral disk that is caudal to the fusion zone (Fig. 2.**144**). In case of double curves, the full corrective potential of anterior techniques (Dwyer, VDS) should generally not be exhausted. The posterior methods are not so effective, as a rule, and thoracic curves are more difficult to correct. The operation should aim to achieve a compensated spinal column, rather than a maximal correction of the lumbar curvature (Figs. 2.**145** and 2.**146**).

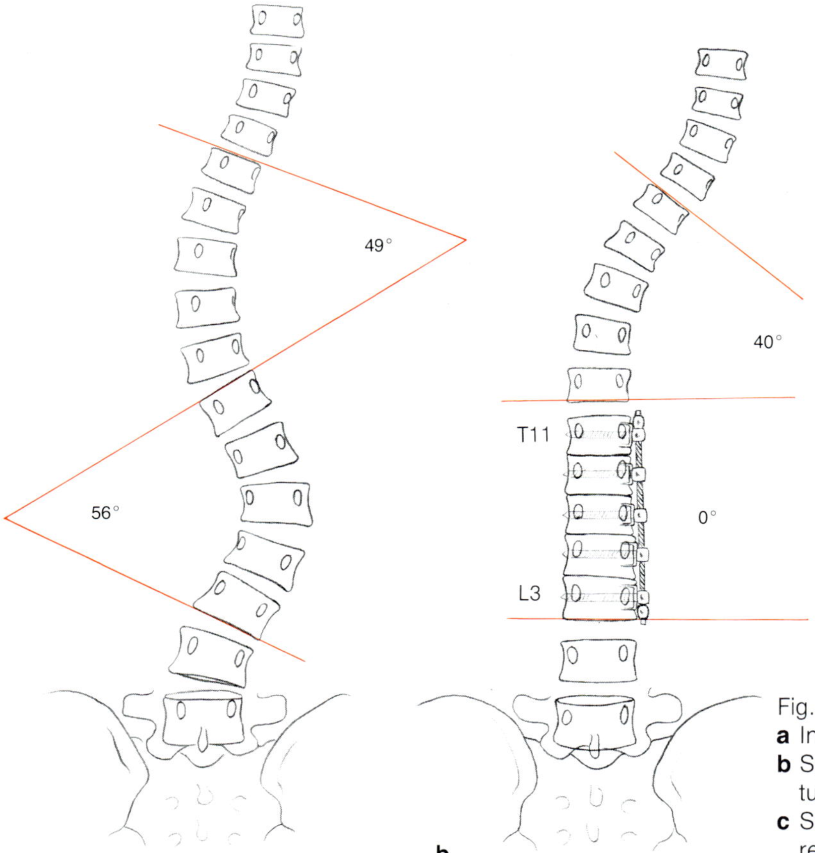

a b

Fig. 2.**144** Available options for spinal compensation.
a Initial status.
b Spinal decompensation after full correction of the caudal curvature.
c Satisfactory spinal compensation with good spontaneous correction of the cranial curvature in combination with moderate postoperative loss of correction.
d Spinal compensation due to tilting-up of the intervertebral disk over the area of fusion with too short a fusion length cranially.
e With appropriate fusion length, compensation by wide opening of the disk space caudal to the fusion.

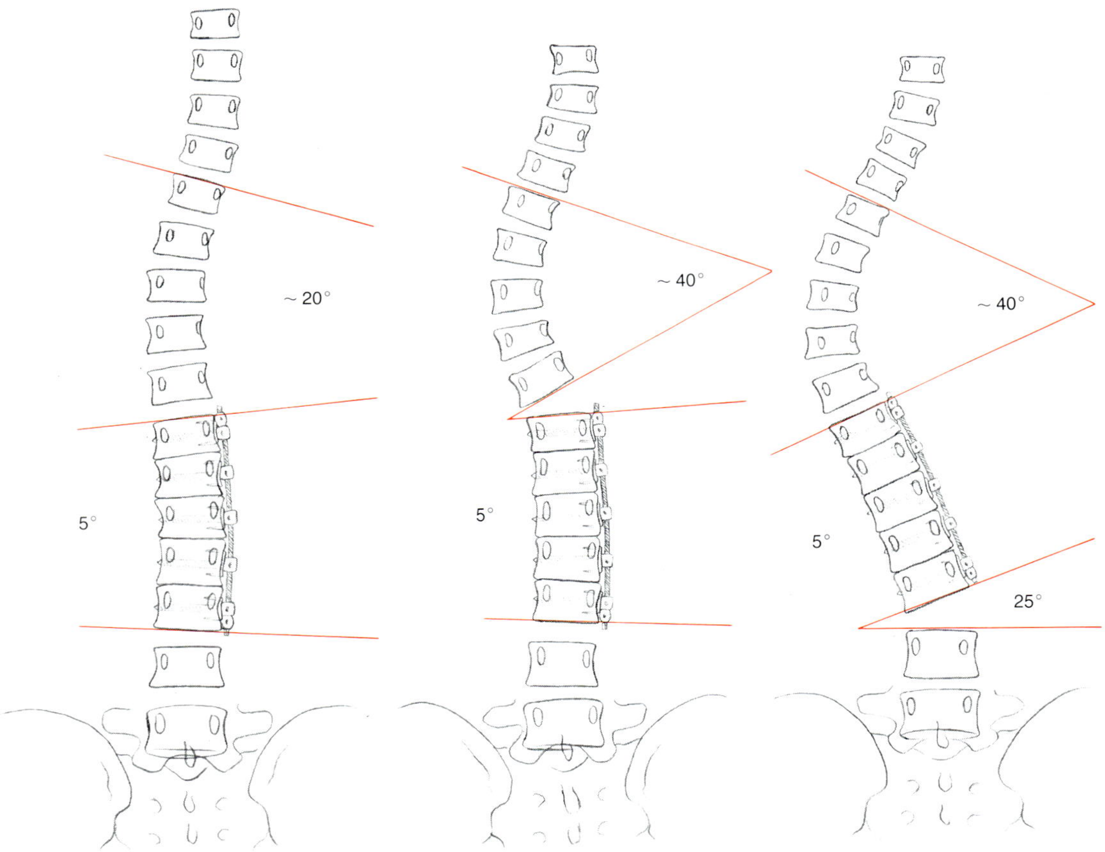

c d e

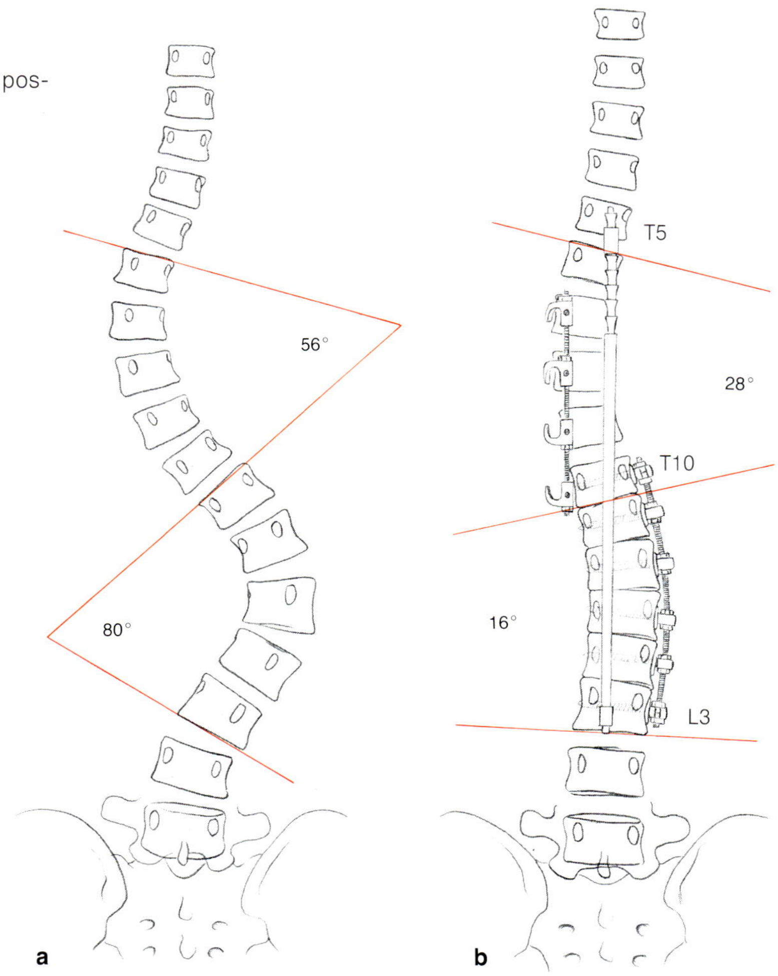

Fig. 2.**145**
a Combined scoliosis.
b Correction through a combination of anterior (VDS) and posterior (Harrington) procedures.

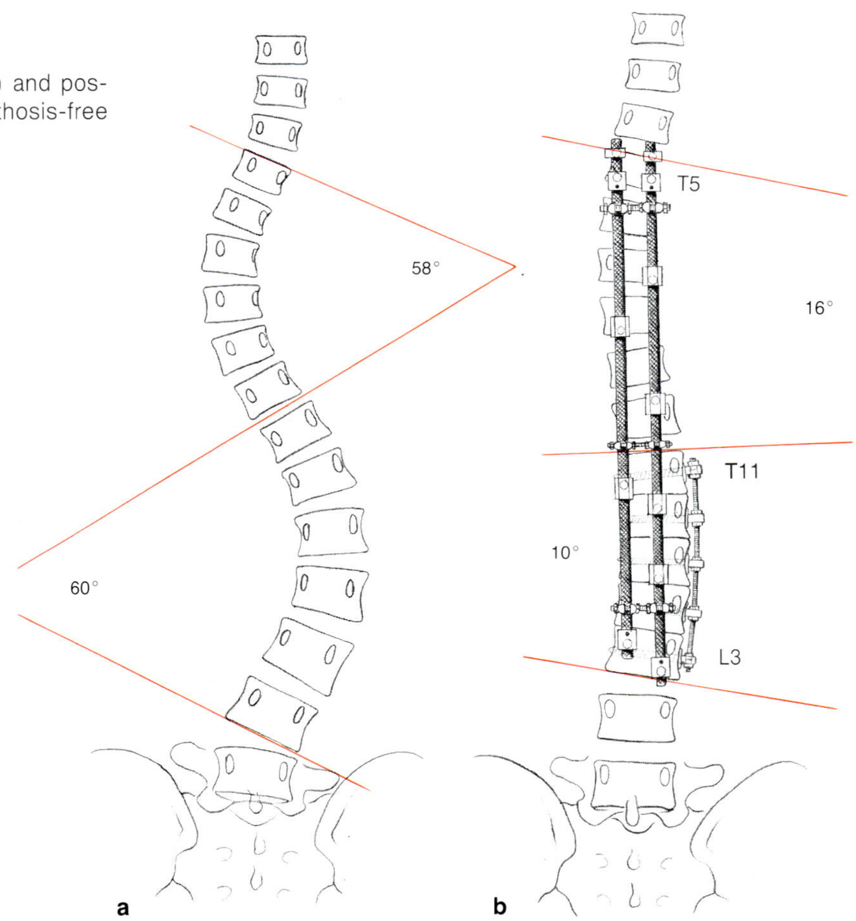

Fig. 2.**146**
a Combined scoliosis.
b Correction through a combination of anterior (VDS) and posterior (Cotrel–Dubousset) procedures, allowing orthosis-free postoperative treatment.

Pelvic Obliquity

(Fig. 2.**147**)

Complete pelvic obliquity has to be distinguished from incomplete pelvic obliquity. In the latter, L5 is obliquely positioned above S1, and also shows different torsion. In incomplete pelvic obliquity (essentially paralytic scoliosis), fusion has to be extended to L5. If this does not succeed in placing L5 and S1 in parallel positions, a posterior fusion including the pelvis should be performed in a second session.

If synostoses of contractures are present in a patient with neuromuscular scoliosis, it is advisable to perform only a mobilizing osteotomy in the lumbar region anteriorly, and to carry out the pelvic fixation, using the Luque technique, for example, from the posterior approach (p. 126).

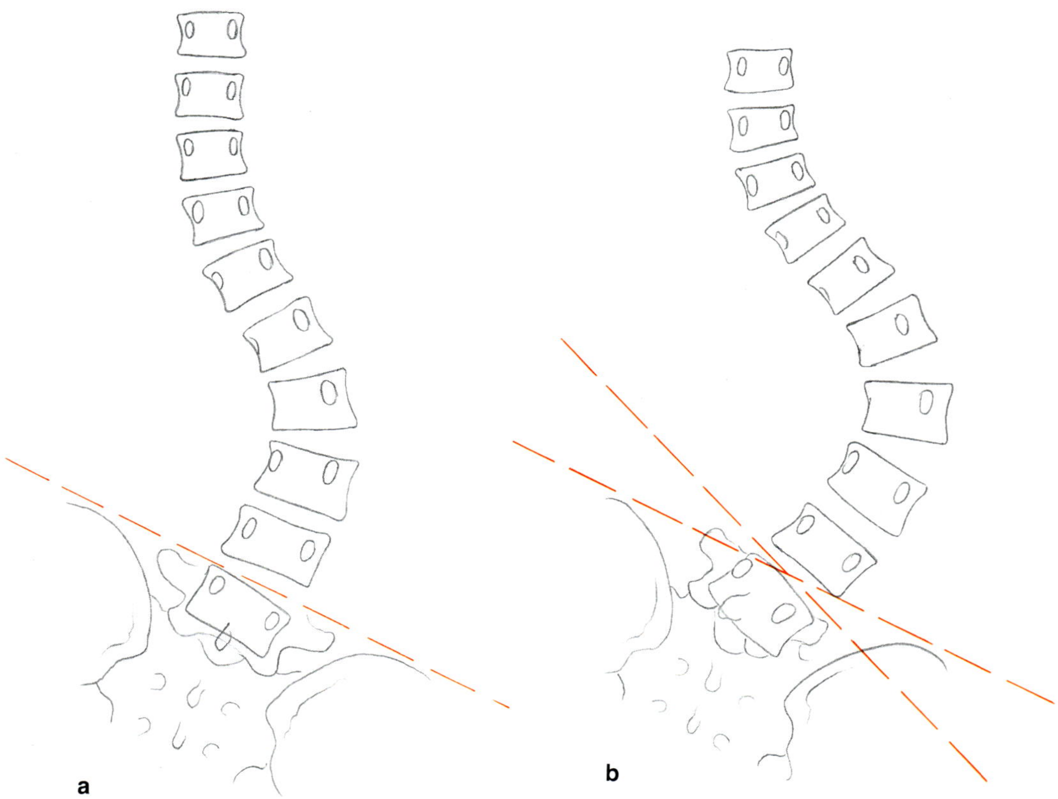

Fig. 2.**147**
a Complete pelvic obliquity (L5 and S1 lie parallel).
b Incomplete pelvic obliquity, with L5 tilted over S1 and torsion.

Instrumentation

(Figs. 2.**148**–2.**159**)

Completion of the spinal dissection from the anterior approach is followed by starting the removal of the intervertebral disks. As a rule, the most readily accessible intervertebral disk at the apex of the curve is removed first. Using a knife, the intervertebral disk is incised at its cranial and caudal borders, the organs posterior to it being protected by a retractor. The intervertebral disk is grasped with clamps and resected, and the remaining tissue is removed with a rongeur, going in a posterior direction as far as the annulus fibrosus or the posterior longitudinal ligament. This ligament is divided only in exceptional cases, when the curves are very rigid. The other intervertebral disks are resected analogously.

The cartilaginous upper plates are now removed with a ring curet until freshly bleeding vertebral cancellous tissue is reached. Following complete debridement of an intervertebral space, this is packed off with a Gelfoam sponge. The remaining intervertebral disks are debrided in the same fashion. Clamps are now placed by the proper technique over the vertebral cortices from the convex side. While effective correction is possible, adjacent clamps will press against each other (thus preventing correction and increasing the risk of pseudarthrosis). We therefore prefer to drive the smallest clamp directly into the vertebral body. The clamps are positioned with the aid of a special clamp placer. Using an awl, the vertebral body is then pierced transversely in the direction of the palpating finger on the contralateral side. It is important to make a correct assessment of the vertebral rotation associated with the scoliosis, so that the screw will not pass too far posteriorly and so possibly enter the vertebral canal.

Warning
Due to the posterior excavation of the vertebral bodies, the screw may be palpable with the finger on the contralateral side and still pierce the vertebral canal tangentially.

The screw length is now determined with a measuring instrument, and screws of the appropriate length are inserted. The titanium cable is passed through the holes of the screwheads. If two screws lie very close to one another, it often proves difficult to introduce the cable. In this case, the adjacent screw can be given a turn of about 45 degrees to facilitate insertion of the cable. Compression of the first segment is now begun. This is done not only with the use of the tensioning device, but by exerting pressure with the applied screwdriver from the convex side of the curve at the same time (Fig. 2.**157**). Pressure is now cautiously applied with the tensioning device, with each marker corresponding to a traction of 10 kg (adjusting screw). A maximum traction of 40 kg is used. If complete matching of the vertebral bodies cannot be achieved, the remaining gap is filled with bone chips. To avoid the tendency to tilt into kyphosis that is inherent in the system (anterior compression), rib segments of the appropriate height are interposed in the lumbar spinal region anteriorly. This serves to counteract a narrowing of the intervertebral space in the anterior region during correction of the scoliosis (Fig. 2.**159**). After maximal tensioning of the cable and compression of the mobile segment, the screwheads are secured with the crimper, thereby locking the cable. In this way, all the segments in the area of fusion are individually placed under tension from cranial to caudal. If there is uncertainty about the effect of the correction, and especially about the extent to which the correction has to be expanded distally, a radiograph can be obtained intraoperatively.

L4 can be reached with the Dwyer instrumentarium with relative ease, but L5 only with great difficulty (mobilization of iliac vessels). The sacrum is accessible only with the use of special techniques. Hall developed a sacral anchor for these cases. This is introduced into the bodies of S1 and S2. The cable is pulled through the sacral anchor, and instrumentation is then performed from caudal to proximal. On the other hand, instrumentation is carried from the cranial end of the fusion to caudal. The link is established with a special clamp that has two holes (Fig. 2.**141**).

Wound Closure

See Chapter 1, p. 35.

Postoperative Treatment

The patient is generally positioned in bed without external supports and is placed in the intensive care unit, where all necessary diagnostic and therapeutic measures are taken.

After removal of the sutures on postoperative days 12–14, a body cast or a spinal orthosis is applied, which should be worn for 7–9 months after the operation.

Pitfalls and Complications

- Complications of thoracic surgery: pneumothorax, hemothorax, chylothorax, pulmonary atelectases.
- System-specific complications: avulsion of clamps, vertebral body fracture, breakage of cable, vascular injury, kyphosis in the fusion zone, pseudarthrosis.
- Neurologic complications: radicular lesion, transverse cord lesions.
- Sympathectomy effect from operations in the lower lumbar spinal region.

Alternative Methods

Ventral derotation spondylodesis (Zielke), while based on the same principles of correction, has an improved technical design. It provides the possibility of derotation and lordosation, and shows increased stability.

Alternative to posterior methods: Cotrel–Dubousset.

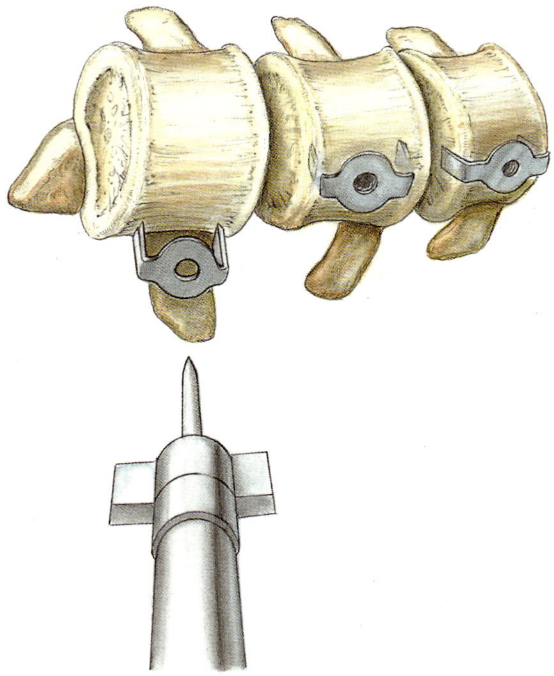

Fig. 2.**148** Insertion of Dwyer clamps with a clamp inserter. In the original method, they are inserted over the lower and upper plates; insertion into the lateral vertebral cortex is recommended.

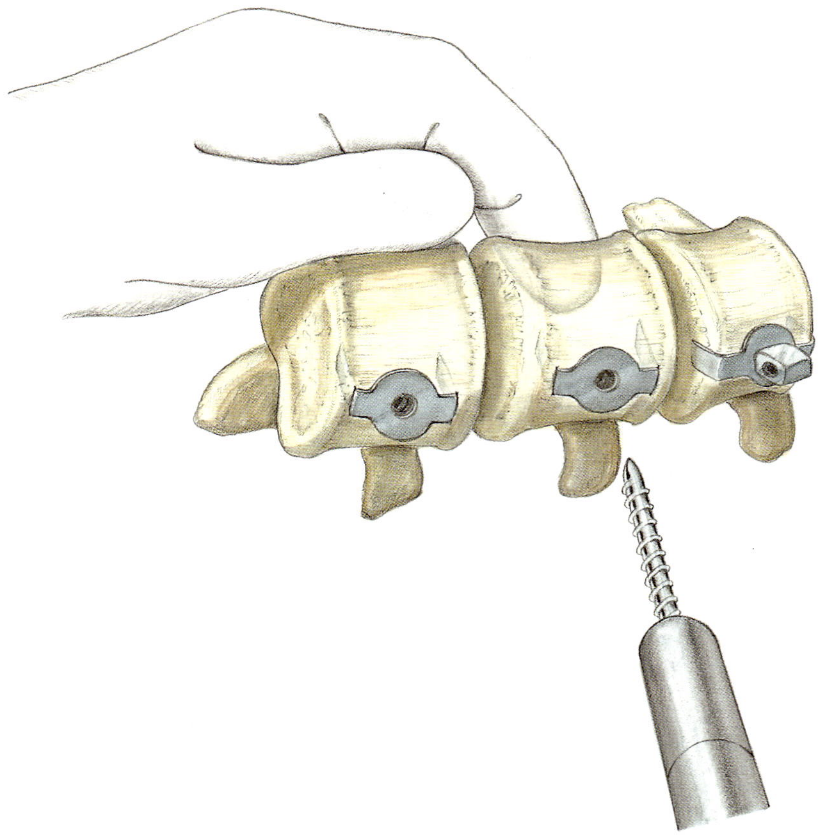

Fig. 2.**149** Insertion of Dwyer screws. The tip of the screw is palpated with the finger from the opposite side.

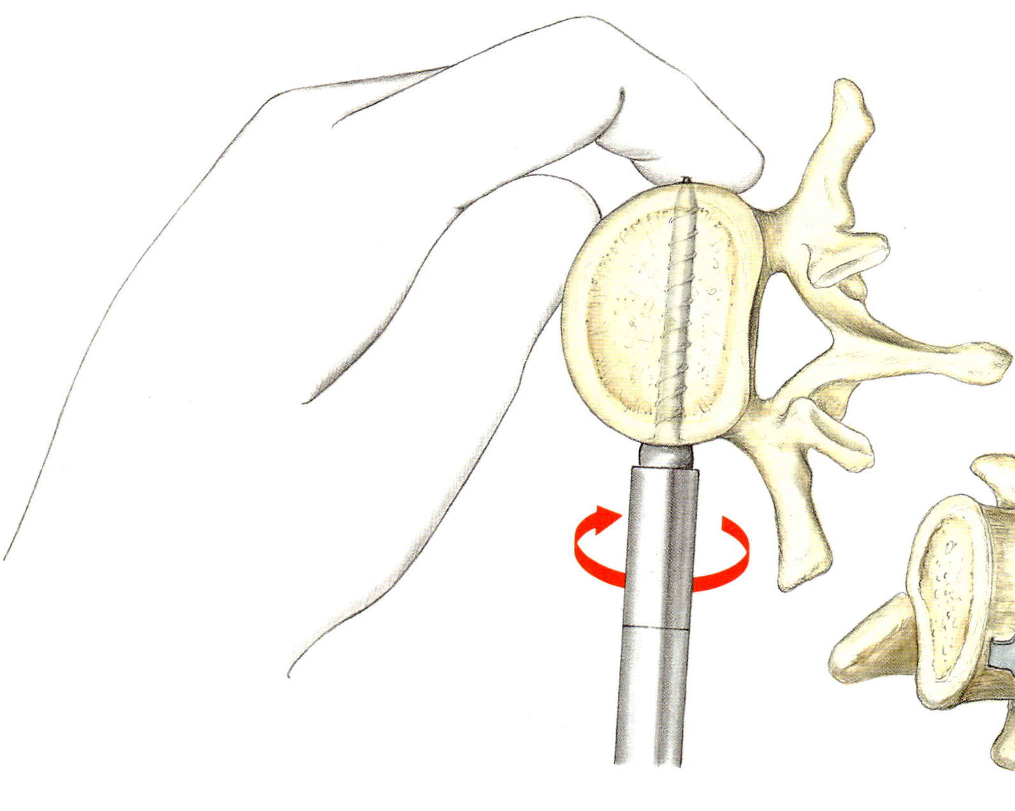

Fig. 2.**150** Correct position of the screw in the vertebral body. Note the vertebral torsion in scoliosis.

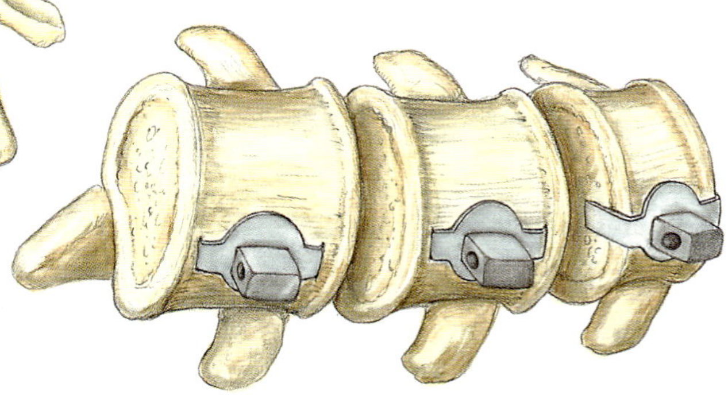

Fig. 2.**151** Status following implantation of clamps and screws.

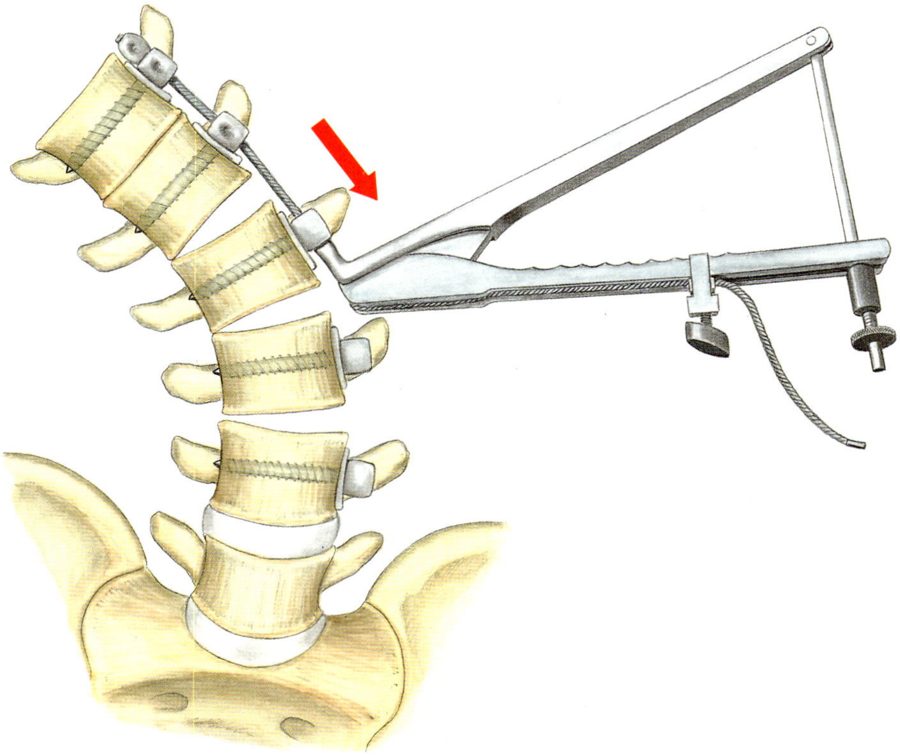

Fig. 2.**152** After removal of the intervertebral disks and insertion of Dwyer clamps and screws, the cable is pulled in, and drawn tight with the cable tensioner.

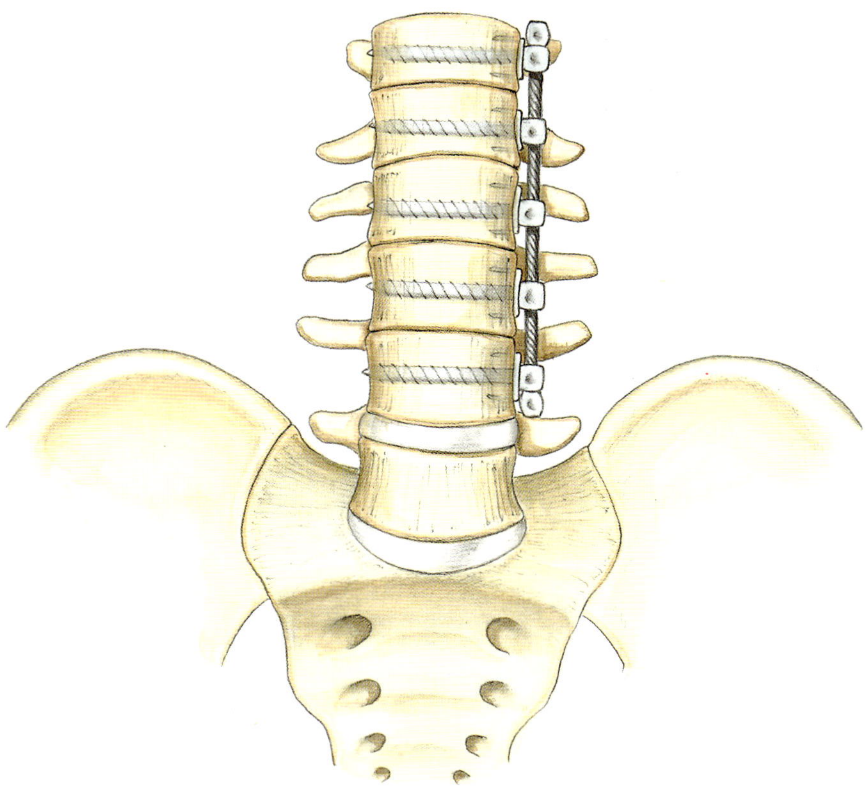

Fig. 2.**153** Dwyer operation. Status after final correction. The cable is fixed in the screwheads by compressing the screwheads with the crimper (Fig. 2.**142**).

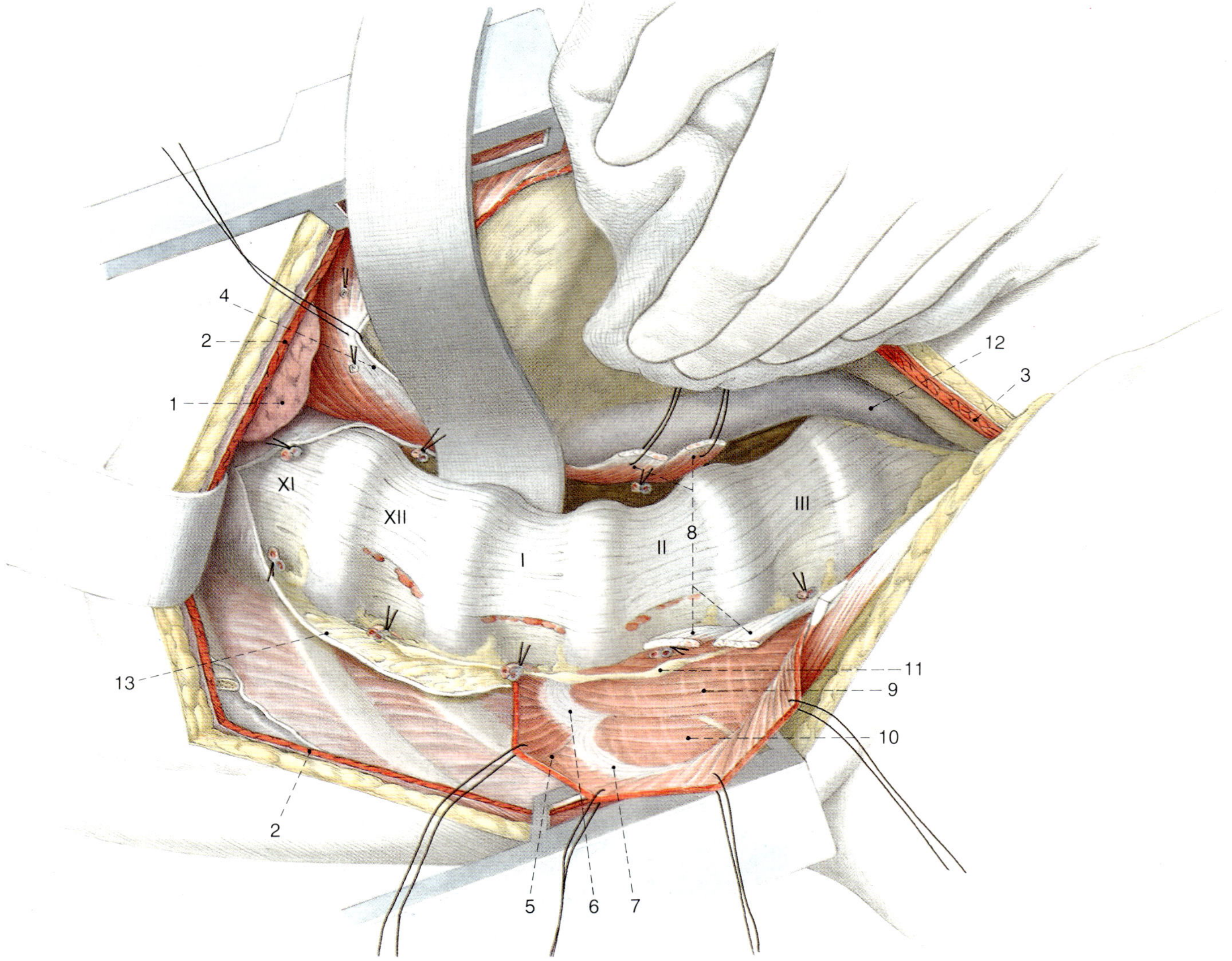

Fig. 2.**154** Exposure of thoracolumbar junction in right convex lumbar scoliosis.

1 Right lung
2 External oblique muscle of the abdomen
3 Internal oblique and tranverse muscles of the abdomen
4 Thoracic diaphragm, tendinous center
5 Thoracic diaphragm, lumbar portion
6 Thoracic diaphragm, medial arcuate ligament
7 Thoracic diaphragm, lateral arcuate ligament
8 Thoracic diaphragm, right medial crus
9 Greater psoas muscle
10 Quadratus lumborum muscle
11 Sympathetic trunk
12 Inferior vena cava
13 Parietal pleura
XI, XII Thoracic vertebrae
I–III Lumbar vertebrae

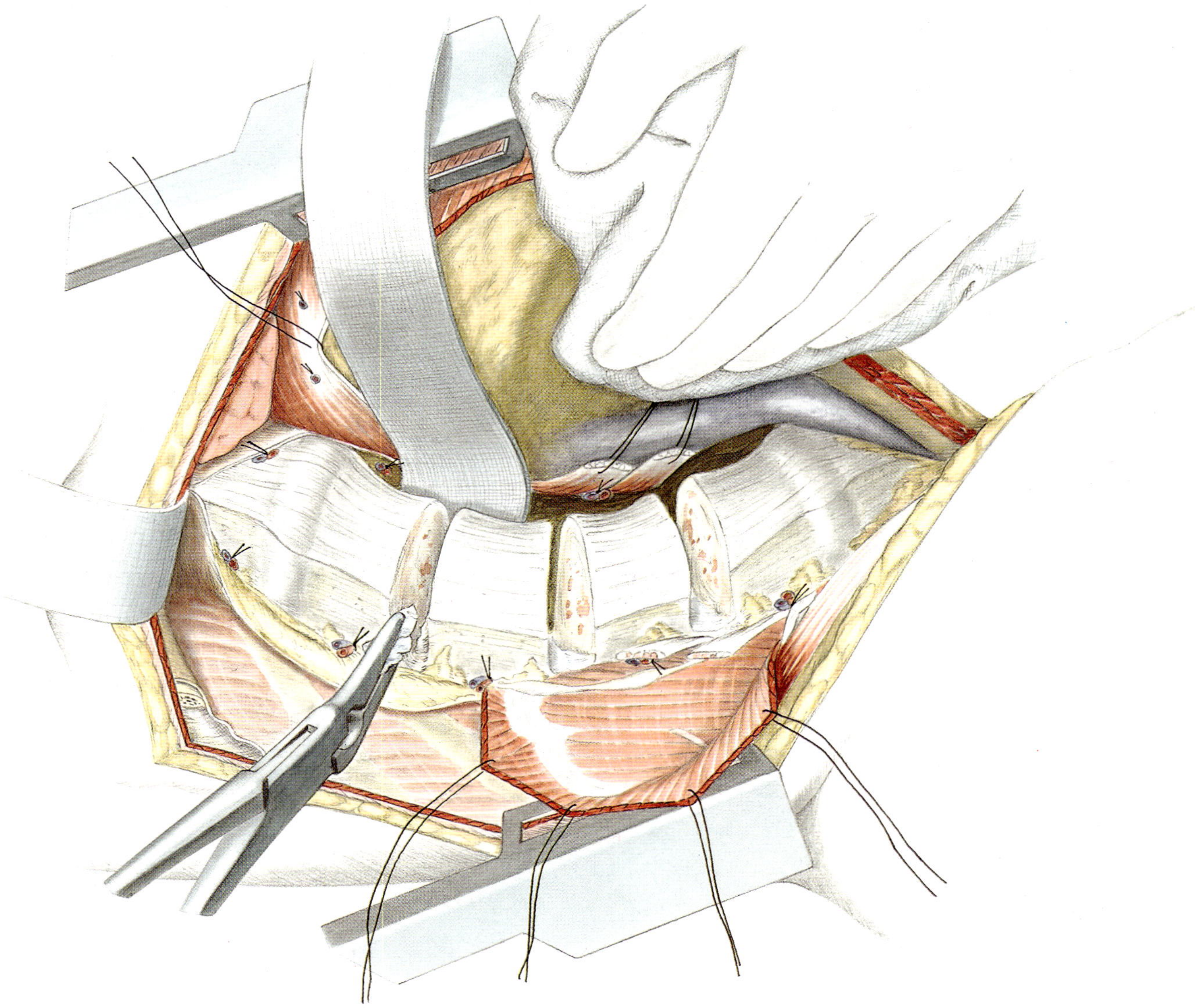

Fig. 2.**155** The intervertebral disks are first excised with a knife and then removed with the rongeur as far as the posterior longitudinal ligament.

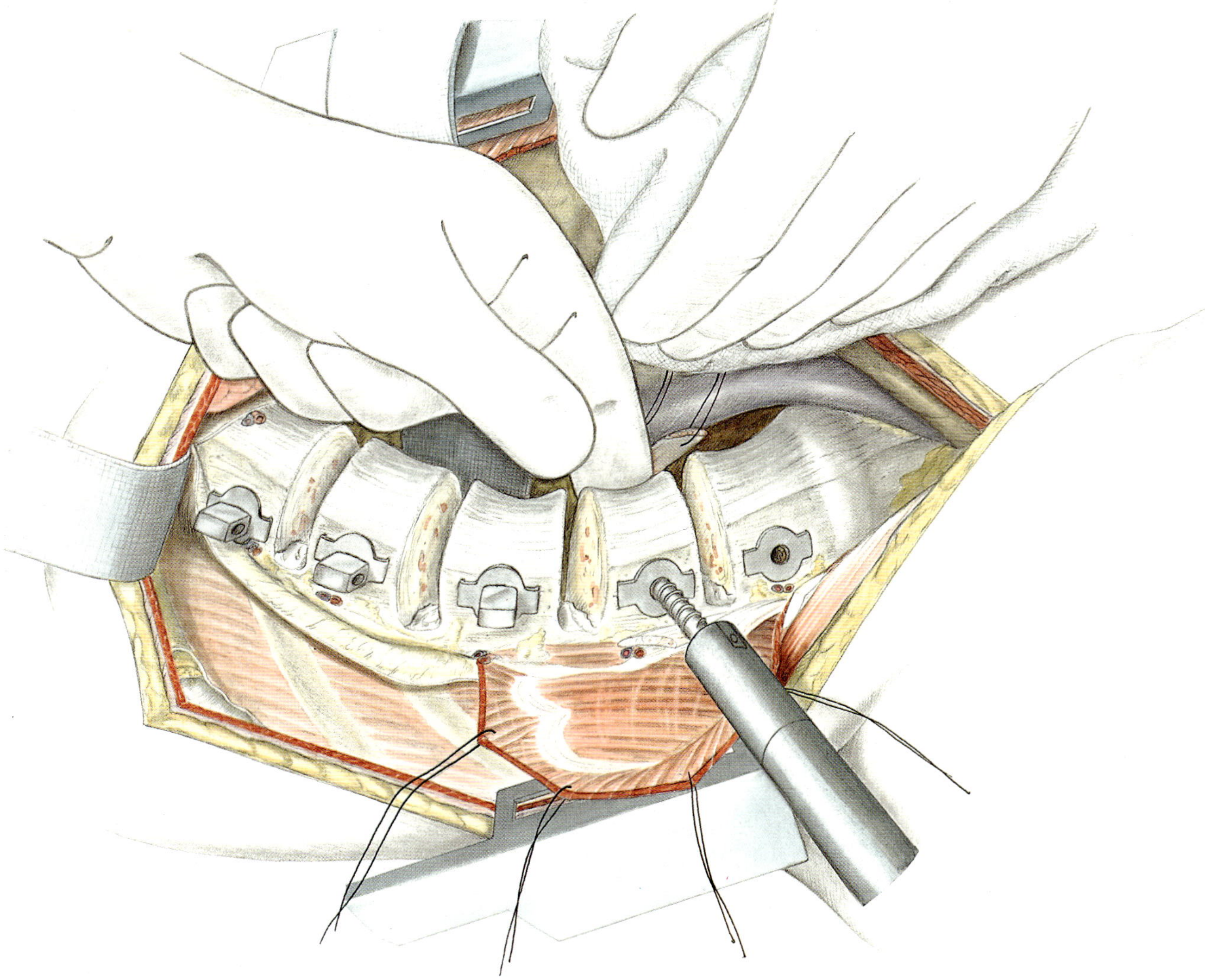

Fig. 2.**156** Insertion of Dwyer clamps and screws, following the preoperative plan.

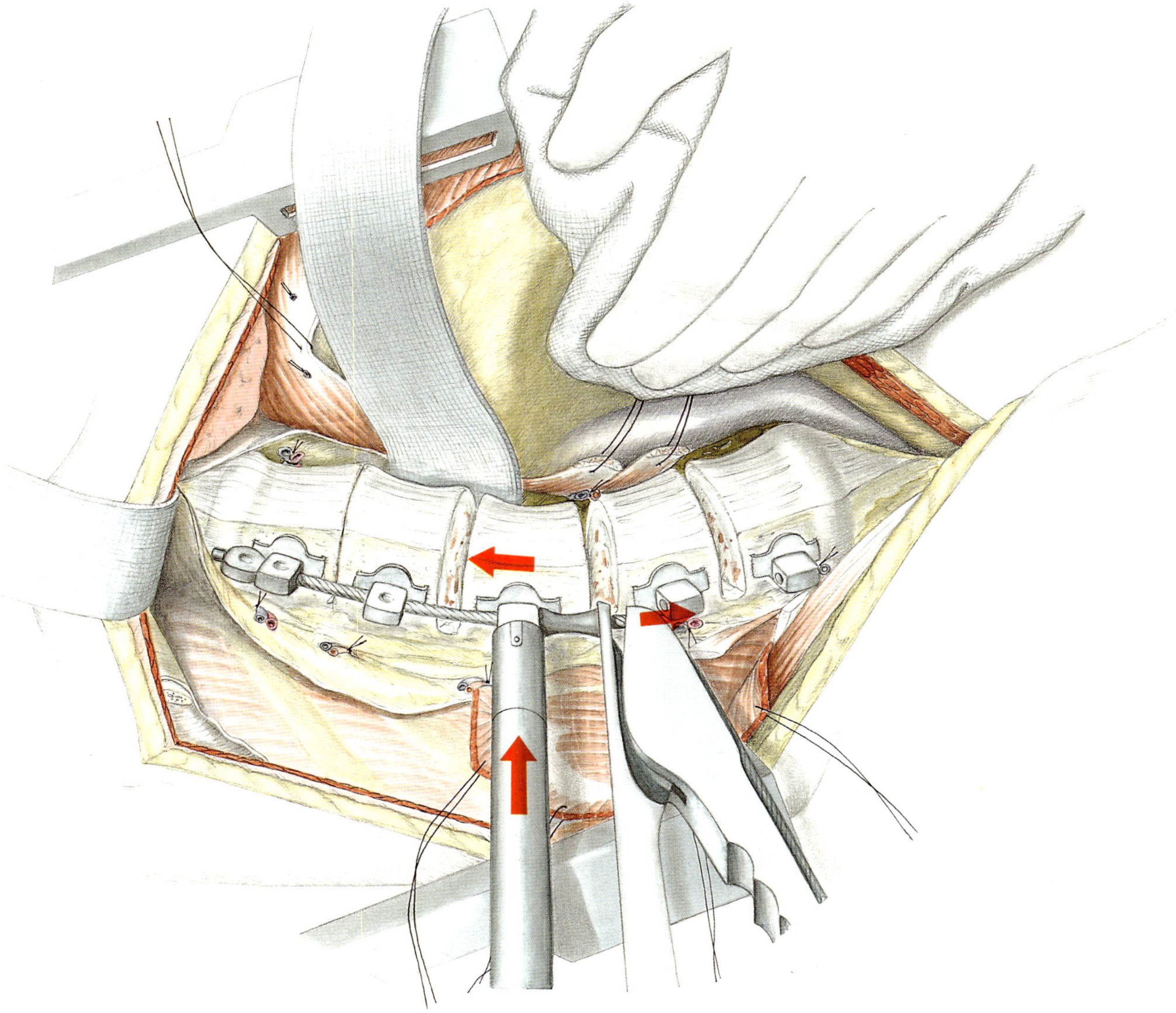

Fig. 2.**157** Correction by tightening the cable with the cable-tensioning device. A screwdriver is used to exert pressure on the cranially-positioned screw.

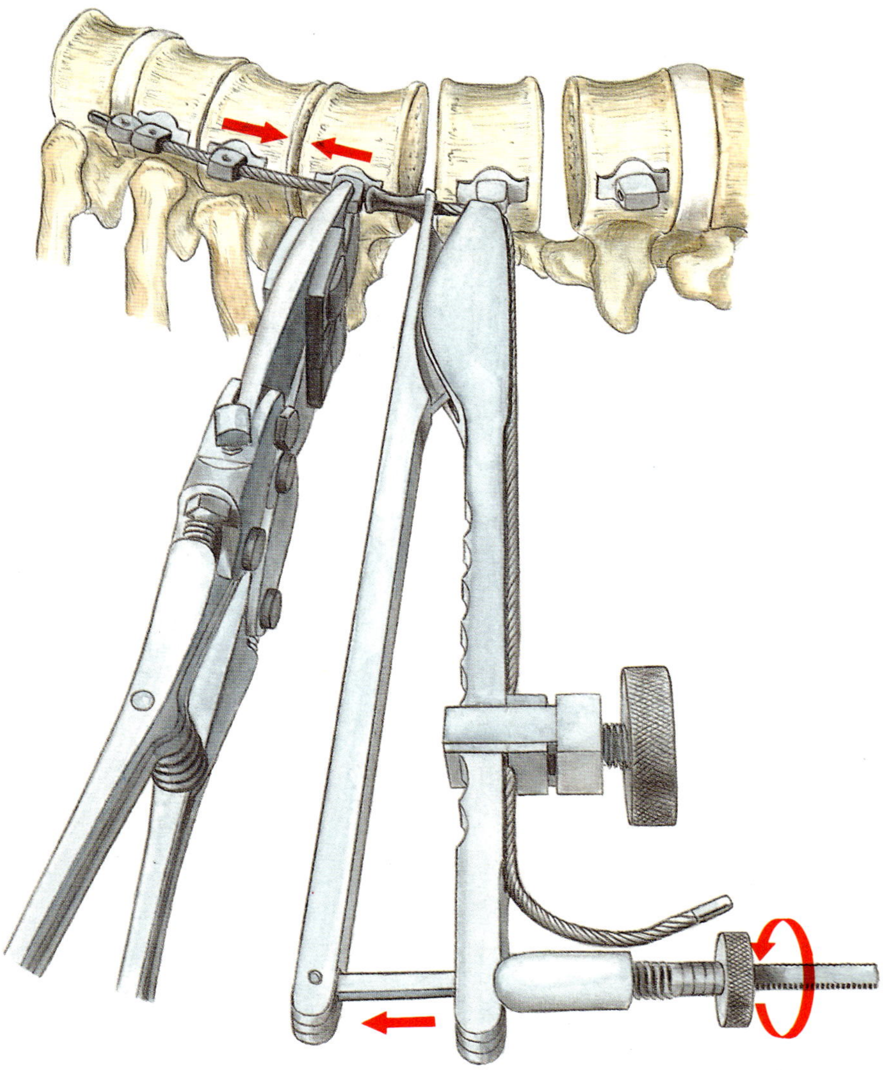

Fig. 2.**158** After maximal segmental correction has been accomplished with the cable tensioner, the screwhead is compressed with the crimper to secure the setting.

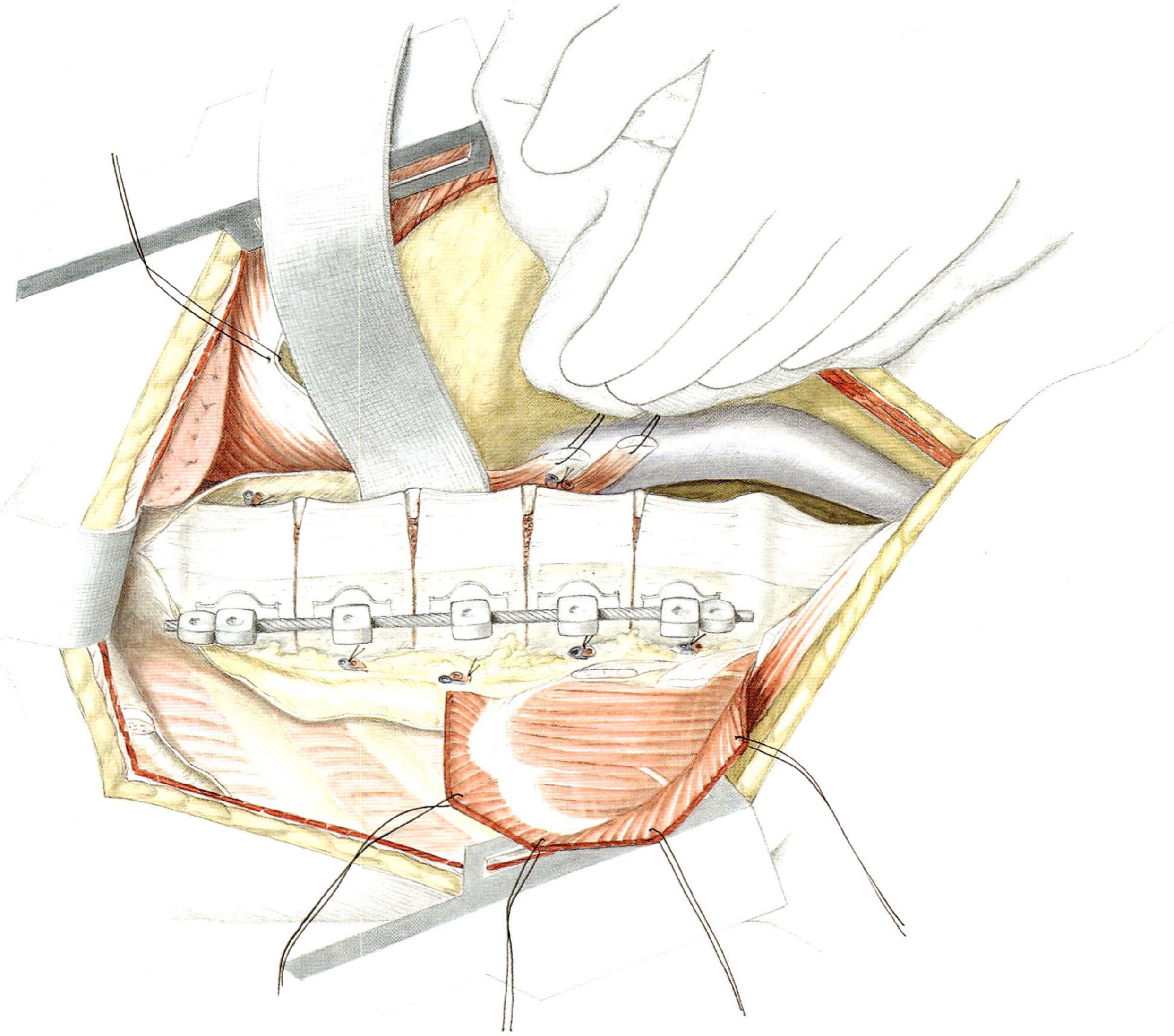

Fig. 2.**159** Status after completion of correction. In the lumbar spinal region, rib cuttings are implanted anteriorly between the vertebral bodies, to prevent kyphosation.

Further Reading

Bauer R. Die operative Behandlung der Skoliose. Berne: Huber, 1979.

Bauer R, Mostegl A, Eichenauer M. An analysis of the results of Dwyer and Zielke instrumentation in the treatment of scoliosis. Arch Orthop Traum Surg 1986;105:302.

Dwyer AF. Anterior instrumentation for scoliosis. Israel J Med Sci 1973a;9:805.

Dwyer AF. Experience of anterior correction of scoliosis. Clin Orthop 1973b;93:191.

Dwyer AF, Newton NC, Sherwood AA. An anterior approach to scoliosis. Clin Orthop 1969;62:192.

Dwyer AF, Schafer MF. Anterior approach to scoliosis: results of treatment in fifty-one cases. J Bone Jt Surg 1974;56-B:218.

Dwyer AP, McDonald C, Shapiro F, Gray JM, Hall JE, Rowell D. Telemetric monitoring of cable tensions following Dwyer spinal instrumentations. 11th Annual Meeting of the American Scoliosis Research Society, Ottawa, Canada, 1976.

Dwyer, AP, O'Brien JP, Seal PP, Hsu L, Yau ACMC, Hodgson AR. The late complications after the Dwyer anterior spinal instrumentation for scoliosis. J Bone Jt Surg 1977;59-B:117.

Hall JE, Gray J, Allen M. Dwyer instrumentation and spinal fusion: a follow-up study. J Bone Jt Surg 1977;59-B:117.

Michel CR, Onimus M, Kohler R. L'opération de Dwyer dans le traitement chirurgical des scolioses. Rev Chir Orthop 1977;63:237.

Onimus M, Michel CR. Evolution des courbures compensatrices après opération de Dwyer. In: Zielke K, ed. Skoliose und Kyphose. Stuttgart: Hippokrates, 1978a:39.

Onimus M, Michel CR. Résultats et indications de l'opération de Dwyer. Int Orthop 1978b;1:323.

Onimus M, Michel CR, Kohler R. L'opération de Dwyer dans le traitement des scolioses paralytiques avec bassin oblique. Rev Chir Orthop 1977;63:257.

Ventral Derotation Spondylodesis (Zielke)

Indications

There are eccentially no basic differences in the indications from those for the Dwyer method (p. 163). Again, thoracolumbar and lumbar scolioses are particularly suitable. Zielke, however, has reported that the ventral derotation spondylodesis (VDS) procedure can also achieve good correction for thoracic curvatures. Special advantages over the Dwyer instrumentation that should be pointed out are the greater stability and the possibility of derotation and lordosation.

Approach

See Chapter 1, pp. 24–36.

Operative Technique

Instrumentarium

(Figs. 2.**160**–2.**162**)

- VDS screws, open on top and on the sides.
- Shim plates (end plates).
- Angle plates.
- Threaded rod with hexagonal nuts.
- Derotator.

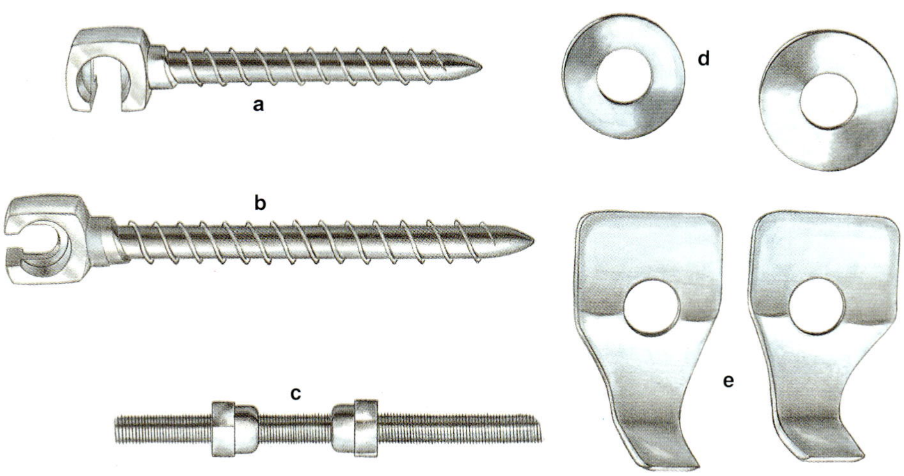

Fig. 2.**160** Zielke implants.
a VDS screw, lateral slit.
b VDS screw, upper slit.
c Threaded rod with nuts (compression rods).
d End plates.
e Angle plates.

Principles of Correction

The scoliotic curvature is corrected by shortening and compressing the convex side using vertebral body screws and the threaded rod (Fig. 2.**163**). The correction proceeds continuously from the periphery toward the apical vertebra.

The special VDS instrument is the derotator. It works on the three-point principle. The sites at which the force is applied are the end screws and the midpoint of the compression rod. The forced lordosation or derotation position is maintained by subsequent compression of one vertebral body against the other.

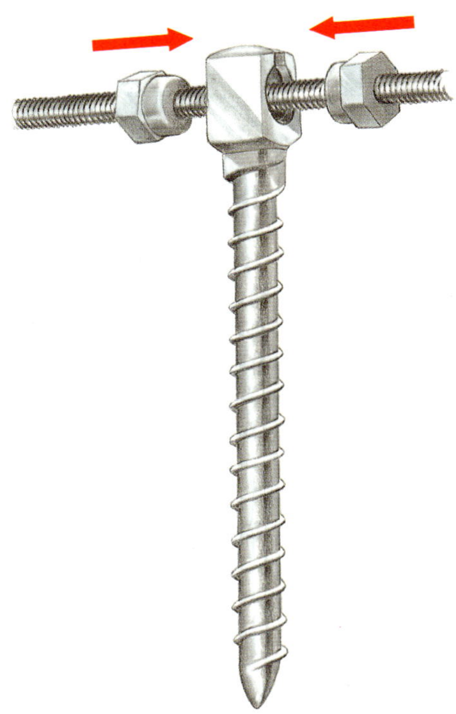

Fig. 2.**161** VDS screw. Angular stability is produced by fixation of both nuts.

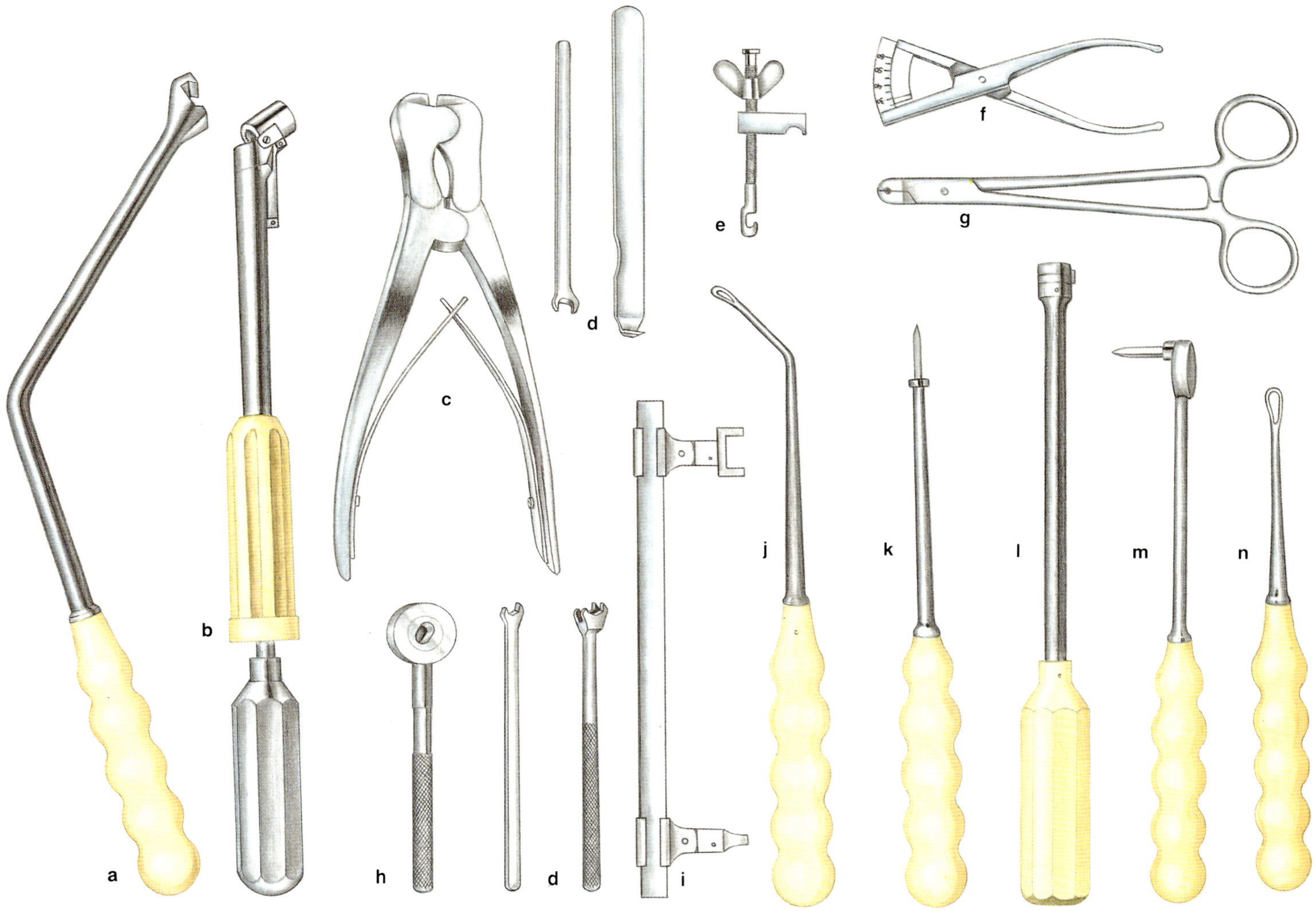

Fig. 2.**162** VDS instruments according to Zielke.
a Derotation lever.
b Cardan screwdriver.
c Cutting forceps for compression rod.
d Various wrenches.
e Tightening screw for derotator.
f Instrument for measuring screw length (vertebral body diameter).
g Rod holder for compression rods.
h VDS wrench.
i Derotating device.
j Intervertebral curet.
k Straight awl.
l VDS screwdriver.
m Rectangular awl.
n Intervertebral curet.

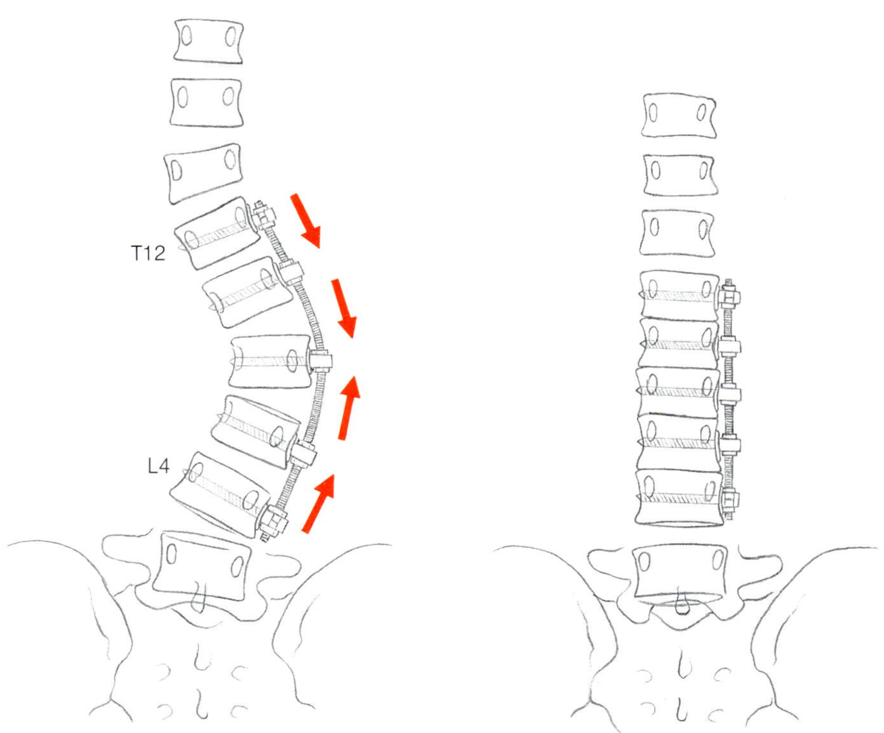

Fig. 2.**163** Correction by compression from the periphery to the apical vertebra.

Area of Fusion

The following radiographs are needed to evaluate the fusion area:

- Standing anteroposterior and lateral film of the entire spine.
- Bending films in the frontal plane.
- Bending films in the sagittal plane (flexion and extension), if there is a deformity in this plane.
- Suspension film.

The area of fusion is the same as in the Dwyer operation. As a rule, the VDS extends from one end vertebra of the curve to the other. On the bending film, the lowest vertebra to be instrumented should show an inclination toward the pelvic axis of no more than 15 degrees and a rotation of no more than 20% (Nash and Moe).

Instrumentation

(Figs. 2.**164**–2.**170**)

The operation is essentially identical to the Dwyer technique, including exposure of the vertebral bodies by ligation of the segmental vessels and resection of the intervertebral disks (p. 172). An awl is now used to make a hole in the middle of the vertebral body (cranial–caudal) as far posteriorly on the convex side as possible. After preliminary measurement (with a special instrument), screws of appropriate length are inserted in the usual way transversely through the vertebral body, in the direction of the palpating finger. The end screws have lateral slits, while the intermediate screws have slits facing upward. The screws are fitted with end plates, with the convex sides facing the screwheads. Alternatively, angle plates can be used. A threaded compression rod, already prepared and fitted with a corresponding number of nuts, is then inserted into

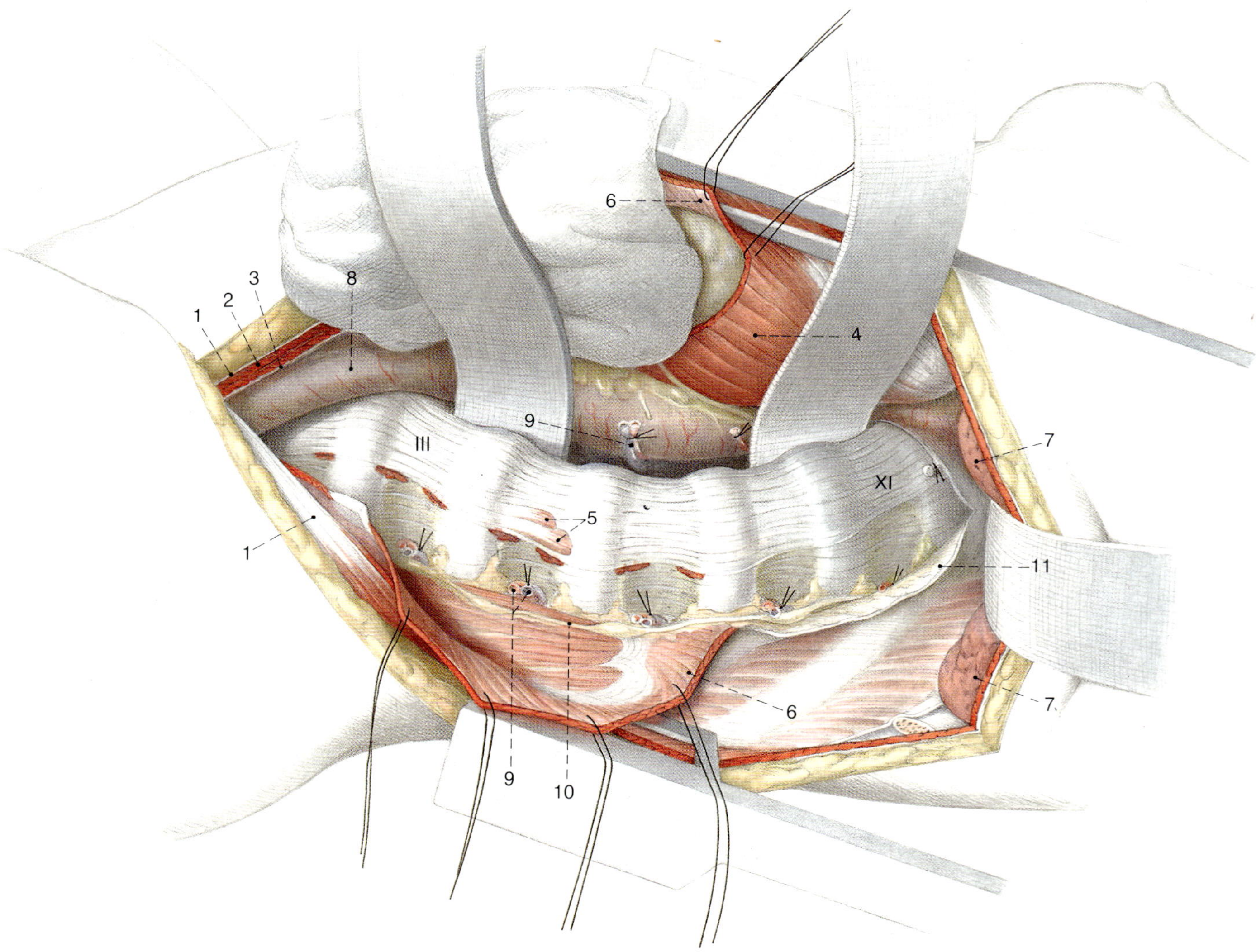

Fig. 2.**164** Exposure of a left convex lumbar scoliosis by the anterior approach.

1 Aponeurosis of the external oblique muscle of the abdomen
2 Internal oblique muscle of the abdomen
3 Transverse muscle of the abdomen
4 Thoracic diaphragm
5 Left medial crus of the thoracic diaphragm
6 Left lateral crus of the thoracic diaphragm
7 Left lung
8 Abdominal aorta
9 Intercostal vessels
10 Sympathetic trunk
11 Parietal pleura
III Lumbar vertebra
XI Thoracic vertebra

the slits of the screwheads, and pretensioning is begun. In this process, the vertebrae cranial to the apical vertebra are subjected to a caudally-directed compression, and those situated caudally to a cranially-directed compression. Before proceeding to final correction of the scoliosis, the derotator is applied to the two end screws in the area. With the aid of the tightening screw, lordosation is now effected, particularly in the lumbar region, and derotation is effected by careful movements of the derotation lever. Here, too, we carry out anterior stabilization in the area of the lumbar lordosis through anterior insertion of rib segments into the disk space. The scoliotic curvature is then corrected by compression in the direction of the apical vertebra. Next, the derotator is removed, and the screws are definitively fixed by pulling the threaded rod nuts light in the opposite direction. The protruding rod ends are clipped off.

Wound Closure

See Chapter 1, p. 35.

Postoperative Treatment

The patient is usually positioned in bed without external support and transferred to the intensive care unit, where the necessary diagnostic and therapeutic measures are carried out. After removal of the sutures on postoperative days 12–14, a body cast or a spinal orthosis is applied, which should be worn for 7–9 months after the operation.

Pitfalls and Complications

- Complications of thoracic surgery: pneumothorax, hemothorax, chylothorax, lung atelectases.
- System-specific complications: screw avulsion, rod fracture, pseudarthrosis.
- Neurologic complications: radicular lesion, transverse cord lesions.
- Sympathectomy effect, particularly with operations in the region of the lower lumbar spine.

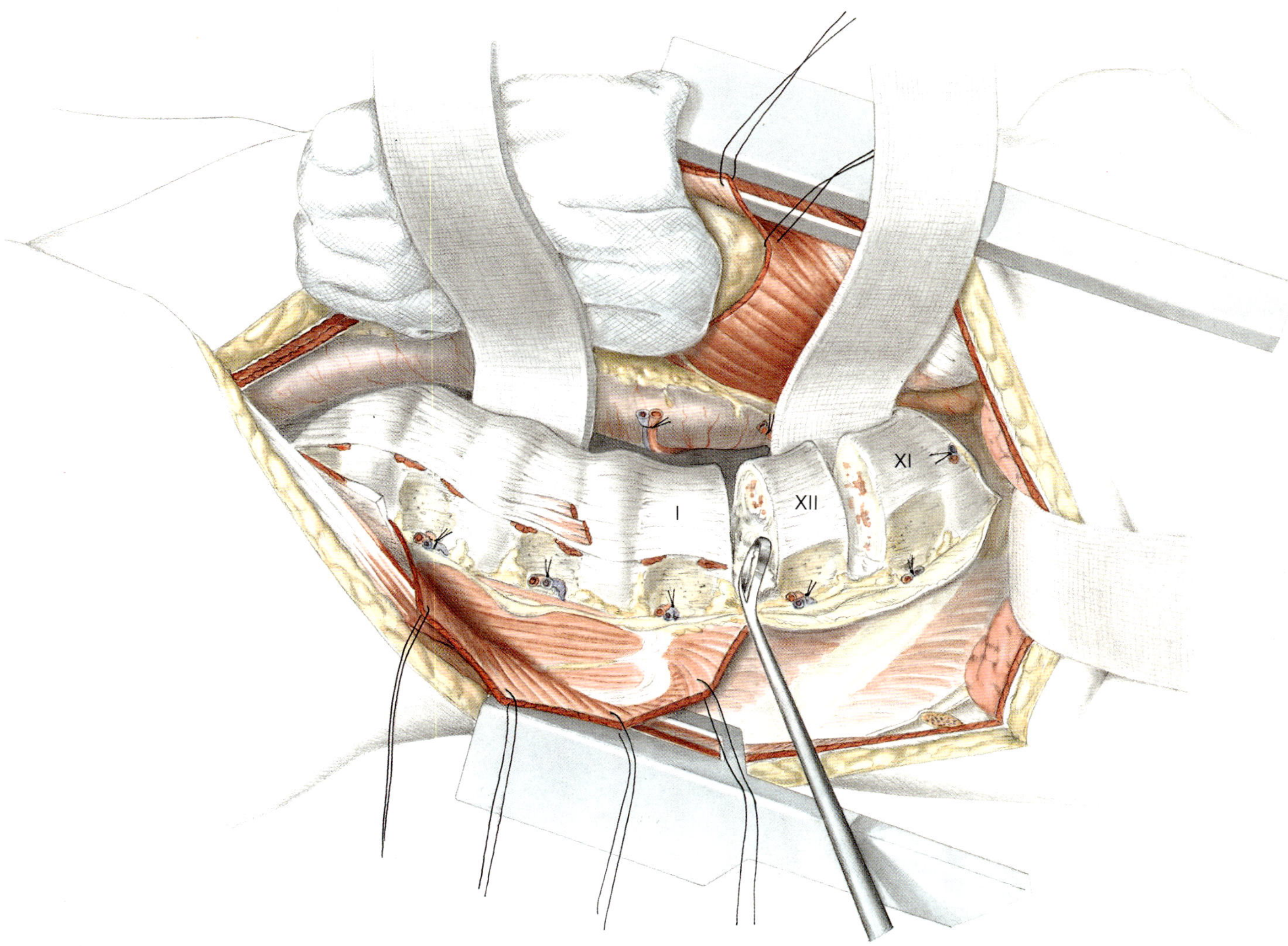

Fig. 2.**165** The intervertebral disks are excised, and the vertebral bodies are debrided with a curet.

I Lumbar vertebra
XI, XII Thoracic vertebrae

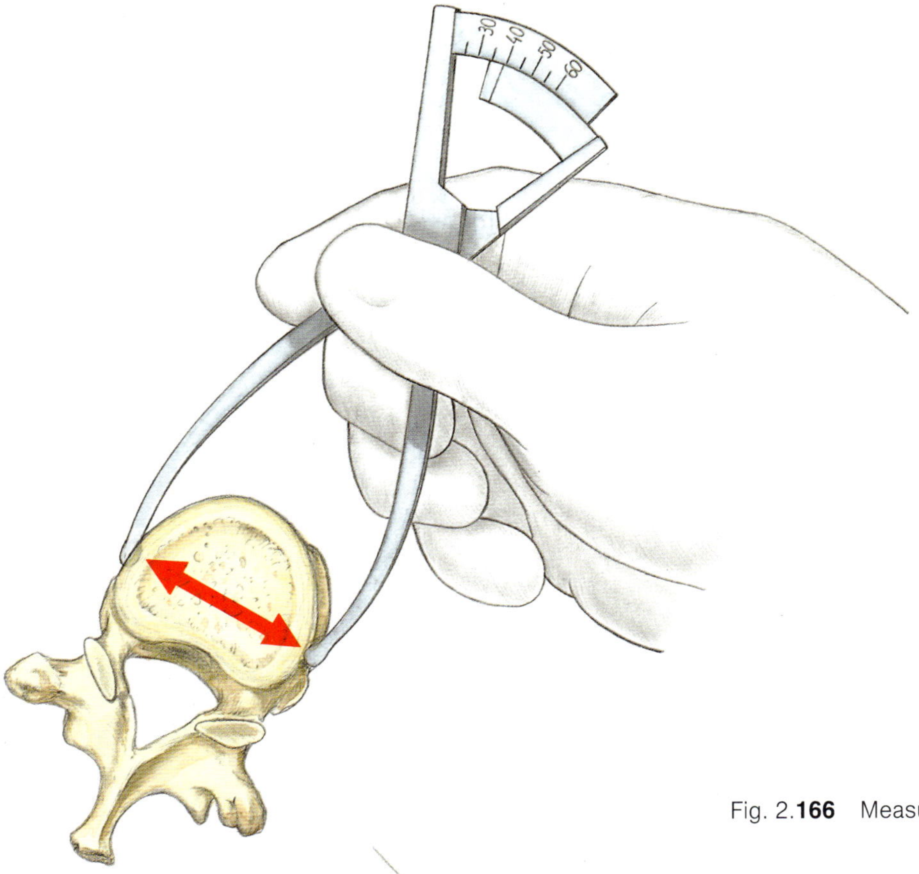

Fig. 2.**166** Measuring the correct screw length.

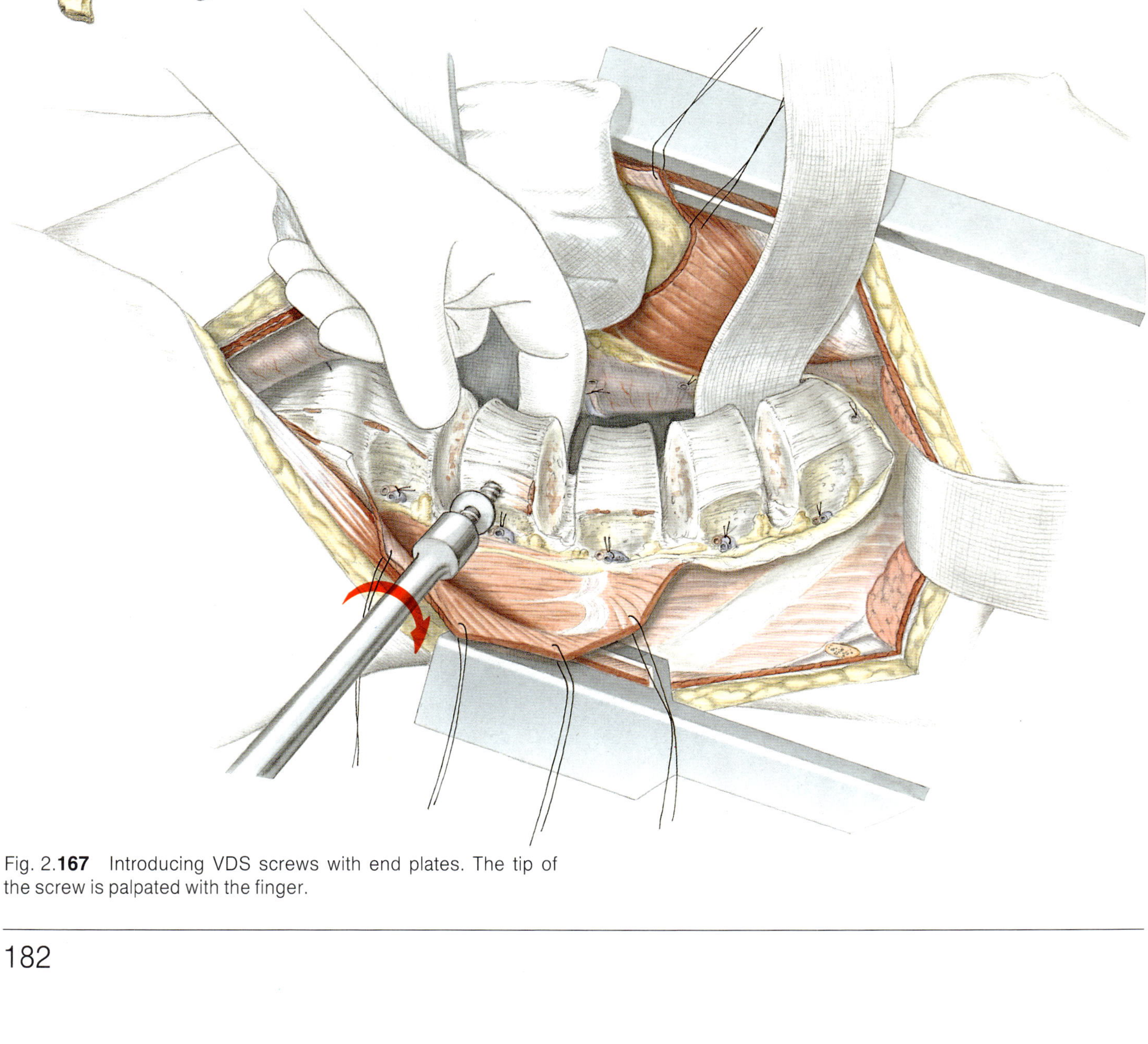

Fig. 2.**167** Introducing VDS screws with end plates. The tip of the screw is palpated with the finger.

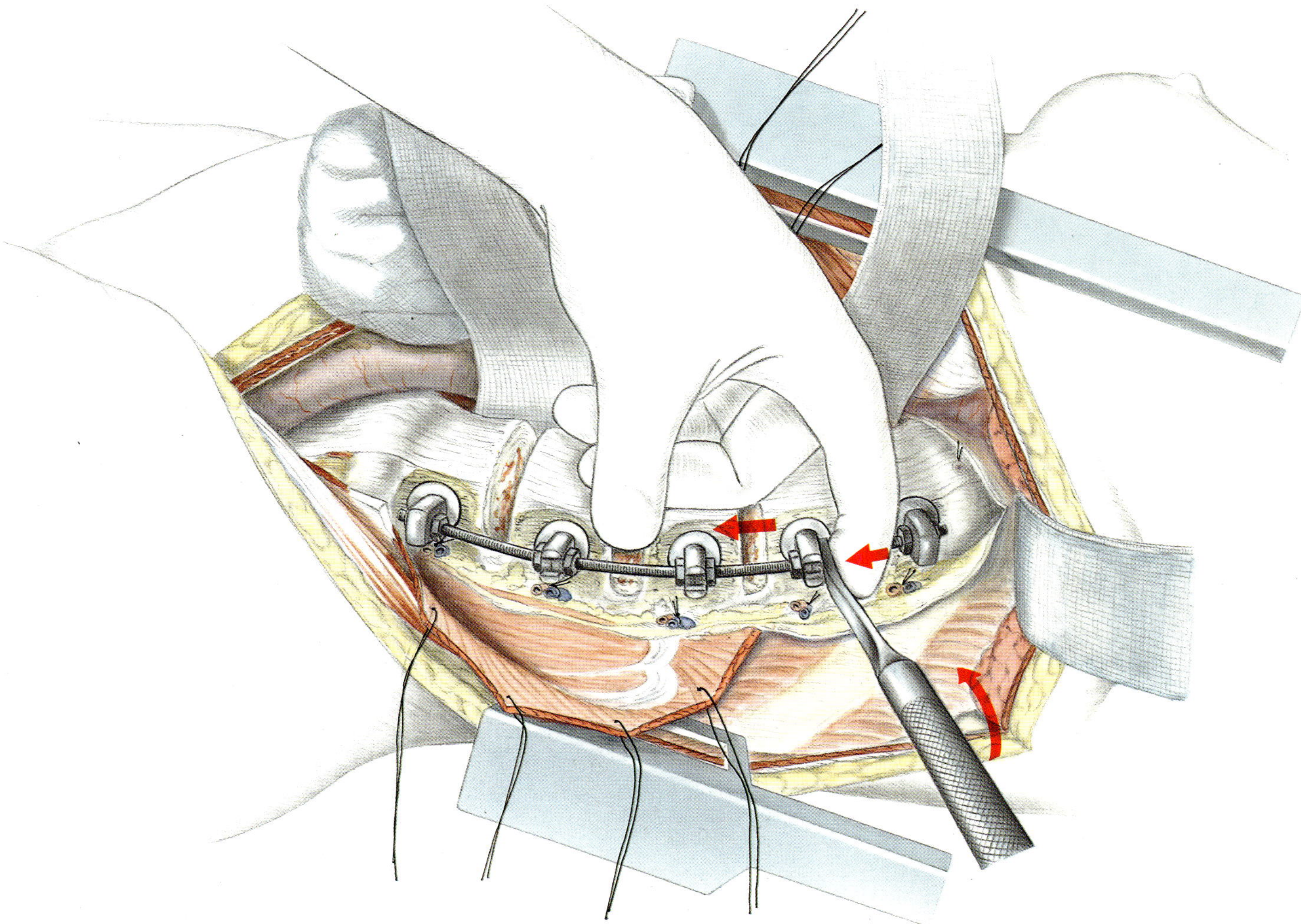

Fig. 2.**168** Status after placement of the compression rod. The correction is made from the ends of the curve to the center.

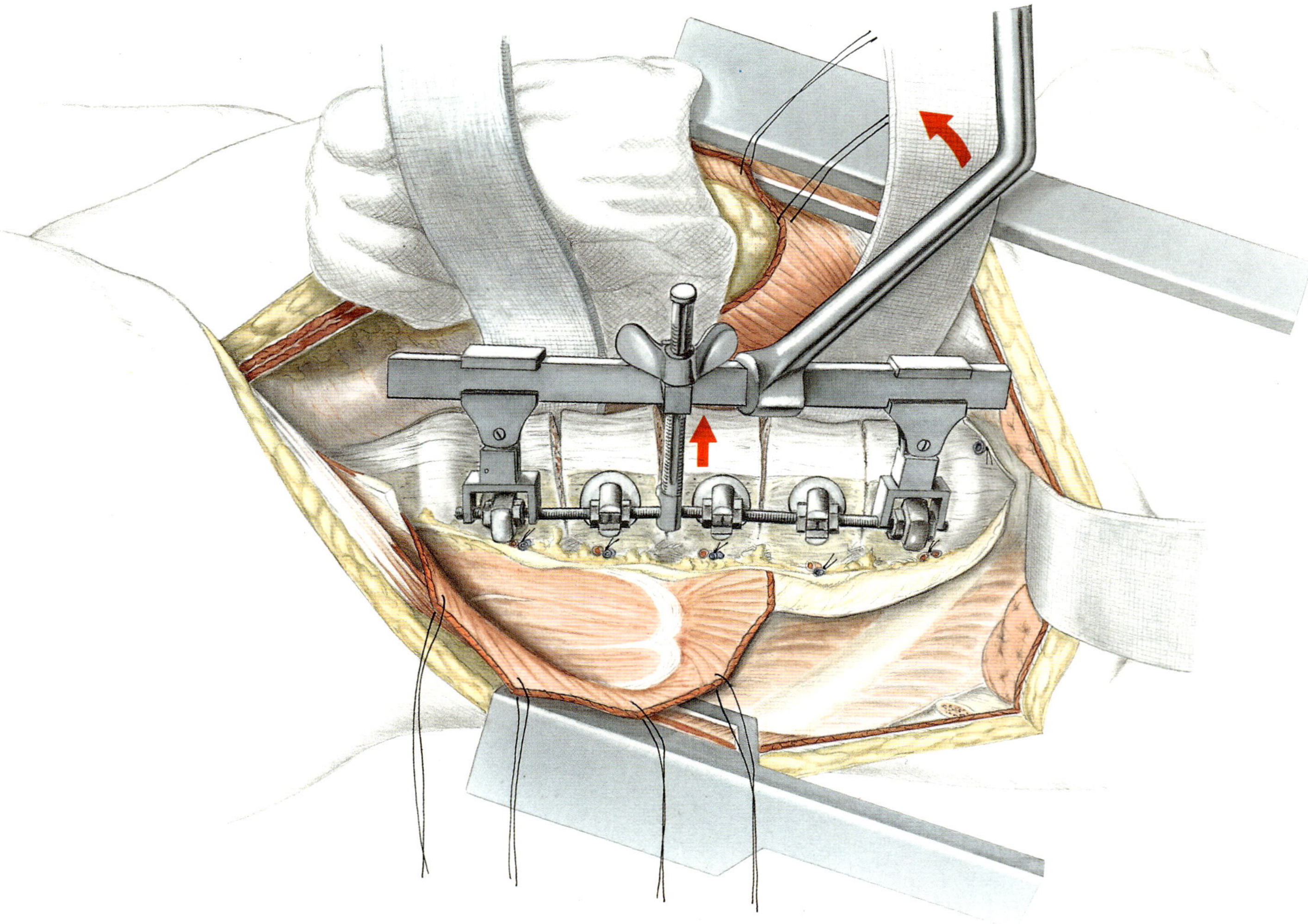

Fig. 2.**169** When enough preliminary tension has been obtained, the tightening screw is used for lordosation and, finally, derotation (arrow).

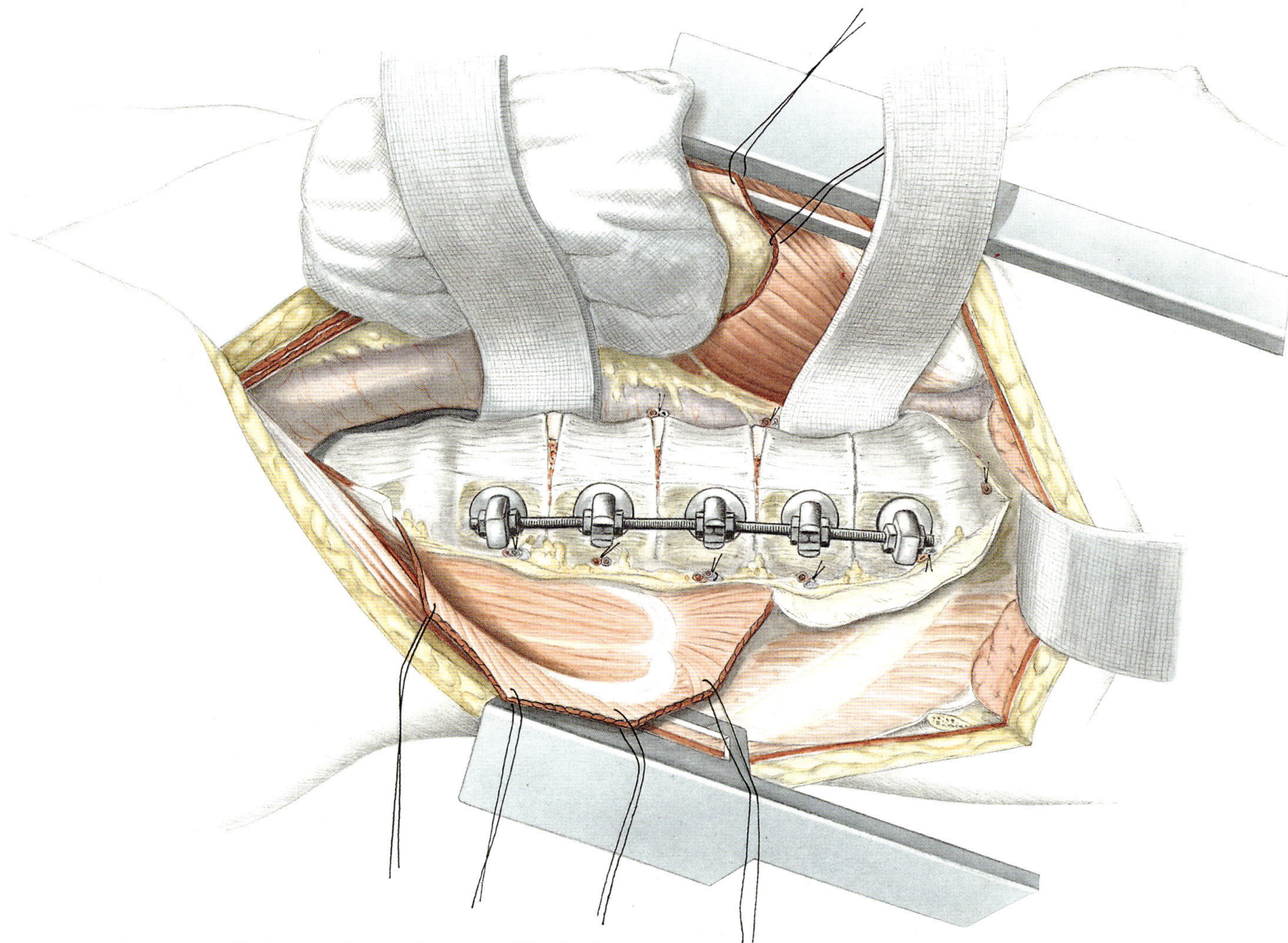

Fig. 2.**170** Status after final correction. In the area of the lumbar spine, the lordosation is maintained using anteriorly implanted rib morsels.

Further Reading

Bauer R, Mostegl A, Eichenauer M. An analysis of the results of Dwyer and Zielke instrumentations of scoliosis. Arch Orthop Traum Surg 1986;105:302.

Giehl JP, Zielke K, Hack HP. Die ventrale Derotationsspondylodese nach Zielke. Orthopäde 1989;18:101.

Zielke K. Indikationen, Ergebnisse und Komplikationen der ventralen Derotationsspondylodese. In: Bauer R, ed. Der vordere Zugang der Wirbelsäule. Stuttgart: Thieme, 1983:109.

Zielke K, Stunkat R. Ergebnisse der ventralen Derotationsspondylodese. In: Zielke K, ed. Skoliose und Kyphose. Stuttgart: Hippokrates, 1978.

Zielke K, Stunkat R, Beaujean F. Ventrale Derotationsspondylodese. Vorläufiger Ergebnisbericht über 26 operierte Fälle. Arch Orthop Unfall-Chir 1976;85:257.

3 Kyphosis

R. Bauer

Treatment Concept

Given the multitude of diseases leading to a kyphotic deformity, it is hardly possible to lay down universally applicable rules for operative therapy. In unisegmental posttraumatic kyphosis, it may be sufficient to remove one or two intervertebral disks by an anterior approach, and to perform an interbody fusion with the help of a laminar spreader after correction of the kyphotic deformity (posttraumatic kyphosis, p. 212). As a rule, however, three basic treatment steps are always required, and can be carried out in one or several operative sessions, depending on the individual case.

1. *Mobilizing osteotomy.* Anterior and/or posterior. In the presence of positive neurologic symptoms, an anterior decompression has to be considered (decompression, p. 198).

2. *Correction*

- Preoperative: halo wheelchair, halo–femoral traction, halo–pelvic apparatus;
- Intraoperative: laminar spreader, distractors developed by Pinto, Slot and others.

3. *Fusion*

- After osteotomy and correction,
- In situ, to prevent progression.

Objective:
- Preparation for osseous fusion.
- Stabilization until bony fusion.

These goals can be achieved by the following techniques:

- A free bone graft, primarily using the fibula, but also the tibia, rib or iliac crest.
- A vascularized pedicle bone graft.
- A bone graft in combination with an *implant.* The bone graft only induces the fusion; temporary stabilization is accomplished by the implant.

4. *Stabilization without osseous fusion*

- Mostly in tumor patients in whom osseous fusion cannot be expected (Chapter 11, Spinal Tumors).
- Vertebral body prosthesis (Polster, Wolter, etc.).
- Internal fixation.
- Cement stabilization.

Anterior Strut Grafting (Free Graft)

Indications

- Severe angular kyphosis of varying etiology, but for the most part congenital kyphosis (p. 205).
- Remote posttraumatic kyphosis.
- Status after postlaminectomy kyphosis.
- Severe kyphoscoliosis.

Approach

In simple kyphosis, a right-sided thoracotomy is performed for anatomical reasons in the area of the thoracic spine. If the deformity is located at the thoracolumbar junction, a left-sided thoracophrenolumbotomy (Hodgson) is carried out. See Chapter 1, pp. 13, 24.

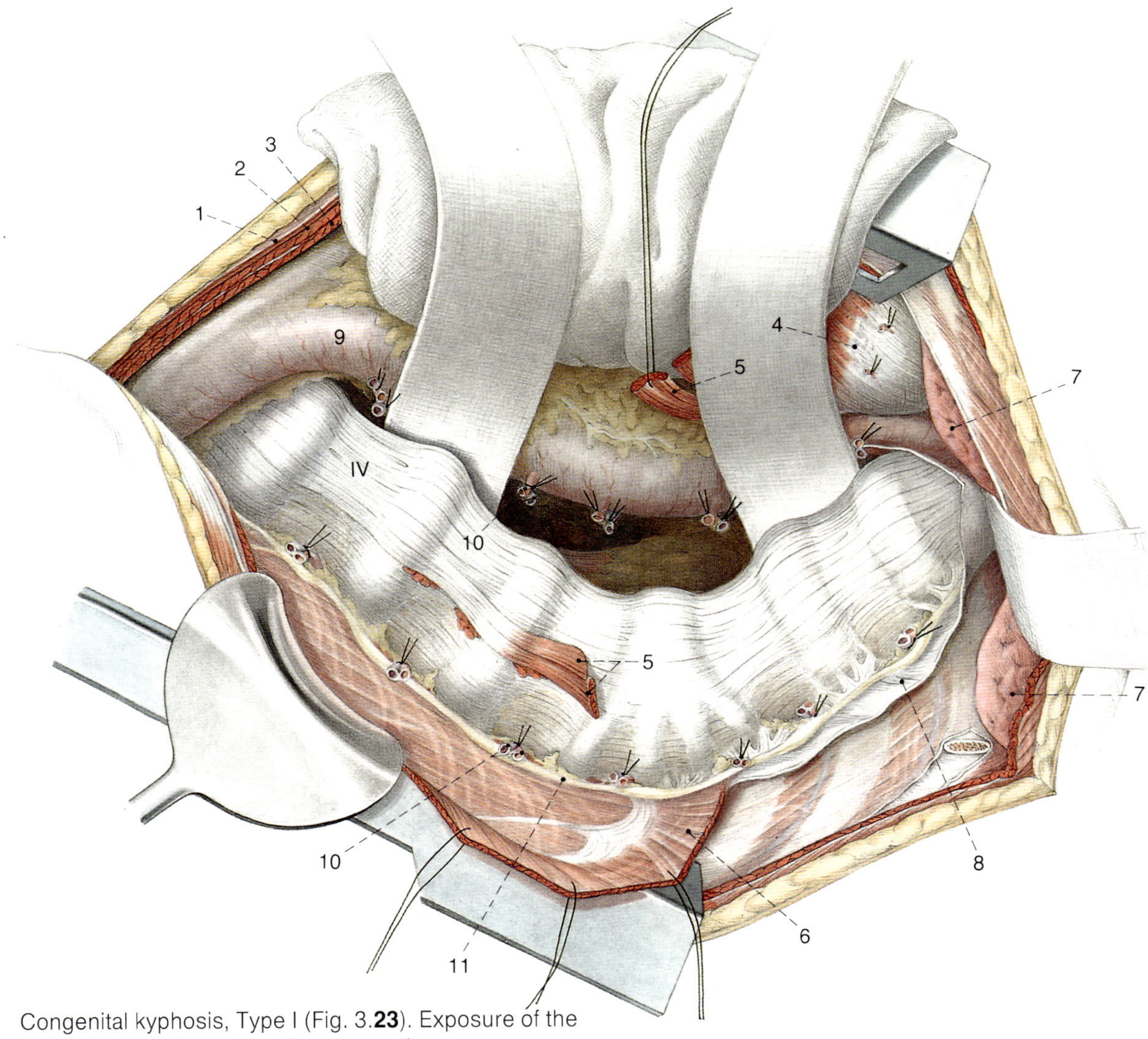

Fig. 3.**1** Congenital kyphosis, Type I (Fig. 3.**23**). Exposure of the spine using the Hodgson thoracolumbar approach.

1 Aponeurosis of the external oblique muscle of the abdomen
2 Internal oblique muscle of the abdomen
3 Transverse muscle of the abdomen
4 Thoracic diaphragm
5 Left medial crus of the thoracic diaphragm
6 Left lateral crus of the thoracic diaphragm
7 Left lung
8 Parietal pleura
9 Abdominal aorta
10 Intercostal vessels
11 Sympathetic trunk
IV Lumbar vertebra

Fusion Area

The following radiographs are required:

- Standing anteroposterior and lateral film of the entire spine.
- Traction film.
- Bending film in the sagittal plane.

Fusion is generally performed from one end vertebra of the kyphosis to the other. The most anterior strut graft—as a rule, several grafts are used—should lie as far anteriorly as possible, near the midline. To begin with, the vertebral bodies in the proposed fusion area are typically exposed over their entire circumference, using the anterior approach. The intervertebral disks are excised, and are removed as far as the posterior longitudinal ligament using pituitary forceps and curets (Figs. 3.**1**, 3.**2**).

After this, two technical options are available: fusion in situ or intraoperative correction of the deformity, followed by fusion.

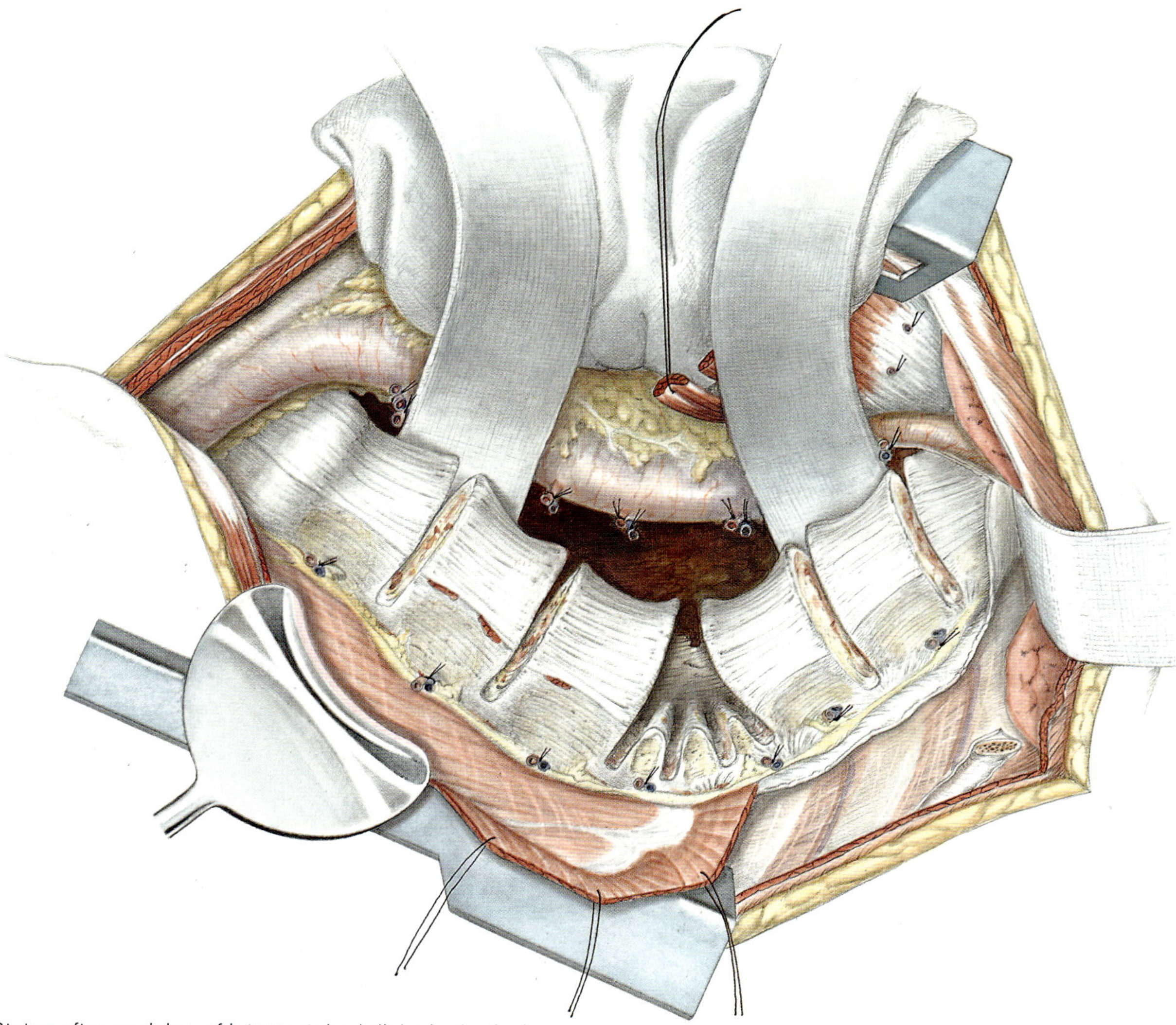

Fig. 3.**2** Status after excision of intervertebral disks in the fusion zone. Three posterior hemivertebrae are visible at the apex.

Fusion in Situ or Fusion with Minimal Intraoperative Correction

(Fig. 3.**3**)

Indications

Severe kyphosis without neurologic deficits, to prevent further progression of the deformity.

Operative Technique

Using a chisel or a ball reamer, anchoring holes for the strut graft are cut in the end vertebrae of the kyphosis. Grafts are used, preferably taken from the fibula, which can withstand a heavy compressive load. Other grafts are used near the spine, for example rib harvested in the course of the thoracotomy, or corticocancellous tibia, or iliac-crest bone chips. The intervertebral spaces or the spaces between the strut grafts are packed with cancellous bone. A certain amount of correction can be obtained by manual pressure on the apex of the kyphosis when the grafts are inserted following mobilization of the vertebral segments.

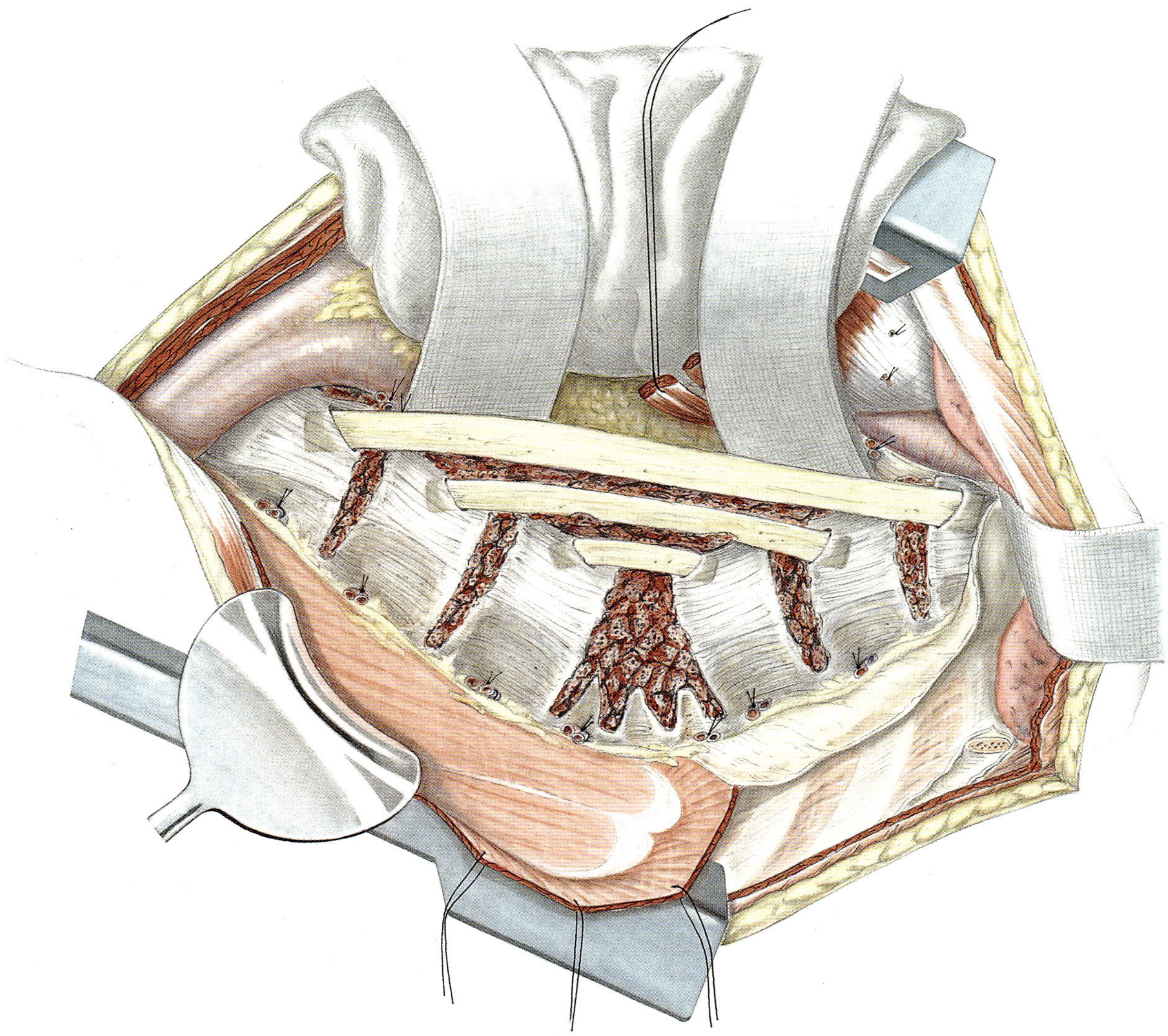

Fig. 3.**3** Status after insertion of anterior strut grafts and moderate correction of the kyphosis. The intervertebral spaces are filled with cancellous bone chips.

Intraoperative Correction Followed by Fusion

(Fig. 3.**4**)

Indications

The primary indication is severe kyphosis with a mobile apex (e.g., congenital kyphosis, Type I, Fig. 3.**23**). There should be no synostoses posteriorly; alternatively, any preexisting synostoses should be osteotomized in a preceding operation. If the kyphotic apex is rigid, distraction carries a high risk of neurologic injury, and is therefore contraindicated.

Operative Technique

Following exposure of the area of fusion, a distractor is applied anteriorly; this is used for a slow, continuous correction of the kyphosis, preferably while evaluating spinal cord function by recording somatosensory evoked potentials. When maximal distraction has been achieved, strut grafts are inserted in the usual way for fusion in situ, and the distractor is removed. It is also possible, however, to replace the distractor by an implant (Fig. 3.**5**). A wake-up test after maximal distraction is mandatory.

Wound Closure

See under thoracotomy or thoracolumbar approach, pp. 22, 35.

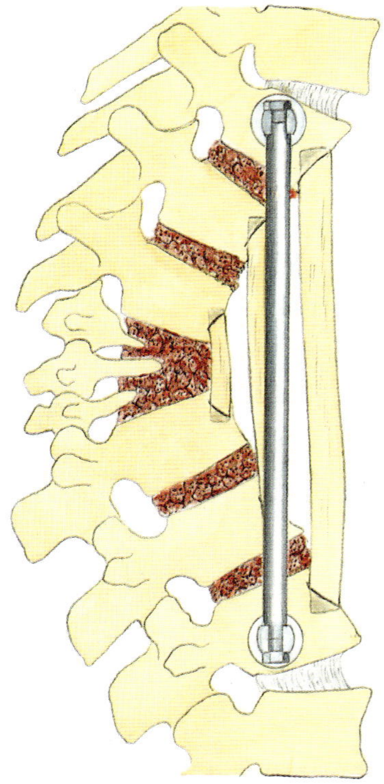

Fig. 3.**5** Same procedure as in Fig. 3.**4**. However, to maintain the correction, an implant (firm rod combined with USIS screws) is placed before removal of the distractor. Added bone-graft fusion is indispensable.

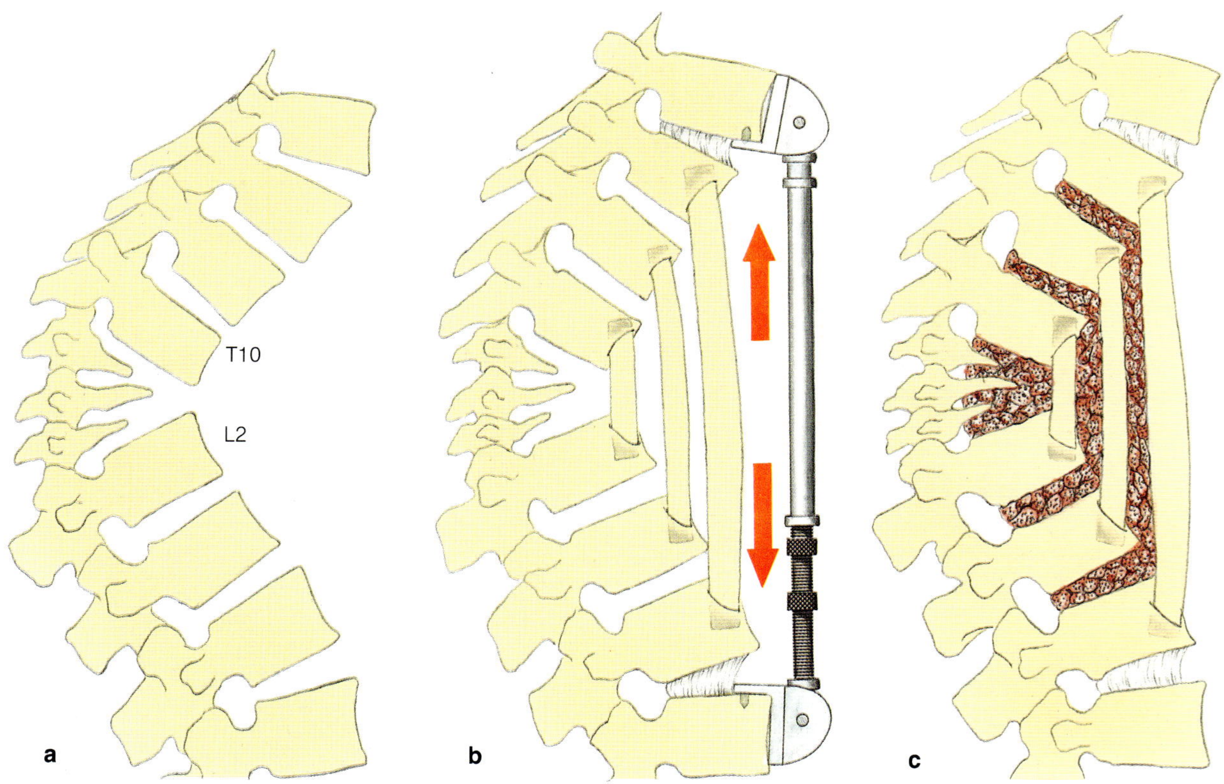

Fig. 3.**4**
a Congenital kyphosis, Type I.
b Intervertebral disk resection is followed by correction with the Slot distractor and insertion of strut grafts.
c Status after removal of distractor and introduction of cancellous bone chips.

Postoperative Treatment

The patient is placed in bed without external orthotic fixation, and is taken to the intensive care unit for postoperative care. A neurologic examination is made immediately after the operation, and the extremities are reassessed, initially at 15-minute, and later at hourly, intervals.

After removal of the sutures 12–14 days postoperatively, a body cast is applied or a spinal orthosis is fitted, which has to be worn for 6–9 months.

Pitfalls and Complications

Complications of thoracic surgery, such as hemothorax, pneumothorax, and pleural effusions, may occur; neurologic complications may be seen, especially after intraoperative correction using distraction devices.

Delayed fusion of the fibular graft; graft fractures; and non-union may occur as well.

Further Reading

See p. 197.

Vascularized Rib Graft

Indications

Severe kyphosis of varying etiology with progression. This is essentially the same indication as for a free fibular strut graft, which has certain disadvantages, however. Osseous incorporation takes about two years, and six months postoperatively there is a distinct risk of fracture, increasingly so as the distance of the graft from the apex of the kyphosis increases. Moreover, ligation of segmental vessels is necessary throughout the fusion site, creating an avascular area.

A vascularized rib graft provides a useful alternative. Firm incorporation is achieved within 6–8 weeks, and ligation of the segmental vessels is unnecessary. From this point of view, kyphoses with preexisting neurologic lesions especially (e.g., postlaminectomy kyphosis) are particularly suitable for this technique.

The low mechanical load capacity of rib grafts is a drawback, and this technique is therefore particularly preferred for a fusion in situ designed to prevent further progression.

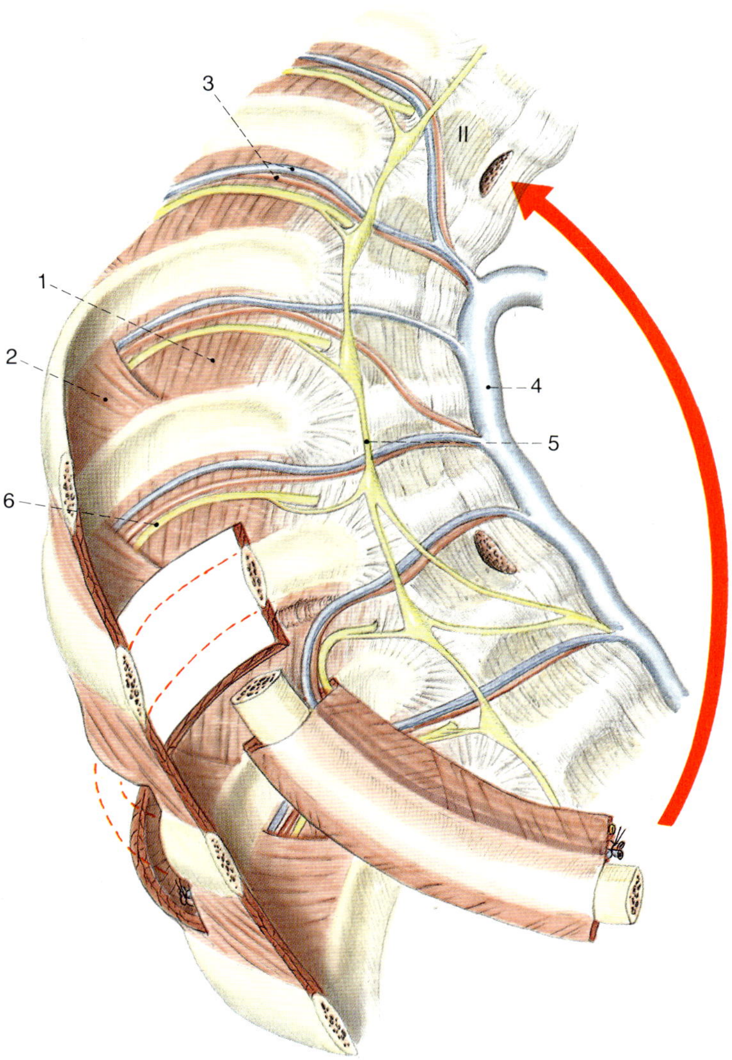

Fig. 3.**6** Grafting a vascular pedicle rib. Operative technique for a high kyphotic apex (T1–T5). The peripheral end of the rib is rotated proximally (arrow).

1 External intercostal muscle
2 Internal intercostal muscle
3 Intercostal vessels
4 Azygos vein
5 Sympathetic trunk
6 Intercostal nerve

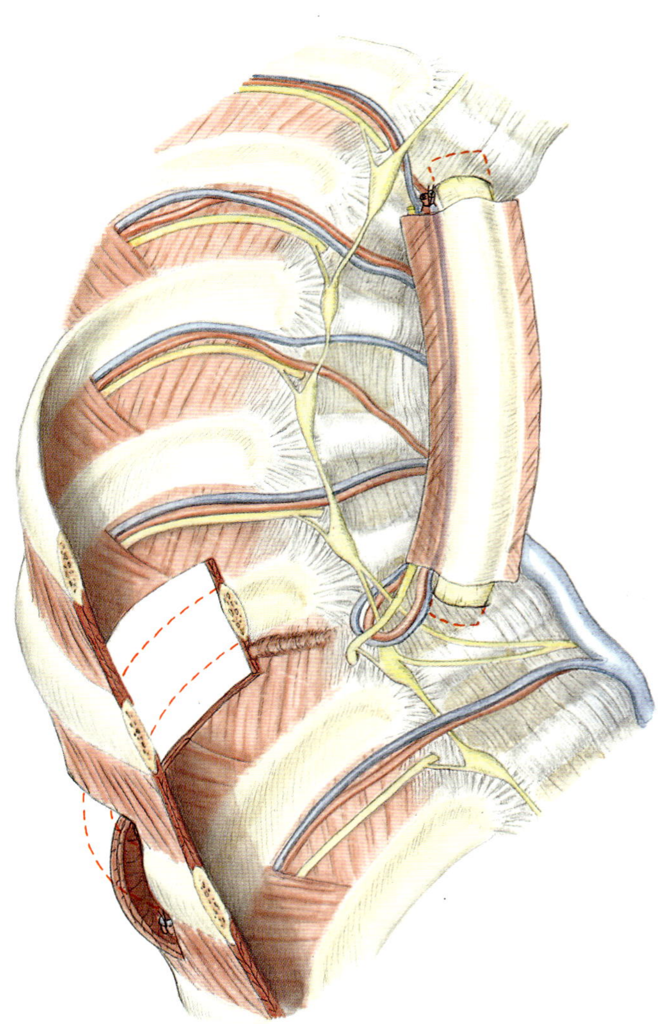

Fig. 3.**7** Status after impaction of rib. *Note:* no ligation of segmental vessels.

Operative Technique

In a kyphosis with an apex between T2 and T5, the rib two or three levels below the apex is used. The peripheral end of the rib is rotated so that it can be driven into the cranial end of the fusion (Figs. 3.**6**, 3.**7**).

In a kyphosis with an apex at T6 or distal to it, a rib two or three levels above the apex is chosen. The peripheral end of the rib graft is here rotated toward the caudal end of the fusion (Figs. 3.**8**, 3.**9**).

The skin incision is made approximately at the level of the rib selected for the fusion; the approach otherwise follows the standard procedure for thoracotomy, involving division of the chest wall musculature. The intercostal musculature cranial to the selected rib is then divided over a grooved dissector. The rib is exposed subperiosteally at the costochondral margin and transected. The intercostal musculature is now divided about 4 mm caudal to the selected rib, sparing the neurovascular bundle. This is ligated and divided at the level of the peripheral resection site. Division of the intercostal musculature is then continued approximately as far as the costal angle, after which a rib spreader can be inserted. Proximally to the costal angle, the chosen rib is exposed subperiosteally; in this region, it is cut off with rib cutters. The neurovascular bundle is followed from the point of the rib division to the intervertebral foramen. However, another possibility is further mobilization of the segmental vessels beyond the vertebral body by transecting the vascular branch to the foramen. As a rule, this is not necessary, however. The rib is cut to the required length; at both ends, a section of at least 1 cm is freed of muscle and periosteum. At the upper and lower ends of the planned strut, a groove is made in the anterior wall of the vertebral body, without dividing the segmental vessels. The vascularized pedicle rib is then rotated, and the free ends of the rib are impacted.

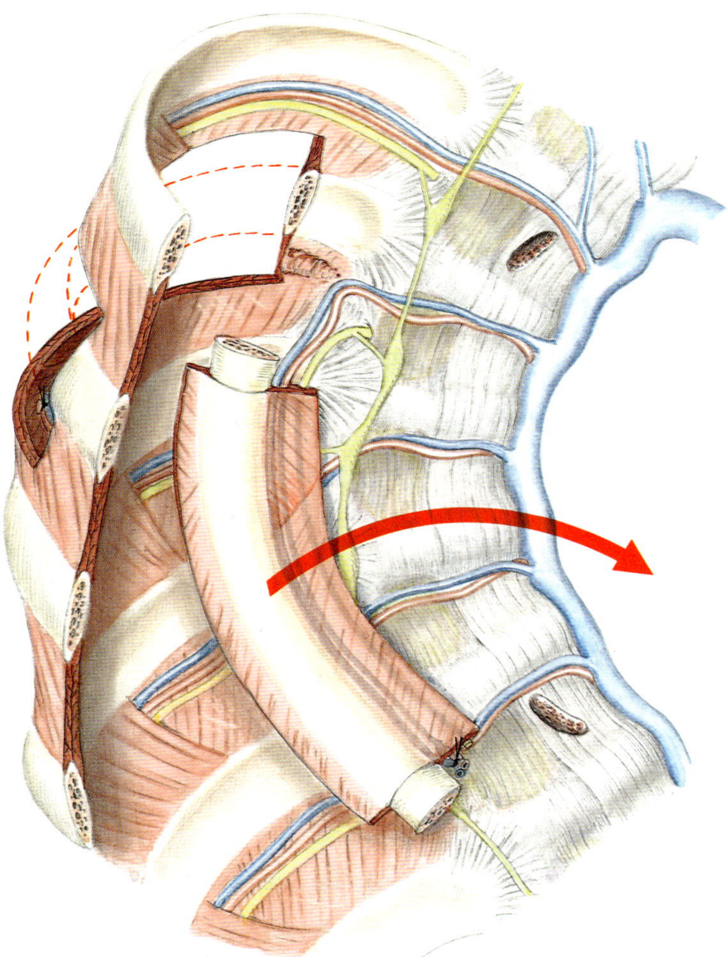

Fig. 3.**8** Grafting of a vascular pedicle rib. Technique for a low kyphotic apex (T6 and below). The peripheral end of the rib is driven in caudally.

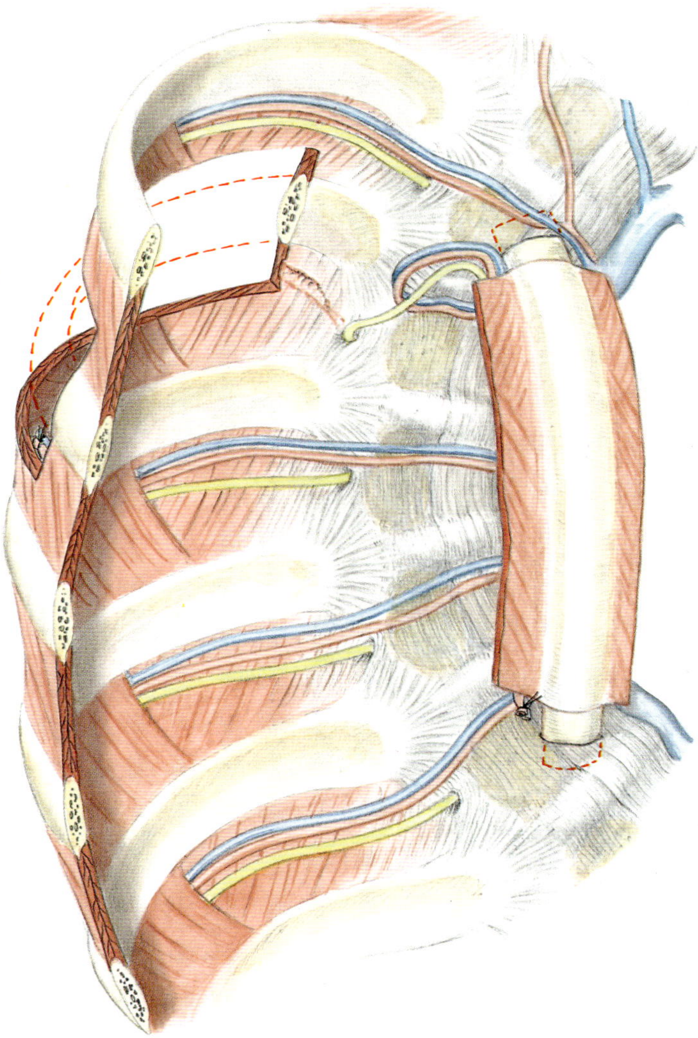

Fig. 3.**9** Status after grafting of rib. *Note:* no ligation of segmental vessels.

Postoperative Treatment

In strut grafting without correction of the kyphosis, it is sufficient for the patient to wear a body cast for about two months.

Note
If this technique is employed before completion of growth, a situation is created which essentially mimics a Type II congenital kyphosis. The operation therefore has to be combined in a second session with an interbody spondylodesis, as well as with a posterior fusion. For the anterior interbody fusion, ligation of the segmental vessels is not absolutely necessary, provided the pleura over the intervertebral disks is incised transversely (epiphysiodesis, p. 160).

Pitfalls and Complications

Possible complications are essentially those of any thoracic surgery, e.g., hemothorax, pneumothorax, pleural effusion, and lung atelectases.

Replacing a Vertebral Body Using a Vascularized Rib Graft (Bradford)

Indication

Posttraumatic kyphosis, with narrowing of the spinal canal and neurologic compromise.

Approach

As a rule, a right-sided thoracolumbar approach (Hodgson) is used. See Chapter 1, pp. 24–36.

Operative Technique

Using the Hodgson approach, the tenth rib is mobilized in the usual way (p. 194) with the neurovascular bundle, by dividing the intercostal musculature from peripheral to central just above and about 5 mm below the costal margin (Fig. 3.**10**). The rib is exposed subperiosteally and divided at the costochondral margin; the neurovascular bundle is mobilized from the central rib stump and traced back as far as the intervertebral foramen. The vascular pedicle is now long enough to allow distal transposition of the mobilized rib as far as the L3–L4 segment if required.

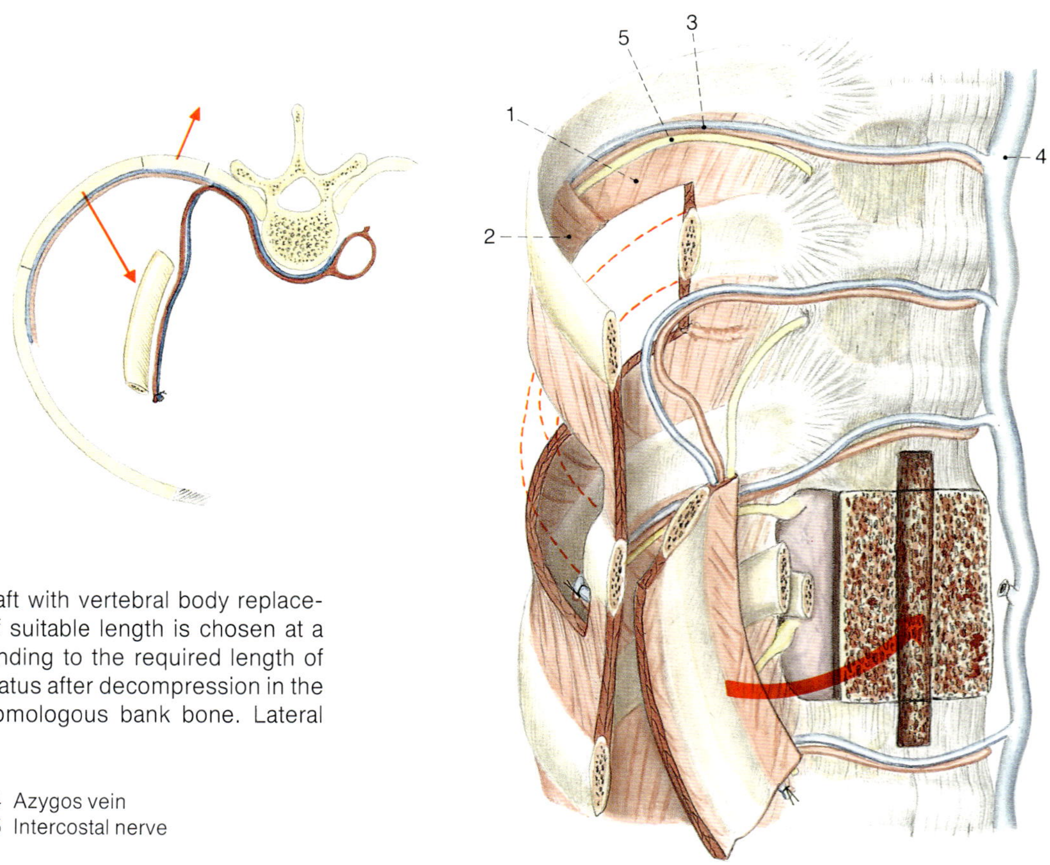

Fig. 3.**10** Vascular pedicle rib graft with vertebral body replacement. A section of the 10th rib of suitable length is chosen at a distance from the spine corresponding to the required length of the vascular pedicle (see inset). Status after decompression in the area of T12 and bridging with homologous bank bone. Lateral groove for insertion of the rib graft.

1 External intercostal muscle
2 Internal intercostal muscle
3 Intercostal vessels
4 Azygos vein
5 Intercostal nerve

Following a typical anterior vertebral body resection (vertebrectomy, p. 156) at the apex of the kyphosis and anterior decompression (p. 198), a femoral head bank graft is impacted, with care being taken to leave at least 5–10 mm of free space for the dura posteriorly. A ball-point drill is then used to fashion a lateral groove through the graft and the two adjacent vertebral bodies.

On the side opposite to the neurovascular bundle, the rib is exposed subperiosteally and inserted into the prepared channel on its denuded side (Fig. 3.**11**). The neurovascular bundle now lies on its surface.

Further Reading

Bauer R. Die operative Behandlung der Kyphose. Arch Orthop Unfall-Chir 1977;87:85.

Bauer R. Der vordere Zugang zur Wirbelsäule. Stuttgart: Thieme, 1983.

Bauer R, Erschbamer H. Technische Möglichkeiten bei der operativen Behandlung der Kyphose. In: Bauer R, ed. Der vordere Zugang zur Wirbelsäule. Stuttgart: Thieme, 1983.

Bauer R, Schwaiger B. Die operative Behandlung der Kyphose. Beitr Orthop Traumatol 1980;27:37.

Bradford DS. Anterior vascular pedicle bone grafting for the treatment of kyphosis. Spine 1980;5:318.

Bradford DS, Daher YH. Vascularized rib grafts for stabilization of kyphosis. J Bone Jt Surg 1986;68-B:357.

Bradford DS, Ganjavian S, Antonius D, Winter RB, Moe JH. Anterior strut-grafting for the treatment of kyphosis. J Bone Jt Surg 1982;64-A:680.

Hack HP, Zielke K. Die ventrale Spanabstützung bei Skoliokyphosen. Indikationen und Ergebnisse. In: Bauer R, ed. Der vordere Zugang zur Wirbelsäule. Stuttgart: Thieme, 1983.

Krismer M, Bauer R. Die operative Behandlung der Kyphose unter besonderer Berücksichtigung der ventralen Spanabstützung. Orthopäde 1989;18:134.

McBride GG, Bradford DS. Vertebral body replacement with femoral neck allograft and vascularized rib strut graft. Spine 1983;8:406.

Moe JH, Winter RB, Bradford DS, Lonstein JE. Scoliosis and other spinal deformities. Philadelphia: Saunders, 1978.

Pinto WC, Avanzi O, Winter RB. An anterior distractor for the intra-operative correction of angular kyphosis. Spine 1978;3:309.

Rose GK, Owen R, Sanderson JM. Transposition of rib with blood supply for the stabilisation of a spinal kyphosis. J Bone Jt Surg 1975;57-B:112.

Slot GH. Correction and fixation of kyphosis with a new distraction method. In: Bauer R, ed. Der vordere Zugang zur Wirbelsäule. Stuttgart: Thieme, 1983.

White AA, Panjabi MM, Thomas CL. The clinical biomechanics of kyphotic deformities. Clin Orthop 1977;128:8.

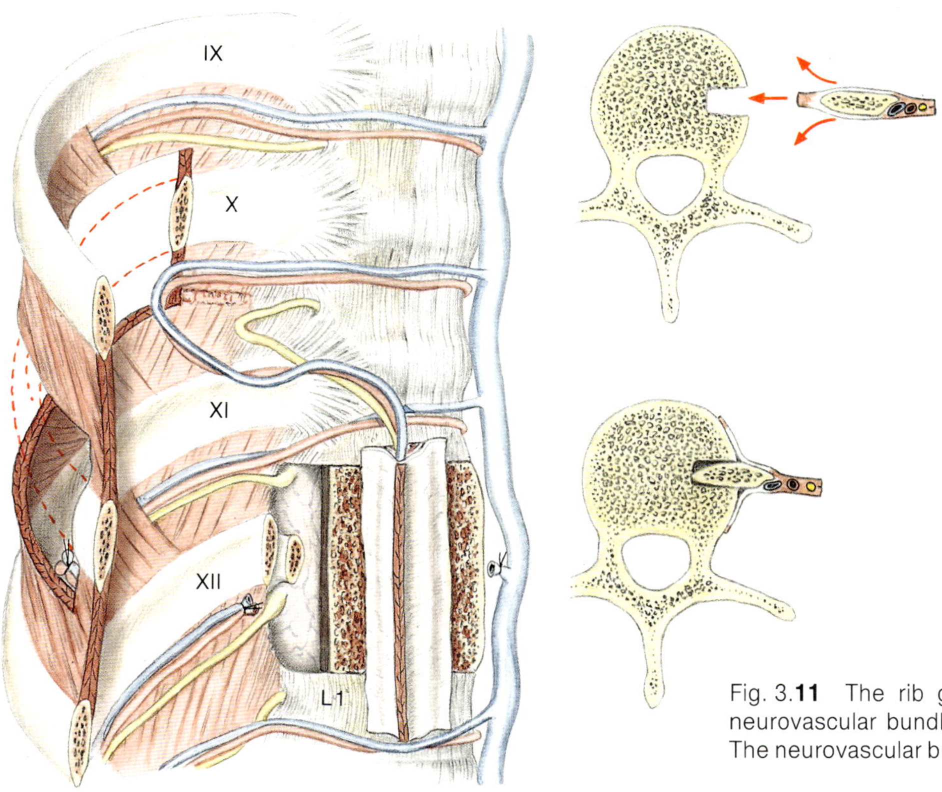

Fig. 3.**11** The rib graft is denuded on the side opposite the neurovascular bundle and is driven into the groove (see inset). The neurovascular bundle courses laterally.

IX–XII Ribs
L1 Lumbar vertebra

Anterior Spinal Cord Decompression

Treatment Strategy

The indications are severe spinal deformities resulting in neurologic deficits.

Precautions
In cases of severe, progressive spinal deformities, early spinal fusion—anterior or posterior or both, depending on the situation—may be indicated in earliest childhood, to prevent secondary neurologic deficits (fusion in situ and congenital kyphosis, p. 205).

However, if a neurologic deficit has already developed in connection with the deformity, an exact radiological assessment is required, using plain radiographs, and flexion and extension radiographs in both planes (important: flexible or fixed apex of curvature?), and possibly also CT, myelography and MRI (mostly for diagnosis, or to rule out a secondary syrinx formation and associated pathology, such as tumors, diastematomyelia, or disk protrusions).

The therapeutic strategy adopted depends to a very large extent on whether the deformity is flexible or fixed in the apical region (Fig. 3.**25**).

If the kyphotic apex is fixed, extension will not result in correction of the deformity. However, the elongation cranial and caudal to the kyphotic apex causes increased compression on the spinal cord in the apical region.

With a flexible kyphosis, the kyphotic deformity is corrected so that the anterior pressure on the spinal cord in the apical region is reduced. Figure 3.**12** gives a summary of the therapeutic measures.

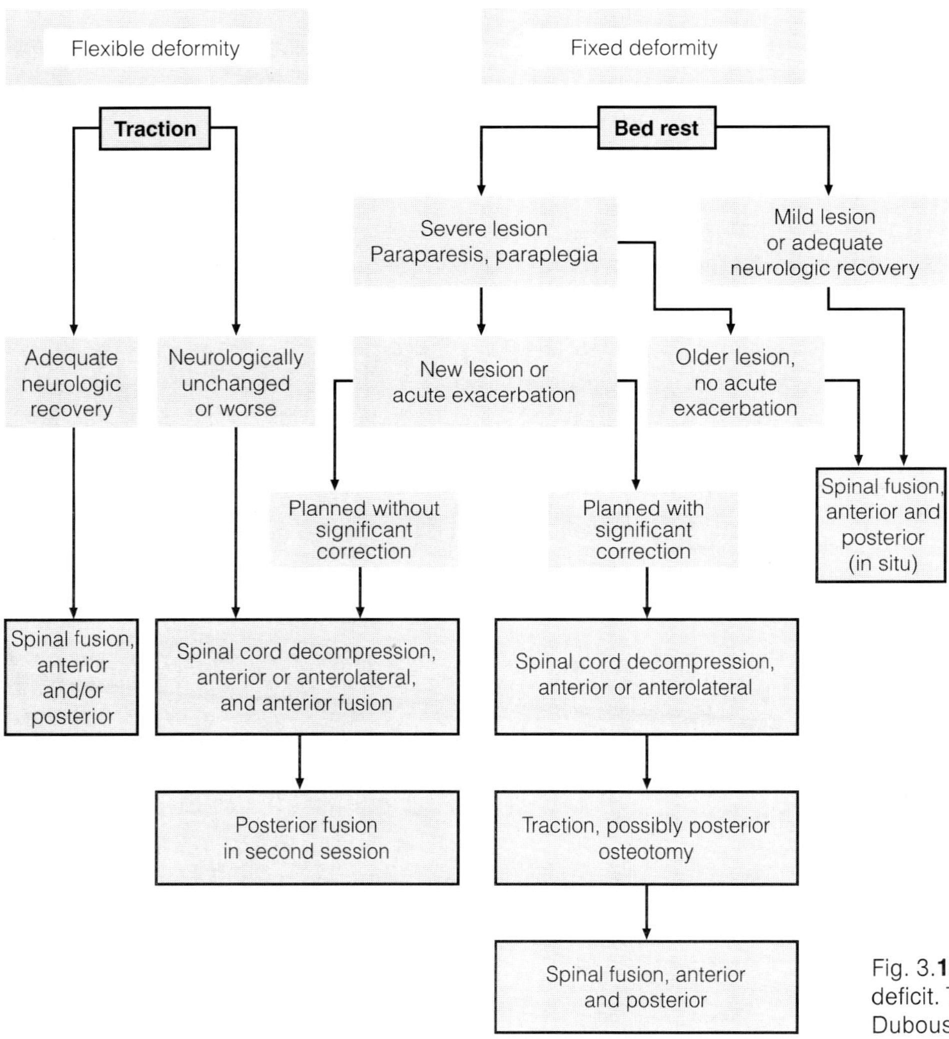

Fig. 3.**12** Spinal deformity with ensuing neurologic deficit. Treatment scheme (according to Lonstein, Dubousset, and Kaneda).

The approach and the operative technique depend on the nature of the deformity, that is, either simple kyphosis or kyphoscoliosis. With the latter, the approach is determined by the scoliosis and the extent of malrotation. This will decide whether thoracotomy on the convex or the concave side is required (see below).

Simple Kyphosis

Approach

In anterior decompression in the thoracic area, anatomical considerations dictate a right-sided thoracotomy; if decompression is required in the area of the thoracolumbar junction, a left-sided Hodgson thoracophrenolumbotomy is chosen. See Chapter 1, pp. 13 and 24.

Operative Technique

(Figs. 3.**13**–3.**19**)

The parietal pleura is split in typical fashion in the proposed area of fusion; the segmental vessels are ligated, and the vertebral bodies are exposed over their entire circumference. To begin with, the intervertebral disks are resected, after which up to three vertebral bodies at the apex of the kyphosis are removed, partially at first, with pituitary forceps. The cancellous bone of the apical vertebral bodies is removed as far as the posterior cortical layer, which can be done effectively with a ball reamer. It is important to hollow out the vertebral bodies in the apical region and posterior parts of adjacent vertebrae before removing the posterior cortical substance. Since the spinal cord is in particularly close apposition to the posterior vertebral wall in the apical region, it is advisable to begin resection of the dorsal vertebral elements from cranial or caudal, and then to advance in the direction of the kyphotic apex. The posterior vertebral elements are removed very cautiously, using bone biters of specially curved small, sharp curets. Serious bleeding from the epidural venous plexus may occur here. After resection of the posterior wall of the vertebral body, the spinal cord is decompressed in the apical region. The decompression should be followed by stabilization with anterior strut grafts (p. 189).

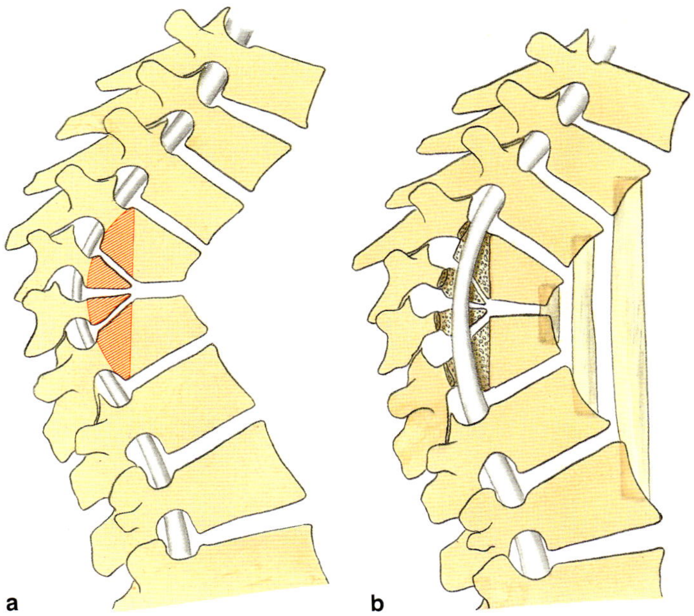

Fig. 3.**13** Anterior decompression in congenital kyphosis.
a Proposed bone resection.
b Status after anterior decompression and anterior strut grafting.

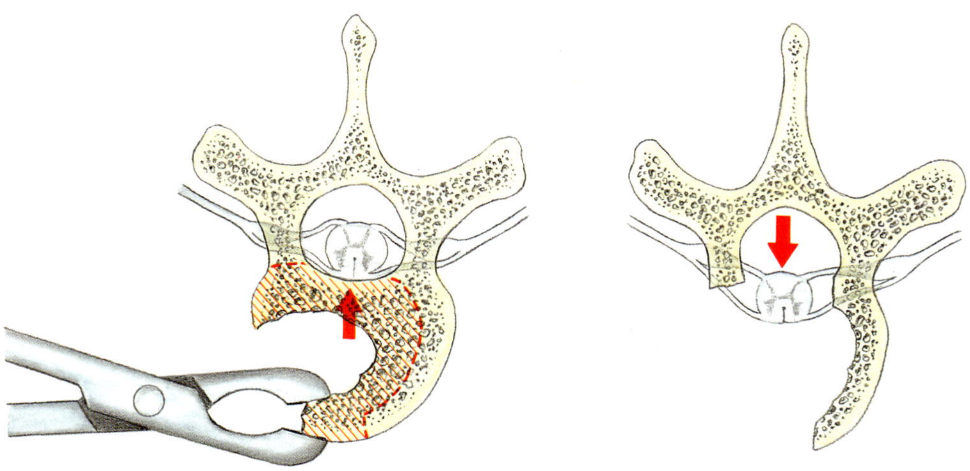

Fig. 3.**14** Anterior decompression in simple kyphosis. The bone parts to be resected (including the posterior wall of the vertebral body) are marked (dashed line).

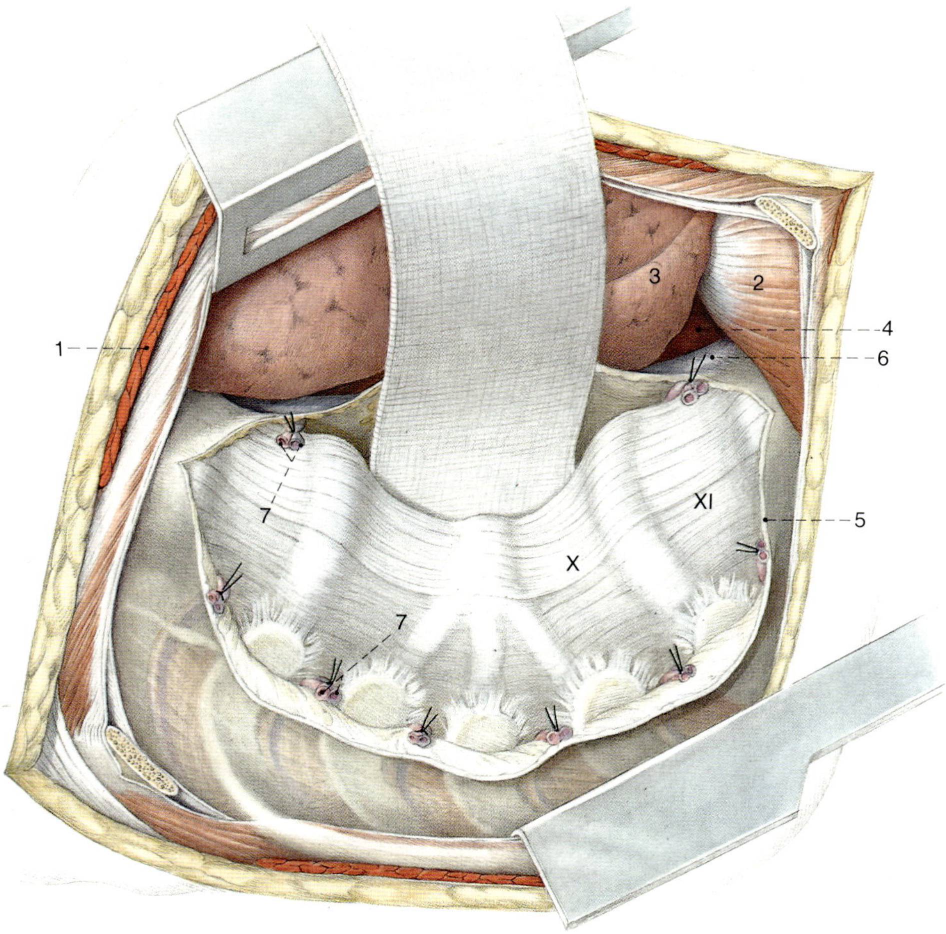

Fig. 3.**15** Congenital kyphosis. The operative site after right-sided thoracotomy. Division of the parietal pleura and ligation of the segmental vessels.

1 External oblique muscle of the abdomen
2 Thoracic diaphragm
3 Right lung
4 Esophagus
5 Parietal pleura
6 Azygos vein
7 Intercostal vessels

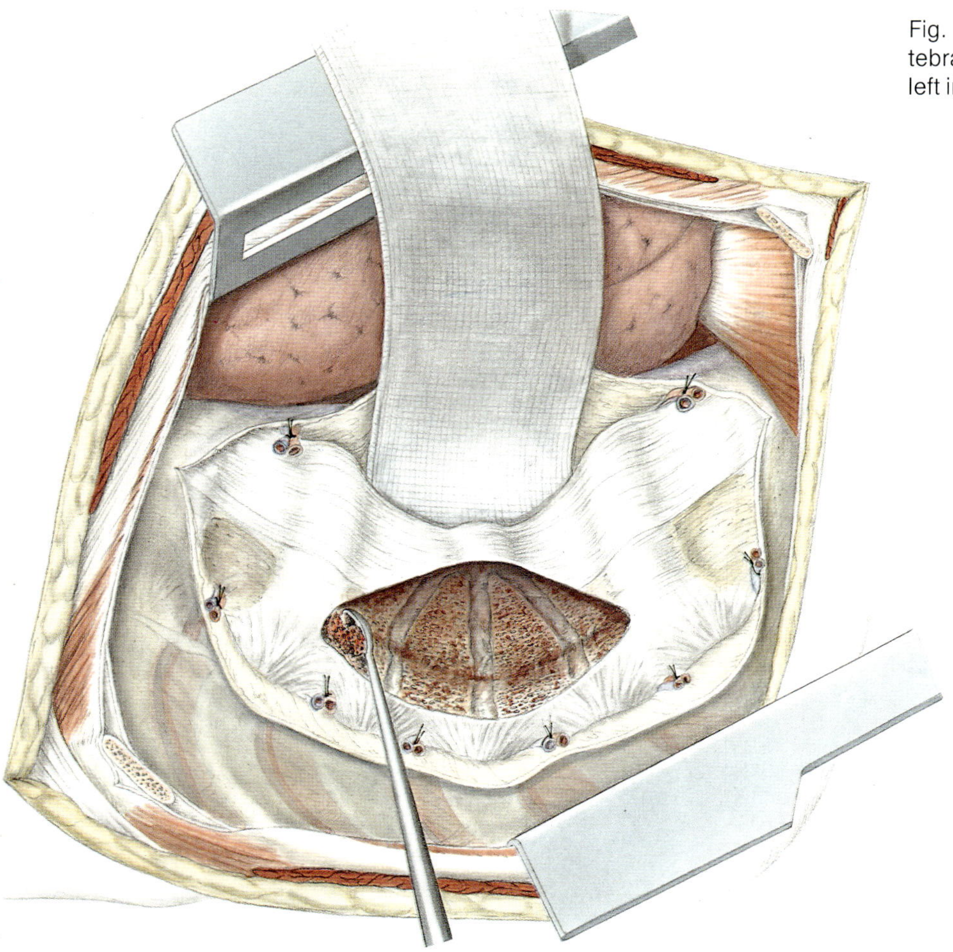

Fig. 3.**16** Subtotal resection of apical vertebrae. Contralateral portions of bone can be left in place.

Fig. 3.**17** The decompression is carried out from cranial or caudal toward the apical vertebra. The posterior parts of the vertebral body are cautiously removed with a bone punch.

1 Spinal ganglion
2 Spinal dura mater

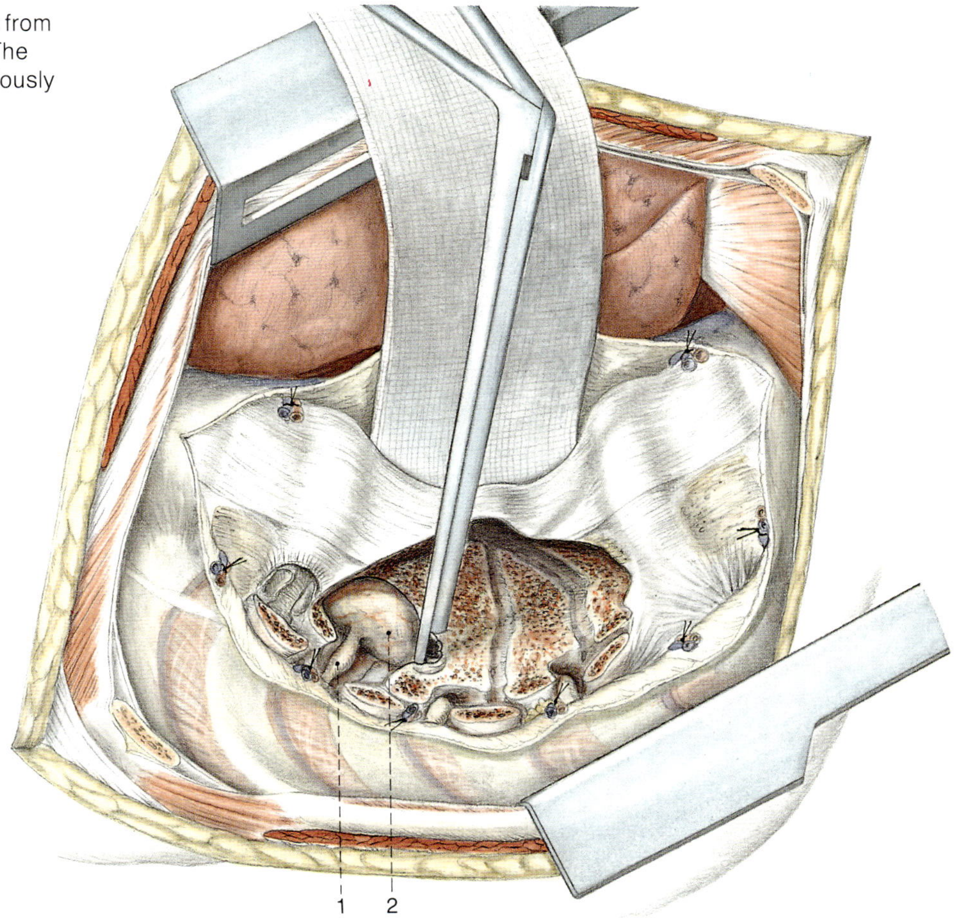

Fig. 3.**18** Status after decompression of the spinal cord in the apical region. The pedicles and the rib resection sites can be seen.

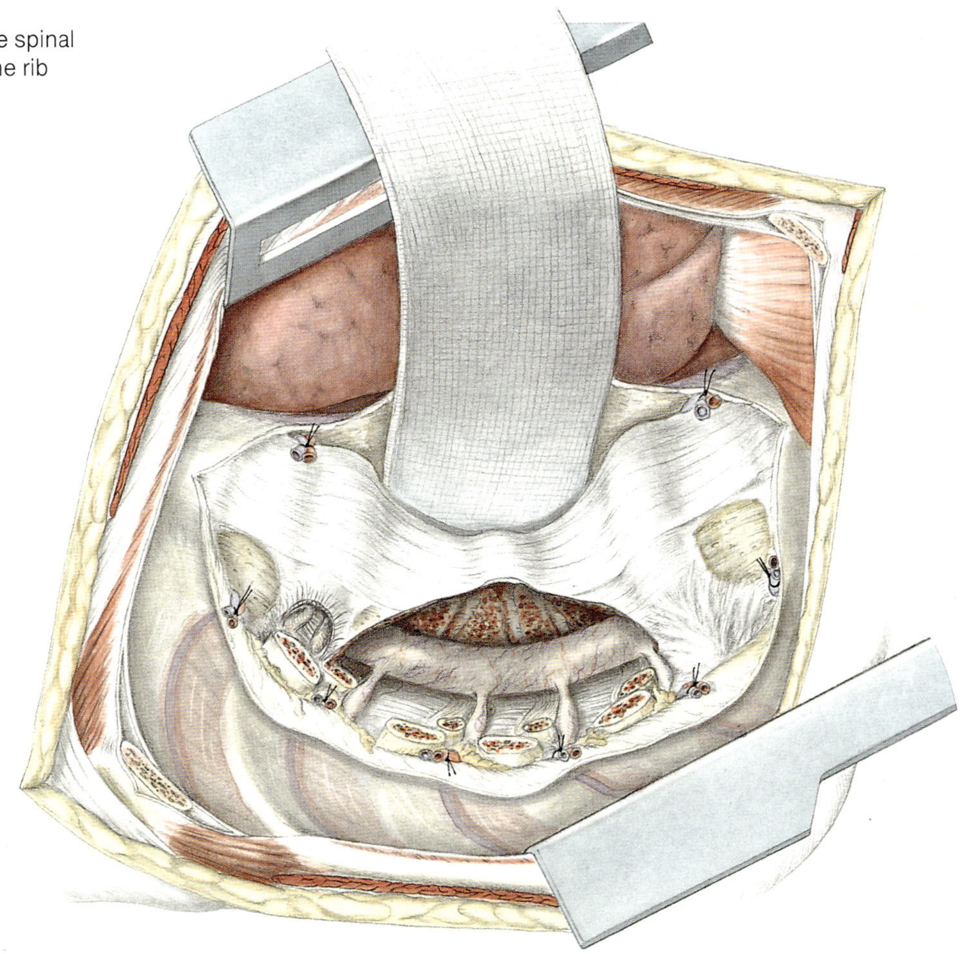

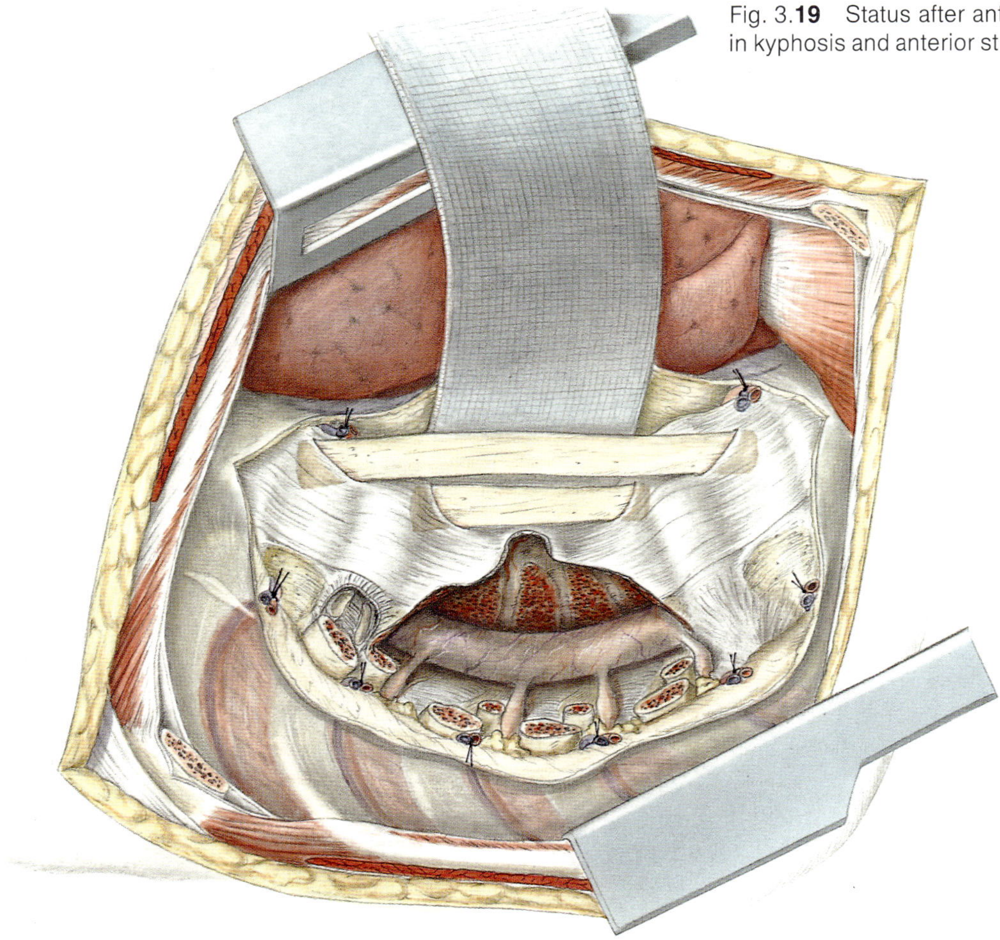

Fig. 3.**19** Status after anterior decompression of the spinal cord in kyphosis and anterior strut grafting.

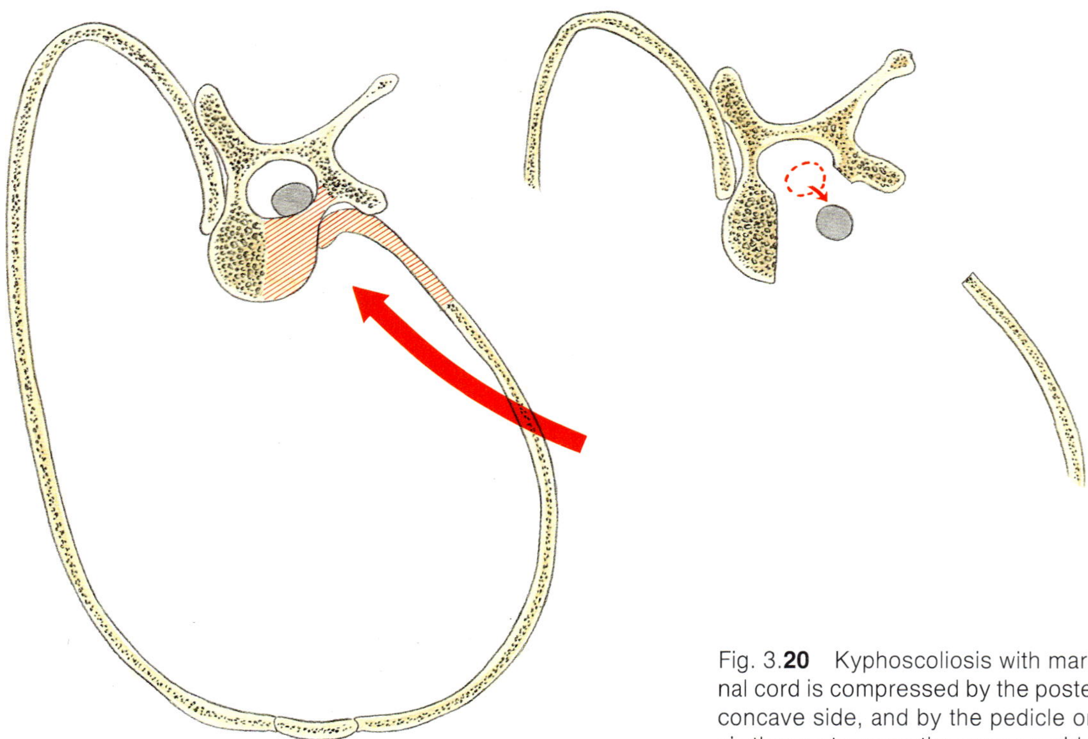

Fig. 3.**20** Kyphoscoliosis with marked vertebral torsion. The spinal cord is compressed by the posterior wall of the vertebra on the concave side, and by the pedicle on the concave side. Approach via thoracotomy on the concave side.

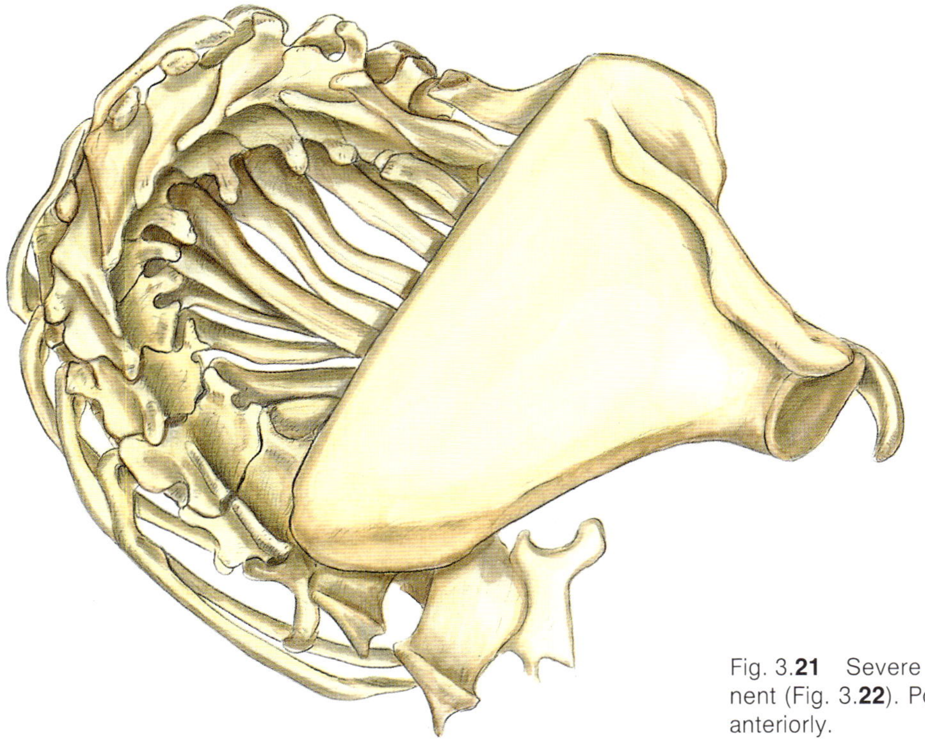

Fig. 3.**21** Severe kyphoscoliosis with a strong rotatory component (Fig. 3.**22**). Portions of the lamina on the concave side face anteriorly.

Kyphosis with a Scoliotic Component and Marked Vertebral Torsion

Because of the pathologic torsion, the spinal cord is compressed by the posterior wall of the vertebral body and the pedicle on the concave side. Thoracotomy on the concave side is recommended here. Parts of the vertebral body and the pedicle on the concave side have to be removed in the course of the operation (Fig. 3.**20**).

Kyphoscoliosis with a Very Severe Rotatory Component

Owing to the profound vertebral torsion, the spinal cord is compressed by the pedicle on the concave side and partially by the lamina (Figs. 3.**21**, 3.**22**). In this situation, it is generally advisable to perform a costotransversectomy as modified by Capener on the concave side. This operation differs from a regular costotransversectomy mainly in that decompression is achieved by resection of the pedicle and of parts of the lamina on the concave side.

Operative Technique

For the operative technique, reference should be made to costotransversectomy (p. 60). The Capener operation is briefly described below (Fig. 3.**22**).

The procedure is carried out in a prone or semilateral decubitus position. A curved paramedian incision is made about 6 cm to the side of the series of spinous processes. A flap is created medially by subcutaneous dissection as far as the spinous processes, and reflected. The trapezius muscle is freed at its origin, and retracted laterally. The intrinsic musculature of the back is transected at the level of the rib leading to the apical vertebra. This group of muscles is dissected free in the cranial and caudal directions, and retracted. The corresponding rib is exposed subperiosteally. To begin with, a segment extending from the costal angle to the transverse process is resected. To gain a better overview, the two adjacent ribs can be removed similarly. The pleura can now be retracted anteriorly from the vertebral body. The central end of the rib is removed after this. Transverse processes and pedicles and, if need be, portions of the concave-sided lamina in the area of the apical vertebrae are also removed. Decompression of the spinal cord can thus be accomplished.

If, as is usual, anterior strut grafting is to be done after the decompression, this operation can be combined with a thoracotomy on the concave side.

Pitfalls and Complications

These are very difficult operations in patients who are in a feeble general condition. Fatal complications have been reported, in addition to further exacerbation of neurologic symptoms ranging up to paraplegia, adult respiratory distress syndrome, pneumonia, pneumothorax, pleural effusion, local infections, and urinary tract infections.

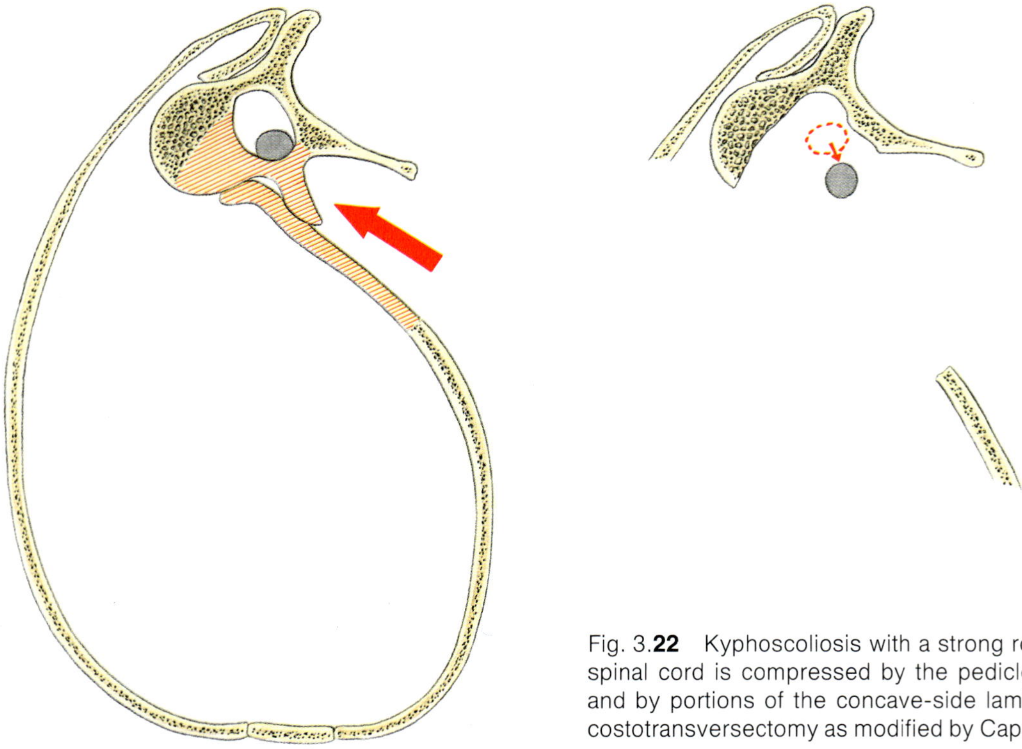

Fig. 3.**22** Kyphoscoliosis with a strong rotatory component. The spinal cord is compressed by the pedicle on the concave side, and by portions of the concave-side lamina. Decompression by costotransversectomy as modified by Capener.

Further Reading

Capener N. The evolution of lateral rhachotomy. J Bone Jt Surg 1954;36-B:173.

Dubousset J. Cyphoses et cyphoscolioses angulaires chez l'enfant. In: Zielke K, ed. Skoliose und Kyphose. Stuttgart: Hippokrates, 1978.

Dubousset J. Congenital kyphosis. In: Bradford DS, Hensigner RM, eds. The pediatric spine. Stuttgart: Thieme, 1985:196.

Dubousset J, Gonon GP. Cyphoses et cyphoscolioses angulaires. S.O.F.C.O.T., Annual Meeting, November 1982. Rev Chir Orthop 1983;69,suppl. II.

Duval-Beaupère G, Dubousset J. La dislocation rotatoire progressive du rachis. Rev Chir Orthop 1972;58:323.

Kaneda K. Spinal cord compression secondary to spinal deformity. In: Bradford DS, Hensinger RM, eds. The pediatric spine. Stuttgart: Thieme, 1985:286.

Lonstein JE, Winter RB, Moe JH, Bradford DS, Chou SN, Pinto WC. Neurologic deficits secondary to spinal deformity. Spine 1980;5:331.

Moe JH, Winter RB, Bradford DS, Lonstein JE. Scoliosis and other spinal deformities. Philadelphia: Saunders, 1978.

Winter RB, Hall JE. Kyphosis in childhood and adolescence. Spine 178;3:285.

Winter RB, Moe JH, Wang JF. Congenital kyphosis. J Bone Jt Surg 1973;55-A:223.

Winter RB, Moe JH, Lonstein JE. The surgical treatment of congenital kyphosis. Spine 1985;10:224.

Congenital Kyphosis

Treatment Strategy

Types of congenital kyphosis (Fig. 3.**23**):

- Type I: Congenital failure of vertebral formation.
- Type II: Congenital failure of vertebral segmentation.
- Type III: Mixture of Types I and II.

Moderate Kyphosis in Early Life

In this situation, the best results are obtained by early posterior fusion, from the first few months of life until three years of age. Essentially, a posterior spinal fusion with resection of the facet joints is carried out (scoliosis, fusion in situ, p. 98). The operation for kyphosis should spare the spinous processes and the interspinal ligament, however. Revision and placement of new grafts will be necessary 4–6 months after the first operation. Orthotic therapy should follow.

Posterior fusion combined with anterior operation. Early anterior fusion is indicated if there is a so-called "empty space" anteriorly owing to a defect in one or more vertebrae. Posterior fusion alone, even with a mild curve, would mean a loss of correction and development of a pseudarthrosis in this situation.

Curvatures of more than 40–50 degrees also require a anterior fusion. The posterior fusion should be extended to at least one segment cranial and caudal to the anterior fusion in order to achieve progressive correction during growth (Fig. 3.**24**).

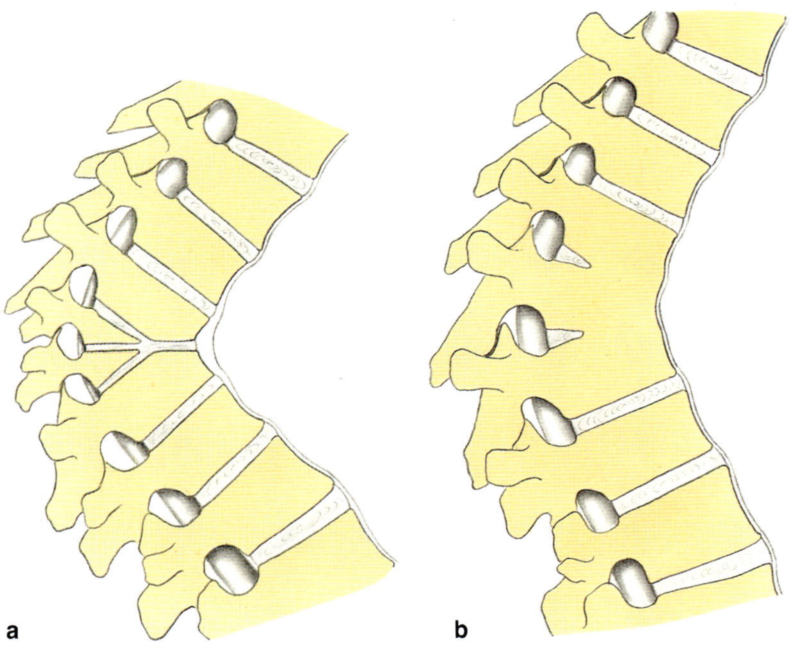

Fig. 3.**23** Congenital kyphosis.
a Type I, anterior vertebral formation defect.
b Type II, anterior segmentation defect.

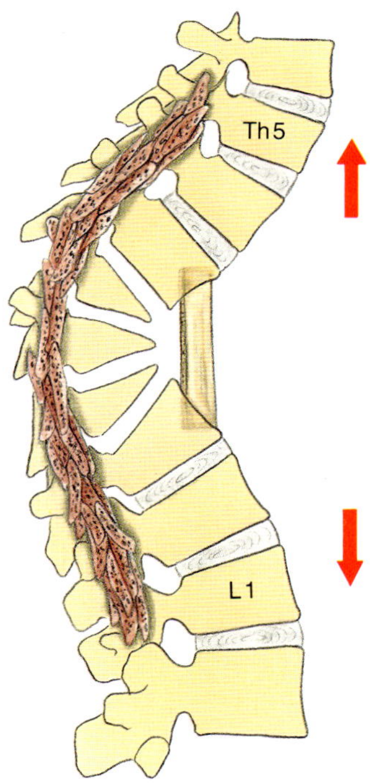

Fig. 3.**24** Congenital kyphosis, Type I. Treatment concept. Early posterior spinal fusion combined with short anterior fusion and anterior bridging of the vertebral body defect. Spontaneous correction due to use of different fusion lengths is possible.

Marked Kyphosis in Older Children

How to treat older children depends on whether the apex of the kyphosis is rigid or mobile (Fig. 3.**25**). For *mobile kyphoses,* traction therapy with careful neurologic monitoring can be employed, to be followed by anterior and posterior fusion.

Rigid Kyphotic Apex
If correction is desirable, an anterior mobilizing osteotomy with decompression is required, to be followed by a posterior mobilizing osteotomy with correction and instrumentation. Further anterior interventions may be necessary in order to enhance stability by means of strut grafts. Up to four operative procedures may be required. These operations are associated with a high neurologic risk. Unless necessitated by a neurological lesion, this procedure is somewhat of a surgical luxury. It seems preferable simply to carry out an anterior fusion to prevent further progression, a slight correction being obtained by mobilization of the intervertebral disks adjacent to the rigid kyphotic apex. Posterior fusion should then follow (anterior strut graft, p. 198).

Type II Congenital Kyphosis
Decision-making is similarly difficult in the presence of a severe Type II deformity. Correction can be accomplished only in combination with an anterior mobilizing osteotomy, which is also associated with a high neurologic risk (p. 149).

Severe Kyphosis with Neurologic Deficit

See p. 198.

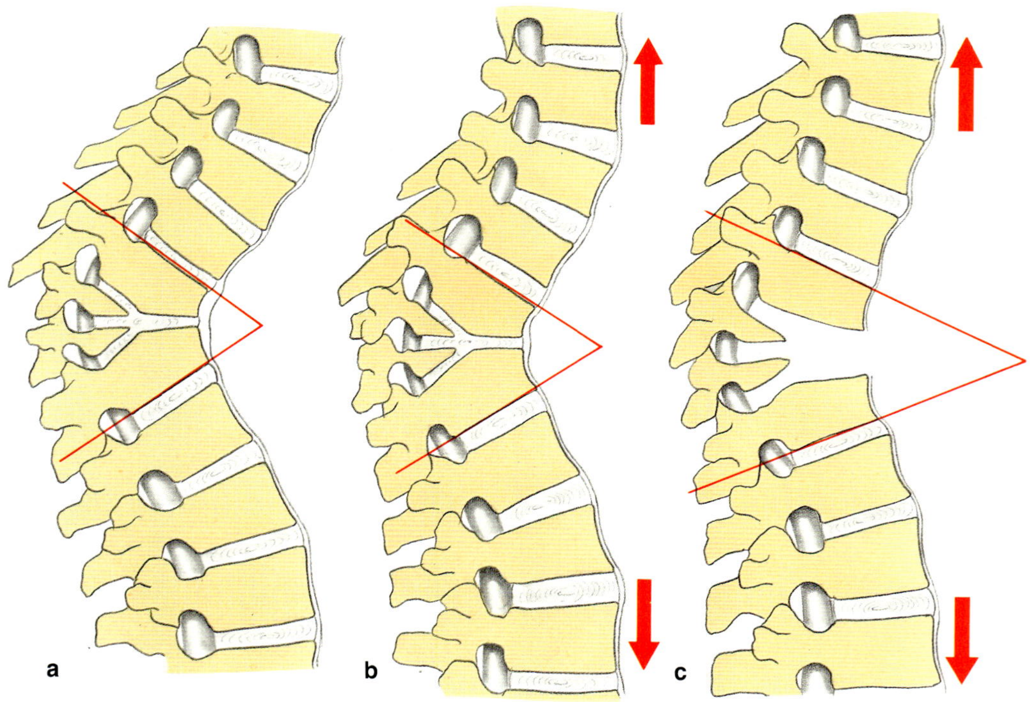

Fig. 3.**25**
a Congenital kyphosis, Type I.
b Rigid kyphotic apex, extension film.
c Mobile kyphotic apex, extension film.

Operation for Kyphosis in Myelomeningocele

Indications

- Mostly skin problems over the kyphotic apex, with decubitus ulcer.
- Repeated infections.
- Compromised sitting posture.

Preparation for Surgery

The preoperative requirements are evaluation of shunt function by the neurosurgeon, urologic assessment of renal function, and catheterization for bacteriologic culture of the urine. All skin lesions should be healed before the operation; intraoperatively, antibiotics should be administered prophylactically, dependent on a positive urine culture where applicable.

Lindseth and Stelzer Operation

This is an operation at an early age; the best results can be obtained when the patient is under 2½ years old.

Operative Technique

The operative technique depends on the patient's age, and varies considerably with the local anatomical conditions. Various possible methods of correction, particularly numerous osteosynthetic techniques, have been described. Relapses are common, and the low capacity for fixation presents a problem.

Essentially, posterior portions of the apical vertebra and one or more of the proximally adjoining vertebral bodies in the lordotic area are resected, followed by anterior portions of the adjacent vertebra (Fig. 3.**26**). Fixation can be effected only by wire cerclage of two contiguous pedicles.

Apart from a longitudinal incision, there is the option of a transverse skin incision over the apex of the kyphosis and at right angles to the scars from the primary closure of the myelomeningocele. The skin is separated from the dura, and an attempt is made to obtain as thick a skin flap as possible. The intrinsic musculature of the back is subperiosteally retracted from the posterior vertebral elements, beginning two vertebrae obove the proposed cranial end of the resection and going as far as the sacrum caudally. The subsequent procedure depends on the neurologic situation. With a complete transverse lesion, the nonfunctioning spinal cord is divided cranially to the proposed osteotomy plane, and the spinal cord is cranially divided further than the dural sac. The dural sac is then closed. It is most important to see that the central canal remains open and in communication with the subdural space (risk of acute hydrocephalus).

Alternatively, the neural sac can be exposed at the lumbosacral junction from the distal side. The segmental nerves are transected, and the neural sac is mobilized cranially to a point above the level of the planned osteotomy. The dural sac itself is not opened. After completed instrumentation, the dural sac is placed over any implants. This reduces the risk of an acute hydrocephalus.

When there is a functionally significant residual neural function, the spinal cord cannot be divided. However, the dural sac has to be mobilized by transecting the segmental vessels and nerves at the level of the apex or one segment above it. After this mobilization, the vertebral bodies in the apical region can be exposed and resected subperiosteally.

Following appropriate dissection, those vertebrae that are to be removed completely are resected first. The posterior third of the apical vertebra is then resected, as is, finally, the anterior third of the vertebrae lying in the area of the lordosis. A new vertebra is then constructed from the remaining parts of these two vertebrae. Fixation can be effected by wire cerclage of the pedicles in the region of the adjacent vertebrae. After this, the intrinsic musculature of the back is sutured over the spine and over the dural sac. If the vertebral canal is wide open, coverage with musculature may be difficult. Occasionally, anteriorly protruding

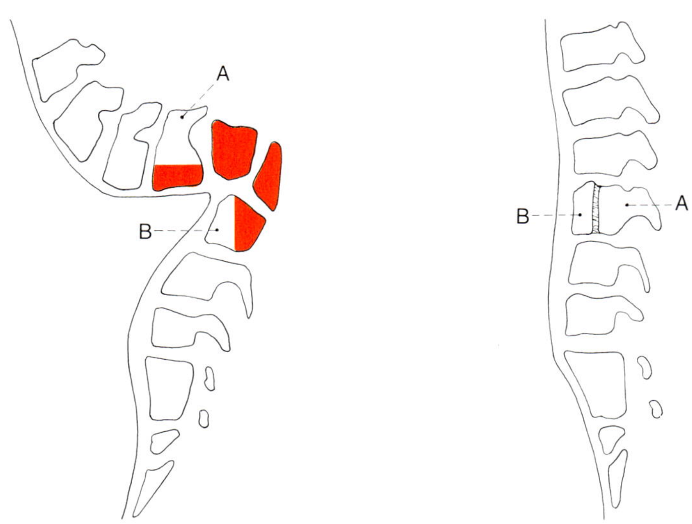

Fig. 3.**26** Correction of kyphosis in younger patients. The anterior longitudinal ligament is left in place and serves as a hinge joint.The red parts are resected; vertebrae A and B are placed in apposition.

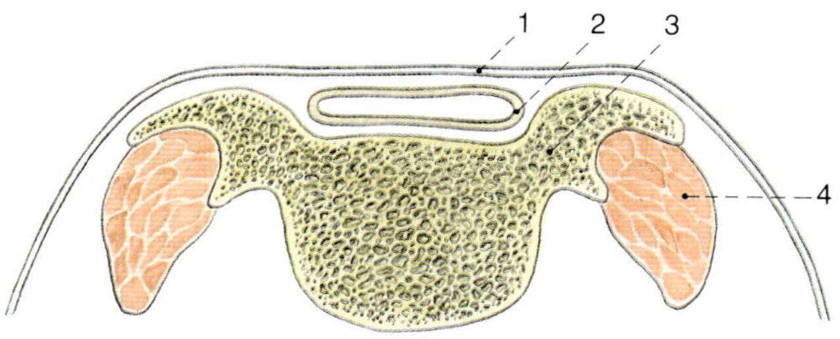

Fig. 3.**27** Vertebral cross-section in myelomeningocele. Note the anterior position of the intrinsic musculature of the back.

1 Cutis
2 Spinal dura mater
3 Pedicle of the vertebral arch
4 Musculature

parts of vertebrae have to be removed to ensure approximation of the muscles. Ablation of bone and closure of the musculature seem to be of particular importance in an operative technique that does not require the use of long osteosynthetic systems, since the erector muscles of the trunk lie lateral to the vertebral bodies and cannot act as extensors (Fig. 3.**27**).

Postoperative Treatment

A body spica including both thighs has to be worn for six months.

Correction of Kyphosis in Older Patients

Instrumentation of the entire spinal column is necessary in adolescence and the immediately subsequent age group.

Operative Technique

(Fig. 3.**28**)

A straight midline incision is made, irrespective of existing scars. The spine is exposed subpoeriosteally as far lateral as the transverse processes. With a complete transverse cord lesion (p. 207), the dural sac is divided above the osteotomy, the spinal cord is transected, and the dural sac is closed again. An osteotomy is then performed at the apex of the kyphosis, and bone material with a posterior wedge is removed. Enough is resected to allow easy correction of the kyphosis, but not so much as to prevent ready approximation of the resection ends. The instrumentation should generally extend to T2 or T3 to avoid kyphotic tilting of the trunk at the upper end of the Luque instrumentation. Also, the pelvis has to be included in the fusion.

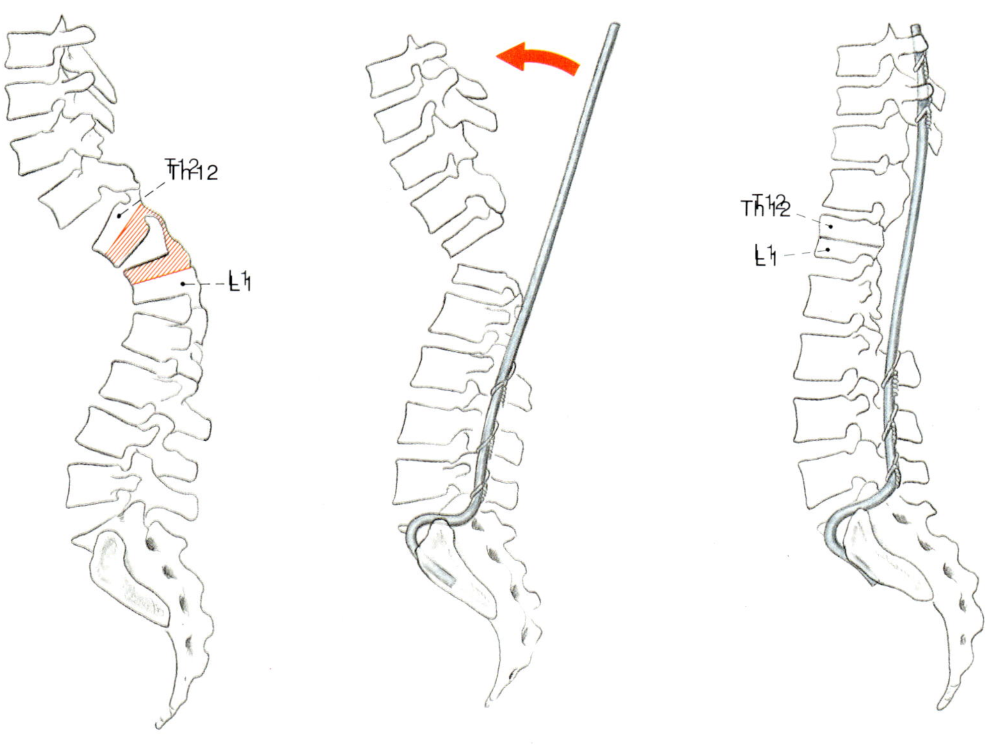

Fig. 3.**28** Correction of kyphosis in myelomeningocele in older patients. Wedge resection via the posterior approach and Luque stabilization. Pelvic fixation (Dunn).

Certain special features are associated with use of the Luque L-rod technique in myelomeningocele. The regular sublaminar fixation cannot be done everywhere in the usual way, due to the defective posterior vertebral elements. If only two or three segments in the lumbar spine are defective, it may be possible to bypass these segments, provided a strong pelvic fixation is feasible. If several levels are defective, the wire generally has to be tied around the pedicles first and then around the Luque rod. In some circumstances, screws can be inserted into the pedicles and the wire cerclages placed around the screws. The wire is attached to the screw head, and is then passed around the Luque rods. Following a suggestion by Luque, a wire can also be pulled transversely through the vertebral body, from pedicle to pedicle, using a suitable awl.

Pelvic fixation poses another problem. The iliac wings are often very soft and osteoporotic, so that the Luque rods may cut out. Sagittal orientation of the wings of the ilia proves difficult in neuromuscular diseases. In the frequently required attempt to correct a lumbar kyphosis, the usual pelvic fixation with the Galveston technique may provide little support; the limb of the rod that is anchored in the ilium slides off in a posterior direction (Figs. 3.**29**, 3.**32**). In this situation, use of the Dunn fixation technique can be recommended.

The Lugue-rods are not anchored in the ilium, but, after appropriate bending, at the anterior surface of the sacral ala. A very good lever arm is then obtained, especially for correction of the arcuate, flexible type of lumbar kyphosis seen in myelomeningocele (Figs. 3.**30**, 3.**31**, 3.**33**).

Pitfalls and Complications

Acute hydrocephalus, cerebrospinal fluid fistula, wound infection, pseudarthrosis, rod fracture.

Warning

Postoperative monitoring for shunt complications is essential.

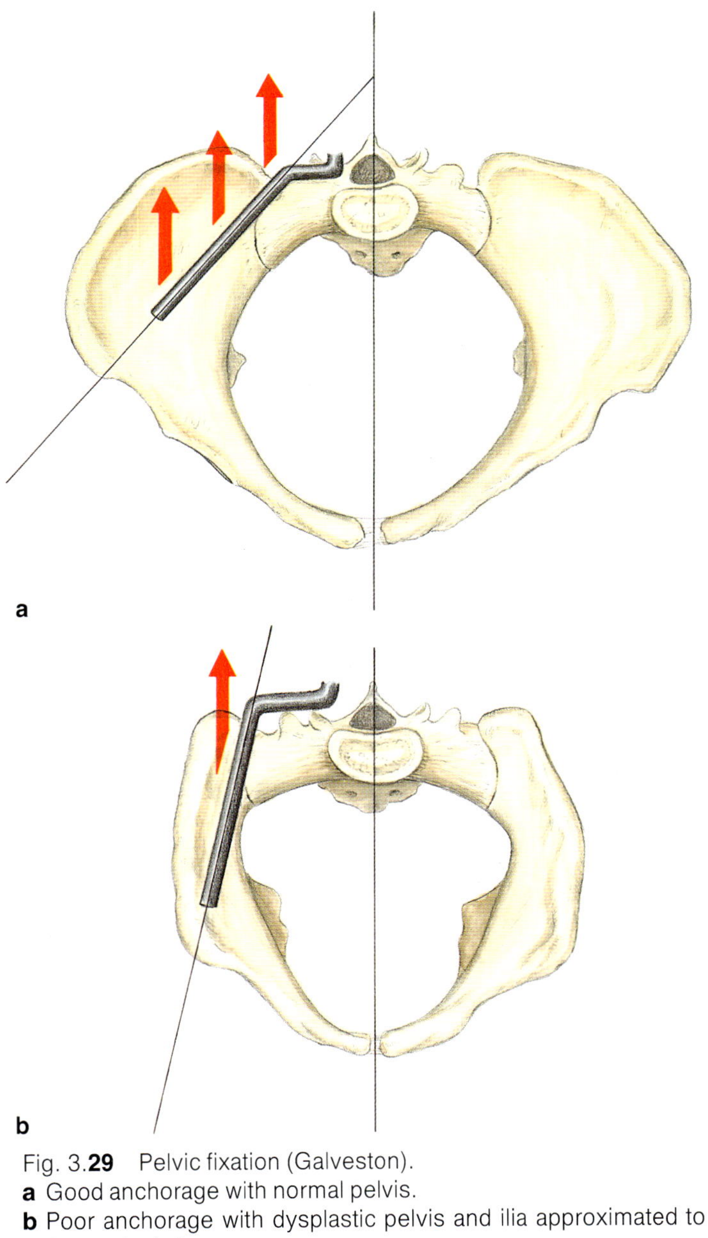

a

b

Fig. 3.**29** Pelvic fixation (Galveston).
a Good anchorage with normal pelvis.
b Poor anchorage with dysplastic pelvis and ilia approximated to the sagittal plane.

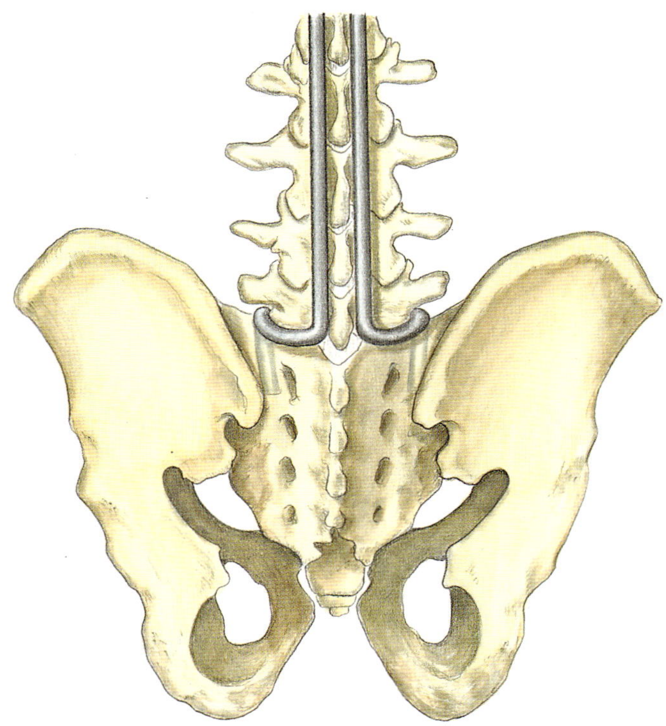

Fig. 3.**30** Lumbosacral stabilization (Dunn), posterior view. The Luque rods curve around the anterior surface of the sacral ala.

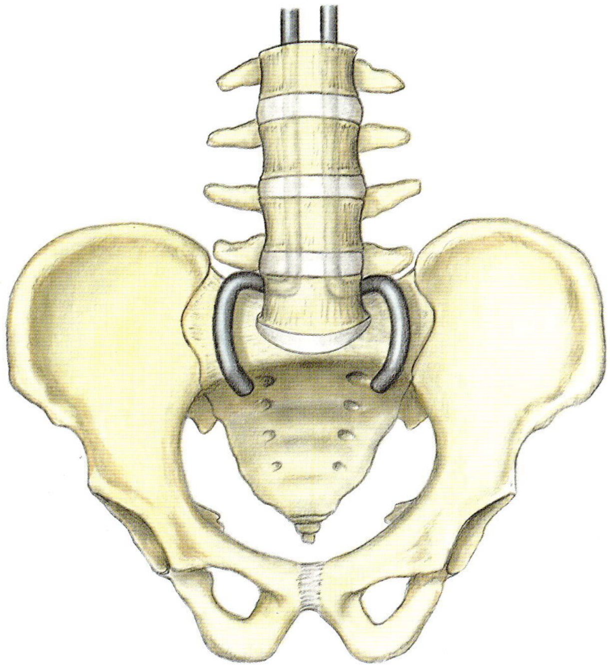

Fig. 3.**31** Lumbosacral fixation (Dunn), anterior view.

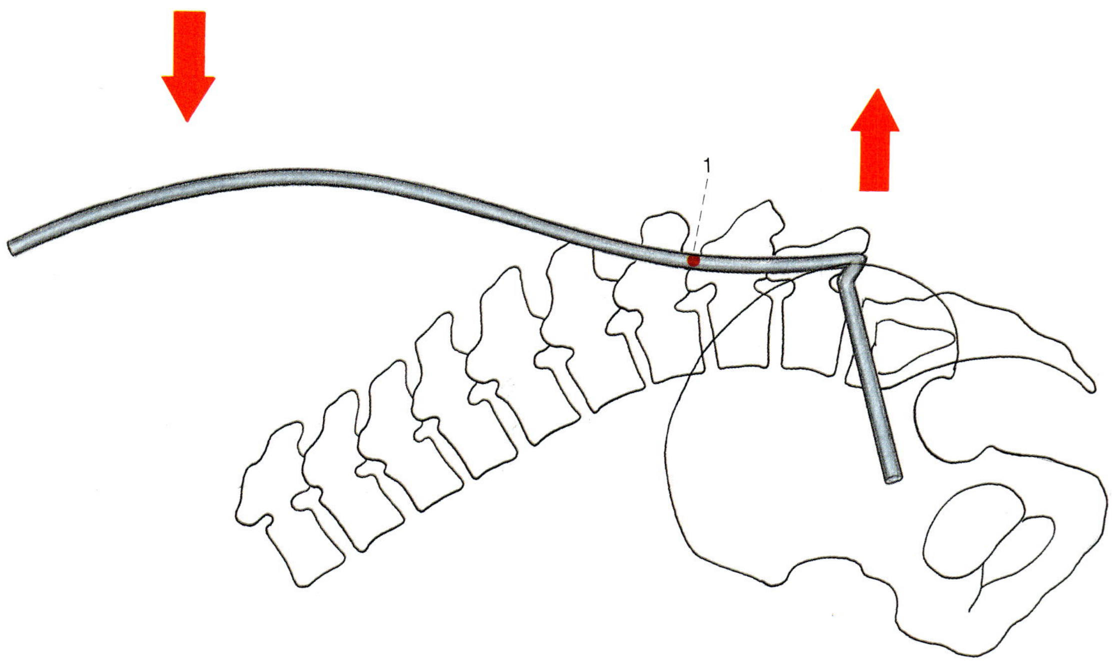

Fig. 3.**32** Pelvic fixation (Galveston). When the ilium is dysplastic and sagittally positioned, applying force to correct a lumbar kyphosis is difficult. The rod is then pulled out of the iliac anchor in a posterior direction.

1 Pivot

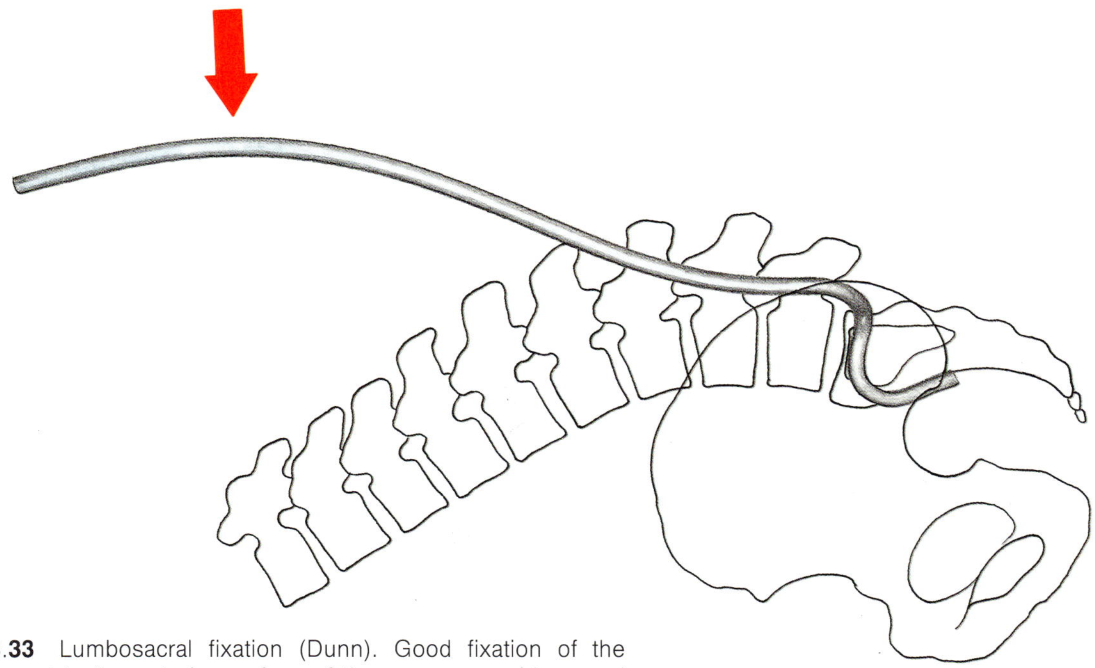

Fig. 3.**33** Lumbosacral fixation (Dunn). Good fixation of the Luque rod to the anterior surface of the sacrum provides good leverage.

Further Reading

Christofersen MR, Brooks AL. Excision and wire fixation of rigid myelomeningocele kyphosis. J Pediat Orthop 1985;5:691.

Heydemann JS, Gillespie R. Management of myelomeningocele kyphosis in the older child by kyphectomy and segmental spinal instrumentation. Spine 1987;12:37.

Leatherman KD, Dickson RA. Congenital kyphosis in myelomeningocele. Spine 1978;3:222.

Lindseth RE, Stelzer L. Vertebral excision for kyphosis in children with myelomeningocele. J Bone Jt Surg 1979;61-A:699.

Stephen JPP, Bodel JG. Luque rod fixation in meningomyelocele kyphosis. Aust NZ J Surg 1983;53:473.

Short-Arc Kyphosis

Indications

A combined anterior–posterior linear osteotomy is generally performed for short-curved (essentially posttraumatic) kyphoses in the thoracolumbar and lumbar regions. Correction and stabilization are effected by the universal spinal instrumentation (USI) system.

No universal guidelines as to whether the posterior or the anterior operation should be performed first can be offered. If spinal mobility is relatively good (demonstrated on bending films), the anterior operation can be done first. A posterior release operation is frequently necessary to begin with, to permit mobilization of the spine. Pedicular screws can already be inserted in this operation. It is inadvisable to connect the pedicular screws to the threaded rod at this stage, because this may hinder the correction in the ensuing anterior operation. The anterior correction is carried out in the second stage, and possibly the decompression as well. Following restoration of compressive stability along the series of vertebral bodies, another operation is performed to connect the previously inserted pedicular screws to the threaded rod from the posterior side, thus producing a tension band effect. This may entail a combined posterior/anterior/posterior procedure, which can be carried out in one or two stages.

Approach

Hodgson's procedure is used in the area of the thoracolumbar junction, which is affected most frequently. See Chapter 1, pp. 24–36.

Operative Technique

(Fig. 3.**34**)

Anterior Operation

Following exposure of the thoracolumbar junction from the left-sided approach with the patient in the lateral position, the vertebrae at the apex of the kyphosis are exposed. The intervertebral disk cranial to the wedged vertebra is resected over its entire circumference. In severe kyphoses, the intervertebral disk below the wedged vertebra has to be similarly removed. The upper plates are freed of cartilage and debrided. Portions of the anterior wall of the wedged vertebra are removed to accommodate an appropriately sized strut graft. VDS screws are now transversely inserted in typical fashion into the vertebral bodies adjoining the wedged vertebra, followed by introduction of the Zielke–Askani system. First of all, rectangular stability is produced by tightening the nuts between the Zielke–As-

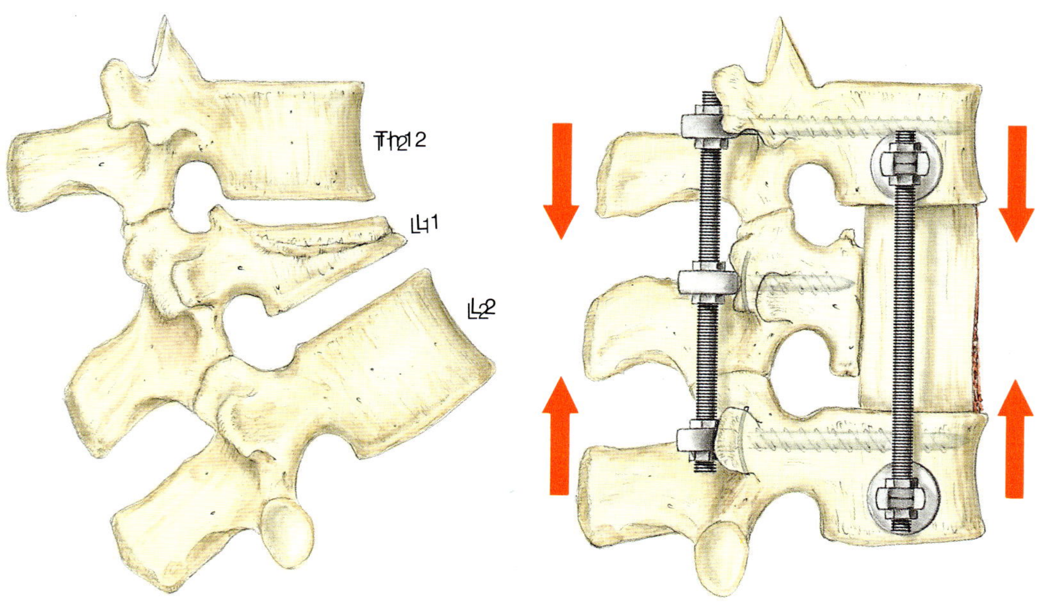

Fig. 3.**34**
a Posttraumatic kyphosis in the area of the thoracolumbar junction.
b Status after correction of kyphosis, anterior/posterior. Removal of two intervertebral disks, partial corpectomy. Anterior strut graft with compression osteosynthesis; posterior transpedicular compression osteosynthesis. The fractured vertebral body is secured by a short pedicular screw. Use of USIS.

kani rod and the VDS screws; the kyphosis is then corrected through manual pressure on the kyphotic apex and elongation of the Zielke–Askani rod. Anteriorly, a corticocancellous bone graft that can be axially loaded is now inserted, and is subsequently placed under pressure by shortening the Zielke–Askani rod. The threaded rod of the USI system can be used in a similar way. The debrided disk spaces are packed with autologous cancellous bone.

If neural structures have been compressed by bony material driven into the vertebral canal, this operation can be used to effect anterior decompression, which essentially involves resection of the wedged vertebra (anterior decompression, p. 198). This requires an extensive osteoplastic reconstruction of the defect (cf. spinal tumors with a good prognosis, p. 396; vascular pedicle grafting, p. 196).

Use of a fibular graft in combination with cancellous bone from the iliac crest is recommended. In this way, posterior-wall stability can be achieved in conjunction with the instrumentation, even when a complete corpectomy has been performed.

Posterior Operation (Second Operative Step)

The posterior intervention that is required for biomechanical stabilization can be carried out in one stage after repositioning of the patient, but may also be performed up to two weeks later.

With the patient in prone position, the appropriate posterior vertebral elements are exposed via a median approach. Cranial and caudal to the kyphotically deformed vertebral body, DCS screws are inserted in the usual fashion, with note being taken of the screw entry sites, and are fixed with a threaded rod, producing rectangular stability and compression. Debridement of the facet joints with graft fusion is carried out in the usual way (see Chapter 11, Spinal Tumors).

Postoperative Treatment

The patient is mobilized about ten days after the operation. If stability requires it, a spinal orthosis should be worn for approximately three months postoperatively.

Alternative Methods

A technical variant, with combined anterior–posterior linear osteotomy for posttraumatic kyphosis in the thoracolumbar or lumbar region, correction of the kyphosis is followed by stabilization with the fixateur interne. In this technique, a posterior metal implant that has angular stability is inserted, so that a bone graft without compression load-bearing capacity will prove sufficient.

In the first operative stage, the patient is in a lateral decubitus position, and the anterior approach is used, as

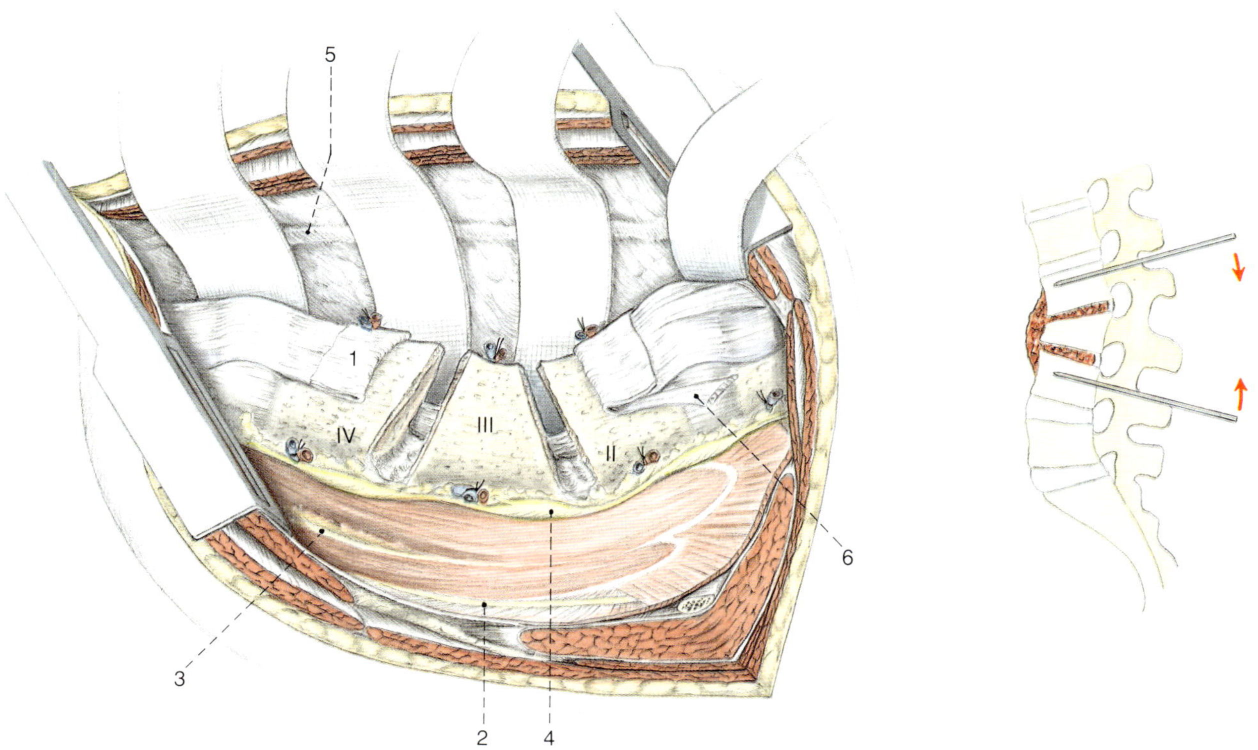

Fig. 3.**35** Posttraumatic kyphosis. The intervertebral disks adjoining the wedged vertebrae have been removed; the vertebral bodies are partially stripped of periosteum. In preparation for the fusion, autologous bone is deposited in the form of a paste. The actual correction is performed from the posterior side with the use of Schanz screws (see inset).

1 Anterior longitudinal ligament
2 Subcostal nerve
3 Ilioinguinal nerve
4 Sympathetic trunk
5 Ureter
6 Left medial crus
II–IV Lumbar vertebrae

described above, to resect the anterior longitudinal ligament. Cranial to the wedged vertebra, the annulus fibrosus on the side of the approach is also resected anteriorly, and as far as possible on the contralateral side as well. In cases of severe kyphosis, the intervertebral disk below the wedged vertebra has to be similarly removed. The upper plates are freed of cartilage and debrided. The adjacent vertebrae are stripped of periosteum up to mid-height on the side of the approach, as well as anteriorly (see Chapter 6, lumbar fusion operations, Figs. 6.**8**–6.**15**, except that for correction of kyphosis, the anterior longitudinal ligament is excised additionally).

As graft material for the anterior spondylodesis, finely morselized autologous bone in the form of bone paste is packed into the space between the upper plates and compressed with a punch. Above all, an ample quantity of bone paste is applied in spindle-shaped deposits to the debrided external aspects of the vertebrae to be fused (Fig. 3.**35**). Fixation is not necessary; the relapsing peritoneal sac and the intra-abdominal pressure following wound closure hold the graft in place.

The second operative stage, which produces the actual correction after the anterior release, can be carried out immediately afterwards, but can also be postponed for as long as 14 days. During this time, the soft paste graft easily adapts to any new vertebral position. With the patient lying prone, the malunited posterior vertebral elements are first mobilized by joint resection via a posterior midline approach, and this is followed by shortening of the curve and resection of the elongated, scarred ligamentum flavum, which might otherwise cause compression of the canal contents upon lordosation. After this, the long Schanz screws of the fixateur interne are inserted transpedicularly (as shown in Chapter 6, Figs. 6.**16**–6.**32**). Correction of the kyphosis is accomplished by compressing the posterior ends of the Schanz screws (Fig. 3.**36**); the posterior border of the vertebral body acts as the pivot. The chucks on the longitudinal threaded rods of the fixateur must be free to move toward one another; the lateral nuts are loose, while the terminal compression nuts are tightened until correction is achieved. The position is then secured by tightening all nuts. Protruding parts of the Schanz screws are cut off.

The construct can be applied to one segment, but is generally carried out bisegmentally.

Further Reading

Dick W. Fixation von Brust- und Lendenwirbelfrakturen. In: Burri C, Harder F, Jäger M, eds. Aktuelle Probleme in Chirurgie und Orthopädie. Berne: Huber, 1984.

Harms J, Stoltze D. Die operative Behandlung der BSW- und LWS-Frakturen mit dem USI-System. In: Stuhler T, ed. Fixateur externe, fixateur interne. Berlin: Springer, 1989.

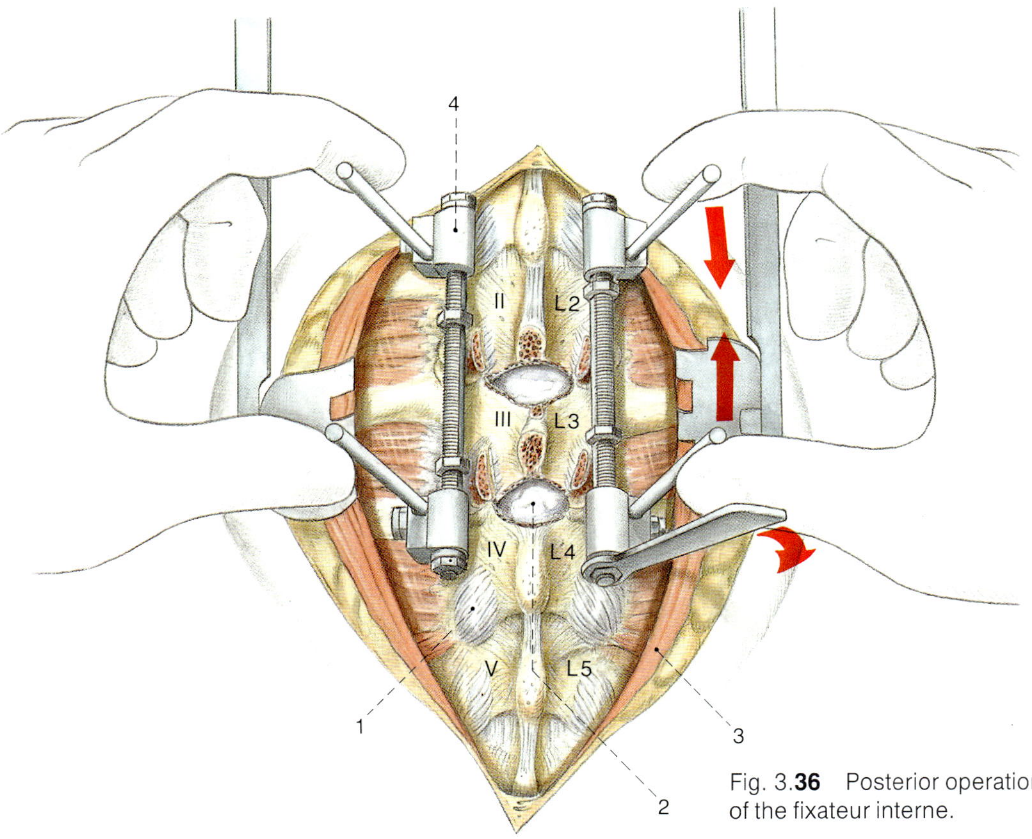

Fig. 3.**36** Posterior operation. Correction of kyphosis with the aid of the fixateur interne.

1 L4–L5 joint capsule
2 Spina dura mater
3 Longissimus muscle
4 Fixateur interne
II–V Lumbar vertebrae

Long-Arc Kyphosis (Scheuermann's Kyphosis)

Indications

The indication for surgical treatment of Scheuermann's kyphosis depends on various factors, and should be established conservatively.

Generally, angles of at least 60–70 degrees are necessary before surgical correction is considered, but the position of the kyphotic apex is also part of the consideration. Caution is advised when the apex lies in the physiologic thoracic region, but even a milder kyphosis at the thoracolumbar junction necessitates an operation.

Other criteria include intractable back pain, cosmetic compromise of the patient and, of course, positive neurologic symptoms related to Scheuermann's kyphosis. Additionally, the patient's age has a bearing on the indication for surgery, as well as on the operative technique.

Risser sign stage 0, I, II: surgical treatment is hardly ever necessary.

Risser sign stage III or IV: in connection with the growth potential remaining in the vertebral area, a posterior fusion of adequate length will suffice.

Treatment Strategy

A combined anterior and posterior procedure is required in skeletally mature patients.

Sequence of operations:

1. Anterior–posterior:
   For a rigid kyphosis with structural changes in the vertebral bodies a primary anterior mobilizing osteotomy seems necessary for good correction of the kyphosis. The posterior operation follows in a second session. Halo traction can be applied immediately after the operation. The second, posterior, operation follows 2–3 weeks later.
2. Posterior–anterior:
   For a relatively mobile kyphosis, comparatively good correction can be achieved with a primary posterior operation. If there is marked gaping of the intervertebral spaces due to the wedge sharpe of the vertebral bodies, particularly in the apical area, an intervertebral spondylodesis should be performed secondarily to maintain the results of the correction.

Area of Fusion

The following radiographs are needed:

- Standing anteroposterior and lateral film of the entire spine.
- Bending film in the sagittal plane.
- Traction film.

As a rule, the fusion is carried out at least from one neutral vertebra to the other. Failures due to loss of correction are attributable to the following factors (Figs. 3.**37**–3.**39**):

- Cranial decompensation:
  The fusion does not include the upper neutral vertebra. Even though the correction may be completely maintained in the fusion zone, a kyphosis develops above it, causing loss of the correction. This type of decompensation can occur particularly with the use of a Luque system (apparently owing to the technically required resection of the yellow ligament and interspinal ligament cranial to the end vertebra).
- Central loss of correction with appropriate fusion length:
  Even with a proper fusion length, central loss of correction can occur over one or several wedged vertebrae. This can be expected when a posterior operation is performed after completion of growth. In this situation, a secondary, anterior operation with intervertebral fusion is indicated in a second session.
- Caudal decompensation:
  This occurs if the fusion is not extended far enough caudally (especially in thoracolumbar kyphosis). In such cases, L1 and possibly L2 should be included in the fusion.

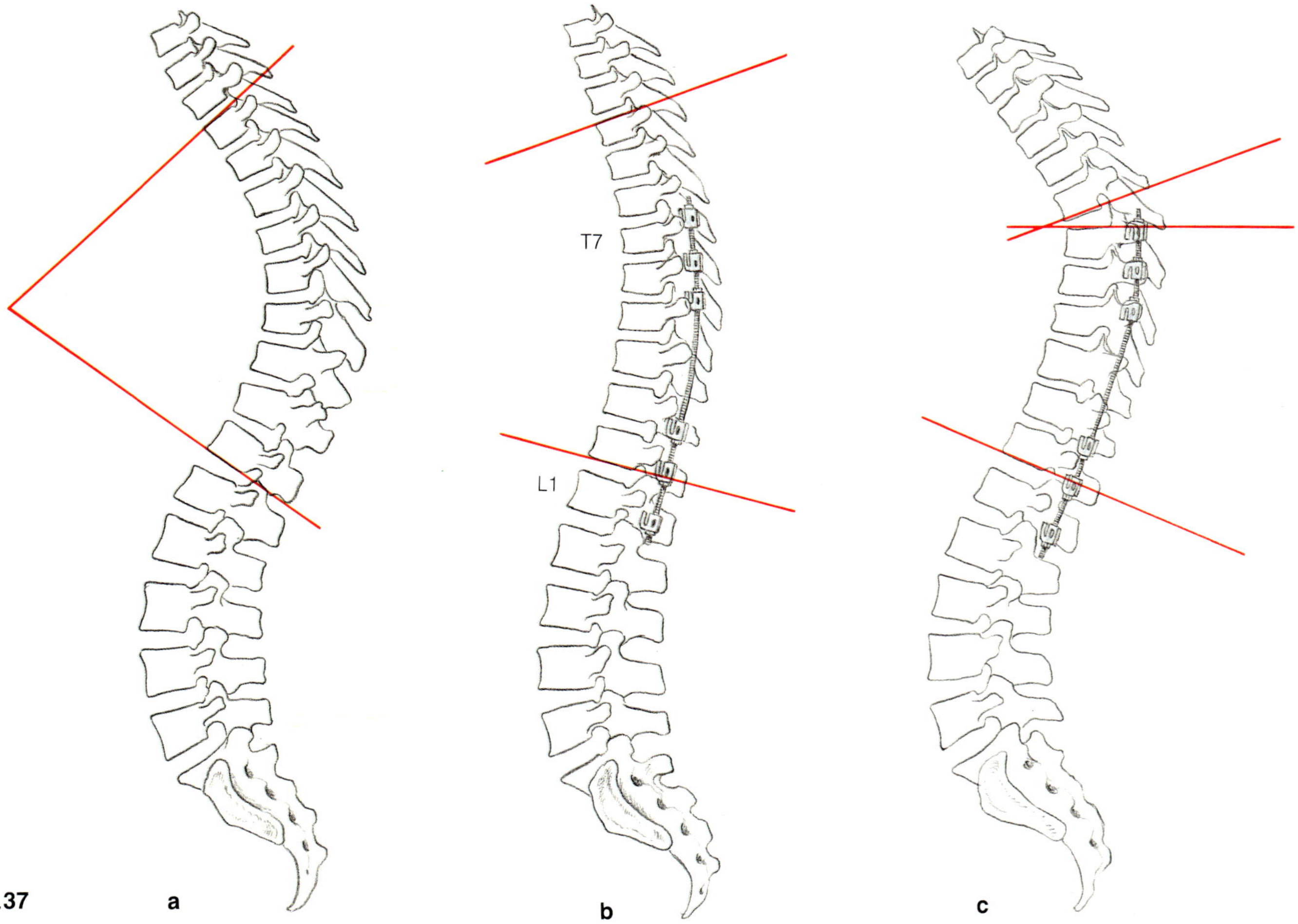

Fig. 3.**37** **a** **b** **c**

Fig. 3.**37**
a Scheuermann's kyphosis.
b Correction using the Harrington compression system. The cranial fusion is too short.
c Increase of kyphosis due to cranial decompensation with no change in fusion length.

Fig. 3.**38**
a Scheuermann's kyphosis.
b Correction with the Harrington compression system. *Note:* there is gaping of the intervertebral spaces at the apex due to wedged vertebrae.
c Loss of correction due to central decompensation. This situation calls for an anterior interbody fusion.

Fig. 3.**39**
a Scheuermann's kyphosis.
b Correction using the Harrington compression system. The fusion is too short caudally.
c Loss of correction due to caudal decompensation.

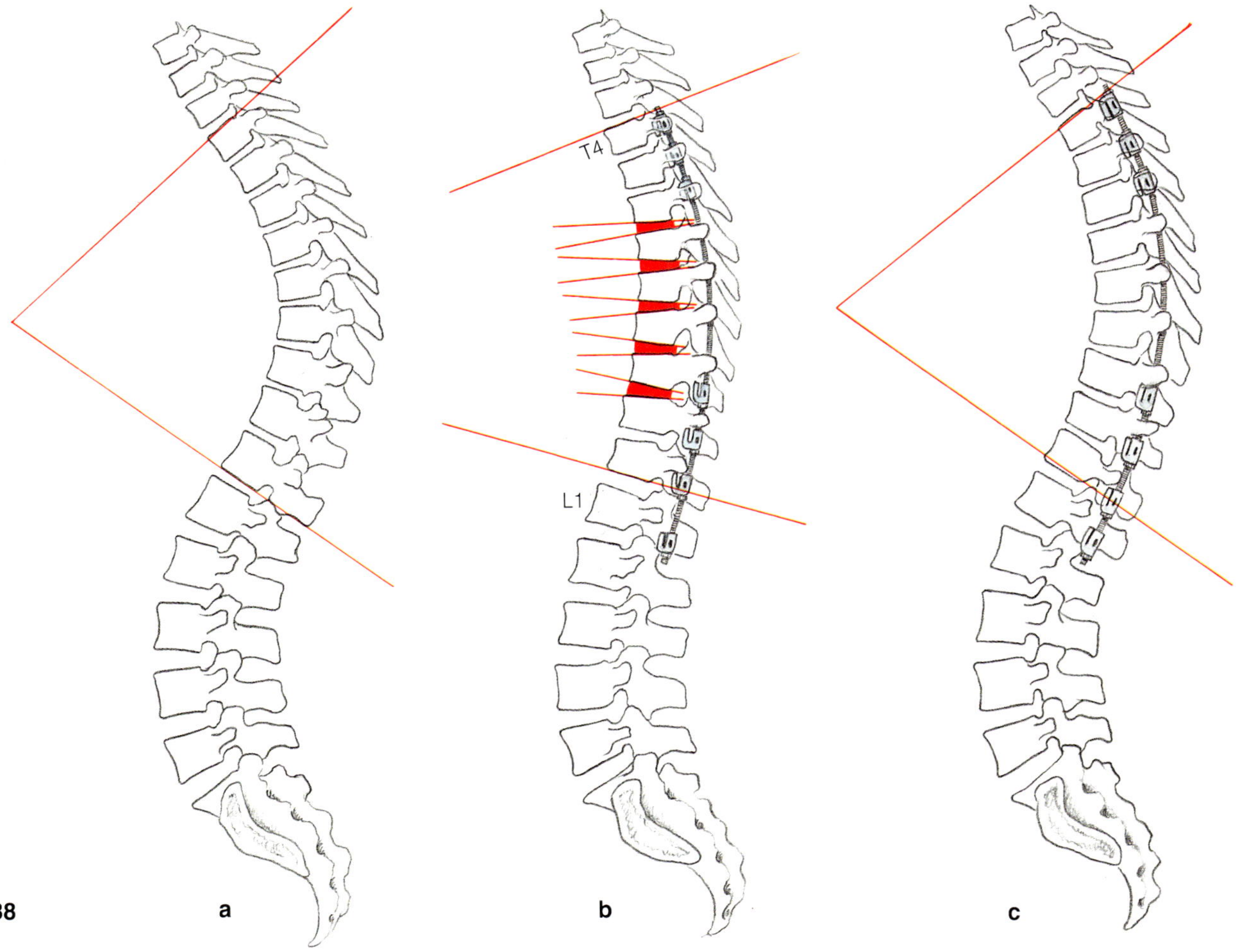

Fig. 3.**38** a b c

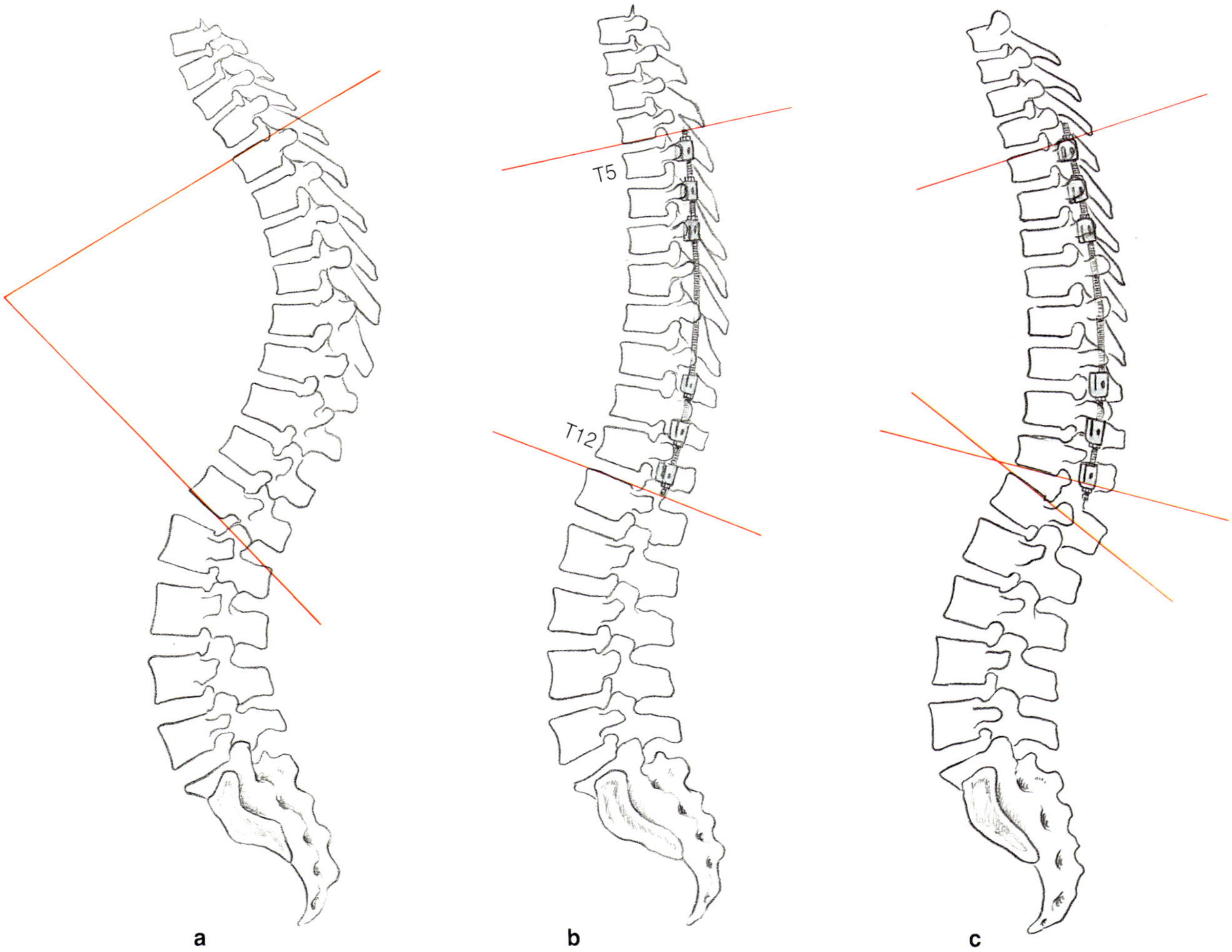

Fig. 3.**39** a b c

Operative Technique

Anterior operation: This is a mobilizing osteotomy, which is generally done via a right-sided thoracotomy (anterior mobilizing osteotomy, p. 147). It is essentially the rigid apical zone that is mobilized. As a rule, five to seven intervertebral disks are removed. The intervertebral spaces are bridged with bone grafts (possibly from the rib obtained in the thoracotomy). The anterior operation can either be performed initially, or can follow the posterior operation (p. 215).

Posterior operation: Various implant systems are used.

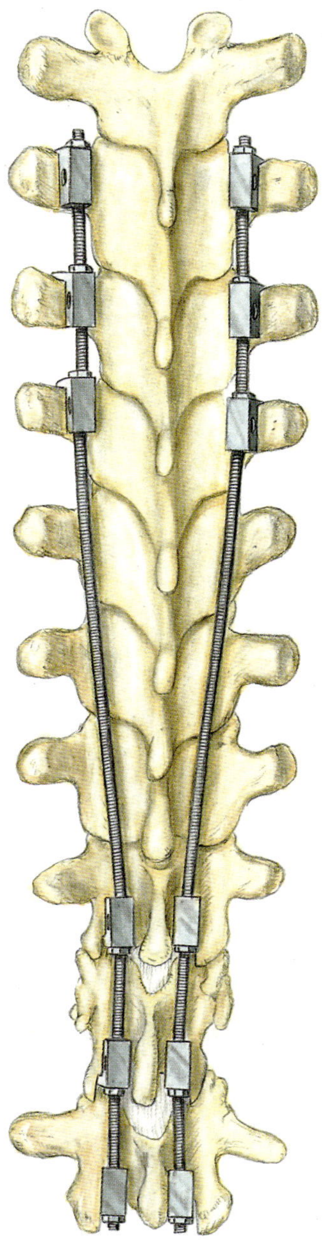

Fig. 3.**40** Scheuermann's kyphosis. Harrington compression hooks bilaterally. *Note* in the area of the thoracolumbar junction, the compression hooks are placed beneath the lamina.

Harrington Compression System

(Fig. 3.**40**)

The procedure substantially conforms to the Harrington operation (p. 92), except that a Harrington compression system is applied bilaterally. The hooks proximal to the apex are placed on the transverse processes and are aligned in a distal direction; the distal hooks are oriented proximally. If the caudal end of the fusion zone lies at the thoracolumbar junction, it is expedient to place the compression hooks beneath the laminae (Harrington operation, p. 93). At least three pairs of hooks are placed cranially and caudally; as a rule, no hooks are placed in the apical region. Correction is then accomplished as usual by alternating continuous tightening of the screws on both sides and at the upper and lower ends of the curve, together with manual correction by pressure on the kyphotic apex. As in the Harrington operation, the facet joints are debrided, and finally an ample quantity of fusion material is introduced. Since the fusion is under tensile stress, a massive graft should be interposed between the two compression rods.

Postoperative Treatment

The patient is placed in bed without external orthotic fixation, and taken to the intensive care unit, where the necessary postoperative diagnostic and therapeutic measures are carried out. Regular neurologic monitoring after the operation is mandatory.

In patients with completed growth and wedge-shaped vertebral deformities, an anterior interbody spondylodesis is indicated two weeks after the operation.

After removal of sutures, the patients are fitted with a body cast or spinal orthosis for 6–9 months.

Luque System

(Fig. 3.**41**)

Via a posterior midline incision, the entire kyphosis—generally from T1 to L2—is subperiosteally exposed in the usual way. Then two L-rods are cut to the length of the spinal segment to be instrumented. With a bending press, the rods are adjusted to the extent of kyphosis that can be expected after the intraoperative correction. Excessive correction should be avoided. This instrumentation is essentially designed to maintain the correction attainable in the course of an anterior and posterior release operation. The pre-bent wires are then pulled through below the lamina in the usual way (Luque operation, p. 118). Two double wires are used for each of the two end vertebrae of the fusion. The subsequent procedure conforms to the Luque technique for the convex side.

The short leg of an L-rod is fixed to the cranial end vertebra of the fusion. The segmental wires are then pulled from the cranial end toward the apex, while at the same time manual pressure is exerted on the kyphotic apex. Next, the second L-rod is affixed to the caudal end vertebra, and wired from caudal to cranial in the direction of the apical vertebra. The kyphosis is additionally corrected by pressure on both rod ends. The fixation of the two rods by wire is now completed, after which the wires are clipped to a length of about 1 cm and curled medially and caudally (p. 121).

Before placement of the cerclage wires and the Luque rods, resection of the facet joints and debridement of the posterior vertebral elements have to be carried out. After completion of the instrumentation, fusion is prepared by application of ample bone graft material.

Postoperative Treatment

After wound closure, the patients are positioned in bed without external orthotic fixation and taken to the intensive care unit. The patients are mobilized without any spinal orthosis 6–10 days after the operation. They are discharged after removal of the sutures. The patients' physical activity has to be reduced for at least six months pending consolidation of the fusion.

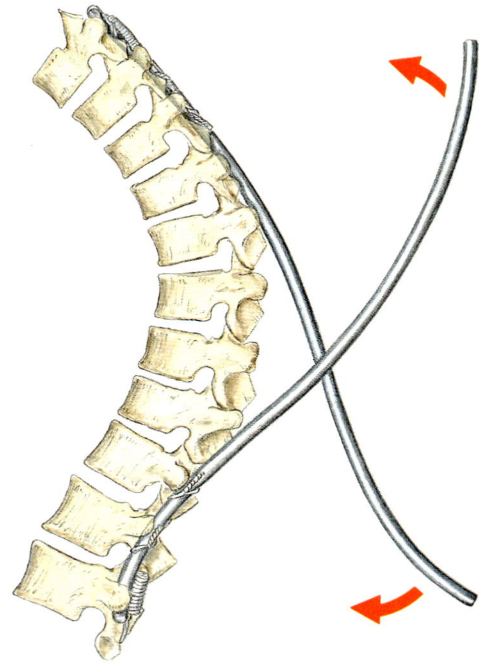

Fig. 3.**41** Luque operation. Correction of kyphosis.

Pitfalls and Complications

The Luque operation is associated with a high rate of neurologic complications (p. 125), and should therefore be reserved for essentially neuropathic spinal deformities. It is hardly ever indicated for Scheuermann's kyphosis.

Cranial decompensation presents another problem. Apparently due to the need for resection of the interspinal ligament and the ligamentum flavum even above the end vertebra, the kyphosis may be aggravated at the upper end of the fusion though the correction in the fusion zone is retained.

Cotrel–Dubousset Technique

(Figs. 3.**42**, 3.**43**)

With the patient in the prone position, the entire kyphotic area is exposed subperiosteally via a posterior midline incision. After appropriate dissection, the facet joints are resected in the usual way, and the posterior vertebral elements are debrided. Two Cotrel rods of appropriate length are then selected and bent to conform to the extent of kyphosis anticipated intraoperatively. The instrumentation and placement of hooks have to be adapted to the type of deformity. A bilateral claw grip with the transverse and pedicular hooks is applied to the superior end vertebra, and another claw grip to the vertebra after the next one caudally. A bilateral claw grip is also used on the caudal end vertebra, this one consisting of a closed laminar hook combined with a blade facing caudally. A hook with a lateral opening can also be used for the purpose. This facilitates the lateral insertion of the rod into its final position without the need for caudal displacement of the rod. With marked kyphosis, this displacement of the Cotrel rod is fairly difficult. Finally, DTTs are attached at least to the two ends of the Cotrel rods to reinforce the assembly. The use of laterally open hooks on the caudal side also prevents the rods from moving out of position laterally.

For long-curved kyphoses, it is possible to use several claw constructs. In addition, compression of the two hooks in opposite directions in the L1–L2 area, for example, can induce lumbar lordosis.

Figures 3.**44**–3.**47** show various possible claw constructs that can be used, depending on the spinal level, the configuration of the lamina, the transverse processes, etc.

Fusion is prepared by applying ample graft material to the debrided posterior vertebral elements.

Postoperative Treatment

After wound closure, the patient is placed in bed without external orthotic fixation, and taken to the intensive care unit. Patients are mobilized without external fixation 6–10 days after the operation, and discharged after removal of sutures. Physical activity has to be reduced until the fusion has consolidated, which generally takes at least six months.

Pitfalls and Complications

See under Cotrel–Dubousset operation for scoliosis, p. 146.

The Universal Spinal Instrumentation System (Zielke)

Transpedicular fixation in conjunction with compression rods (Zielke) can be used in principle to achieve a very effective posterior correction (p. 233). Because of the complexity of the operation, however, this procedure is reserved primarily for ankylosing spondylitis kyphosis.

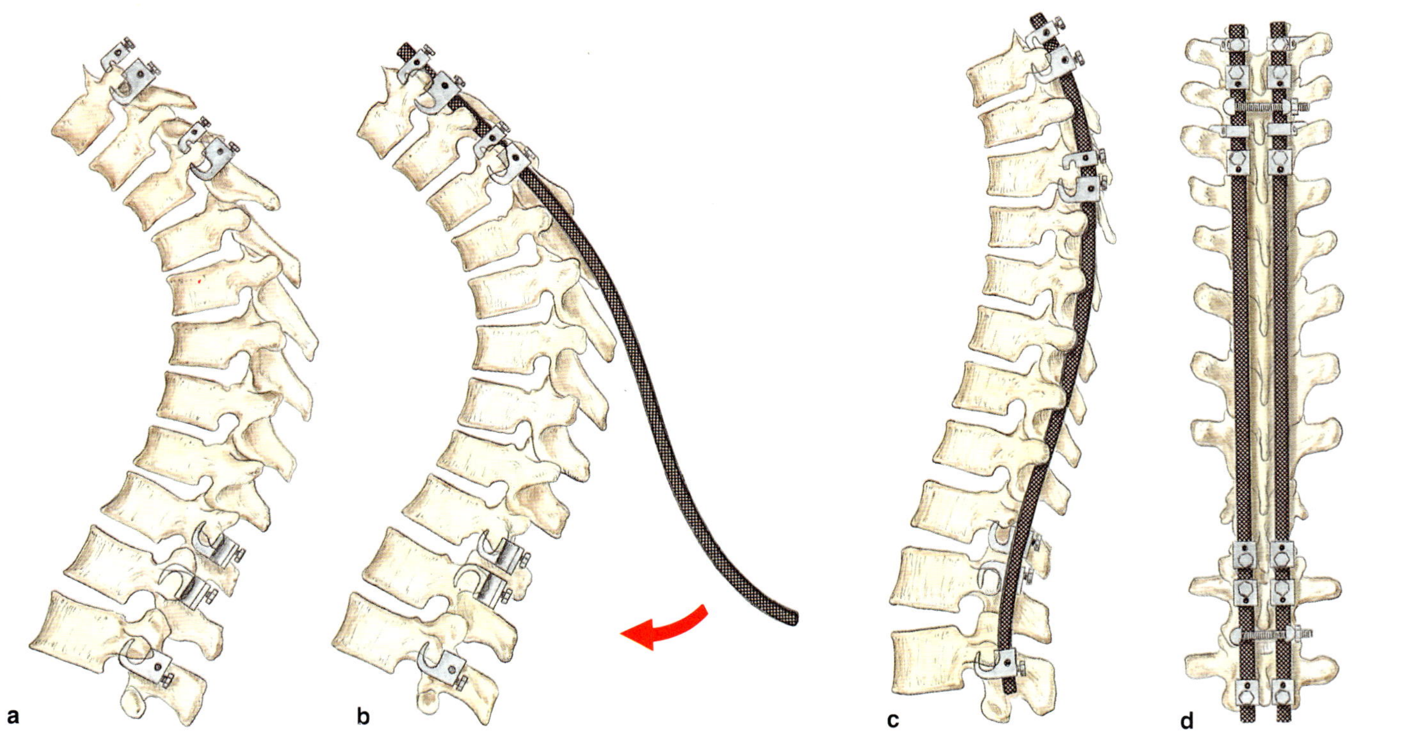

Fig. 3.**42** Correction of kyphosis using the Cotrel–Dubousset system.
a Claw grip at the cranial and caudal ends of the curve. *Note:* opposite placement of the laminar hooks at L1 and L2 allows induction of lumbar lordosis.
b Correction of kyphosis with an appropriately bent Cotrel rod. *Note:* induction of lumbar lordosis by caudal bending of rod.
c, d Correct implant seating in both planes. Restoration of physiological curvatures. Stabilization with a DTT.

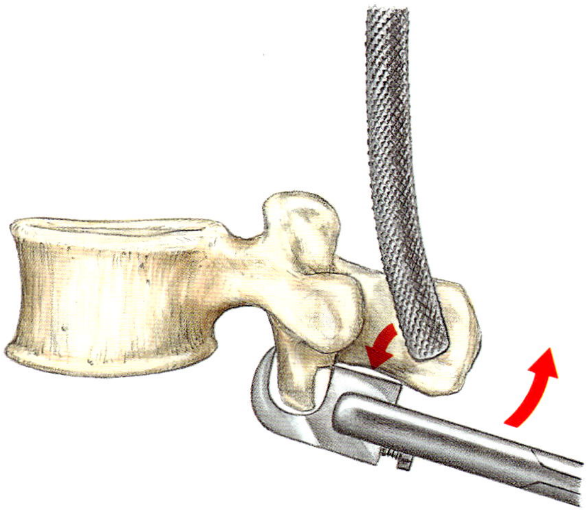

Fig. 3.**43** Insertion of a Cotrel rod into the caudal hook. A rod length is chosen that allows the rod to pass into the lowest hook without appreciable displacement (later displacement is very difficult in kyphosis operations). After slight tilting of the hook with the hook holder, the rod can be inserted into the hook opening by adequate pressure. *Note:* induction of lumbar lordosis at the lower end of the rod.

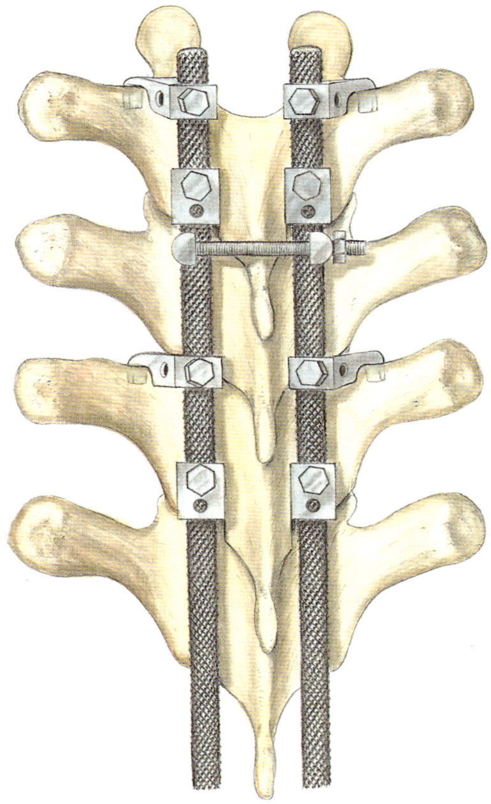

Fig. 3.**44** Double-claw construct at the cranial fusion end (pedicular–transverse hook combination applied twice).

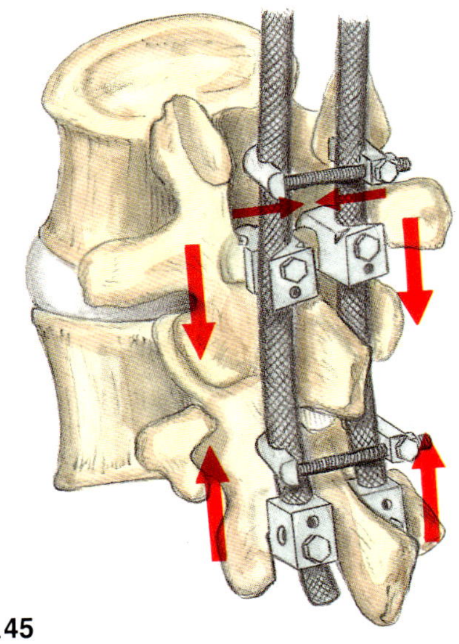

Fig. 3.**45**

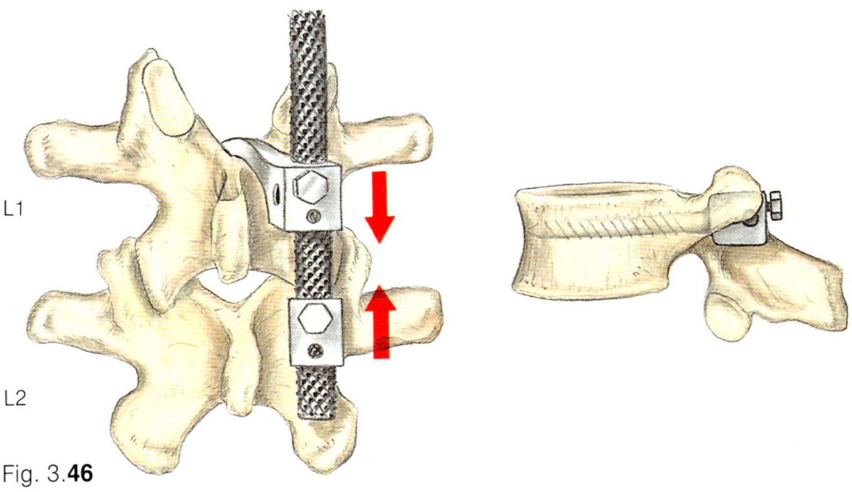

Fig. 3.**46**

Fig. 3.**45** Claw grip at the caudal end of the curve. Lumbar lordosis is induced by compression. A DTT is used for stabilization, particularly with a laterally open hook (facilitating insertion of rod).

Fig. 3.**46** Claw grip with a pedicular screw. A pedicular screw with an angulated laminar hook is applied to the next higher vertebra.

Fig. 3.**47** Claw grip with a pedicular screw. A pedicular screw combined with a specially angulated hook below the lamina is applied to the same vertebra.

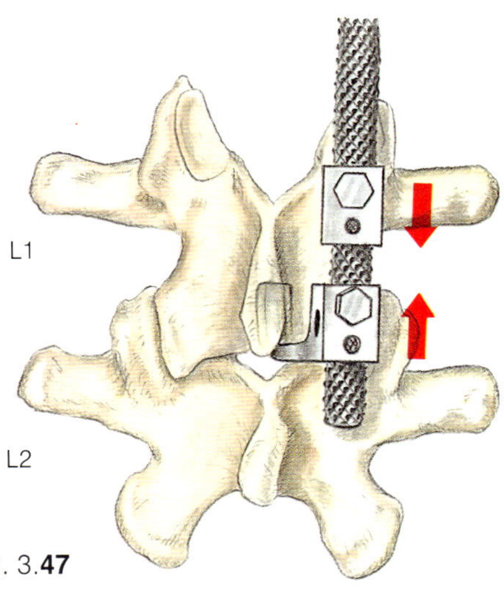

Fig. 3.**47**

Further Reading

Bradford DS, Garcia A. Neurological complications in Scheuermann's disease. J Bone Jt Surg 1969;51-A:567.

Bradford DS, Moe JH, Montalvo FJ, Winter RB. Scheuermann's kyphosis. J Bone Jt Surg 1975;57-A:439.

Bradford DS, Ahmed KB, Moe JH, Winter RB, Lonstein JE. The surgical management of patients with Scheuermann's disease. J Bone Jt Surg 1980;62-A:705.

Dubousset J, Cotrel Y. Die CD-Instrumentation in der Behandlung von Wirbelsäulendeformitäten. Orthopäde 1989;18:118.

Griss P, von Andrian-Werburg H. Mittelfristige Ergebnisse von dorsalen Aufrichtungsoperationen juveniler Kyphosen mit dem Harrington-Instrumentarium. Arch Orthop Traum Surg 1978;91:113.

Griss P, Pfeil J. Aufrichtungsoperationen bei juvenilen Kyphosen. Z Orthop 1983;121:665.

Heine J, Stauch R, Matthiass HH. Ergebnisse der operativen Behandlung des Morbus Scheuermann. Z Orthop 1984;122:743.

Lowe TG. Double L-rod instrumentation in the treatment of severe kyphosis secondary to Scheuermann's disease. Spine 1987;12:336.

Nerubay J, Katznelson A. Dual approach in the surgical treatment of juvenile kyphosis. Spine 1986;11:101.

Ogilvie JW, Coscia MF, Bradford DS. Scheuermann's kyphosis treated with Luque instrumentation. AOA meeting, Hot Springs, 1988.

Rodegerdts U, Gisbertz D, Zielke K. Untersuchung zur dorsalen Aufrichtungsosteotomie der Kyphose. Z Orthop 1985;123:374.

Speck GR, Chopin DC. The surgical treatment of Scheuermann's kyphosis. J Bone Jt Surg 1986;68-B:189.

Taylor TC, Wenger DR, Stephen J, Gillespie R, Bobechko WP. Surgical management of thoracic kyphosis in adolescents. J Bone Jt Surg 1979;61-A:496.

Thoracic Lordosis

Indications

The Cotrel–Dubousset technique is a major contribution to the management of mobile thoracic lordoscoliosis, in that the lordosis is relieved and the scoliotic curve is converted to a physiological kyphosis by rotation of the Cotrel rod. This, however, is possible only with mobile curves with maximum Cobb angles of 60–70 degrees. With pronounced lordosis, the mobility of the thoracic lordosis has to be verified by bending films in the sagittal plane. If the lordosis is rigid, an anterior mobilizing osteotomy is required to begin with.

For simple thoracic lordosis (without a scoliotic component), an operation may be indicated in skeletally mature patients with severe structural curvatures in excess of −25 to −30 degrees and marked pulmonary dysfunction.

Operative Technique

(Figs. 3.**48**–3.**50**)

Anterior Operation

Thoracotomy is performed on the convex side if there is a scoliotic component. The vertebral bodies are exposed in the usual way after ligation of the segmental vessels (Chapter 1, p. 13).

The intervertebral disks are excised and completely resected as far as the posterior longitudinal ligament (anterior mobilizing osteotomy, p. 147). If the latter is greatly foreshortened and thickened, it has to be removed as well. Using a chisel, a narrow bone wedge with an anterior base is then cut from the adjacent vertebral bodies. No bone graft should be introduced into the intervertebral spaces in preparation for fusion; this would hinder the correction. However, in preparation for the fusion, a ball reamer can be used to tunnel through the lateral vertebral body wall, and the resulting groove is packed with bone graft (harvested either from the resected rib or from resected anterior vertebral elements).

In the presence of a simple thoracic lordosis without a scoliotic component, correction via the posterior approach can be facilitated by a rib osteotomy, following a suggestion by Bradford. First of all, sections of rib about 0.5 cm wide lying 10 cm lateral to the spine are resected subperiosteally during the thoracotomy (mobilizing anterior osteotomy) at several levels of the apical region. A corresponding rib resection is performed contralaterally as part of the posterior operation.

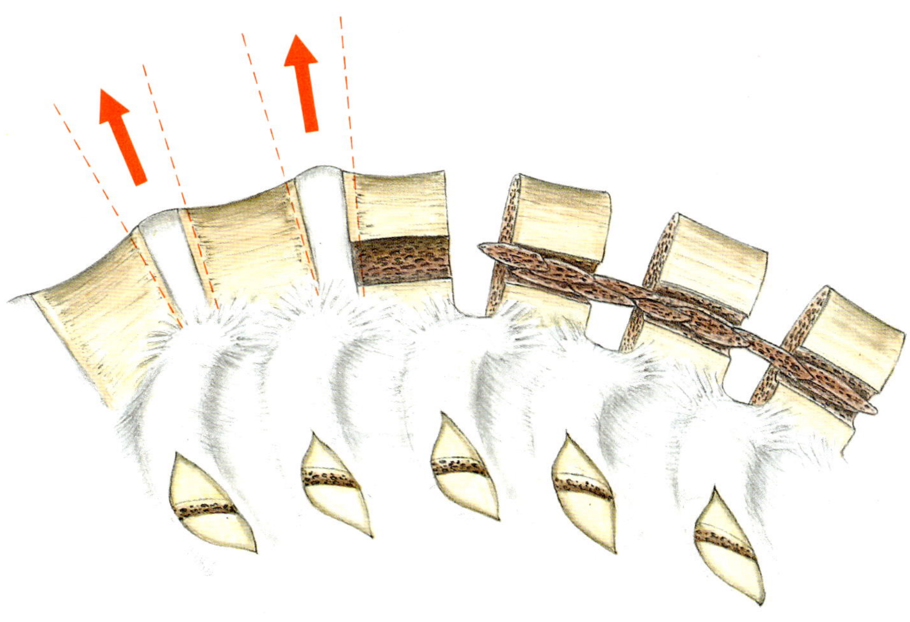

Fig. 3.**48** Anterior mobilizing osteotomy in thoracic lordosis (Bradford). Resection of intervertebral disks, possibly together with anterior portions of the vertebral bodies (dashed line). In preparation for fusion, a lateral groove is cut into the vertebral bodies. Resection osteotomy of the ribs in the apical region in the side of the thoracotomy.

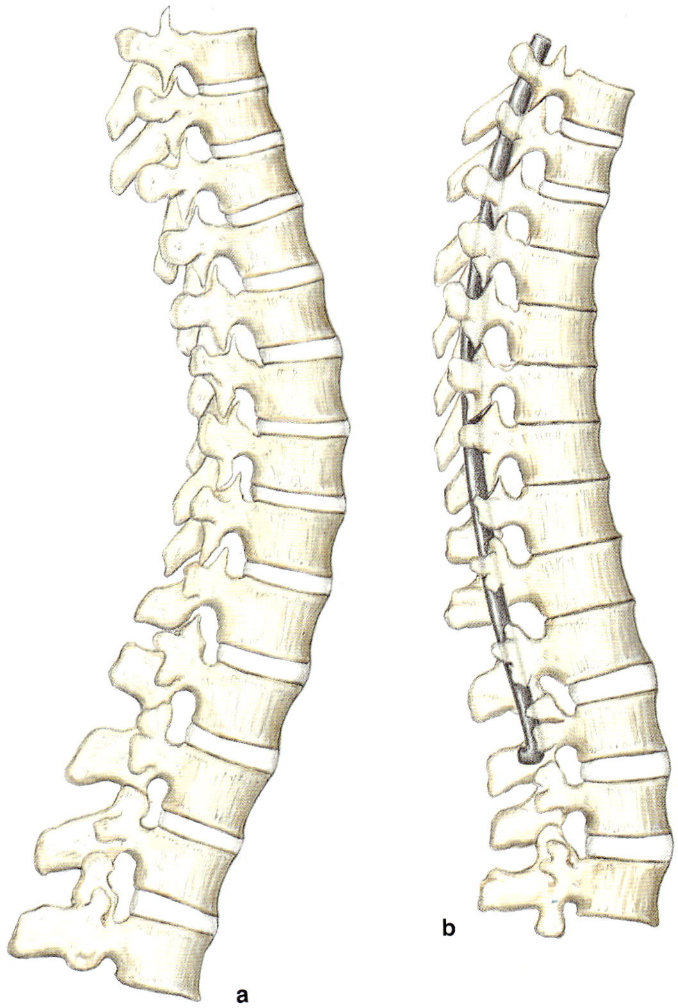

Fig. 3.**49**
a Pronounced thoracic lordosis.
b Status after correction using the L-rod technique. *Note:* firm closure of intervertebral spaces after correction of lordosis.

Posterior Operation (Second Session)

There are a number of technical options:

– Cotrel–Dubousset technique. In the presence of a mobile lordoscoliosis (with or without anterior mobilizing osteotomy), the correction can be effected by the customary Cotrel–Dubousset technique (derotation, p. 135).
– Harrington technique.
– L-rod technique (Luque).

The two last-mentioned techniques are suitable for correction of a simple thoracic lordosis mobilized from the anterior side. With the Harrington system, use is made bilaterally of two Harrington distraction rods combined with sublaminar wires (Harrington–Luque system, p. 129). The Harrington rod has to be pre-bent according to the planned thoracic kyphosis; the correction is accomplished by means of the sublaminar wires. Since a rotatory component is involved, rectangular rods with rectangular hooks (Moe) have to be used.

The L-rod technique is used in corrections involving Luque rods (p. 120). The short legs of two L-rods are then fixed at the cranial and caudal ends of the lordotic curve. The kyphosis is corrected by approximating the spine to the corresponding pre-bent Luque rods by means of sublaminar wires.

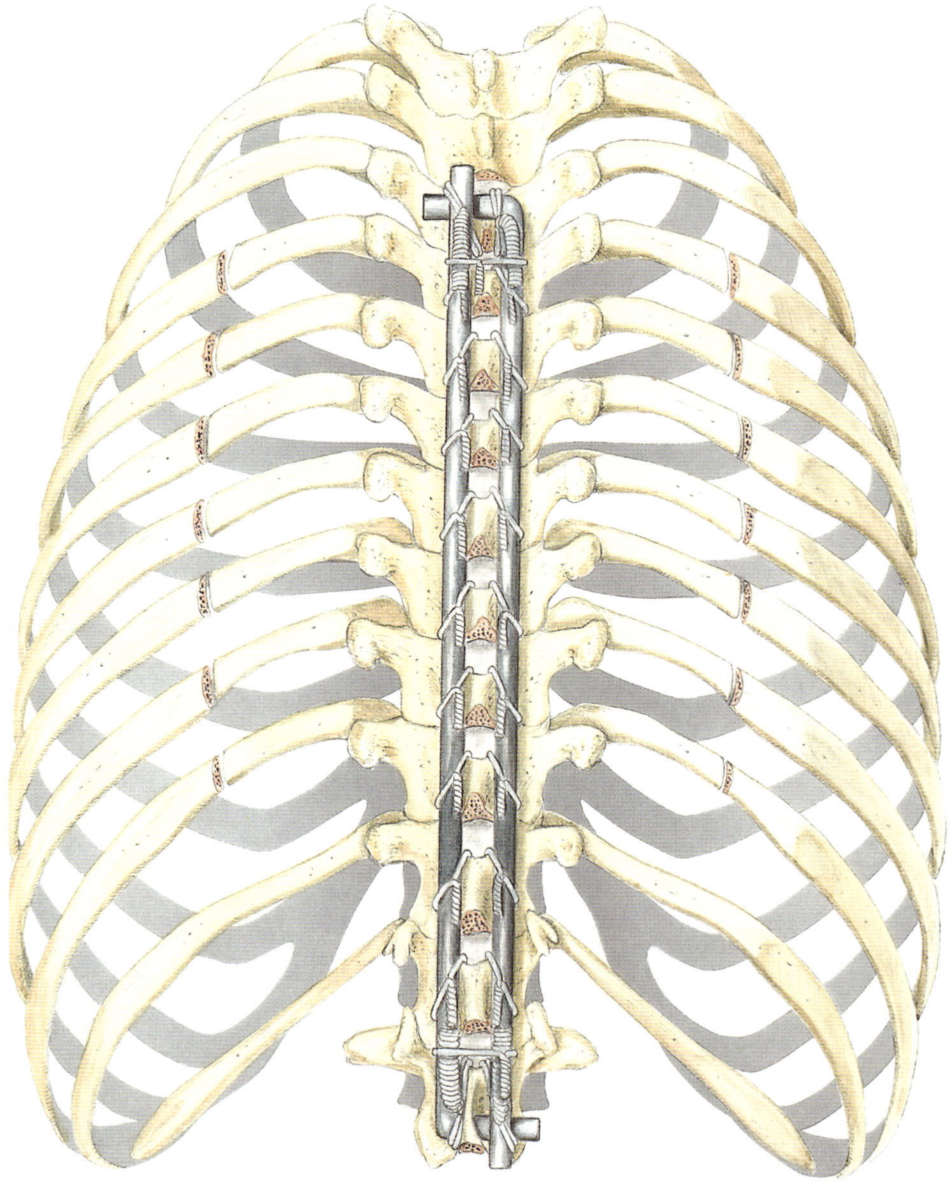

Fig. 3.**50** Correction of thoracic lordosis after anterior mobilization, bilateral rib resection osteotomy, and stabilization with the double L-rod technique.

Further Reading

Bradford DS, Blatt JM, Rasp FL. Surgical management of severe thoracic lordosis. Spine 1983;8:420.

Bradford DS, Lonstein JE, Ogilvie JW, Winter RB. Scoliosis and other spinal deformities. Philadelphia: Saunders, 1987.

Hall JE, Millis MB, Lipton H, Gebhardt M. Treatment of hypokyphotic scoliosis, non-operative and operative. 18th Annual Meeting of the American Scoliosis Research Society, 1983.

4 Ankylosing Spondylitis

H. J. Hehne
K. Zielke

Operations for Kyphotic Deformity

Zielke Technique (Polysegmental Lumbar Lordosation Spondylodesis)

Indications

Principal indication: Long-curved or thoracic kyphotic deformities of at least 70 degrees, and lumbar kyphotic deformities of at least 20 degrees with ankylosis of the spine.

Secondary indication: Kyphotic deformities of less than 70 degrees with uncontrollable vertebrogenic pain (early spondylodesis) or with spondylodiskitis (Andersson lesion).

Note
The Zielke method can also be employed to correct the kyphotic deformity in Scheuermann's disease. The instrumentarium used in anterior derotation spondylodesis can in principle be applied in scoliosis, kyphosis, spondylolisthesis, spondylodiskitis, tumors, fractures, instabilities, and degenerative changes of the spinal column.*

* Universal Spinal Instrumentation System (USIS), Zielke; Ulrich Co., Ulm.

The operation in ankylosing spondylitis can generally, in a second session, be combined with a cervical lordosation spondylodesis following Mason–Urist (p. 241).

Positioning

The patient is placed in a prone position. The operating table, which must be adjustable, has to be flexed so that the table surfaces conform to the kyphosis (Fig. 4.**1**).

During the correction, the table should be continuously adjustable by remote control. The patient's lower pelvis lies near the apex of the table. Padding is placed under the sternum and the pubic bone, to prevent compression of the abdomen (Fig. 4.**1**). The head is held in place with a neurosurgical head-holder.

Note
Immobile cervical kyphoses may, in rare cases, hinder or prevent intubation. Nasal or bronchoscopic intubation is an alternative. Tracheotomies are required extremely seldom (fewer than 0.5% of cases).

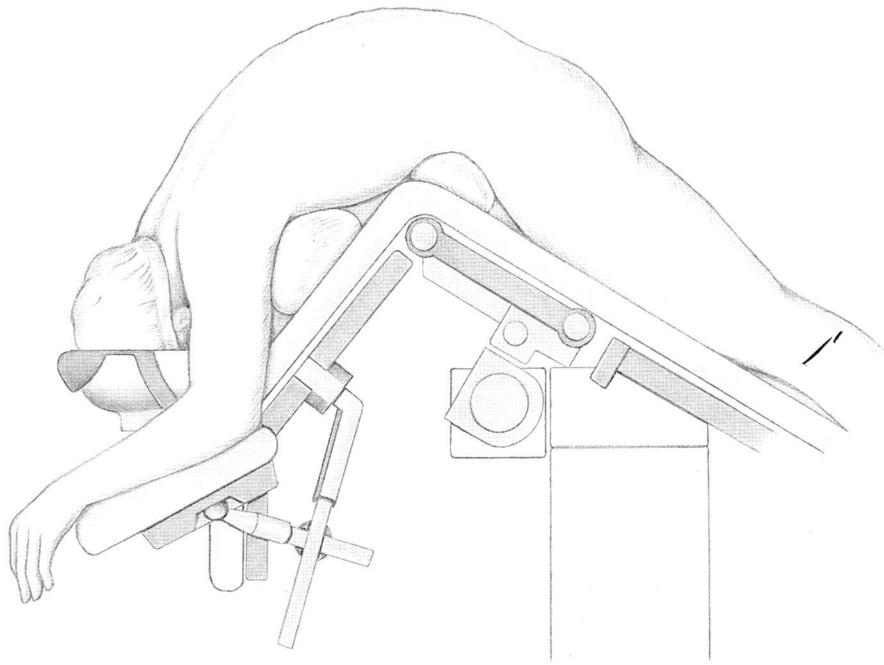

Fig. 4.**1** Positioning on flexed operating table.

Incision and Exposure of the Spine

The procedure is the same as for a posterior scoliosis operation (pp. 64–69). However, in accordance with the most commonly used instrumentation levels, from T10 to S1, exposure from T8–T9 to S2 is sufficient (Fig. 4.**2**).

The dissection is preferably started at the apex of the kyphosis. From here, it continues caudally and cranially. Due to the exposure of the lumbosacral junction, identification of the levels is not difficult.

The site is characterized by the following features (Fig. 4.**2**).

The facet joints, including their capsules, are nearly always completely ossified, as are the yellow and interspinal ligaments. This compact bony block of the posterior vertebral elements may make orientation difficult. It is therefore advisable to expose the bases of the transverse processes.

Note
Separation of layers sometimes proves difficult in ankylosing spondylitis as a result of muscular metaplasia and osteoporosis.

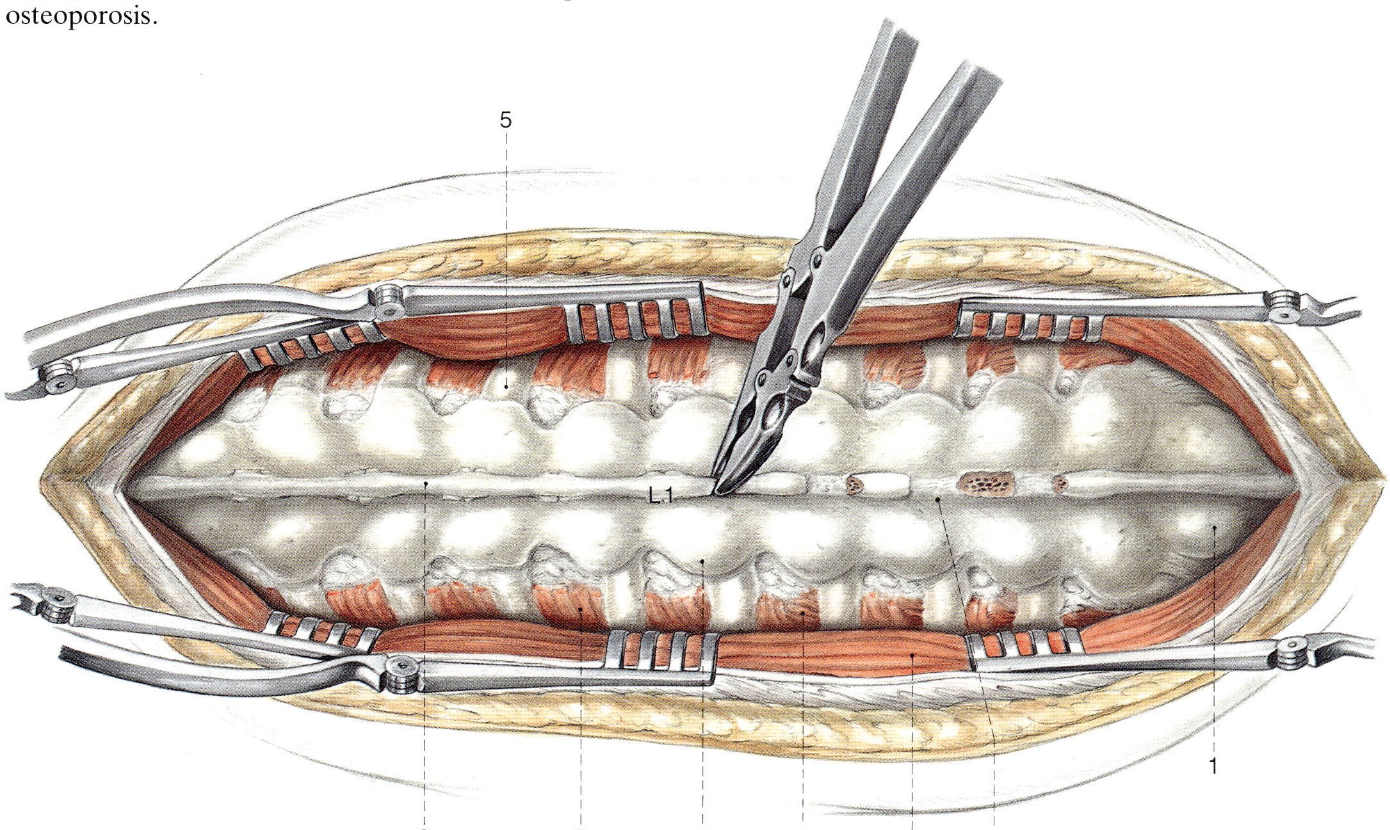

Fig. 4.**2** Operative site after subperiosteal exposure of the posterior vertebral elements from T9 to S1, with resection of the ossified interspinal ligament L1–L2. These ligaments have already been removed from L2–L3 to L4–L5, as has the spinous process at L4.

1 Sacrum
2 Multifidus muscles
3 Medial intertransverse lumbar muscles
4 Longissimus muscle of the thorax
5 Transverse process
6 Ossified interspinal ligament
7 Ossified joint capsule
8 Ossified yellow ligament
L1 Spinous process of the first lumbar vertebra

Operative Technique

Instrumentarium

Zielke USIS implants (Fig. 4.**3**; see also p. 178).

Threaded rod: Manually flexible rod 3 mm thick, with a fine-pitch thread and hexagonal nuts that are rectangularly beveled on one side.

Pedicular screws: Cancellous bone hollow-head screws with a transverse bore in the screw head for insertion of the rods. For this purpose, superior apertures are provided in the screw heads. Screw heads with lateral openings may be used as well. The boreholes are beveled to permit an angularly stable engagement of the nuts. In addition, washers are provided.

Instruments include pituitary forceps, gouges, punches, dissectors, an awl, a 3.2 mm drill, a depth gauge, screwdrivers, rod holders and grasping forceps, various wrenches, and possibly also burrs.

Principles of Correction

The spine is osteotomized at multiple levels in the region of the vertebral arches, and a long-curved harmonious lordosis is induced by posterior compression on the convex side (Fig. 4.**4**). The goal is a horizontal visual axis. The correction is carried out with threaded rods that are fixed by pedicle screws (Fig. 4.**4d**). Two rods are needed. The correcting forces are applied by centripetal tightening of the nuts in the direction of the central screw of each row of rods. The compression almost invariably breaks the anterior syndesmophytes (Figs. 4.**4c**, **d**). Closure of the osteotomies completes the correction. The operating table has to be successively straightened out during the correction.

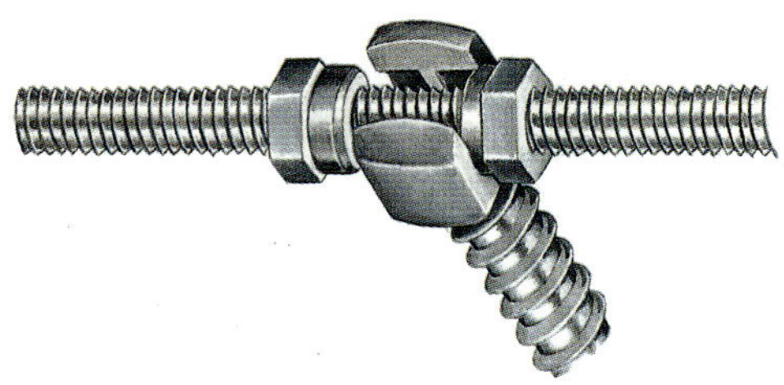

Fig. 4.**3** Detail of Zielke USIS implant. The slotted screw and the rectangular bevels on the nuts ensure right-angle stability between the threaded rod and the screw.

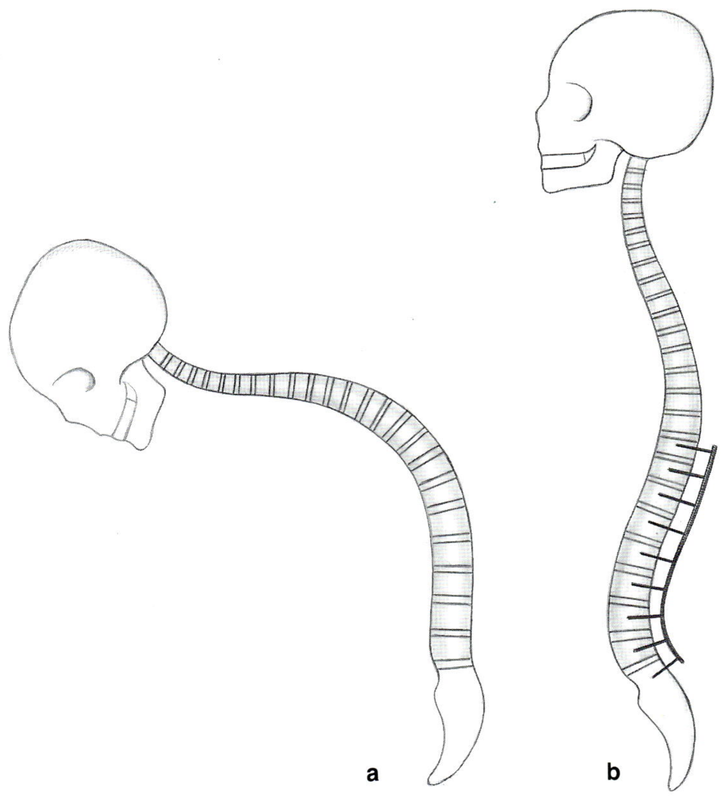

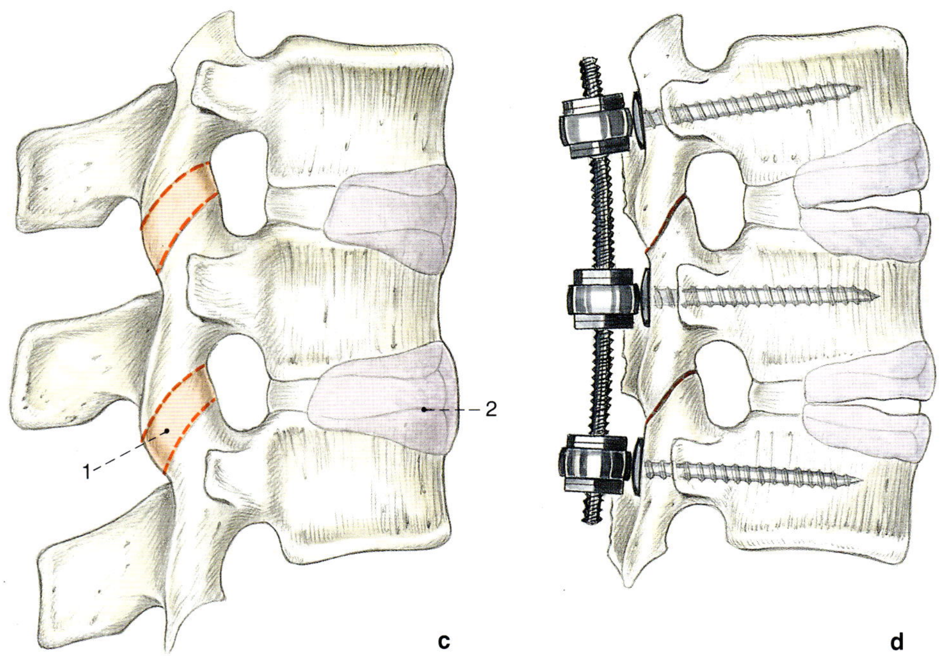

Fig. 4.**4** Principle of correction.
a The spine before correction.
b The spine after correction.
c Lumbar segments before correction.
d Lumbar segments after correction.

1 Osteotomy
2 Syndesmophytes

Depending on the extent of the kyphotic deformity, 4–6 osteotomies are generally sufficient, whereas the implantation for counterbalancing the pressure on the end screws is carried 1–2 segments beyond the osteotomies. This permits a correction of approximately 40–60 degrees. The extent per segment is approximately equal to the physiological range of movement. Possible additional scoliotic curves can be corrected at the same time through increased compression unilaterally.

Choice of Segments

The correction is done in the lumbar and lower thoracic areas, and should include the kyphotic apex, if at all possible. This has the following advantages: leverage for raising the head is maximized. The stability of the lumbar vertebrae allows large correction forces to be applied. Fixed ribs do not interfere with the correction. The screws can be inserted more easily and safely. The risk of paralysis is lowest in the lumbar region.

The osteotomies are carried out between T12–L1 and L4–5. Optionally, L5–S1 or T11–12, or both, can be included, depending on the location and extent of the kyphosis.

The screws are placed between T9 or T10 and S1 or S2.

Osteotomy Technique

The ossified interspinous ligament and the adjoining spinous processes are resected with a rongeur (Fig. 4.**2**). At the center of the interlaminar space, the ossified ligamentum flavum is opened far enough with pituitary forceps or burrs to allow dissectors to be inserted into the opening, so that the dura which usually adheres to the lamina in ankylosing spondylitis can be stripped off. The epidural fatty tissues are nearly always absent. Using punches, the hole is expanded to the original size of the ligament (Fig. 4.**5**). The anterior borders of the adjacent arches are resected with punches.

Any remnants of the ligamentum flavum are resected at the same time, so that neither thery nor the edges of the arches will compress the dura after the lordosation.

Starting from the midline osteotomy, lateral osteotomies are carried out bilaterally, through the original joints, in the direction of the interspinal foramina (Fig. 4.**6**). These osteotomies are directed laterocranially, with an angle of 30–40 degrees to the horizontal. The desired slot width of 5–7 mm is obtained by using suitably wide rongeurs. If there is a lateral overhang, the osteotomies are made slightly larger on the convex side. Closely anterior to the foramen, the cortical substance on the anterior side is

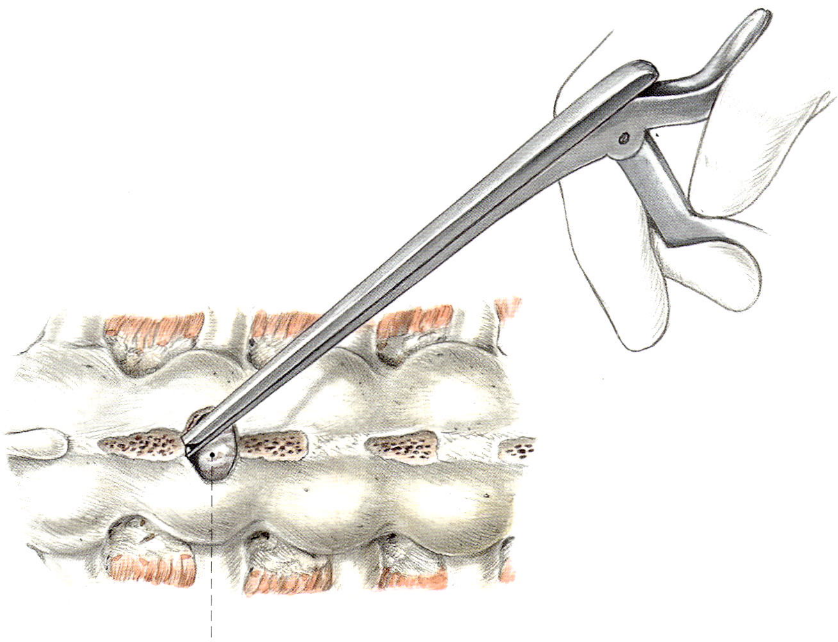

Fig. 4.**5** Median interlaminar osteotomy by resection of the ossified yellow ligament.

1 Spinal dura mater

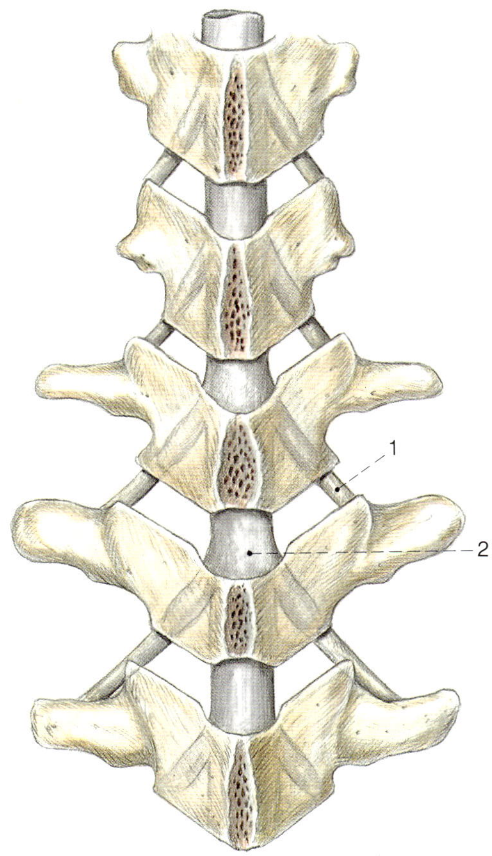

Fig. 4.**6** Position of osteotomies in relation to the posterior vertebral elements and the neural structures.

1 Spinal nerve
2 Spinal dura mater

resected with punches to prevent injury to the dura and roots (Fig. 4.**7**). The latter are further protected by dissectors.

Beginning at the kyphotic apex, the remaining segments are osteotomized in a similar way.

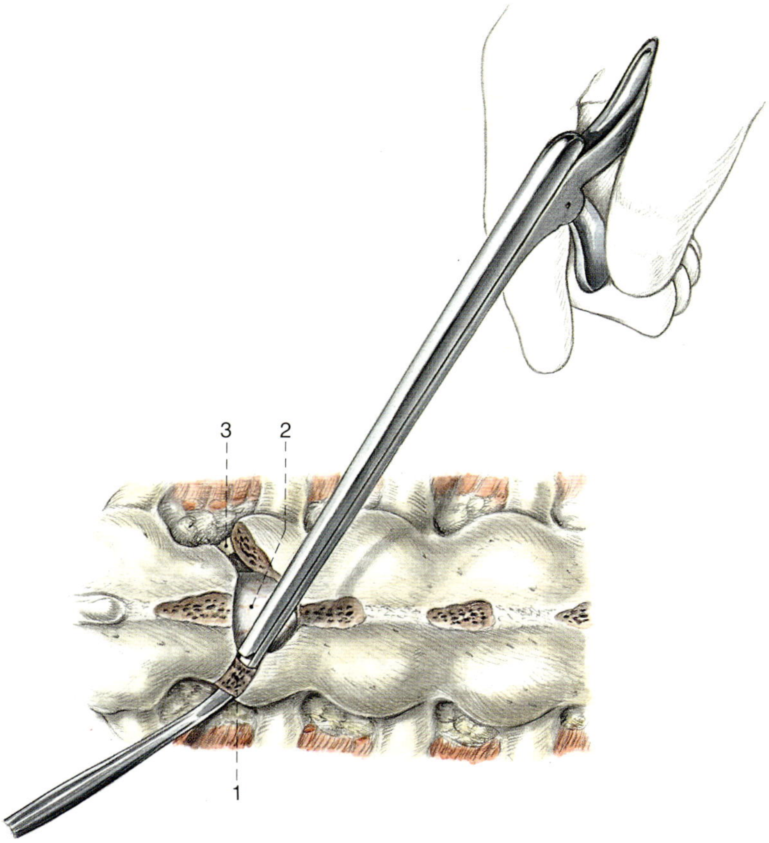

Fig. 4.**7** Oblique lateral osteotomy shortly before completion.

1 Remaining osseous bridge in front of the intervertebral foramen, the spinal nerve being protected by a dissector
2 Spinal dura mater
3 Spinal nerve

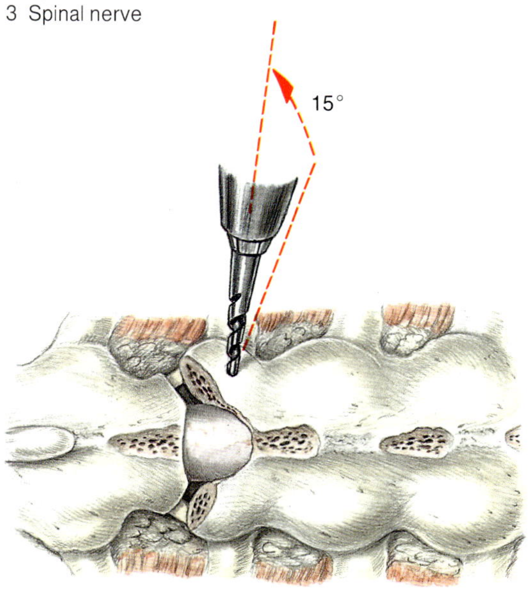

Fig. 4.**9** Drilling of a hole for screw implantation in anteromedial direction at an angle of 15 degrees to the sagittal plane.

Implantation of Screws

The pedicular axis passes posteriorly across the intersection between the sagittal joint plane and the horizontal axis along the transverse process (Fig. 4.**8**). The hole for the screw is drilled 2–3 mm lateral to the point of intersection of these lines, after it has been marked with an awl; the drilling is done in anteromedial direction at an angle of about 15 degrees to the sagittal plane, to avoid perforation of the lateral wall of the vertebral body (Figs. 4.**9**, 4.**10**).

For exact placement of the screws, the pedicles of the next lower vertebra can also be palpated with dissectors. The drilling should be done as close to the anterior wall of the vertebral body as possible, but should not perforate it (Fig. 4.**10**). The length of the hole is generally 45–55 mm. It is advisable to check the integrity of the drill canal with the depth gauge. Self-tapping screws are then inserted.

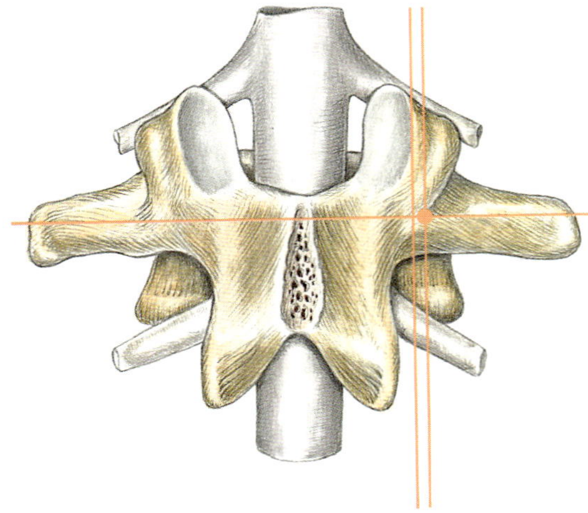

Fig. 4.**8** Position of the drill hole in the direction of the pedicular axis 3 mm lateral to the intersection of the joint plane with the axis of the transverse process.

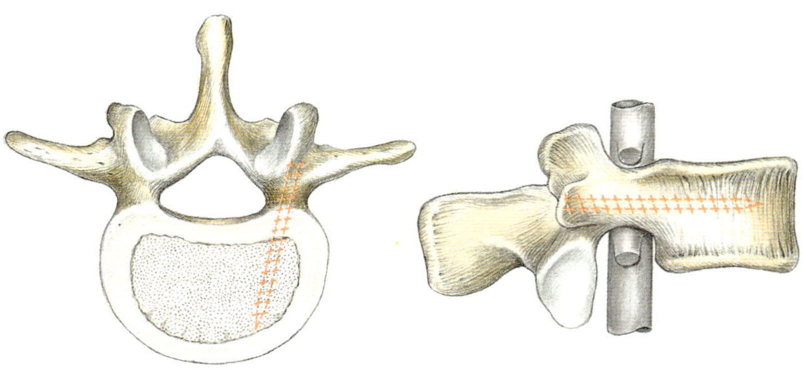

Fig. 4.**10** Position of the pedicular screw in the pedicle and vertebral body.
a Horizontal plane
b Sagittal plane

If these do not grip because of the frequently present osteoporosis, a small portion of bone cement can be inserted into the vertebral body through the pedicle hole. For better support of the screws, washers are applied. The holes in the screw heads are aligned vertically (Fig. 4.**11**). Slotted screw heads offer the greatest security against disengagement of the rods. However, since it may be difficult to implant the rods into these screws, and we have never seen rod dislocations with top-slotted screws, we use the latter exclusively (Fig. 4.**11**). As a rule, 16–20 screws are required.

Implantation of Rods

The two threaded rods that have already been fitted with nuts are placed into the screw heads from below upward, using two rod-holding forceps (Fig. 4.**11**). Two nuts are needed for each screw. These are turned down far enough to cause their cylindrical portions to engage the screw heads loosely, thus aligning the screw and the rod during the correction. At this point, the rod is firmly fixed to the screw that is positioned centrally (usually L2 or L3) (Fig. 4.**11**).

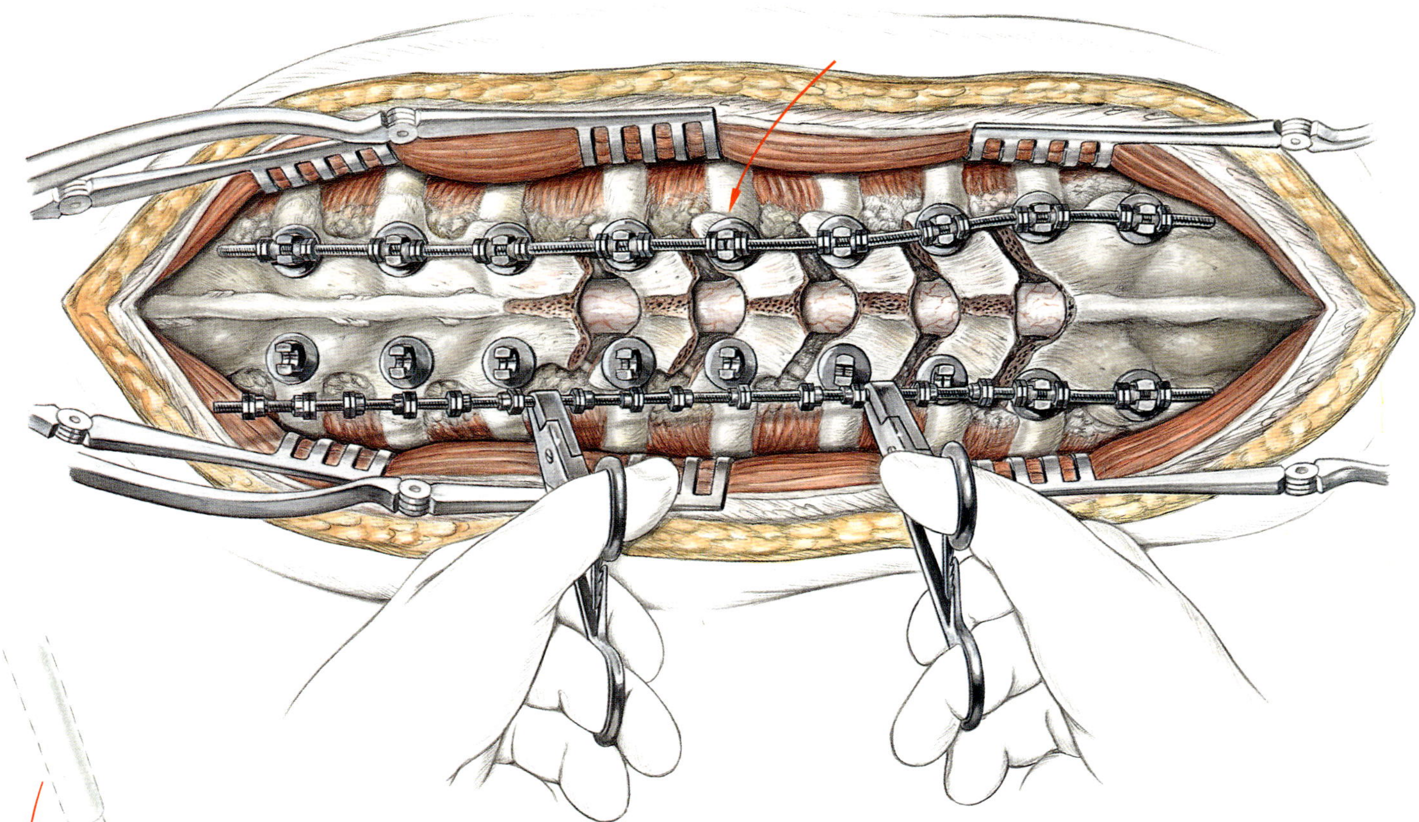

Fig. 4.**11** Site after insertion of the right threaded rod between T10 and S1. Fixation of nuts on the central screw at L2 (see arrow), and insertion of the left threaded rod.

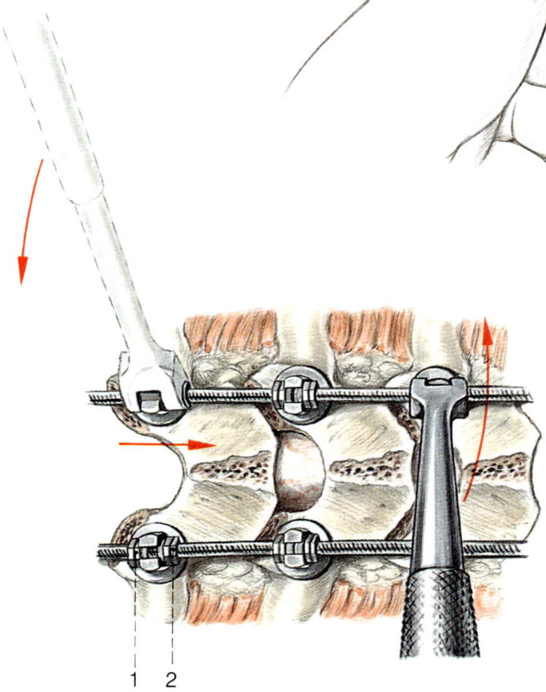

Fig. 4.**12** Correction of the nuts peripheral to the central screw by centripetal tightening. The counternuts loosely seated in the screw hole are moved simultaneously with the Zielke double-key Haifaa wrench.

1 Correcting nut
2 Counternut

Correction Technique

Using the selfengaging double-key system Haifaa by Zielke, the nuts are turned toward the central screw (Fig. 4.**12**). This is done successively on both sides for each pair of screws, starting with the more centrally located ones. The peripheral nuts are used for correction, but the central counternuts should remain engaged. If there are scoliotic curves, they can be corrected at the same time.

To this end, the nuts on the convex side are appropriately tightened for greater compression after somewhat wider osteotomies have been carried out on this side.

The lateral osteotomies close during the correction (Fig. 4.**13**). At the same time, the table has to be straightened out slowly. Once this has been done, and any additional deviations have been corrected by greater unilateral compression, the nuts and counternuts are firmly tightened with regular keys and the rod tips are clipped off. This completes the correction (Fig. 4.**13**).

Spondylodesis

The spinous processes, vertebral arches, and articular elements in the area of the instrumentation zone are decorticated using the Risser–Hibbs technique for scoliosis surgery (p. 91). This decortication is carried out just between the rods. Resected bone from the osteotomies and the spinous processes serves as graft material (Fig. 4.**14**). No additional graft material has to be harvested.

Wound Closure

This is done by the same technique as in any scoliosis surgery (p. 96).

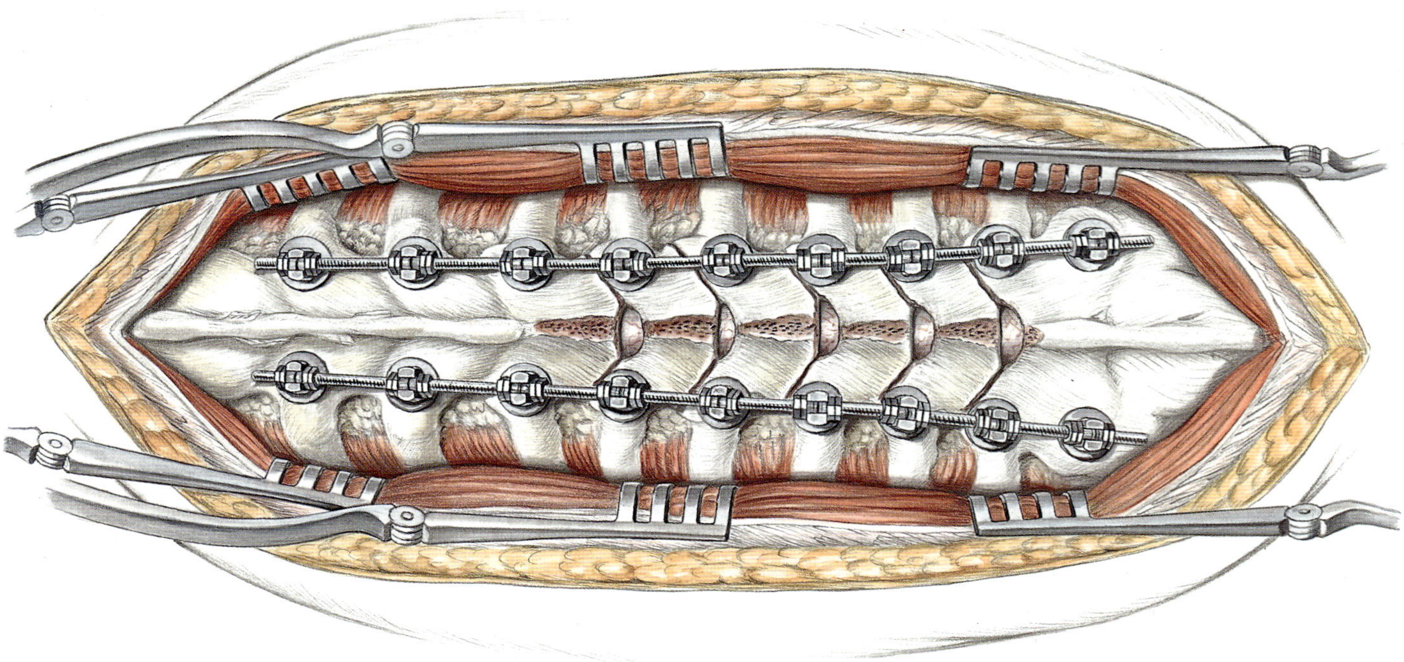

Fig. 4.**13** Site after correction. The lateral osteotomies are closed.

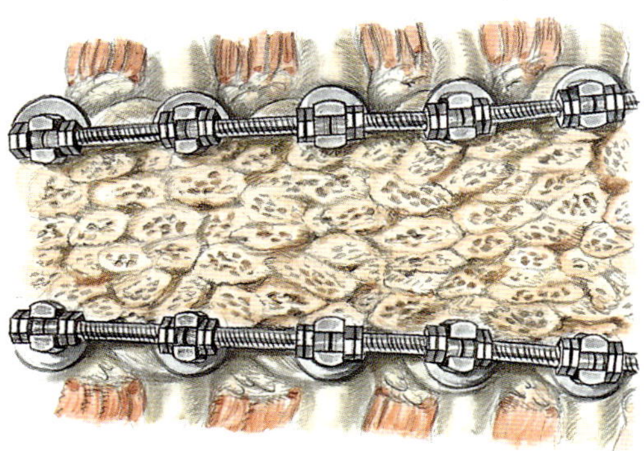

Fig. 4.**14** Detail of site after grafting. It is important to apply the large chips from resection of the spinous processes to the median osteotomies.

Postoperative Treatment

In order to provide compression against possible wound hematomas, a simple posterior plaster shell is molded to the patient while he or she is still on the operating table, and is left in place for 1–3 days. The patient rests in a regular bed, remaining in the intensive care unit for about three days.

Neurologic monitoring is performed, first at 30-minute intervals, and later every hour. The patient immediately undergoes repeated daily chest physiotherapy to prevent atelectasis, using Zielke's breathing technique.

Seven days after the operation, a body cast is fitted on a Risser frame, and the patient is mobilized. The cast is worn for four months, and is then replaced by a Stagnara brace for another four months.

Radiographs are obtained immediately after the operation (spondylodesis zone), in the plaster jacket (standing films of the whole spine), and before replacement and removal of the braces, with full-length films of the spine and added oblique views of the area of spondylodesis.

Note
Owing to the increased spontaneous ossification characteristic of the underlying disease, fusion is accomplished rapidly and reliably.

Pitfalls and Complications

Specific risks in this operation are neurologic complications due to dura or root injuries caused by improper osteotomy or misplacement of the pedicular screws. The risk varies between one and two percent. Mild, almost exclusively sensory symptoms of root irritation, reversible within a few days, occur somewhat more frequently. They are most likely due to hematoma compression.

Greater monosegmental corrections can take place if the anterior ossifications are present in only one segment. Screw fixation failure or screw migration is possible during the operation when porotic bones are subjected to excessive forces.

Immediately after the operation, patients at risk are more susceptible to pneumonia (1–2%).

Alternative Methods

Monosegmental corrections using the Smith–Petersen, Hsu and Leong, and Ziwjan methods are feasible, but result in more neurologic, vascular, and abdominal complications because of the short-curve lordotic kink and possible subluxations. Long-curve harmonious lordoses obviously cannot be obtained by monosegmental correction. We only employ the monosegmental osteotomy procedure of Hsu and Leong, and then solely in cases of excessive anterior ossification and concomitant osteoporosis. In these cases, the syndesmophytes may not rupture, or it may not be possible to apply sufficiently strong forces to the spine.

Note
Although it is in principle possible to use the Herbert method to cut through the syndesmophytes in the segments to be osteotomized by an anterior intervention 2–3 weeks before the posterior operation, this not only means additional surgery, but also poses a serious risk of instability in the interim, when the patient is totally confined to bed, as well as during the later surgical manipulations, especially after the dorsal osteotomies have been made. Complete dislocations of one vertebral body relative to another may occur immediately after the posterior osteotomy.

Hsu–Yau–Leong Technique as Modified by Zielke (Monosegmental Lumbar Lordosation Spondylodesis)

Indications

Global or thoracic kyphotic deformities of 70 degrees or more, and lumbar kyphotic deformities of at least 20 degrees, with ankylosis of the spine and excessive syndesmophytosis of the ostotic type according to Hehne.

Note
In cases of excessive ostotic syndesmophytosis, the syndesmophytes cannot be expected to break using Zielke's polysegmental technique. They could in principle be osteotomized by an anterior operation using the Herbert technique, but this not only means an additional operation which has to be performed 12 weeks before the posterior operation, but also requires strict bed rest for the patient during the interval, and creates an appreciable risk of dislocation during the posterior procedure.

Positioning

The positioning is the same as for the Zielke operation (p. 228).

Incision and Exposure of the Spine

The procedures are the same as for posterior scoliosis operations or the Zielke operation (p. 228). However, exposure from L1 to L5 is sufficient, as the correction is most frequently done at L3 (Fig. 4.**22**).

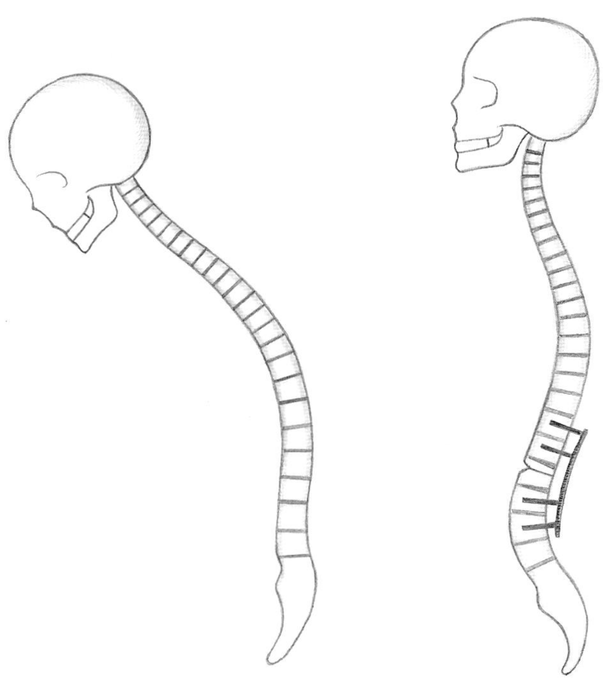

Fig. 4.**15** Position of spine before and after the correction.

Operative Technique

Instrumentarium

This is the same as for the Zielke operation (p. 230).

Principles of Correction

The spine is posteriorly osteotomized monosegmentally by resection of a vertebral arch, including the pedicles and a part of the posterior wall of the vertebral body, and a short-curved lordosis is induced by posterior compression on the convex side (Figs. 4.**15**, 4.**16**). The vertebral body is posteriorly shortened as a result. It then assumes a wedge shape in the sagittal plane, with an anteriorly open angle. The center of rotation of the lordosis lies in the center of the vertebral body. This prevents excessive lordotic kinking or gaping of its front wall. It also means that—in contrast to the Smith–Petersen monosegmental arch osteotomy—the large vessels and the sympathetic trunk are minimally stretched.

For the correction, use is made of Zielke pedicular screws and threaded rods (p. 230). The correcting forces are produced by centripetal tightening of the nuts. They are sufficient to compress the vertebral body posteriorly. The correction is completed by closure of the vertebral body osteotomy (Fig. 4.**16**). As a rule, the degree of correction is approximately 30 degrees, and therefore smaller than in the Zielke polysegmental osteotomy. The operating table has to be straightened in the course of the correction.

Choice of Segment

The correction is carried out in the lumbar region, for the same reasons as in the Zielke operation (p. 228). It is performed at the apex of the kyphosis, that is, usually at L3 and occasionally at L2.

Osteotomy Technique

After resection of the adjacent, generally ossified, interspinal ligaments L2–L3 and L3–L4, the L3 spinous process, and portions of the adjoining spinous processes, a midline osteotomy and a V-shaped lateral osteotomy are made through the upper part of the L2–L3 articulation, proceeding exactly as in the Zielke operation (p. 231; Fig. 4.**7**). The median osteotomy is at the level of the ligamentum flavum, L2–L3. From here, the L3 lamina, following continued stepwise dissection of the dura from the posterior elements, is resected in a caudal direction using bone punches or, optionally, burrs (Fig. 4.**17**). This resection is at first done between the pedicles.

After this, the inferior part of the lamina and, optionally, the cranial portions of the ossified yellow ligament L3–L4 are similarly resected, and the inferior margin of the resection is undermined. This prevents the bony edges from pressing on the dura after the correction.

Starting from this extended medial osteotomy, the inferior articular L3 processes, which form the posterior boundary of the L3–L4 foramen, are resected, also with the bone punch. The upper quarters of the L3–L4 joints are usually

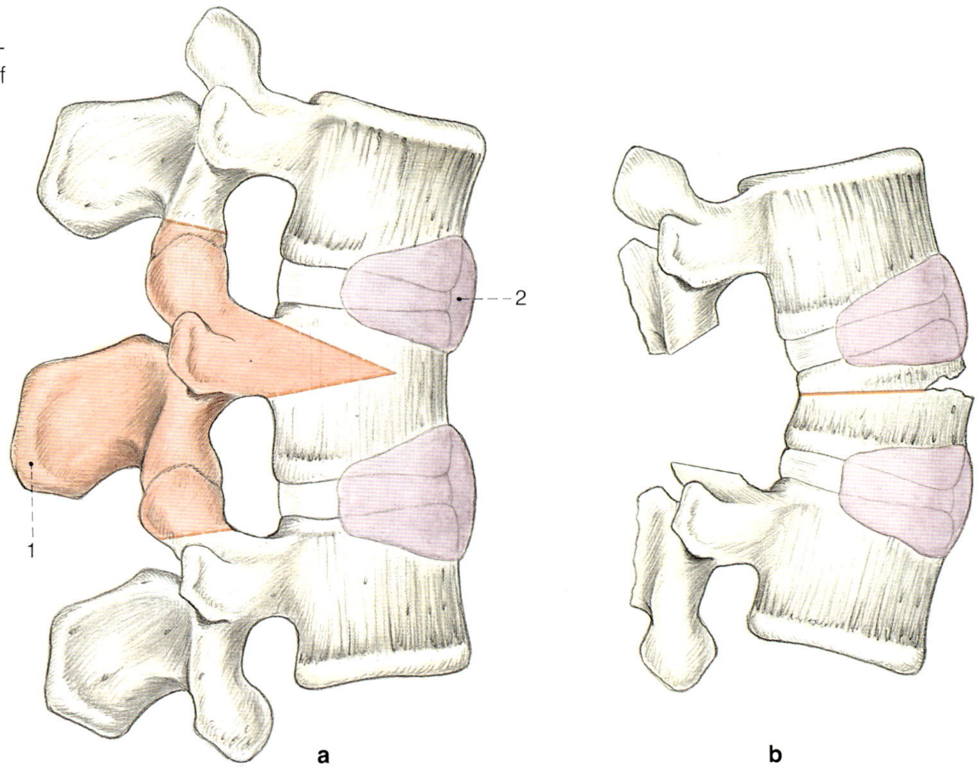

Fig. 4.**16** Principle of correction.
a Lumbar segments with resected posterior portions and partial osteotomy of the vertebral body.
b Lumbar segments after correction.

1 Resected bone
2 Syndesmophytes

removed at the same time. The L3–L4 foramen, with the L3 roots, should now be fully visualized (Fig. 4.**18**).

Of the posterior vertebral elements, only the pedicles, the transverse processes, and the articular portions of L2–L3 remain. These are removed step by step using pituitary forceps. The transverse processes are therefore isolated and subsequently elevated from the surrounding muscles. From the now posteriorly opened pedicles, the cancellous bone can be removed, and the pedicles successively removed down to the base with the aid of small pituitary forceps or rongeurs (Fig. 4.**19**). From here, the cancellous bone on the posterior side is scooped out of the vertebral body (Fig. 4.**19**). Following blunt exposure of the posterior halves of the side walls of the vertebral bodies, these side walls, starting from the pedicle base, are now osteotomized down to the middle and interpedicular portions of the posterior wall to a width of 10–15 mm, using punches or right-angle pituitary forceps (Figs. 4.**20**–4.**21**). Alternatively, the posterior wall can be osteotomized with narrow chisels, and the resected portion packed into the vertebral body cavity.

Throughout the osseous resection, the dura and the spinal nerves are protected with dissectors and Krayenbühl retractors.

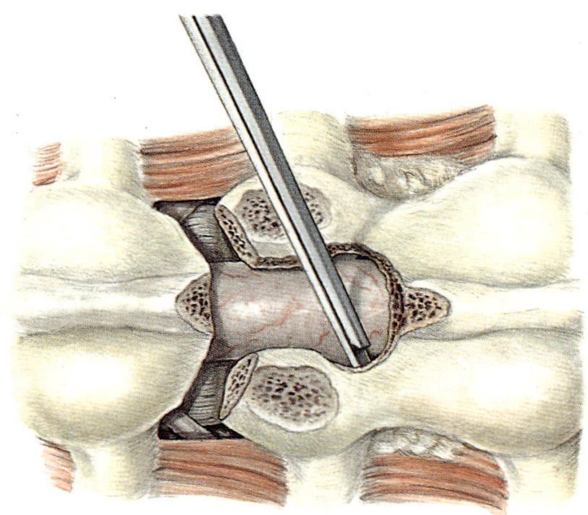

Fig. 4.**17** Detail of the site after the lateral osteotomies and laminectomy. Resection of the upper articular process of the next lower vertebra.

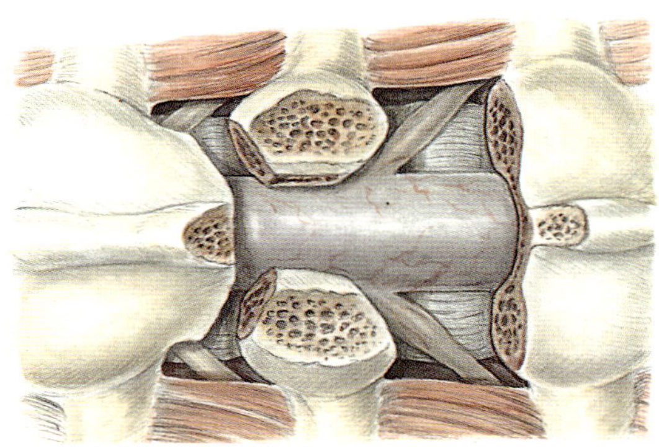

Fig. 4.**18** Detail of the site after lateral and median osteotomies. The articular components are still partly intact, and the transverse processes and pedicles are completely intact. The dura and the four adjacent spinal nerves are visualized.

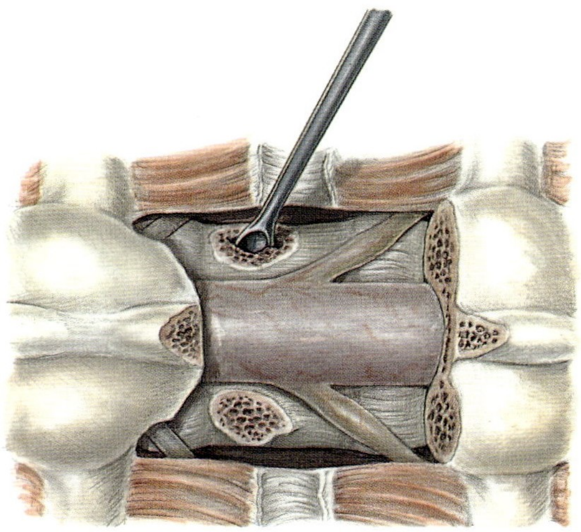

Fig. 4.**19** Cancellous bone is scooped out of the vertebral body from the base of the right pedicle. The left pedicle is still intact. The transverse processes have been resected together with the articular components.

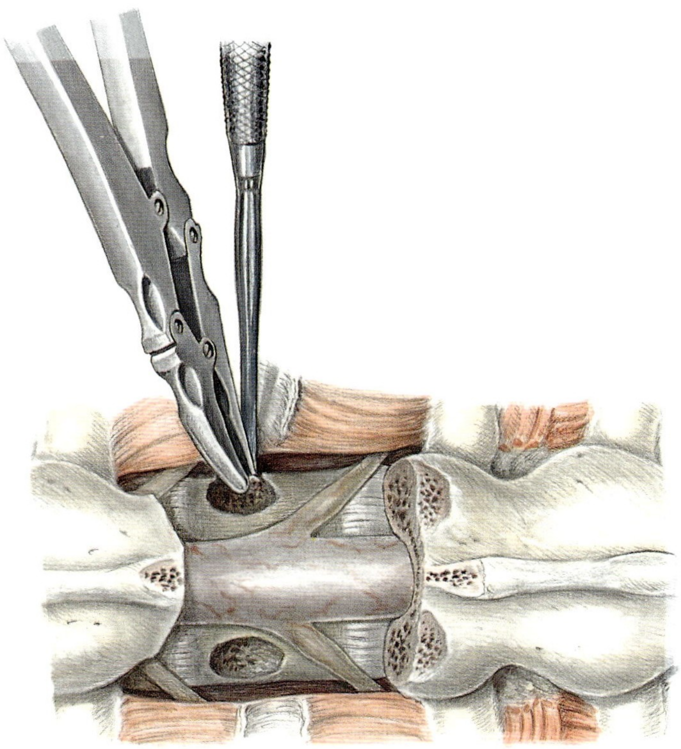

Fig. 4.**20** Osteotomy of the left wall of the vertebral body from the base of the pedicle.

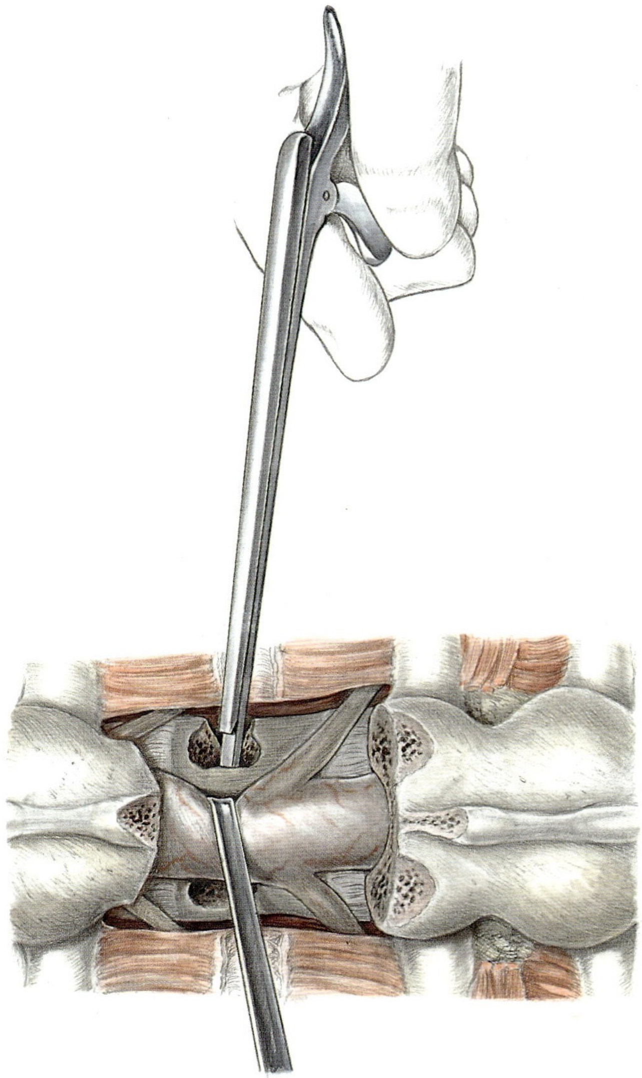

Fig. 4.**21** Osteotomy of the posterior wall of the vertebral body.

Implantation of Screws

The technique is the same as in the Zielke operation (p. 232). The osteotomized segment remains free, of course. Two segments above and below the osteotomy, that is, generally L1 and L2 as well as L4 and L5, are instrumented (Fig. 4.**22**).

Implantation of Rods

This is done as in the Zielke operation (p. 233 and Fig. 4.**22**).

Correction Technique

The correction produced with the nuts and threaded rods also follows the Zielke technique (p. 233). The rods completely bridge the osteotomized segment on the posterior side. The central point at which the forces are directed is the free portion of the rod above the osteotomy. During the correction, the vertebral body is posteriorly compressed until closure of the osteotomy. This completes the correction (Fig. 4.**23**).

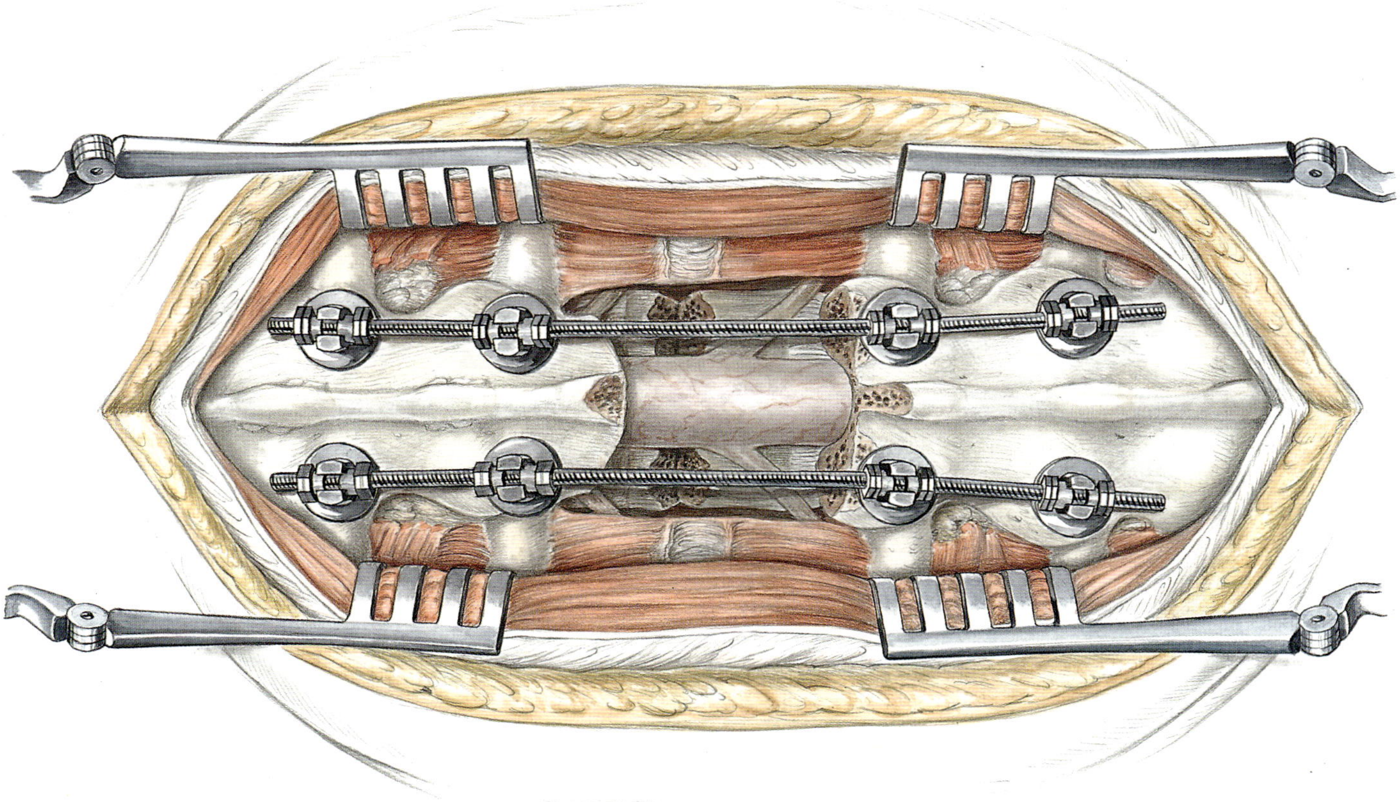

Fig. 4.**22** Site after implantation of the complete USI system.

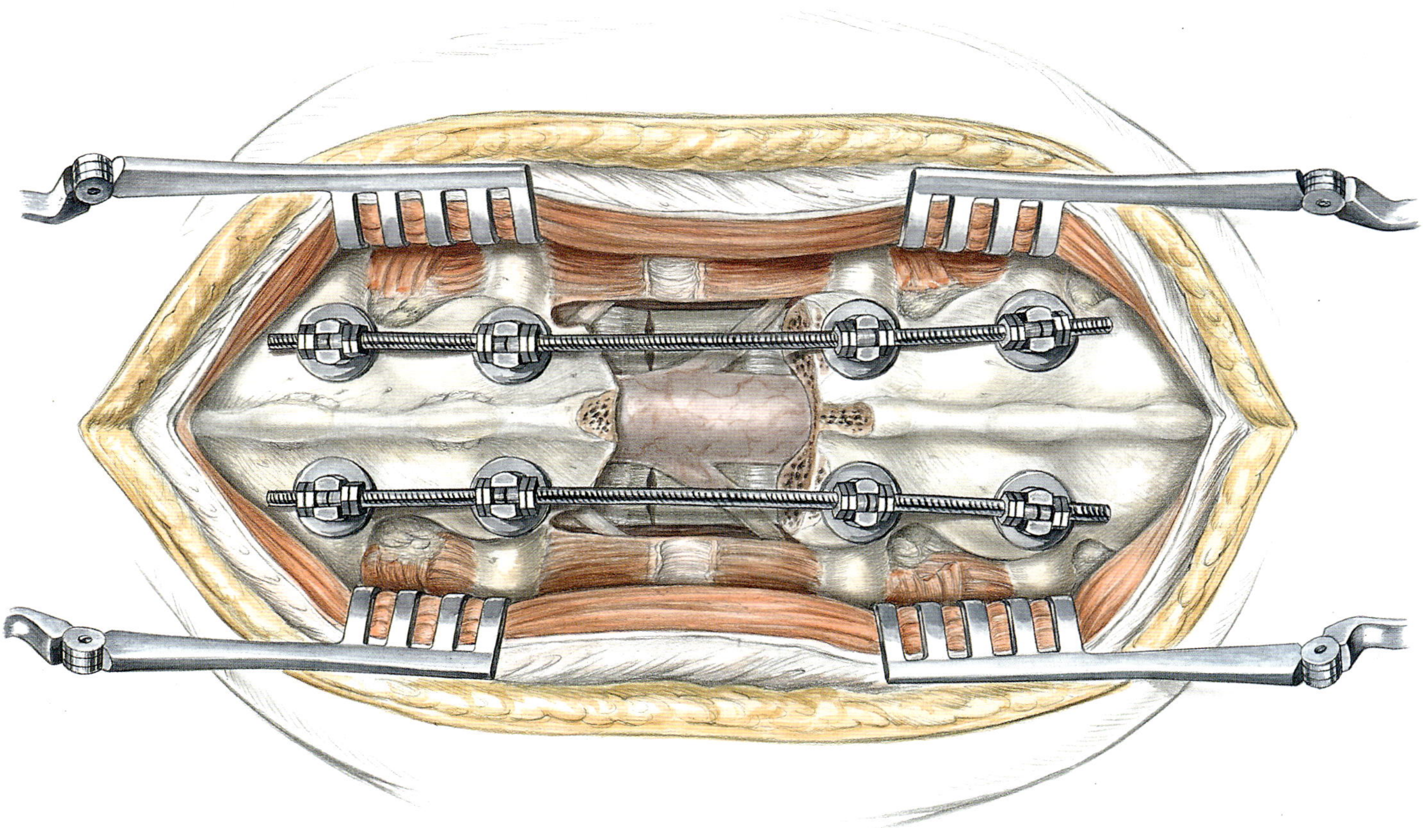

Fig. 4.**23** Site after correction and fixation of the correcting nuts and counternuts. The vertebral body osteotomy has been closed.

Spondylodesis

The adjacent arches are posteriorly decorticated with gouges, and are bridged by posterior application of large corticocancellous iliac crest grafts between the threaded rods. The grafts are fixed with two heavy sutures that are passed around the rods (Fig. 4.**24**).

Wound Closure

This is done using the technique for scoliosis operations (p. 96).

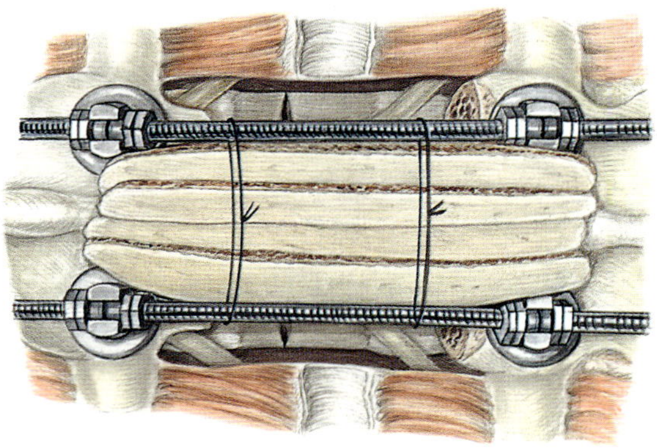

Fig. 4.**24** Detail of the site after application of corticocancellous iliac crest chips to the adjacent decorticated laminae. The chips are attached to the threaded rods with sutures.

Postoperative Treatment

This follows Zielke's method (p. 235).

Pitfalls and Complications

The risks are the same as these in the Zielke operation (p. 235). However, because of the monosegmental lordotic kink, the large vessels on the anterior side are subjected to a somewhat greater strain. For this reason alone, the correction ought not to exceed 30 degrees. Results from a larger series of cases are not yet available.

Alternative Methods

The alternative methods include the Zielke polysegmental correction, and Smith–Petersen or Ziwjan monosegmental correction. Polysegmental correction is always preferable in the absence of syndesmophytosis, or in cases of annular or mild osteogenetic syndesmophytosis, since the anterior column is then certain to yield to the lordosis-inducing forces.

The Smith–Petersen correction only involves an arch osteotomy, so that the disk space is opened wide anteriorly due to the more posteriorly positioned center of rotation. Added anterior osteotomy of syndesmophytes with Herbert's method is today considered obsolete in view of the added inherent risks.

Technique of Mason and Urist (Monosegmental Cervical Lordosation Spondylodesis)

Indications

Short-curved cervical or high-thoracic kyphotic deformities with complete ankylosis, particularly those impeding opening of the mouth owing to insufficient distance between the chin and the sternum.

Note
As a general rule, the operation can be combined with a lumbar lordosation spondylodesis. It is advisable to perform the cervical operation about 14 days after the lumbar surgery.

Preoperative Preparation and Positioning

The patient wears a halo ring and a body jacket before the operation (Fig. 4.**25**). In the thoracic and posterior regions, two aluminium plates with threaded screw holes are incorporated into the jacket. Perforated metal hoops are attached to them and passed over each shoulder (Fig. 4.**25**).

During the operation, before the correction, the hoops and the halo ring are each joined by two threaded rods (Fig. 4.**36**). The reduction and fixation are carried out with the aid of these rods.

The patient is seated during the operation (Fig. 4.**25**). The halo and hoops are draped posteriorly, so that an assistant can carry out the correction during the operation, using the threaded rods, from the front. The surgeon sits behind the patient, while the assistant stands on his left.

The operation is performed under local anesthesia, so that the patient himself can help to determine the ideal position of the visual level and raise the alarm for potential neurological symptoms.

Incision and Exposure of the Spine

The skin incision is made in the midline posterior to the spinous processes C4–T2 (Fig. 4.**26**). The prominent vertebra, C7, serves as a landmark.

If this is not palpable, which may occasionally be the case in patients with ankylosing spondylitis, an image converter should be used. The nuchal septum is divided with a knife in the same direction as the incision. Next, the sides of the spinous processes are exposed with the knife for several millimeters. This frees the origins of the trapezius, rhomboid, serratus posterior superior, and splenius cervicis and capitis muscles.

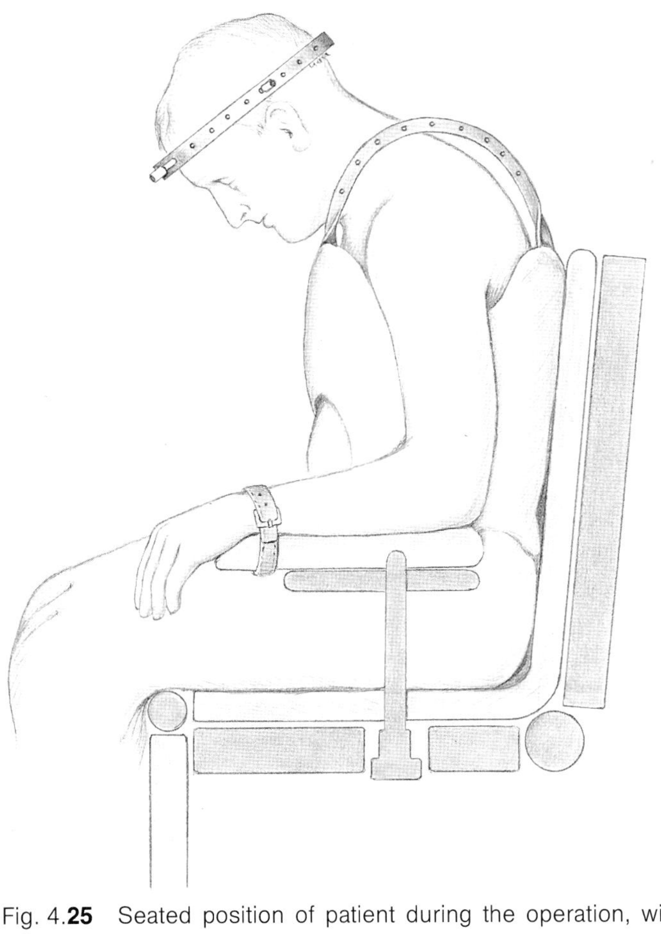

Fig. 4.**25** Seated position of patient during the operation, with halo and torso plaster casts.

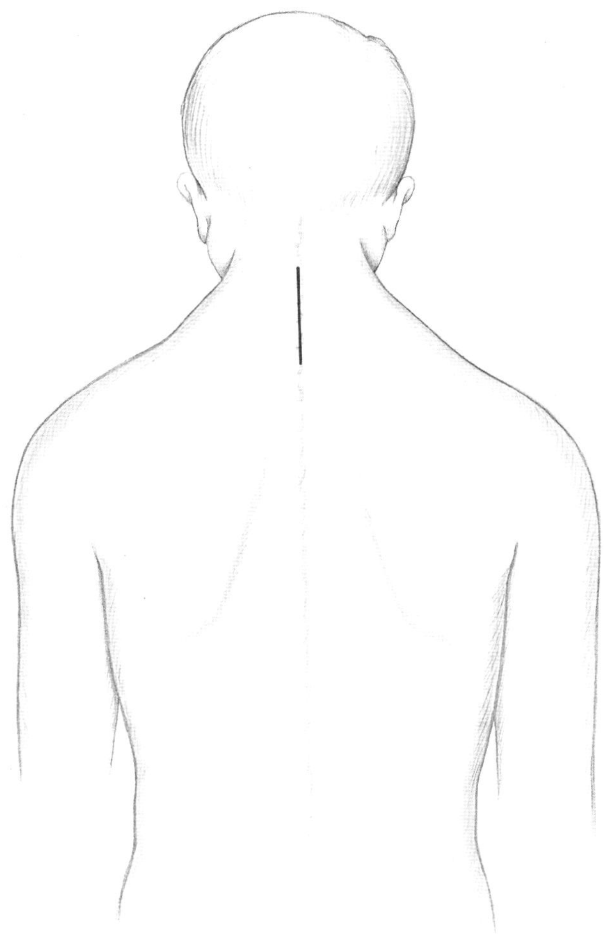

Fig. 4.**26** Incision for monosegmental cervical lordosation spondylodesis.

They are retracted to the side, together with the medial parts of the semispinalis capitis muscle (Fig. 4.**27**). The intrinsic back muscles, interspinalis, multifidus, and semispinalis cervicis, are now discernible in the depth (Fig. 4.**27**). Using a Cobb elevator, they are sharply freed subperiosteally from medial to lateral from the spinous processes and vertebral arches C6–T2. The wound is subsequently packed with gauze strips between the vertebral arches and the musculature, and the retractor is repositioned after removal of the gauze (Fig. 4.**28**).

The origins of the semispinalis capitis and longissimus muscles can now be seen at the lateral borders of the articular elements. They are sharply detached with a knife from the C7 and T1 articular and transverse processes. For identification of the level, it is best to use the sixth cervical vertebra as a guide. Its spinous process, in contrast to that of C7 and the other cervical vertebrae, is bifid (Figs. 4.**29**, 4.**30**). If there is any doubt, the first rib can be palpated laterally to T1 (watch for cervical rib) or, preferably, a radiograph can be taken intraoperatively.

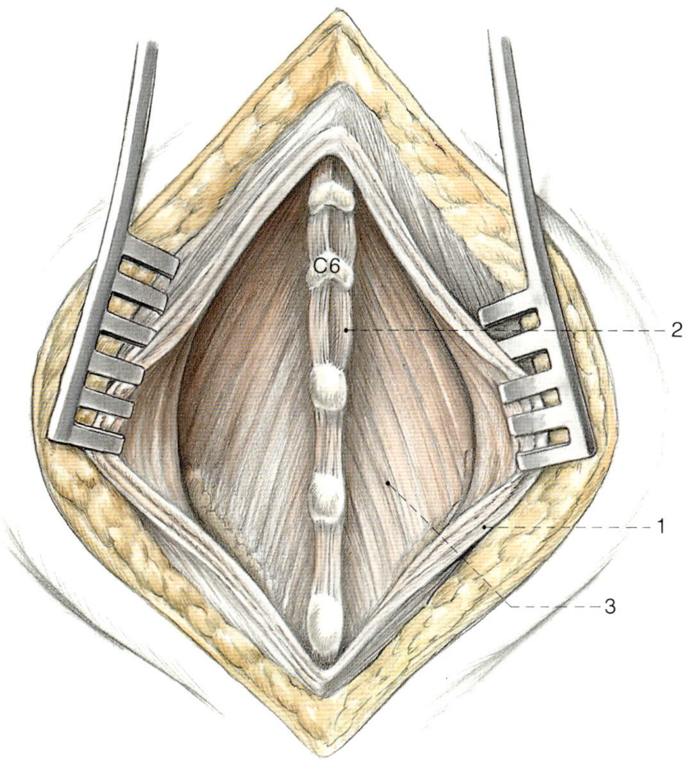

Fig. 4.**27** The operative site after incision of the nuchal septum and detachment of the splenius muscles. The medial portions of the semispinalis capitis muscle are retracted laterally, together with the splenius muscles and the trapezius. The C6 spinous process, in contrast to C7, still has two spikes on the posterior side.

1 Trapezius muscle, splenius capitis and cervicis muscles, and the semispinalis capitis muscle
2 Interspinal muscles
3 Multifidus muscles and semispinalis cervicis muscle
C6 Spinous process of the 6th cervical vertebra

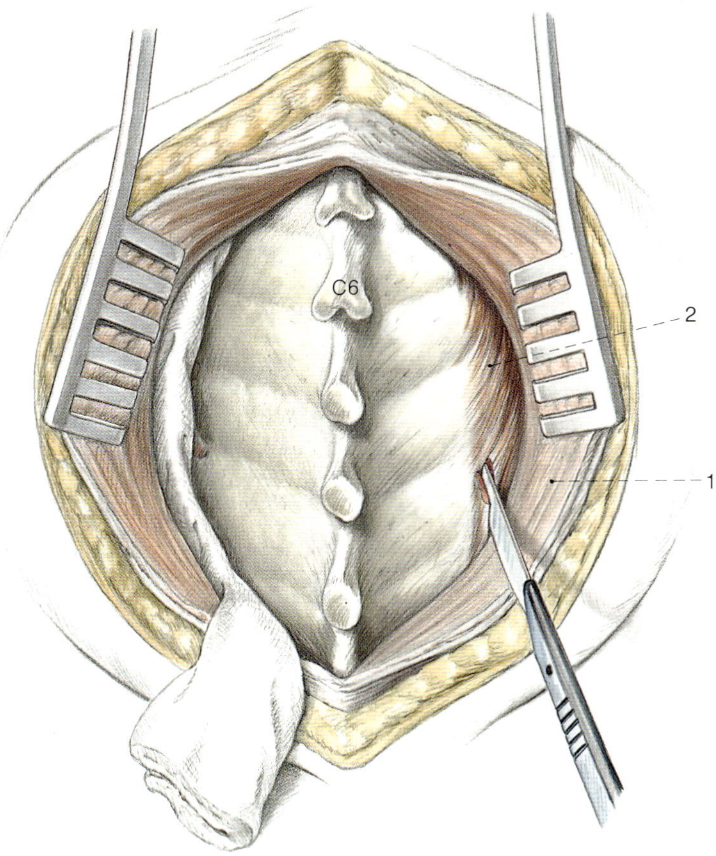

Fig. 4.**28** The operative site after subperiosteal exposure of the posterior vertebral elements by detachment of the multifidus muscles and the semispinalis cervicis muscle, as well as resection of the interspinal muscles and ligaments. The semispinalis capitis muscle and the longissimus capitis muscle are detached at the lateral portions of the articular processes and at the transverse processes.

1 Multifidus and semispinalis cervicis muscles
2 Semispinalis capitis and longissimus capitis muscles
C6 Spinous process of the 6th cervical vertebra

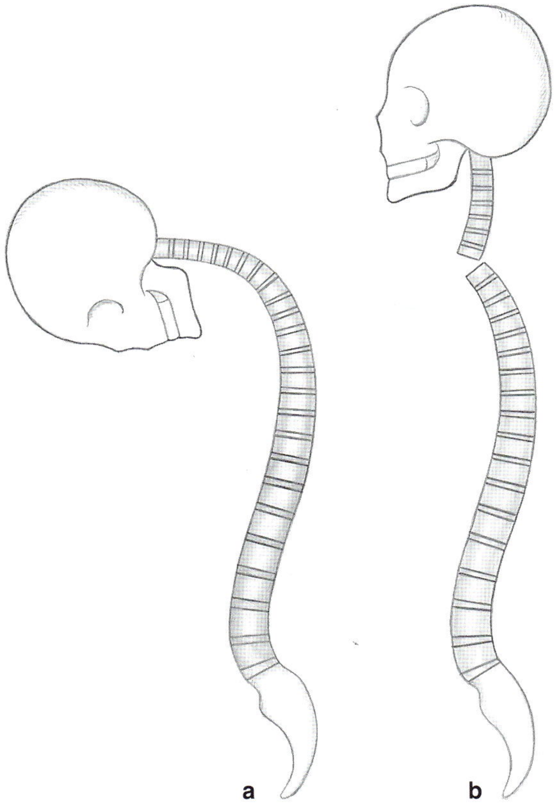

a b

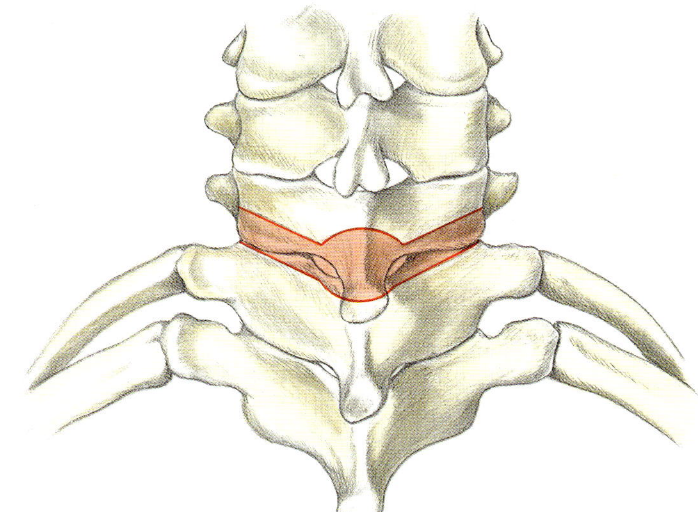

c

Fig. 4.**29** Principle of correction.
a The spine before correction.
b The spine after correction.
c Segment C7–T1 after the osteotomy, posterior view.
d Segment C7–T1 after the correction, lateral view.

1 Vertebral artery
2 Syndesmophytes

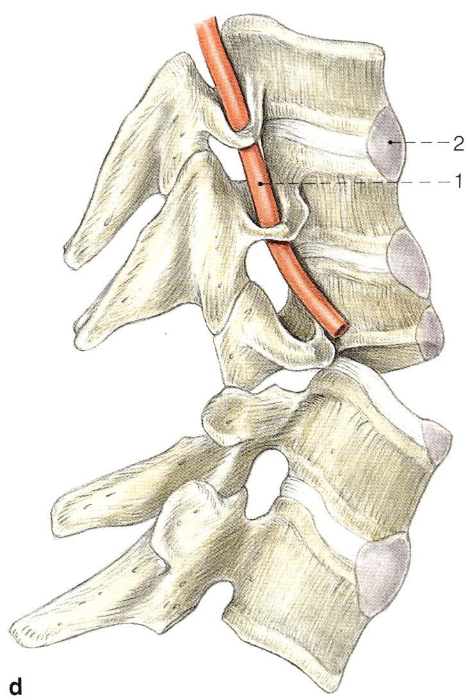

d

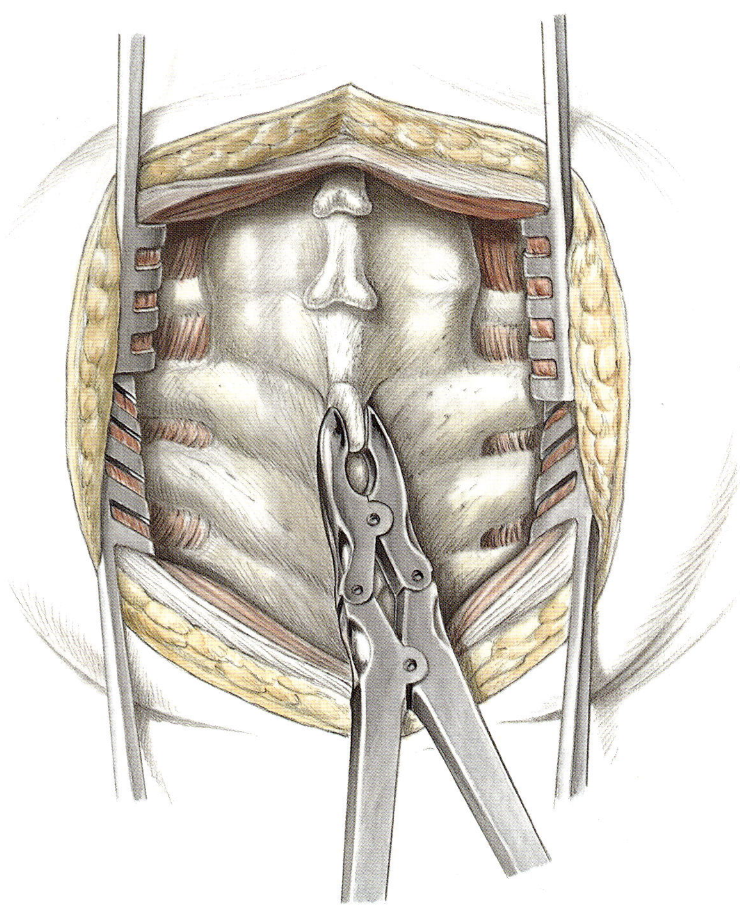

Fig. 4.**30** Resection of the C7 spinous process after removal of the usually ossified interspinal ligaments.

Operative Technique

Instrumentarium

Implants are not used, since correction and immobilization are carried out via the halo cast. Small pituitary forceps or a burr, and punches, are required for the osteotomy.

Principles of Correction

The spine is only mobilized posteriorly in segment C7–T1 by an osteotomy in the area of the ossified interlaminar portion, the laminae, and the articular portions of C7–T1, and short-curve lordosation is induced by way of the threaded rods between the halo and the body jacket (Fig. 4.**29a–d**). Closure of the osteotomy completes the correction (Fig. 4.**29d**). External fixation is used for the correction and for postoperative immobilization, so that no osteosynthesis material is needed. The correcting forces are large enough in most cases to cause the anterior syndesmophytic ossifications to rupture.

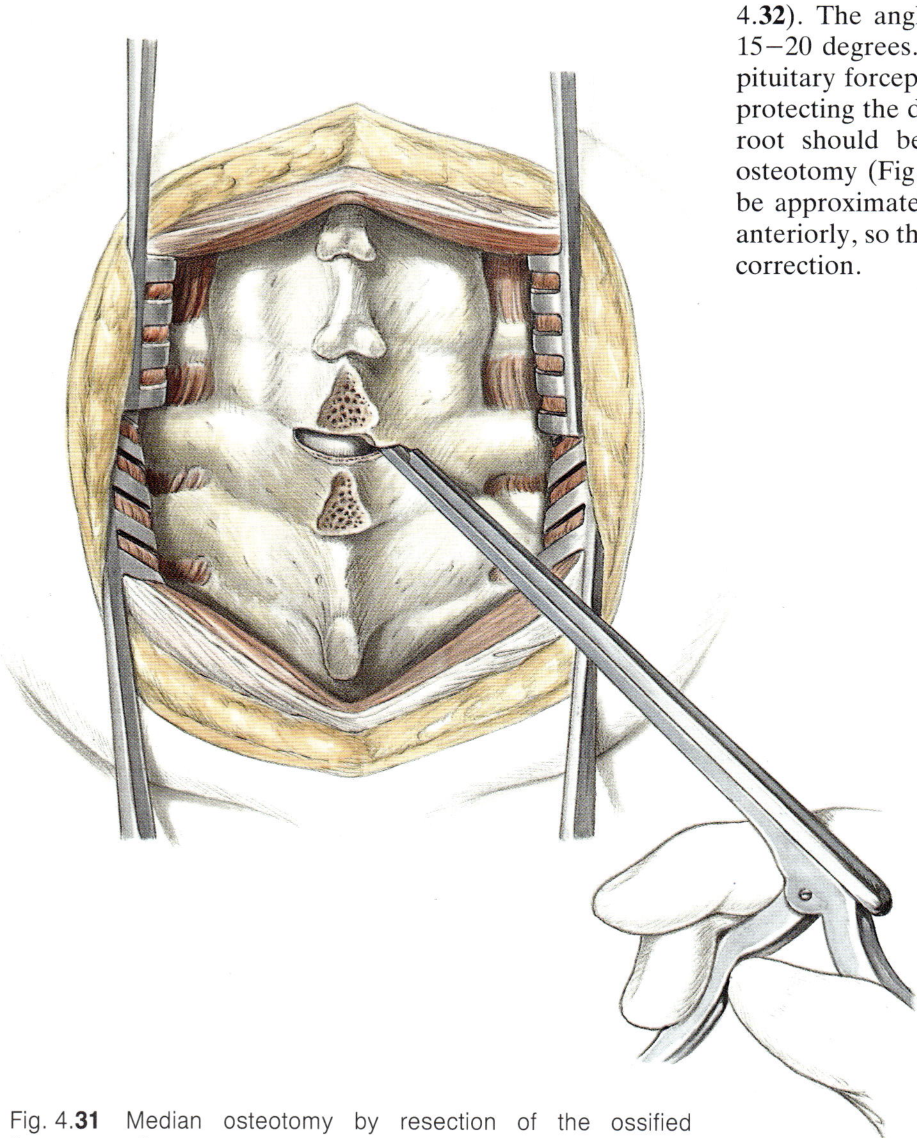

Fig. 4.**31** Median osteotomy by resection of the ossified ligamentum flavum.

Choice of Segment

Only segment C7–T1 should be chosen, since here the vertebral artery still takes an extravertebral course (Fig. 4.**29d**), and the correction cannot be hindered by the fixed ribs. Variations in the course of the vertebral artery and cervical ribs that may be present therefore need to be ruled out preoperatively.

Osteotomy Technique

The generally ossified C6–C7 and C7–T1 interspinal ligaments, as well as the C7 spinous process and, optionally, that of T1 as well, are resected with a pituitary forceps (Fig. 4.**30**). Occasionally, the C6 spinous process also has to be resected to obtain a better view. After this, the usually ossified yellow ligament is resected with a pituitary forceps, burr, and punch, as in lumbar osteotomies (Fig. 4.**31**). These median osteotomies are widened by resecting 3–4 mm each of the adjacent vertebral arches and undermining their borders after prior dissection of the dura.

From the midline osteotomy, the lateral arch osteotomies are carried out bilaterally through the lower portions of the arch of C7 and the previous joint components of C7–T1 in the direction of the intervertebral foramina C7–T1 (Fig. 4.**32**). The angle of the osteotomy with the horizontal is 15–20 degrees. The osteotomy is performed with a small pituitary forceps and a punch or, optionally, a burr, while protecting the dura and the C8 nerve root (Fig. 4.**32**). The root should be readily visible laterally after a proper osteotomy (Fig. 4.**33**). The lateral osteotomy gaps should be approximately 7 mm wide, and should expand slightly anteriorly, so that the foramina are not constricted after the correction.

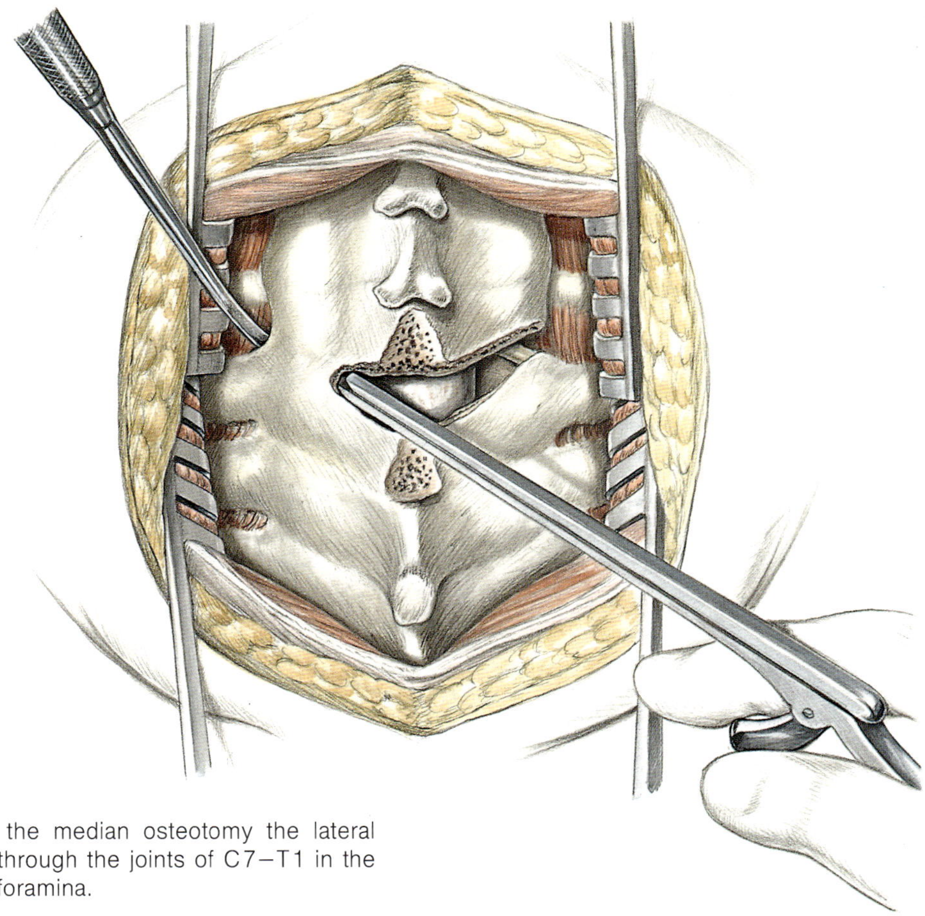

Fig. 4.**32** From the site of the median osteotomy the lateral osteotomies are carried out through the joints of C7–T1 in the direction of the intervertebral foramina.

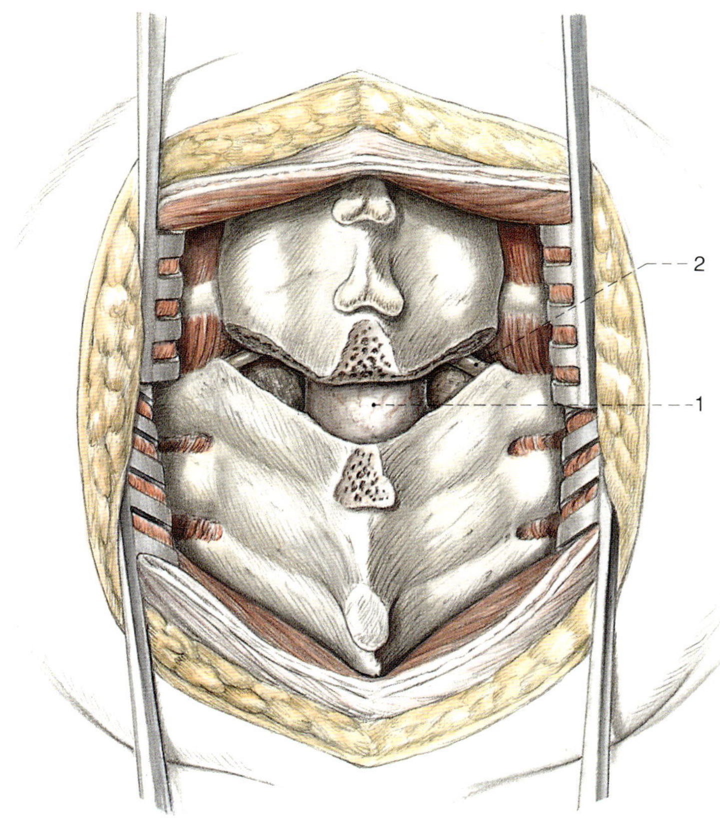

Fig. 4.**33** Site after complete osteotomy.

1 Spinal dura mater
2 Spinal nerve C8

Correction Technique

After completion of the osteotomy, an assistant working on the anterior side, tilts back the head and the neck slowly, by shortening the distance between the halo and the corset posteriorly and correspondingly increasing it anteriorly with the aid of the upper nuts on the posterior threaded rods. Slight deviations to the side can also be corrected in this way through greater unilateral advancement, but this requires a somewhat wider osteotomy on the convex side.

During the correction, the osteotomies and spinal nerves need to be observed by the surgeon. If a nerve compression threatens, further freeing with the punch on the lateral side is necessary, followed by further correction. Closure of the lateral osteotomy gaps completes the correction (Fig. 4.**34**), ideally so that the patient achieves a horizontal visual level (Fig. 4.**36**).

Spondylodesis

After completed correction, the resected spinous processes and the osteotomy materials are deposited on the partly decorticated C7 and T1 laminae. The graft of the C7 spinous process then covers the partly open medial osteotomy (Fig. 4.**35**).

Wound Closure

This is done in accordance with the posterior scoliosis operations (p. 68).

Postoperative Treatment

The patient can be mobilized at once (Fig. 4.**36**). No special care is required immediately after the operation. Neurologic assessments are important, and should be done every half-hour on the first day and every hour on the two following days. Should deficits develop, minimal distraction or rekyphosation, or both, can be performed through the halo cast on the affected side. It should be borne in mind, however, that initial paresthesias, probably due to the hematoma, generally disappear within a few days.

Radiographic documentation should be done—as preoperatively—by tomography performed immediately after the operation, before discharge, and before removal of the plaster jacket. The cast is worn for six months, and should be checked every four weeks.

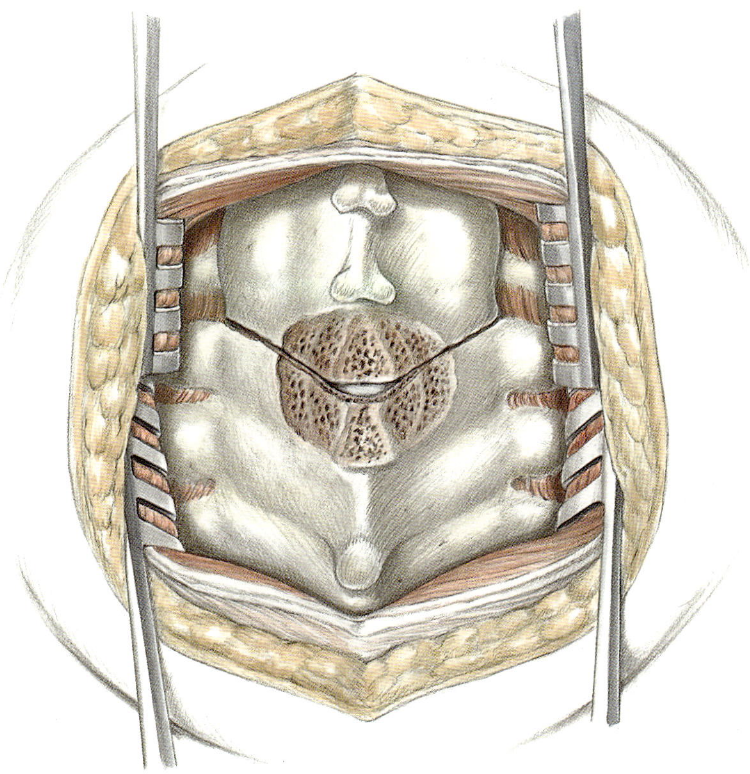

Fig. 4.**34** The operative site after correction.

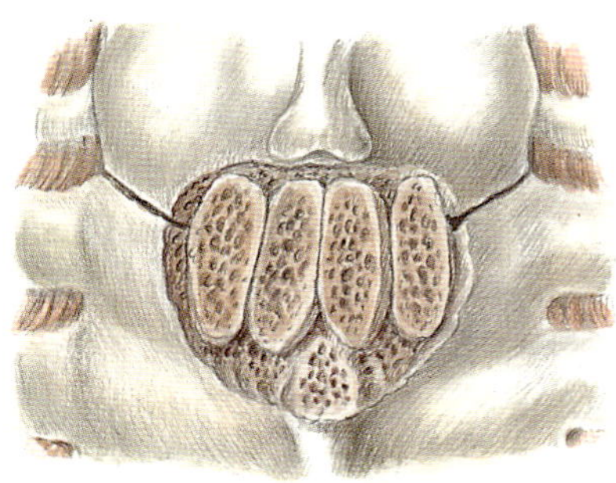

Fig. 4.**35** Posterior spondylodesis. The median osteotomy is covered with material resected from the spinous processes.

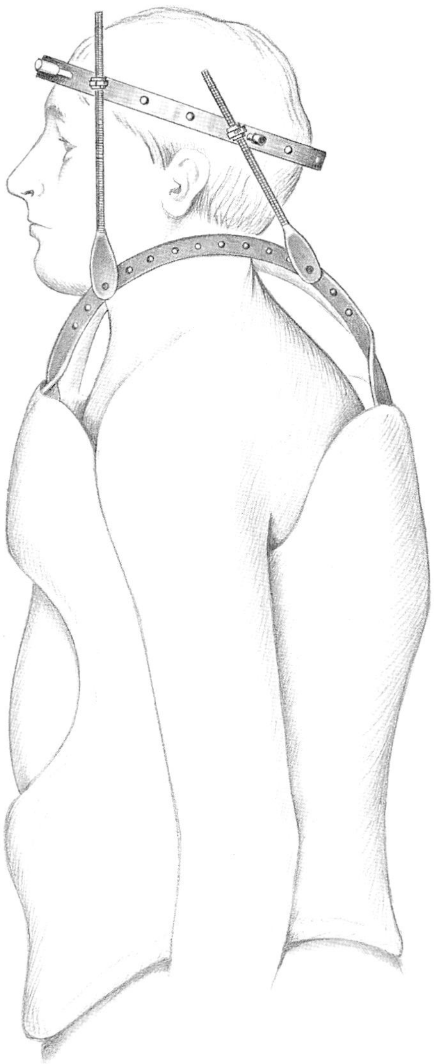

Fig. 4.**36** A patient in a halo vest after the operation.

Pitfalls and Complications

Specific risks in the operation include complications due to dura or root injuries during the osteotomy, or constriction of the foramen as a result of insufficiently wide lateral osteotomy gaps. The risk amounts to approximately 5–10%. However, since the center of rotation induced by the halo cast does not necessarily coincide with the level of the osteotomy during the correction, the correction being enforced rather through the osseous weakening in the osteotomized segment, mechanically induced subluxations may occur. This has been observed in two out of 30 cases. The correction should therefore be carried out very slowly and cautiously. Mild paresthesias and brachialgia, which are probably caused by the hematoma, occur frequently, but are reversible within a short time.

Alternative Methods

No other surgical methods are known. In principle, gradual traction in the halo cast over a period of several weeks is a possibility. In the presence of excessive bony ankylosis, however, this method is of very limited usefulness.

Operations for Spondylodiscitis (Andersson Lesion)

Anterior Interbody Spondylodesis

The indications, which are rare, include long-standing pain that cannot be controlled conservatively, and progression of osteolyses or of frequently ensuing monosegmental kyphotic kinking, or both.

The operation does not differ from interbody spondylodesis carried out for reasons. The approach is transthoracic (up to T12–L1), lumbar (L1–L2 to L4–L5), or transperitoneal (L5–S1), depending on the localization.

The operation consists of clearing the affected intervertebral space, including resection of the upper and lower plates, packing with corticocancellous bone graft, and segmental osteosynthesis with Zielke implants, following the procedure used in ventral derotation spondylodesis (p. 178), with the help of which any correction by distraction that is required can also be effected. The postoperative care is the same as for any lumbar corrective surgery in kyphotic deformities (p. 212).

Note
If there is a kyphotic deformity requiring correction besides the spondylodiskitis, a local resection of the lesion is unnecessary. Spondylodiskitis completely heals spontaneously within a year after the posterior surgery with static correction and the resulting stabilization.

The lesion thus corresponds functionally to a pseudarthrosis.

Operations for Fractures

Because of the complete ankylosis, lack of compensation, and the osteoporosis due to the underlying disease, the spinal column is at high risk of fracture in ankylosing spondylitis, particularly in its late stage. Fractures of the lower cervical spine as a result of whiplash injuries occur most frequently. Since the external impact is usually small, however, neurologic lesions occur only rarely. If the vertebrae are not deformed, an operation is seldom indicated, as the ossifying tendency of the underlying disease favors bony union.

Secure immobilization by a well-fitting Minerva or body jacket, or an appropriate plastic brace, is a prerequisite. Without it, there is a risk of pseudarthrosis due to the monosegmental mobility. Even pseudarthrosis, however, usually heals spontaneously as a result of the external immobilization.

If the vertebra is deformed—usually kyphotically—an operation is indicated, since this short-curve kyphosis markedly increases the kyphotic deformity that is either already present or can be expected to develop in ankylosing spondylitis. The choice of operative procedure is the same as for any other fracture. As a general rule, however, the following procedure is recommended:

- A kyphotic deformity has existed even before the injury. A lumbar vertebra or a thoracic vertebra below T8 is fractured. In such a case, Zielke's polysegmental lumbar lordosation spondylodesis (p. 228) with osteotomy and instrumentation of the fractured vertebra, should be considered. If the form of the fracture precludes transpedicular screw fixation of the fractured vertebra, this has to be bridged without screws. If there is marked gaping of vertebral bodies or intervertebral disk spaces after the correction, the space should be curetted by an anterior operation, packed with bone graft, and bridged by additional VDS instrumentation using threaded rods 4 mm thick (USIS, p. 212).
- If there is any traumatic kyphotic deformity, a posterior–anterior combined approach is recommended, since the correction and a secure spondylodesis can be performed better from the anterior side. In case of a dislocated posterior wall, a secure decompression may additionally be possible from the anterior side. Here again the USI system proves effective. The spine is then additionally stabilized from behind by transpedicular screw implantation using the USIS or the fixateur interne. The procedure is similar to the correction of short-curved kyphoses due to other causes, or to the resection of tumors (p. 212).

Further Reading

Brussatis F. Zervikale Aufrichtungsosteotomie bei Morbus Bechterew. Orthopäde 1981;10:178.

Dihlmann W. Die sog. Spondylitis anterior, Discitis und Spondylodiscitis bei Morbus Bechterew. Schlüssel zum Verständnis dieser Erkrankung. Fortschr Röntgenstr 1966;104:699.

Hehne HJ, Zielke K. Aufrichtungsosteotomien an der Wirbelsäule bei Spondylitis ankylosans – Ergebnisse und Erfahrungen nach 146 Operationen. Orthop Prax 1987;23:552.

Hehne HJ, Zielke K. Die zervikale Aufrichtungsosteotomie an der Wirbelsäule nach Mason und Urist bei Spondylarthritis ankylopoetica. Akt Rheumatol 1987;12:126.

Hehne HJ, Zielke K. Die Kyphotische Deformität bei Spondylitis ankylosans. Klinik, Radiologie und Therapie. Stuttgart: Hippokrates, 1990.

Hehne HJ, Zielke K, Püschel J. Aufrichtungsoperationen an der Wirbelsäule bei Spondylarthritis ankylopoetica. In: Albrecht HJ, ed. Neues für die Praxis aus konservativer und operativer Rheumatologie. Basel: Colloquia Rheumatologica, 1986.

Herbert JJ. Vertebral osteotomy: technique, indications and results. J Bone Jt Surg 1948;30-A:680.

Herbert JJ. Vertebral osteotomy for kyphosis, especially in Marie–Strümpell arthritis. J Bone Jt Surg 1959;41-A:291.

LaChapelle EH. Osteotomy of the lumbar spine for correction of kyphosis in a case of ankylosing spondylarthritis. J Bone Jt Surg 1946;28:851.

Law WA. Osteotomy of the cervical spine. J Bone Jt Surg 1959;41-B:640.

Law WA. Osteotomy of the spine. J Bone Jt Surg 1962;44-A:1199.

Leong JCY, Yau AC, Hsu LCS. Transpedicular decancellization osteotomy for correction of kyphosis in ankylosing spondylitis. 16th International Congress Rheumatology, Sydney, 1985.

McMaster MJ, Coventry MB. Spinal osteotomy in ankylosing spondylitis: technique, complications, and long-term results. Mayo Clin Proc 1973;48:476.

McMaster PE. Osteotomy of the spine for fixed flexion deformity. Pacif Med Surg 1965;73:314.

Mason C, Cozen L, Adelstein L. Surgical correction of flexion deformity of the cervical spine. Calif Med 1953;79:244.

Moll JMH. Ankylosing spondylitis. Edinburgh: Churchill Livingstone, 1980.

Morscher E, Müller W. Operative Korrektur fixierter Kyphosen. Orthopäde 1973;2:192.

Osgood C, Martin LG, Ackermann E. Fracture-dislocation of the cervical spine with ankylosing spondylitis. J Neurosurg 1973;39:764.

Püschel J, Zielke K. Korrekturoperation bei Bechterew-Kyphose. Indikation, Technik, Ergebnisse. Z Orthop 1982;120:338.

Rodegerdts U, Gisbertz D, Zielke K. Untersuchung zur dorsalen Aufrichtungsosteotomie der Kyphose. Z Orthop 1985;123:374.

Roy-Camille R, Demeulenaere C. Ostéosynthèse du rachis dorsal lumbaire et lumbo-sacré par plaques métalliques vissées dans les pédicules vertébraux et les apophyses articulaires. Presse Méd 1970;78:1447.

Schilling F. Spondylitis ankylopoetica. In: Diethelm L, et al., eds. Handbuch der medizinischen Radiologie VI/2. Berlin: Springer, 1974.

Schöllner D. Ein neues Verfahren zur Reposition und Fixation bei Spondylolisthesis. Orthop Prax 1975;11:270.

Simmons EH. The surgical correction of flexion deformity of the cervical spine in ankylosing spondylitis. Clin Orthop 1972;86:132.

Simmons EH. Kyphotic deformity of the spine in ankylosing spondylitis. Clin Orthop 1977;128:65.

Smith-Petersen MN, Larson CB, Aufranc OE. Osteotomy of the spine for correction of flexion deformity in rheumatoid arthritis. J Bone Jt Surg 1945;27:1.

Urist MR. Osteotomy of the cervical spine: report of a case of ankylosing rheumatoid spondylitis. J Bone Jt Surg 1958;40-A:833.

Yau ACMC, Chan RNW. Stress fracture of the fused lumbodorsal spine in ankylosing spondylitis. J Bone Jt Surg 1974;56-B:681.

Zielke K, Stunkat R, Beaujean F. Ventrale Derotationsspondylodese. Vorläufiger Ergebnisbericht über 26 operierte Fälle. Arch Orthop Unfall-Chir 1976;85:257.

Ziwjan JL. Die Behandlung der Flexionsdeformitäten der Wirbelsäule bei der Bechterewschen Erkrankung. Beitr Orthop Traumatol 1982;29:195.

5 Fusion of the Cervical Spine

W. Dick

Anterior Fusion (Robinson)

Indications

- Monosegmental osteochondrosis in segments C3 to T1, most commonly at C5–C6 and C6–C7.
- Cervical herniated disk operation.

Contraindications

- Gross instability of the segment (traumatic, inflammatory).
- Extensive stiffness of adjacent segments, as in ankylosing spondylitis, for example; in such cases, added stabilization with implants is required.

Approach

See Chapter 1, pp. 4–12.

The skin incision is made transversely; division of the omohyoid muscle is generally unnecessary.

Operative Technique

Instrumentarium

A narrow spreader that can be inserted into the intervertebral space is required, or a Caspar spreader that can be screwed into the vertebral bodies (Fig. 5.**1**).

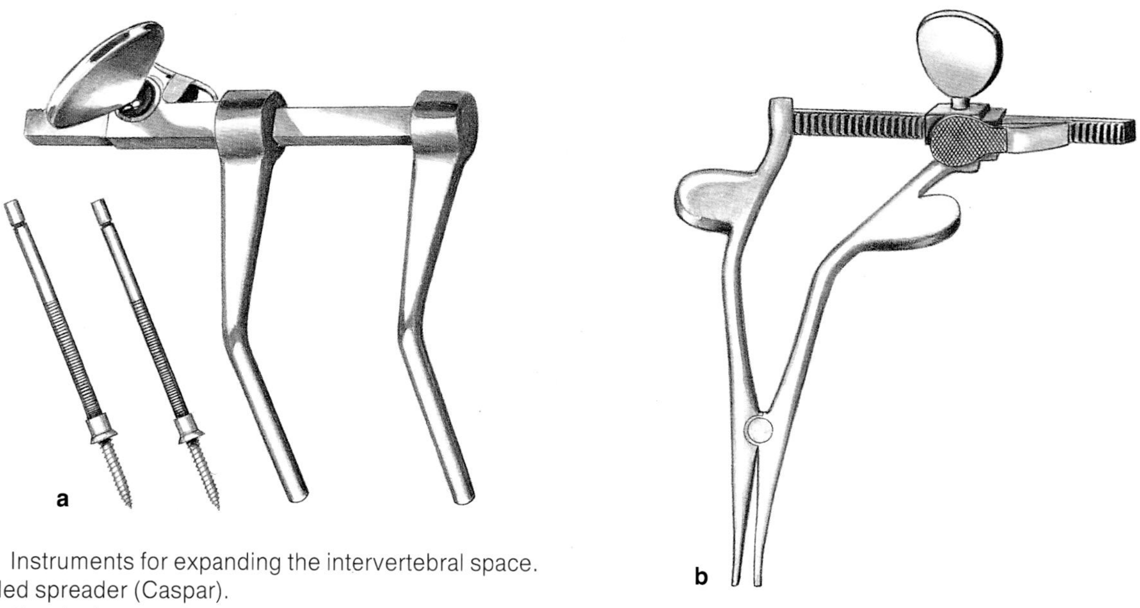

Fig. 5.**1** Instruments for expanding the intervertebral space.
a Threaded spreader (Caspar).
b Small arthrodesis spreader.

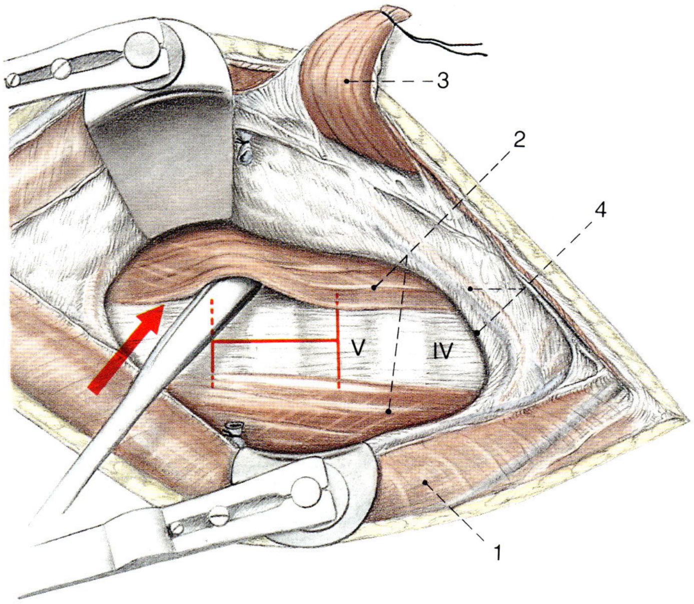

Fig. 5.**2** Lateral retraction of the longus colli muscle and H-shaped incision of the anterior longitudinal ligament. Any injury to the inbound fibers of the next higher and next lower anulus fibrosus must be avoided.

1 Sternocleidomastoid muscle
2 Longus colli muscle
3 Omohyoid muscle
4 Superior thyroid vessels
IV–V Cervical vertebrae

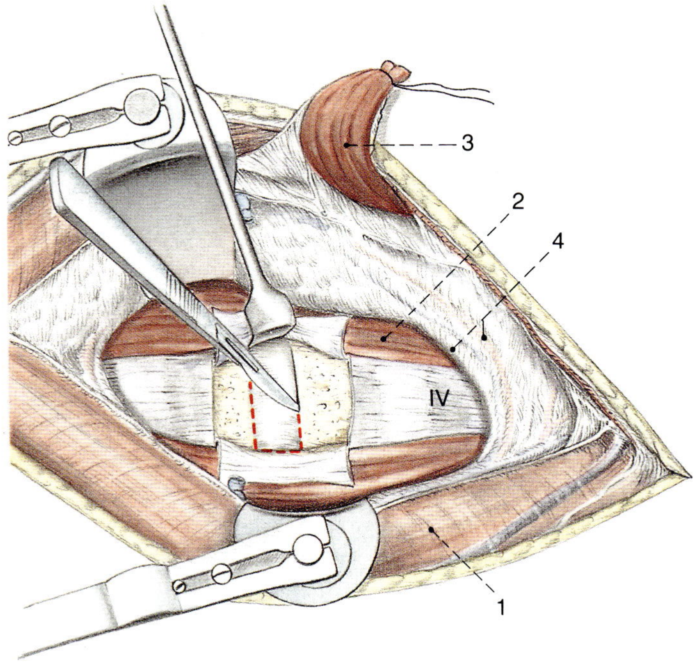

Fig. 5.**3** Excision of the anterior portion of the annulus fibrosus for a width of at least 15 mm.

1 Sternocleidomastoid muscle
2 Longus colli muscle
3 Omohyoid muscle
4 Superior thyroid vessels
IV Cervical vertebra

Preparation of Graft Bed

Following mandatory level identification using an image intensifier, the anterior longitudinal ligament is opened by an H-shaped incision over the two corresponding vertebrae (Fig. 5.**2**), the nearest intervertebral disk areas remaining untouched. If the long muscle of the neck overlaps too far from the side, it should first be retracted over a width of at least 18 mm. The anterior portion of the annulus fibrosus of the selected segment is excised with a knife over a width of at least 15 mm (Fig. 5.**3**). Removal of the intervertebral disks with a rongeur can be carried out by expanding the intervertebral space. The upper and lower plates of the adjacent vertebrae are carefully dechondrified with a small, sharp spoon, but the subchondral bone plate is left intact. Posteriorly, the posterior portion of the annulus fibrosus is also left intact in simple osteochondrosis without herniated disk. Large anterior osteophytes are trimmed, but the original cortical edge, which is used for fixation of the graft, is retained (Fig. 5.**4**). If the end plates are sclerosed to a high degree and seem avascular, they can be perforated at individual points with a ball-pointed drill, but should not be chiseled out. The surface area prepared in this way now averages 15 × 15 mm.

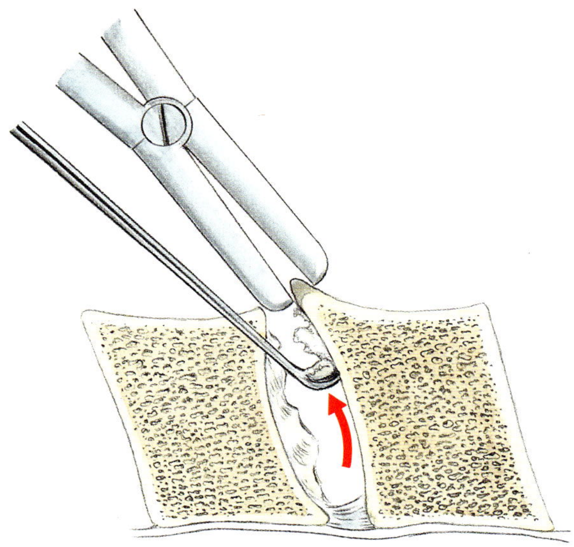

Fig. 5.**4** Debridement of end plates and sparing resection of anterior osteophytes. The original anterior border of the vertebra should be preserved.

Bone Graft

An autologous tricortical bone graft is harvested from the iliac crest in Robinson's method. With the cortical surfaces placed vertically, the graft is wedged into the intervertebral space like a posteriorly open horseshoe. Its height should be measured at the maximal expansion, and its length, too, should be exactly measured (Fig. 5.**5**), so that, when driven in, it can be countersunk just behind the anterior edges of the vertebrae without protruding posteriorly (Figs. 5.**6**, 5.**7**). After removal of the spreader, the graft should be firmly lodged in place. If it is movable, plate fixation is indicated.

Wound Closure

The wings of the H-incised anterior longitudinal ligament are approximated by suture if possible. After insertion of a deep suction drain, the wound is closed by suture of the platysma and the skin.

Postoperative Treatment

The patient can be mobilized immediately with a semirigid neck orthosis. The collar may be removed since radiographs show consolidation of the fusion.

Pitfalls and Complications

Specific risks of the operation include injuries to the posterior longitudinal ligament due to too deep dissection; anterior migration of the graft in instability resulting from insufficient impaction; break-in of the graft into the vertebral bodies, causing loss of the expanding effect because of excessive weakening of the end plates; and pseudarthrosis.

Alternative Methods

Added fixation with anterior plates (see below).

Other graft configurations without fixation (Cloward dowel graft or anteriorly reamed-in Bailey and Bagley graft) have proved less satisfactory.

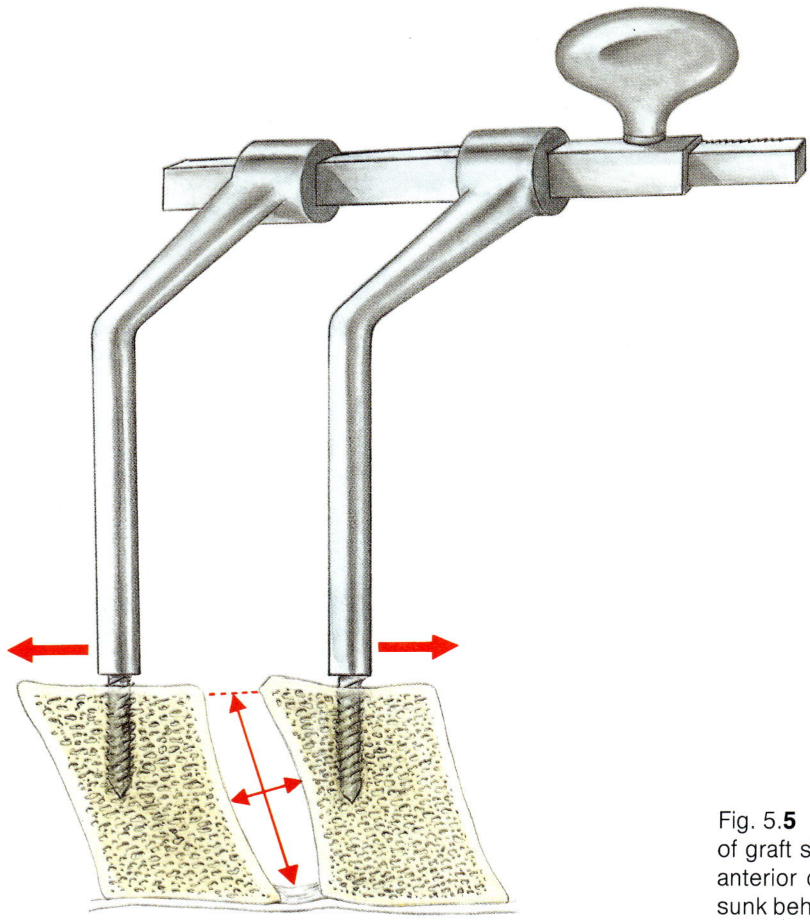

Fig. 5.**5** Expansion of the intervertebral space and measurement of graft size. The graft should not protrude anteriorly beyond the anterior contour of the vertebral bodies, but should be countersunk behind the marginal lip.

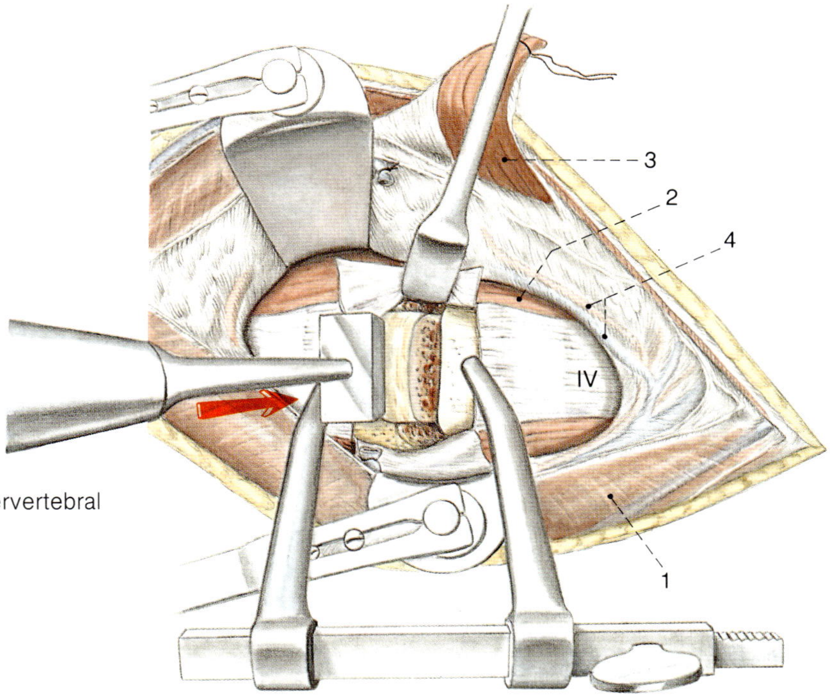

Fig. 5.**6** The graft is wedged into the expanded intervertebral space. Note the shaping and course of the graft cortex.

1 Sternocleidomastoid muscle
2 Longus colli muscle
3 Omohyoid muscle
4 Superior thyroid vessels
IV Cervical vertebra

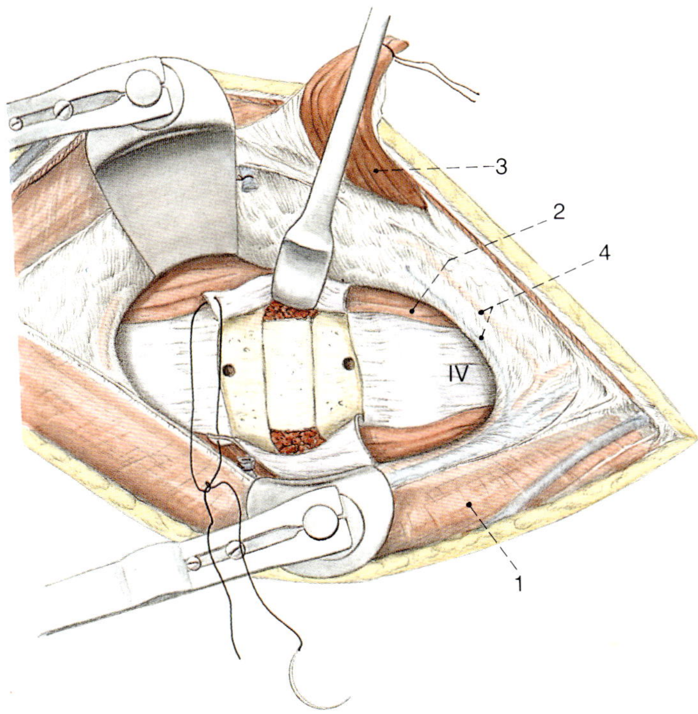

Fig. 5.**7** Correct graft seat without anterior protrusion. The space remaining on the side of the graft is packed with cancellous-bone graft. Approximation suture of the anterior longitudinal ligament.

1 Sternocleidomastoid muscle
2 Longus colli muscle
3 Omohyoid muscle
4 Superior thyroid vessels
VI Cervical vertebra

Interbody Fusion with Anterior Plate, Monosegmental or Polysegmental

Indications

- Instability of the cervical spine.
- Corpectomy (tumor, anterior spinal-cord decompression, inflammation).
- Posttraumatic kyphosis.

Approach

Anterior approach, see Chapter 1, pp. 4–12. A transverse skin incision suffices for the instrumentation of three vertebrae in the C5 to T1 segment; for more extensive revisions, and for C3 to C5, a longitudinal incision at the anterior border of the sternocleidomastoid muscle is recommended.

Operative Technique

A bisegmental fusion, corresponding to longer extensions in surgery for metastases, is presented below. In a monosegmental operation, placement of the plate follows the Robinson fusion described above.

Preparation of the Graft Bed

Following the mandatory identification of the level using the image intensifier (Fig. 5.**8**), the anterior wall of the cervical vertebrae to be fused is exposed over a width of at least 18 mm, which may require lateral retraction of the longus colli muscle.

The anterior longitudinal ligament and the annuli fibrosi of the two intermediate intervertebral disks are excised with a knife to a width of 15 mm (Fig. 5.**9**). Using a rotary burr drill and rongeur, a groove 15 mm wide is now cut out of the middle vertebra until contact is made with the posterior cortical layer (Fig. 5.**10**). When a rotary drill is used, the soft tissues of the neck have to be protected against any contact, to avert the risk of their being wound up and lacerated. Bleeding from the walls of the groove in the vertebral body can be minimized by impressing a Gelfram scrub.

If the underlying disease necessitates removal of the posterior wall of the vertebral body as well, a fine probe is used, from the side of the disk space, to undermine the wall and separate it step by step from the posterior longitudinal ligament, after which it is removed with a small punch (Fig. 5.**11**).

Similarly to the procedure in Robinson fusion, the lower plate of the cranial end vertebra and the upper plate of the caudal end vertebra are carefully dechondrified and debrided (Fig. 5.**12**). The subchondral bone remains. It is in these vertebrae that the plate screws are to be placed.

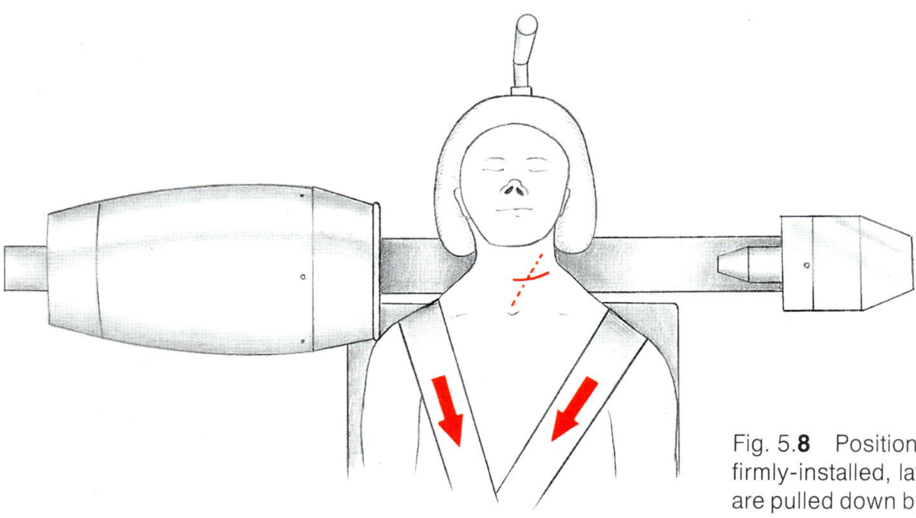

Fig. 5.**8** Positioning of the patient for anterior plate fusion, with a firmly-installed, laterally-directed image intensifier. The shoulders are pulled down by adhesive strap traction.

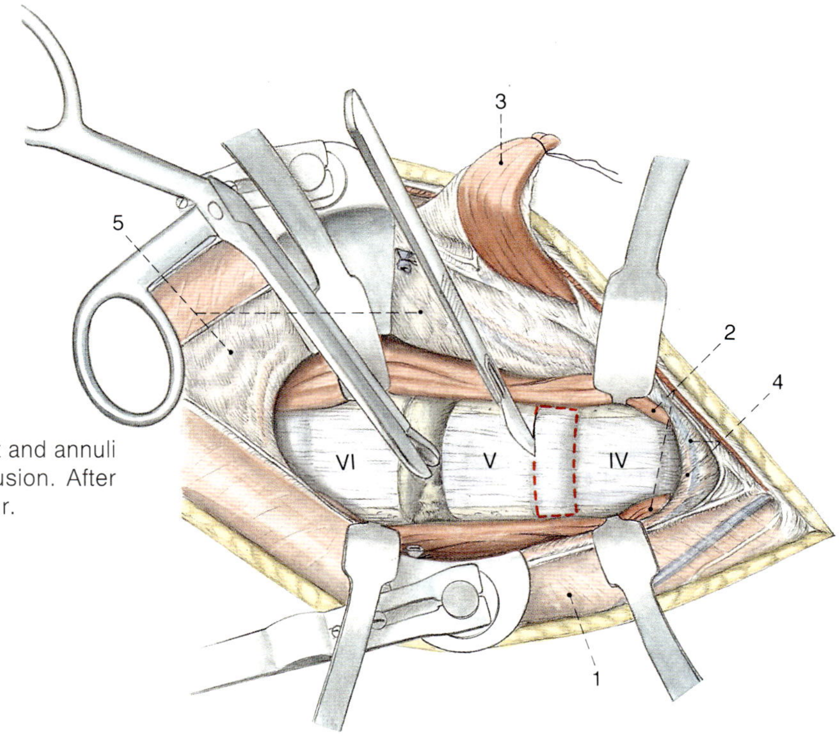

Fig. 5.**9** Excision of the anterior longitudinal ligament and annuli fibrosi of both intervertebral disks for bisegmental fusion. After this, the intervertebral disks are removed with a rongeur.

1 Sternocleidomastoid muscle
2 Longus colli muscle
3 Omohyoid muscle
4 Superior thyroid vessels
5 Thyroid gland
IV–VI Cervical vertebrae

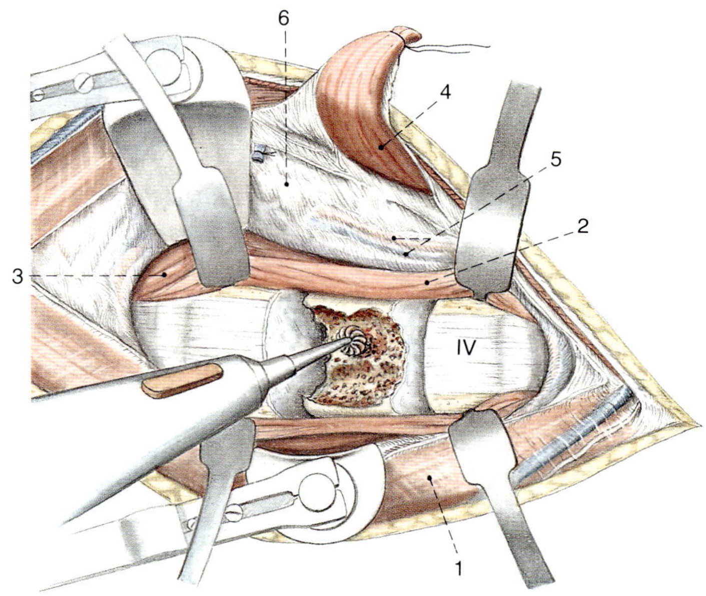

Fig. 5.**10** A longitudinal groove 15 mm wide is cut into the intermediate vertebral body. If a rotary burr is used, the jarring caused by a chisel and hammer is avoided. Watch for laceration of the soft tissues by coiling around the rotary burr. Take care to protect the soft tissues.

1 Sternocleidomastoid muscle
2 Longus colli muscle
3 Longus capitis muscle
4 Omohyoid muscle
5 Superior thyroid vessels
6 Thyroid gland
IV Cervical vertebra

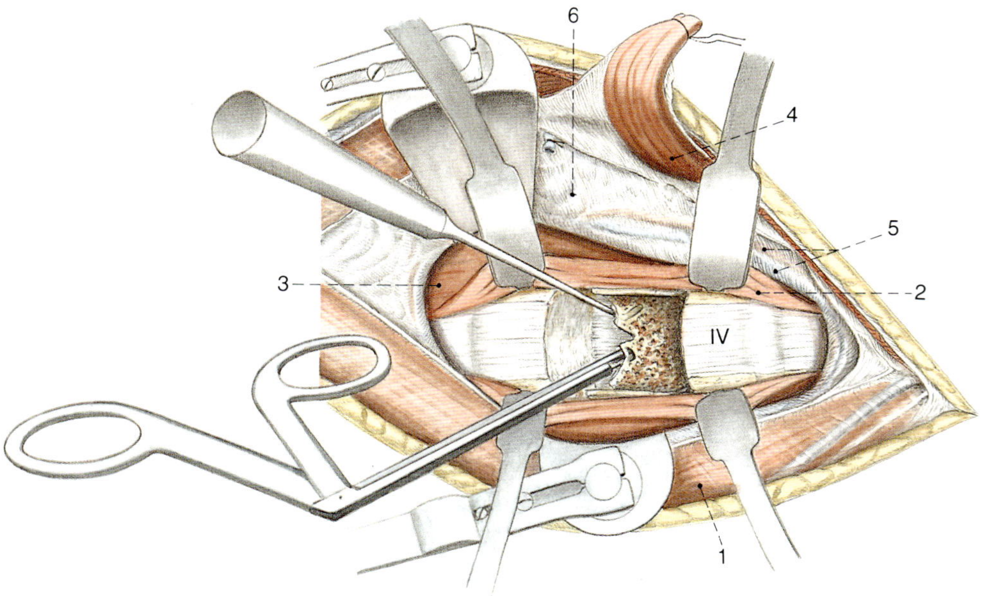

Fig. 5.**11** Resection of the posterior wall of the vertebral body if required by the underlying disease. The posterior cortical layer is undermined step by step with a small dissection hook, and is then detached and resected with a fine punch forceps.

1 Sternocleidomastoid muscle
2 Longus colli muscle
3 Longus capitis muscle
4 Omohyoid muscle
5 Superior thyroid vessels
6 Thyroid gland
IV Cervical vertebra

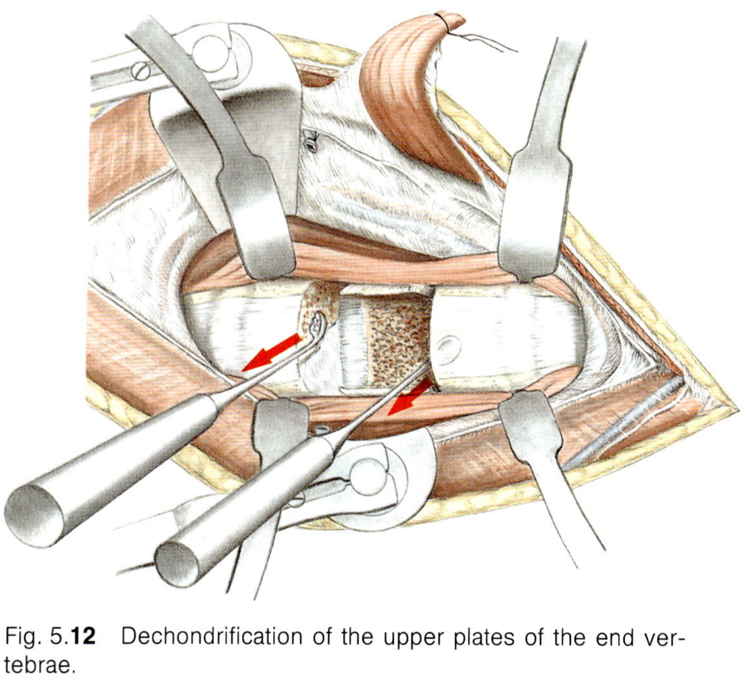

Fig. 5.**12** Dechondrification of the upper plates of the end vertebrae.

Bone Graft

A corticocancellous autologous iliac crest graft is trimmed to the required dimensions. When shaping its ends, care should be taken to ensure an oblique ascent of the lower and upper plates on the cervical spine (Fig. 5.**13**). The cortical side should face forward.

Since the graft is protected against dislocation by the plate, its ends do not need to be sunk into the end vertebrae (Fig. 5.**14**).

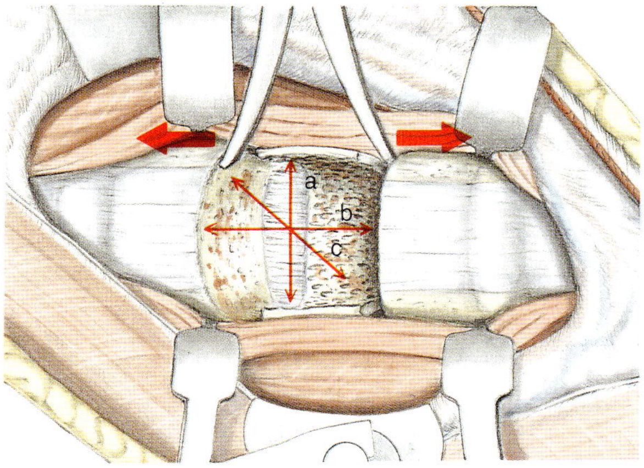

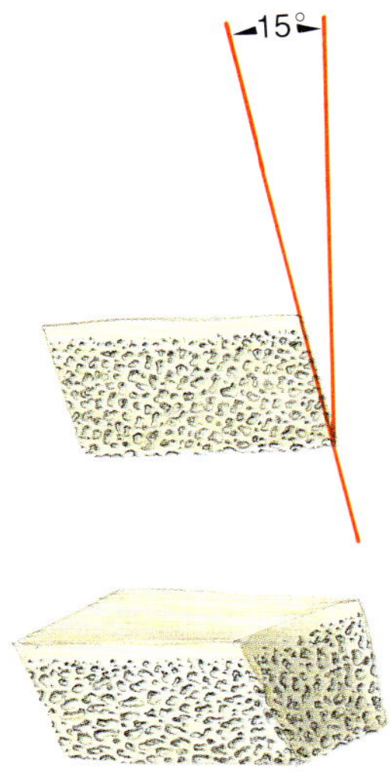

Fig. 5.**13** Measuring the size and shape of the graft for expanded intervertebral spaces. Note the ascending course of the upper plates.

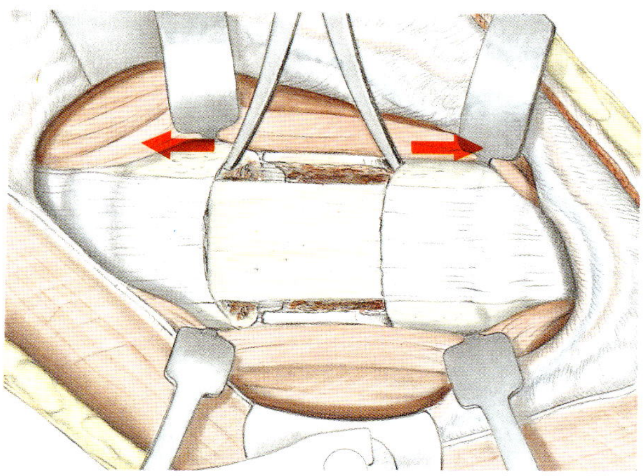

Fig. 5.**14** Implantation of corticocancellous graft, with forward-facing cortex and the spreader in place. Since the graft is fixed here by the anterior plate, dovetailing into the end vertebrae is not necessary.

Plate Fixation

Fundamentals

For plate osteosynthesis of the cervical vertebrae, various implant types are available in the assortment of sizes required; each is fastened with two screws per vertebra. They can be divided into two main groups: simple plates with separate screws, and "plate fixators," in which the anchoring screws are locked into the plate to provide angular stability (Fig. 5.**15**).

A bisegmental fixation with the Orozko plate is shown as an example of the first group in Chapter 11, Figures 11.**17**–11.**20**. This implant is also available for one segment and, with a greater length, for extensive tumor stabilizations. It can be readily fitted to the physiologic lordosis of the cervical spine.

An example of the group of "plate fixators" is shown below.

Instrumentarium

The head of the screw is cylindrical, and provided with a "rim stop." The screw head is cross-split down to the vicinity of the thread, and can be firmly locked into the plate hole using a conical expansion bolt (Figs. 5.**15c**, 5.**16**).

Advantages

- Angular stability between screw and longitudinal support.
- Security against disengagement of the screws.
- Other than with simple plates, penetration of the posterior cortex by the screw tip is unnecessary, so that there is
- reduced operative risk due to reduced depth of drilling.

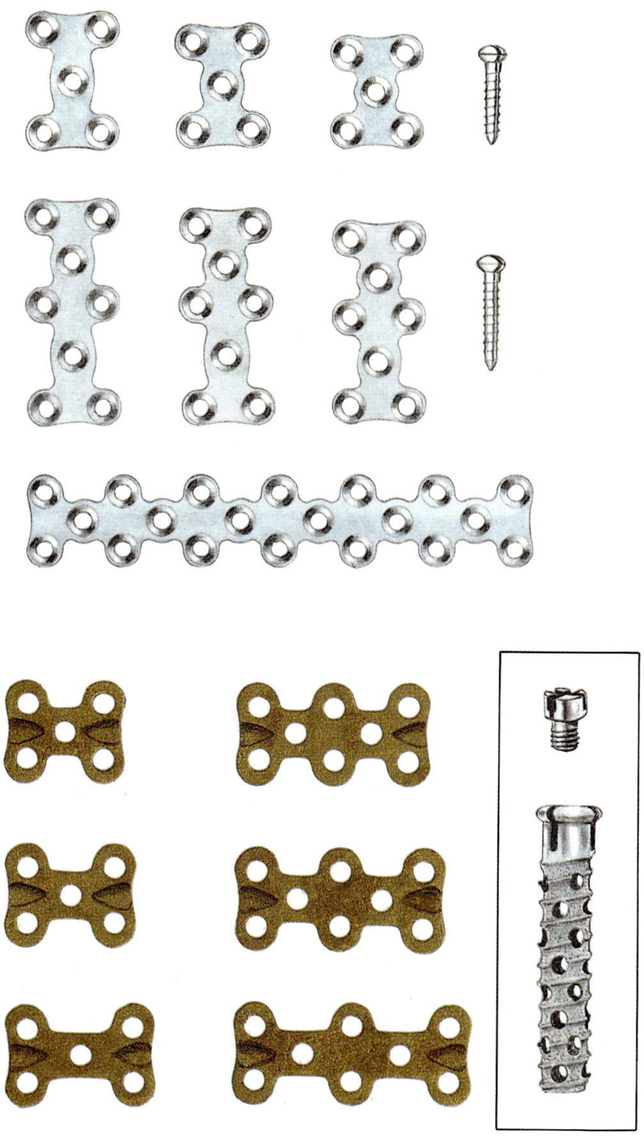

a

c

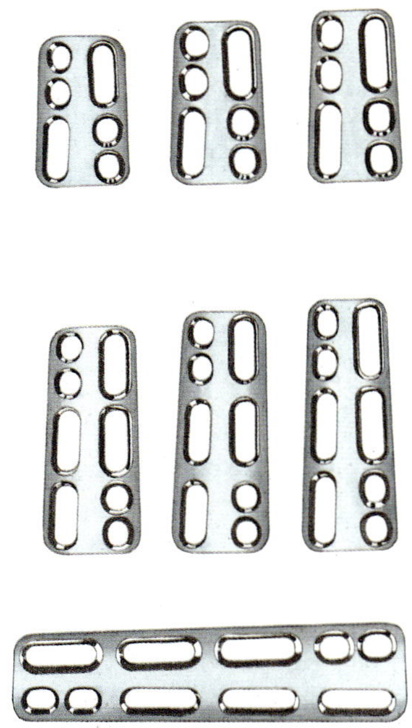

Fig. 5.**15** Implants. Simple plates with loose screw-plate connection, **a** Orozco, and **b** Caspar. Plates for fixation of one or two segments are available in various lengths. For unusual indications, they can also be supplied in longer sizes. **c** Plate fixator with a rigid screw–plate connection and a safeguard against disengagement of the screw by impacting the cross-split screw head into the plate hole with an expansion bolt (Morscher cervical-spine locking plate, made of titanium).

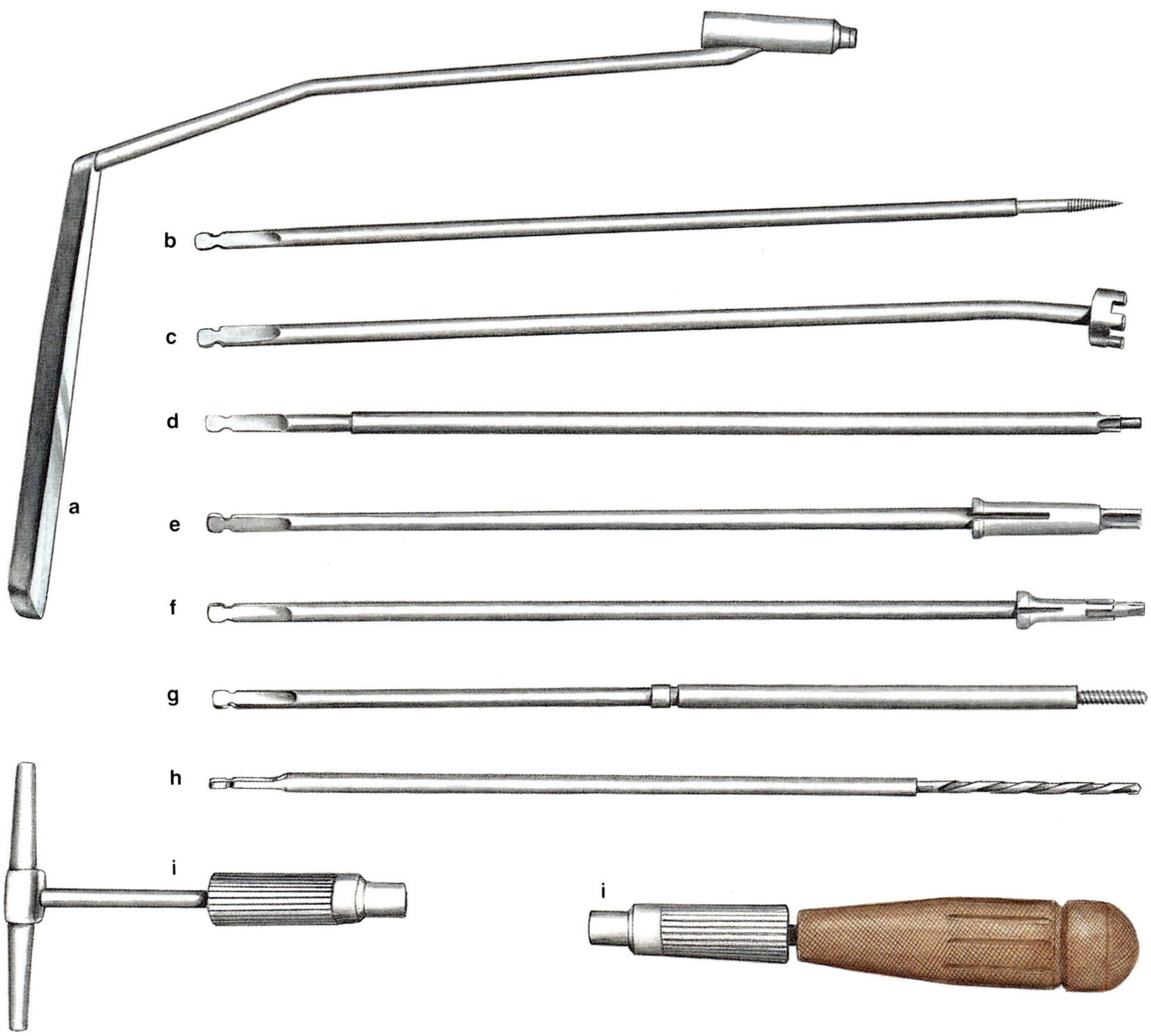

Fig. 5.**16** Instrumentarium for cervical-spine locking plate.
a Drill guide.
b Screw-removing mandrel.
c Plate holder.
d Countersinking tool.
e Screwdriver for plate screw.
f Screwdriver for expanding bolt.
g Thread tapper with depth-limiting stop.
h Drill with depth limitation by drill guide.
i Handles.

Since the posterior cortex does not need to be perforated in this system, the screws have a standard length of 16 mm. The drill and the tap are provided with a stopcock device. Special screwdrivers are necessary for the anchoring and expanding screws (Fig. 5.**16**).

Insertion of the Plate

After placement of the graft, the proper plate size is selected, and the plate is slightly pre-bent if necessary. The plate is held down in the correct position with the plate holder. With regard to the entry sites of the screws, it should be borne in mind that the upper plates ascend posteriorly on the cervical spine, so that the rectangularly-placed screws must not be inserted more caudally than in the middle of the anterior wall. The holes are drilled in the plate after attachment of a drill guide (Fig. 5.**17**); the instruments have a stopcock that allows a depth penetration of only 16 mm.

Subsequently, the tapping is carried out using a stop-protected soft-tissue guide (Fig. 5.**18**). When the screw is applied, a sleeve on the special screwdriver prevents premature expansion of the screw head until it has entered the plate hole. After the final tightening, the anchoring screw is locked into the plate by tapping the conical expanding screw (Fig. 5.**19**).

The autologous graft bridged by the plate can now also be affixed to the plate with a screw.

If there is still room in the disk spaces next to the graft, it is filled with small cancellous-bone chips.

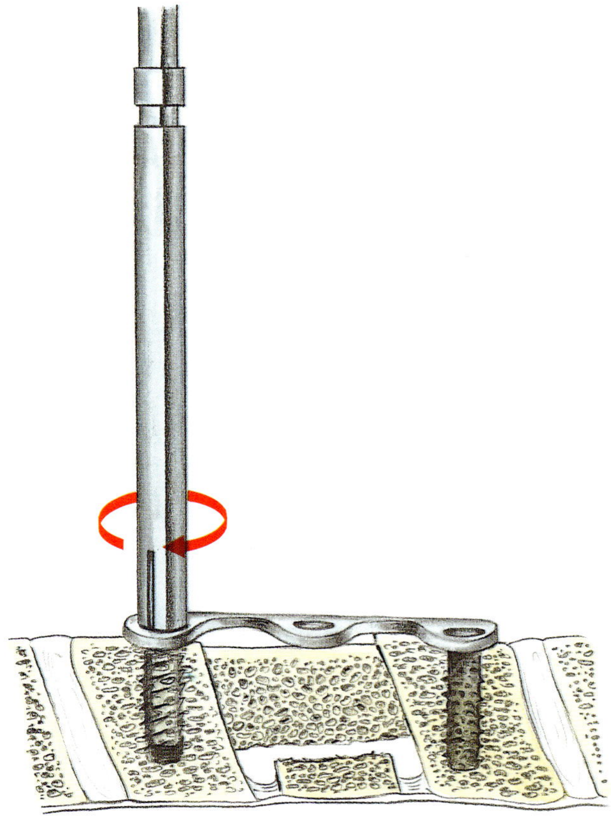

Fig. 5.**18** During threading, too, a stop limits the depth of penetration.

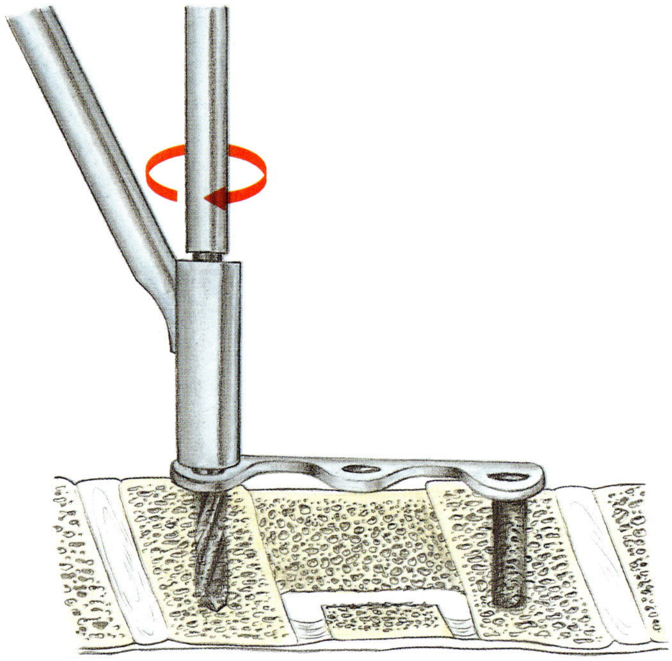

Fig. 5.**17** The screw holes are drilled through the fitted plate with the attached drill guide. A stop limits the penetration to 16 mm. The posterior cortex is not perforated.

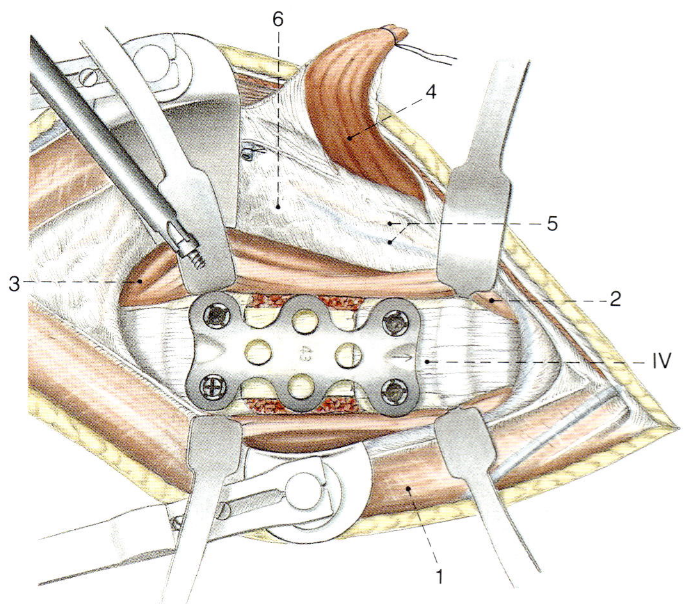

Fig. 5.**19** When all the anchoring screws have been tightened, they are locked by inserting the conical expansion bolts into the screw heads. The graft, too, can be screwed to the plate so that it cannot shift in either anterior or posterior direction. If free space remains next to the graft at the level of the previous intervertebral disks, it is packed with small chips of cancellous bone.

1 Sternocleidomastoid muscle
2 Longus colli muscle
3 Longus capitis muscle
4 Omohyoid muscle
5 Superior thyroid vessels
6 Thyroid gland
IV Cervical vertebra

Wound Closure

After introduction of a Redon drain, the wound is closed by suturing the platysma and skin.

Postoperative Treatment

The patient is immediately mobilized, and wears a soft plastic foam collar for six weeks.

Pitfalls and Complications

The specific risk inherent to all anterior plate fixations on the cervical spine consists of degeneration of the adjacent intervertebral disks, particularly if the longitudinal ligament in that location is compromised during dissection, or by the edge of a plate that is slightly too long. There is also a risk of injury to the esophagus (a wide stomach tube should always be passed during the operation); and a risk of difficulty in swallowing owing to protrusion of the plate.

Alternative Methods

Posterior fusion.

Posterior Fusion

Indications

- Instability of disk and ligament below C3.
- Fusion following laminectomy.
- Additional complementing of an anterior fusion (in ankylosing spondylitis, pseudarthroses, tumors).

Contraindication

In the absence of an intact anterior column (comminuted fracture, tumor), the procedure should not be used alone, but at best as an adjunct to anterior spondylodesis.

Approach

Positioning and Incision

The shoulders are pulled down with adhesive straps. A laterally-placed image intensifier should be installed in a fixed position and included in the draped area (Fig. 5.**20**).

Exposure of the Spine

The approach is the same as that described in Chapter 1, pp. 56–59, but as a rule the arches of the three uppermost cervical vertebrae do not need to be exposed for posterior fusion of the medial and lower cervical spine. This removes the risk of injury to the vertebral artery or the suboccipital and greater occipital nerves. The subperiosteal dissection is carried as far as the lateral border of the articular-process masses (Fig. 5.**21**).

Operative Technique

Instrumentarium

Magerl hook plates for posterior fusion of two or three cervical vertebrae are available in seven sizes (Fig. 5.**22**). They are used bilaterally, and can easily be shaped with the aid of narrow flat pliers. The hook is applied caudally to the arch of the lower end vertebra; at the upper end vertebra, fixation is effected by screws inserted into the articular-process masses.

Technique of Plate Fixation

Radiography to identify the segment level is mandatory. To determine the entry point for the screw, the middle point between the superior and inferior joint surfaces is identified. The drilling site lies in the medial half of the articular-process mass (Fig. 5.**23**).

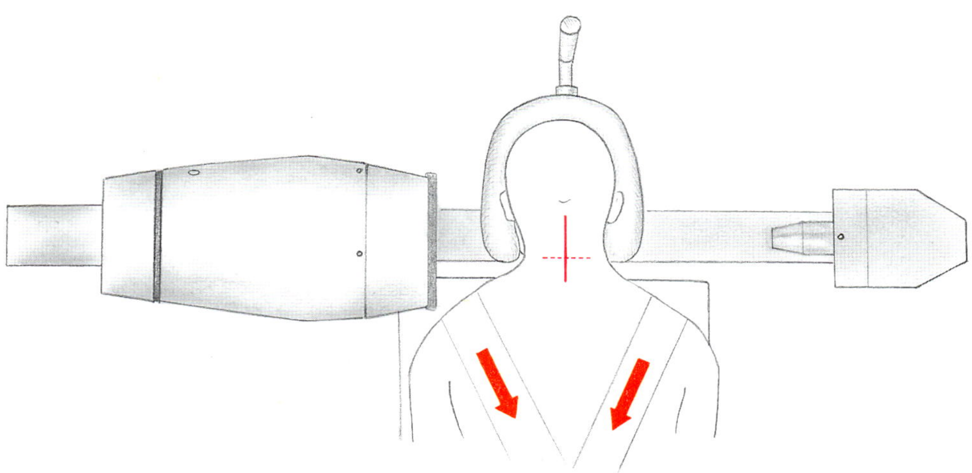

Fig. 5.**20** Posterior approach to the cervical spine. Positioning with a firmly-installed image intensifier. The shoulders are pulled down by adhesive strap traction. Incision: longitudinal; for exposure of at most three vertebrae, a transverse skin incision can be made at the level of the spinous process tip of the lowest vertebra to be accessed. In either case, the subcutaneous dissection is performed in a longitudinal direction, as shown in Figs. 1.**98**–1.**102**.

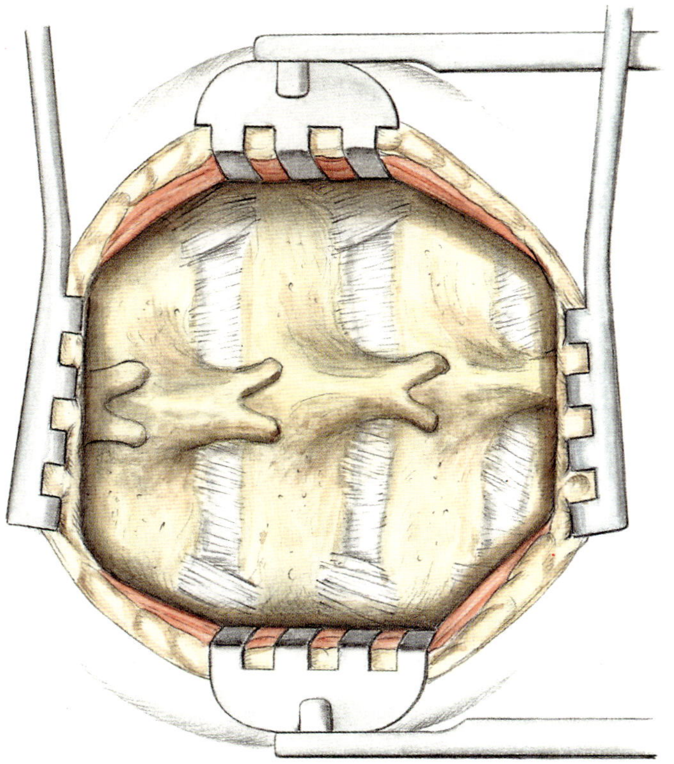

Fig. 5.**21** The cervical spine is exposed from the fifth to the seventh cervical vertebra, and the articular-process masses are visualized.

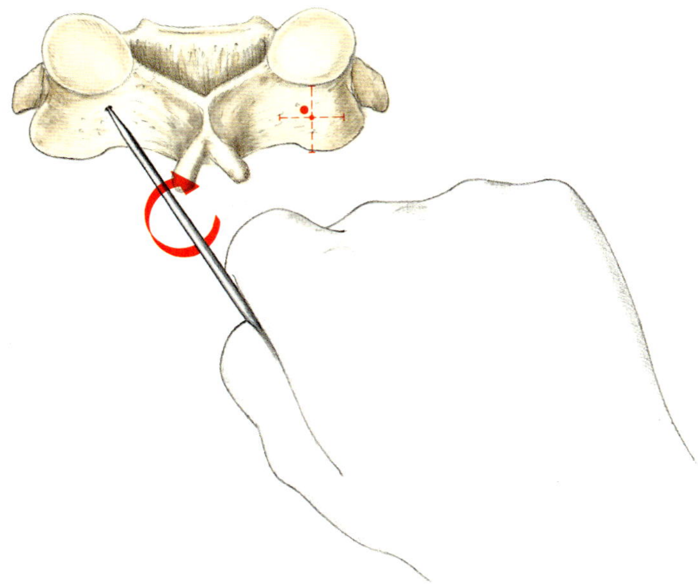

Fig. 5.**23** Determination of the entry point for the anchoring screw. The entry point is marked with an awl or Kirschner wire perpendicularly to the surface, to prevent slippage of the drill.

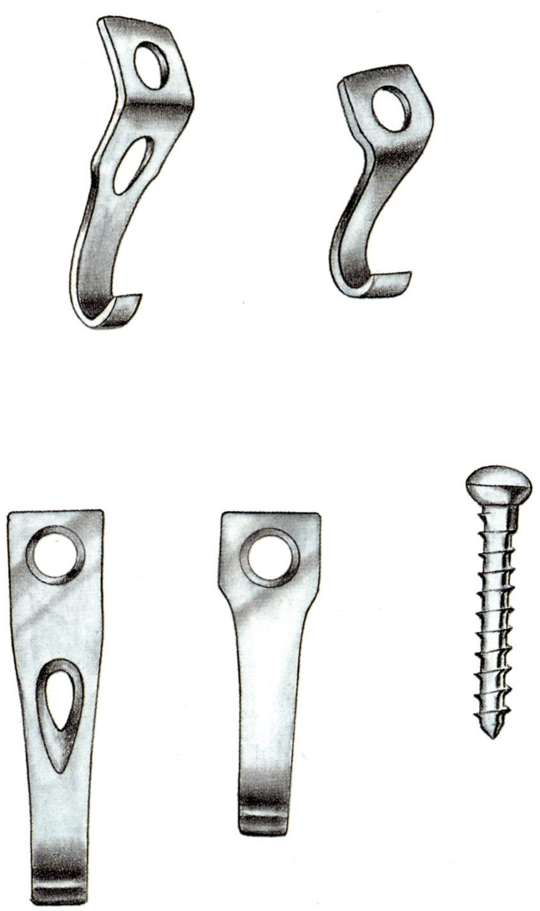

Fig. 5.**22** Posterior hook plates for the cervical spine (Magerl).

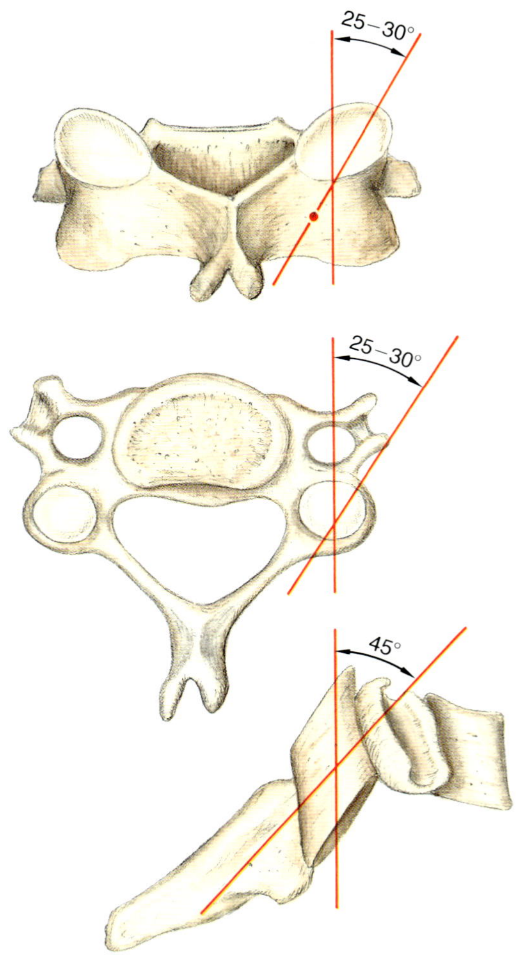

Fig. 5.**24** The correct drill direction is approximately 30 degrees lateral and 45 degrees cranial, which means that, in the lateral projection, it runs parallel to the joint surfaces. Dangerous proximity to the vertebral artery and the spinal nerve is thus avoided.

In Magerl's technique, the direction of the drill is 30 degrees lateral and about 45 degrees cranial; that is to say, laterally projected it runs parallel to the joint surfaces (Fig. 5.**24**). The direction of the these can be determined by inserting a fine dissector into the caudally adjacent joint space (Fig. 5.**26**).

Drilling process

- The entry site is marked with an initially perpendicularly applied drill, awl, or Kirschner wire: given the oblique course, the drill would otherwise slip off (Fig. 5.**23**).
- Use a specially long 2-mm drill.
- Make room sparingly with the small rongeur if a spinous process tip is in the line of advance of the drill (Fig. 5.**25**).
- Prevent the drill, which is fitted with a tissue-protector sleeve, from sliding off laterally. The drill position and direction are verified using a lateral image intensifier.
- Carefully perforate the far anterior cortex.

With this direction of the drill canal, the drill or the screw tip emerges at a very safe distance, lateral to the vertebral artery and lateral–cranial to the spinal nerve (Fig. 5.**24**).

Measurement of length. This is made through the applied plate (Fig. 5.**29**).

Threading. Only as far as the anterior cortex.

Hook seat. A suitably narrow notch is made at the caudal border of the lamina of the lower end vertebra, directly medial to the intervertebral joint, which is not touched (Fig. 5.**27**). The hook is thus prevented from sliding into the intervertebral joint.

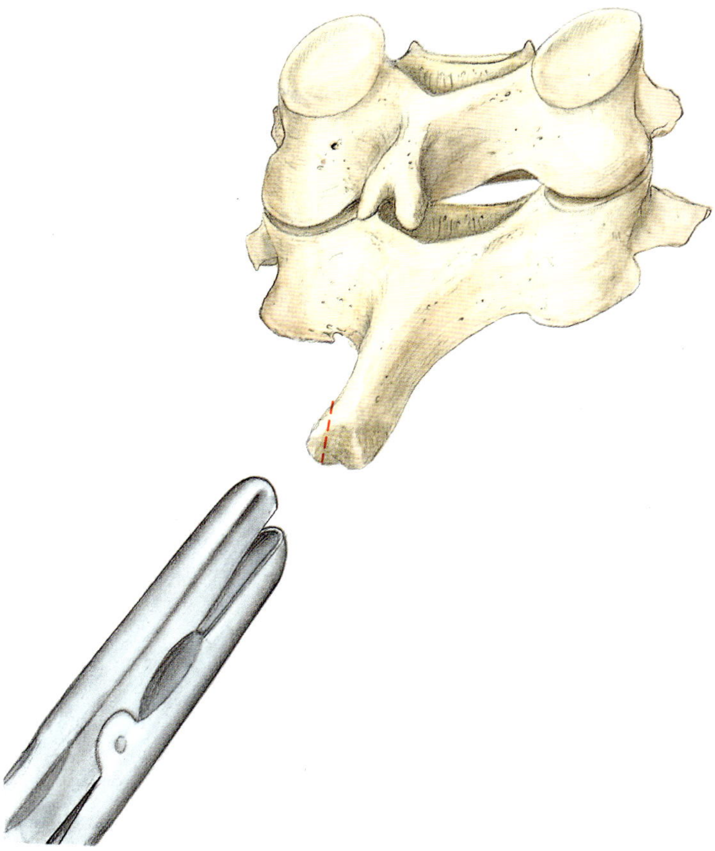

Fig. 5.**25** If a spinous process obstructs application of the drill in the right direction, it is sparingly trimmed with the Luer forceps.

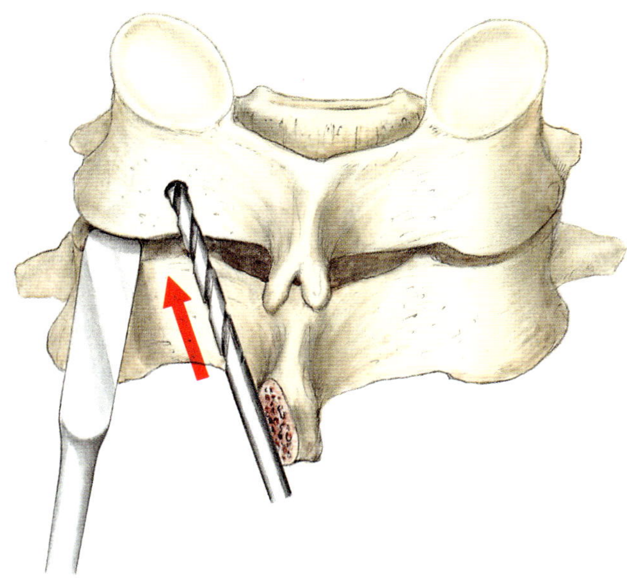

Fig. 5.**26** A small, flat rasp in the joint space helps to keep the drill aligned in the sagittal plane parallel to the joint surfaces. *Note:* For greater clarity, the tissue-protector which helps prevent slippage of the drill in vivo has been omitted from the illustration.

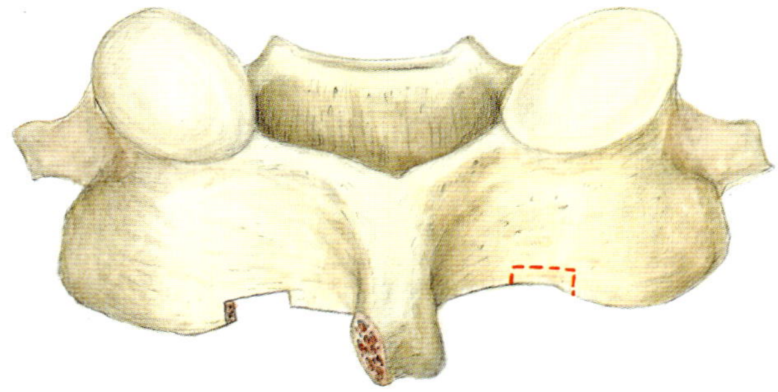

Fig. 5.**27** A small notch to serve as hook seat is cut into the lamina of the caudal vertebra directly medial to the joint facet; this prevents the hook from being pulled laterally into the joint.

Fitting of plate. The length of the plate to be selected is suitable if it still compresses the segment when the screw is tightened. This means it is not too long. It has to be contoured by torsion, and the hook, too, usually has to be adjusted in its curvature (Fig. 5.**28**).

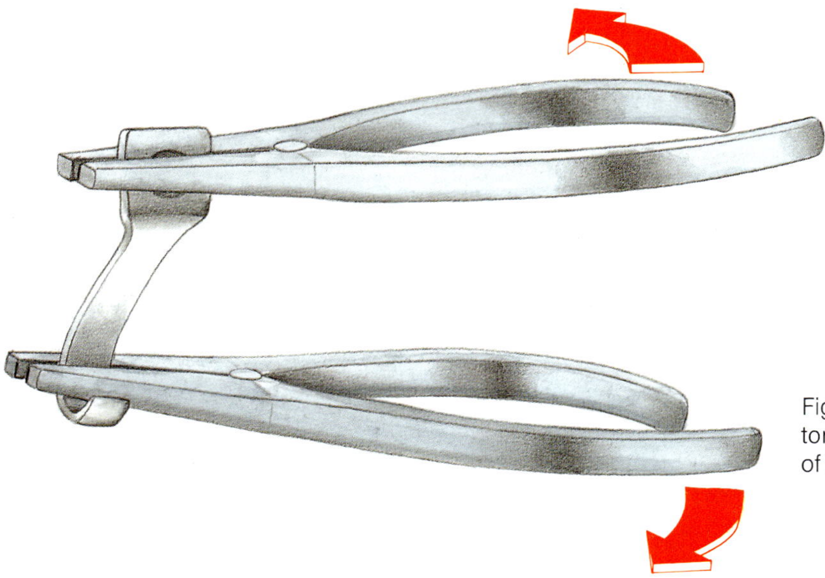

Fig. 5.**28** The hook plate always has to be contoured by torsion, and usually has to be bent more sharply in the area of the hook.

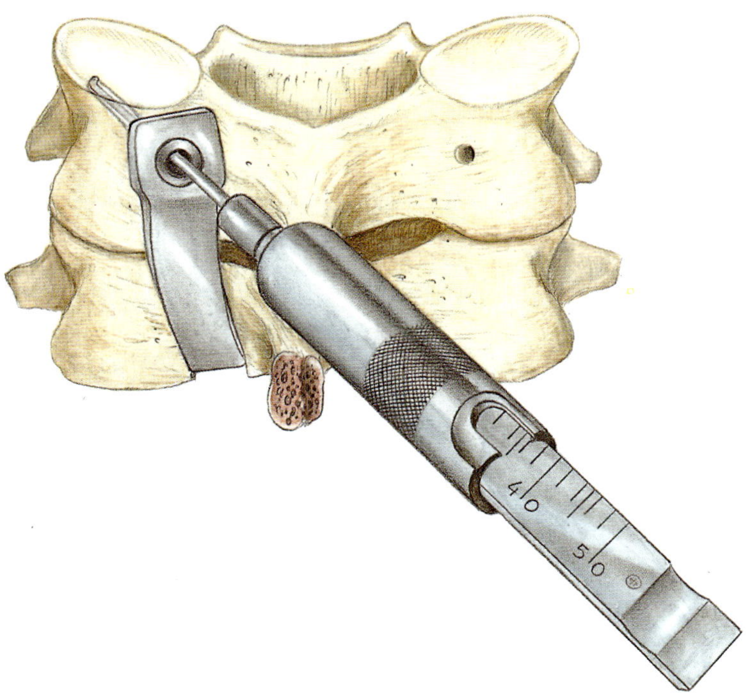

Fig. 5.**29** Measurement of length through the screw hole of the fitted plate.

Graft and Graft Bed

A flat, horizontal step is cut into the oblique superior border of the spinous process of the caudal end vertebra, to prevent slippage of the graft. It should not be too deep, so that the spinous process will not break off, and anteriorly it should not extend to the canal (Fig. 5.**30**). For the fusion of three vertebrae, the medial spinous process is completely ablated.

An autologous corticocancellous H-graft from the posterior iliac crest is dovetailed in the normal position of the vertebrae before the plate screws are tightened.

As the plate screws are tightened, the graft is compressed and firmly wedged in. Since the plates lie between the graft and the two articular process columns, these three pressure-resistant struts are pretensioned; the resultant interlocking system is stable in all directions.

The spondylodesis is completed by applying small cancellous-bone chips to the periosteum-free laminae and articular-process masses (Fig. 5.**31**).

For the fusion of three vertebrae, the articular mass of the middle vertebra is finally similarly secured with a screw that is passed through the medial plate hole (Fig. 5.**32**).

Note
In cervical plate fusion, the intervertebral joints are not dechondrified.

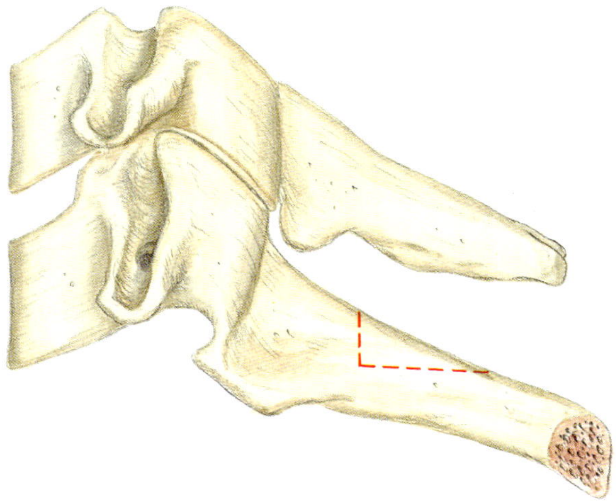

Fig. 5.**30** A straight excision is made at the oblique superior border of the caudal spinous process for improved seating of the spondylodesis graft. Watch out for opening of the vertebral canal or rupture of the spinous process.

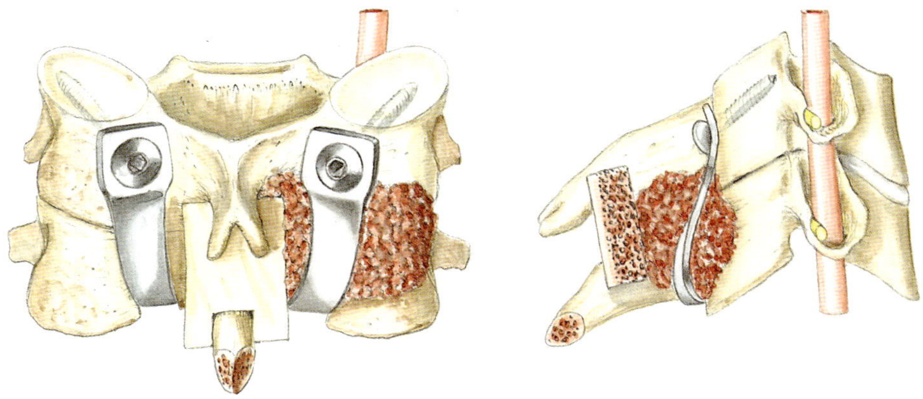

Fig. 5.**31** After insertion of the autologous H-graft, the screws are tightened on both sides. Small cancellous-bone chips are placed between and alongside the plates for fusion.

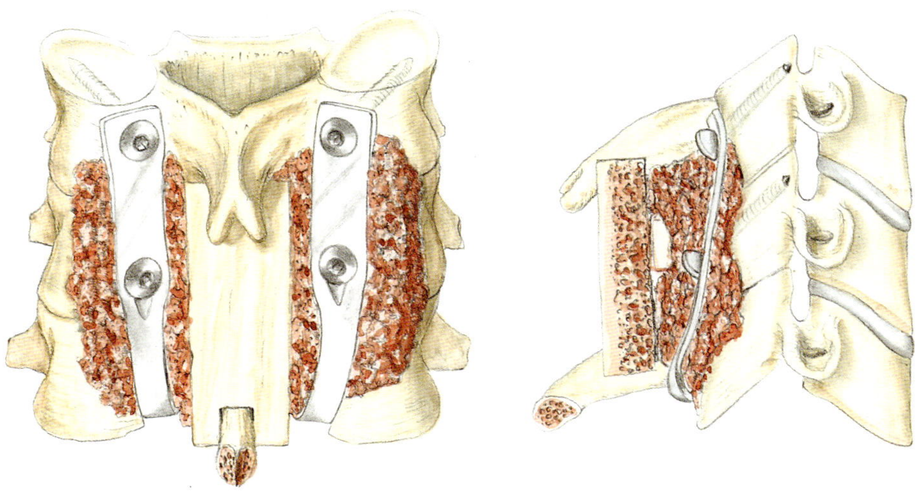

Fig. 5.**32** Example of bisegmental fusion.

Wound Closure

The wound is closed by suture of the musculature and the nuchal ligament after insertion of a suction drain.

Postoperative Treatment

For postoperative care, a semifirm plastic foam collar, to be worn for eight weeks, is sufficient and allows immediate mobilization of the patient.

Pitfalls and Complications

In the technique with a divergent screw direction, there is less risk of injury to the vertebral artery or a spinal nerve than in plate spondylodeses, in which the screws enter the lateral mass in a sagittal direction.

Breakage of the spinous process is possible if the step is made too deep or the screw is tightened excessively, and disengagement of the hook ends may also occur.

Alternative Approach

The skin incision can be made transversely at the level of the tip of the spinous process of the lowest vertebra to be accessed (Fig. 5.**21**) (better cosmetic result); further dissection is then performed in the longitudinal direction, as usual.

Alternative Methods

Fusion on the medial and lower cervical spine can also be performed with suitable straight plates using exactly the same screw channel, which diverges 30 degrees laterally and ascends cranially parallel to the joint surfaces. Such plates are appropriate if only strutting but no intervertebral pressure is to be applied, because of rupture or resection of an articular process by the implant.

Wire cerclages around the spinous processes represent the oldest form of implant. However, in the medial and lower cervical spine, they are decidedly less stable than plate fusions, because the spinous processes may easily be severed or break off.

Further Reading

Bailey RW, Bagley CE. Stabilization of the cervical spine by anterior fusion. J Bone Jt Surg 1960;42-A:565.

Caspar W. A new metal plate for stabilization of unstable fracture dislocations of the cervical spine. In: International College of Surgeons, Austrian Section, First Viennese Workshop, Vienna, October 3–6, 1982:88.

Cloward RB. Treatment of acute fractures and fracture-dislocations of the cervical spine by vertebral body fusion. J Neurosurg 1961;18:201.

Magerl F, Grob D. Dorsal fusion of the cervical spine with the hook plate. In: Kehr P, Weidner A, eds. Cervical spine. 2nd ed. Berlin: Springer, 1987.

Morscher E, Sutter F, Jenny H, Olerud S. Die vordere Verplattung der Halswirbelsäule mit dem Hohlschrauben-Plattensystem aus Titanium. Chirurg 1986;57:702.

Orozco Delclos R, Llovert Tapies J. Osteosintesis en los fracturas de raquis cervical. Rev Ortop Traumatol 1970;14:285.

Rathke FW, Schlegel KF. Wirbelsäule und Becken. In: Hackenbroch M, Witt AN, eds. Orthopädisch-chirurgischer Operationsatlas. Vol. 3. Stuttgart: Thieme, 1974.

Robinson RA. Fusions of the cervical spine. J Bone Jt Surg 1959;41-A:1.

Robinson RA, Walker E, Ferlic DC, Wiecking DK. The results of anterior interbody fusion of the cervical spine. J Bone Jt Surg 1962;44-A:1569.

Robinson RA. Anterior and posterior cervical spine fusions. Clin Orthop 1964;35:34.

Smith GW, Robinson RA. The treatment of certain cervical-spine disorders by anterior removal of the intervertebral disk and interbody fusion. J Bone Jt Surg 1958;40-A:607.

6 Fusion of the Lumbar Spine

W. Dick

Anterior Monosegmental Fusion L5–S1

Principal Indications

- Osteochondrosis L5–S1
- Spondylolisthesis L5–S1, grades I–II
- Spondylodiskitis

Approach

See Chapter 1, pp. 52–55.

Objective of the Operation

The goal is to achieve a firm osseous union, over as large an area as possible, between the fifth lumbar vertebra and the sacrum by means of a bone graft, as well as to restore the original height of the intervertebral space, which usually has been narrowed by the pathological process.

Operative Technique

Preparation of Graft Bed

Before dissection of the intervertebral space is started, radiography for identification of the lumbosacral intervertebral disk is mandatory. Orientation by palpation may be deceiving. Using a knife, the anterior longitudinal ligament is now excised over its entire width, together with the anterior portion of the annulus fibrosus (Fig. 6.**1**), and the accessible intervertebral disk tissue is removed with a rongeur. Further dissection is facilitated by inserting a laminar spreader into one half of the intervertebral space. In the other half, the two end plates are carefully dechondrified and debrided with the use of a sharp curet and chisel (Fig. 6.**2**). Posteriorly, the most posterior portion of the annulus fibrosus is preserved. It is stretched tight by the expansion. If the intervertebral space is steep, it may be necessary to chisel off the inferior anterior border of L5 to obtain access (Fig. 6.**3**). The upper plates of L5 and S1 should not be completely resected down to cancellous bone, so that the expanding graft will not penetrate into the cancellous tissue later on.

The laminar spreader is then shifted to the dissected half, and the other half is prepared in the same way.

Subsequently, the anterior border of L5 and S1 is removed with the rongeur. Here, poorly vascularized fibers entering the bone were left in place during resection of the annulus fibrosus, and should now be completely removed. Using an elevator and proceeding from the edge, the periosteum is stripped from the anterior surface of the fifth lumbar vertebra over approximately one-quarter of the vertebra's height, and the vertebral surface is debrided (Figs. 6.**4**, 6.**5**). The same procedure is applied to the anterior surface of the first sacral vertebra; as a variation, the periosteum can here be chiseled off, together with a thin bone splinter. By this means, the area available for vascularization of the graft is considerably enlarged, and a bone bridge can form over the anterior surfaces of L5 and S1 as well.

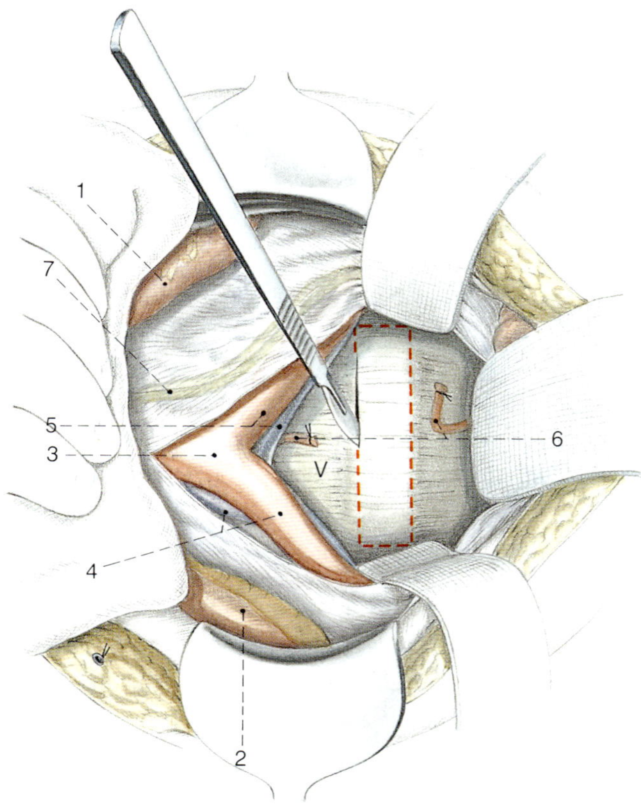

Fig. 6.**1** Resection of the anterior longitudinal ligament and of the anterior portion of the annulus fibrosus of the lumbosacral intervertebral disk.

1 Sigmoid colon
2 Ascending colon
3 Aortic bifurcation
4 Right common iliac vessels
5 Left common iliac vessels
6 Median sacral artery
7 Superior hypogastric plexus
V Lumbar vertebral body

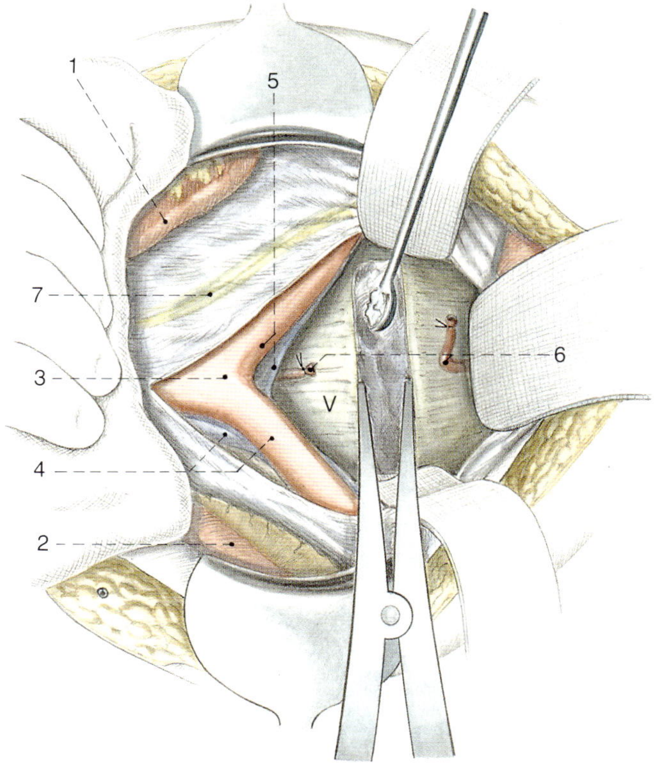

Fig. 6.**2** Dechondrification of the end plates next to the off-center spreader.

1 Sigmoid colon
2 Ascending colon
3 Aortic bifurcation
4 Right common iliac vessels
5 Left common iliac vessels
6 Median sacral artery
7 Superior hypogastric plexus
V Lumbar vertebral body

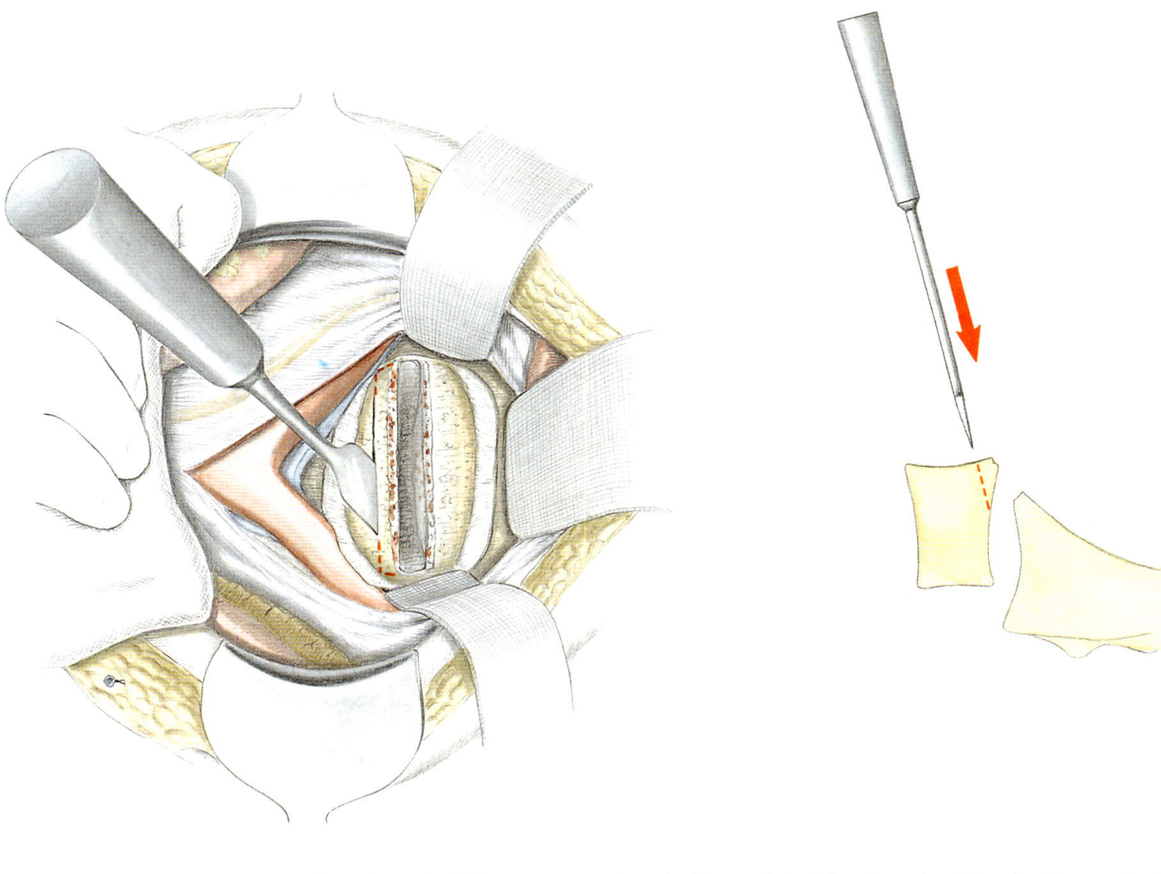

Fig. 6.**3** The inferior anterior edge of L5 is chiseled off if necessary because of a sharp rise of the end plates, in order to reach the intervertebral space; in the middle of the vertebra the subchondral bone is left in place (graft bed). The posterior portion of the annulus fibrosus, which has been tightened by the expansion, is preserved.

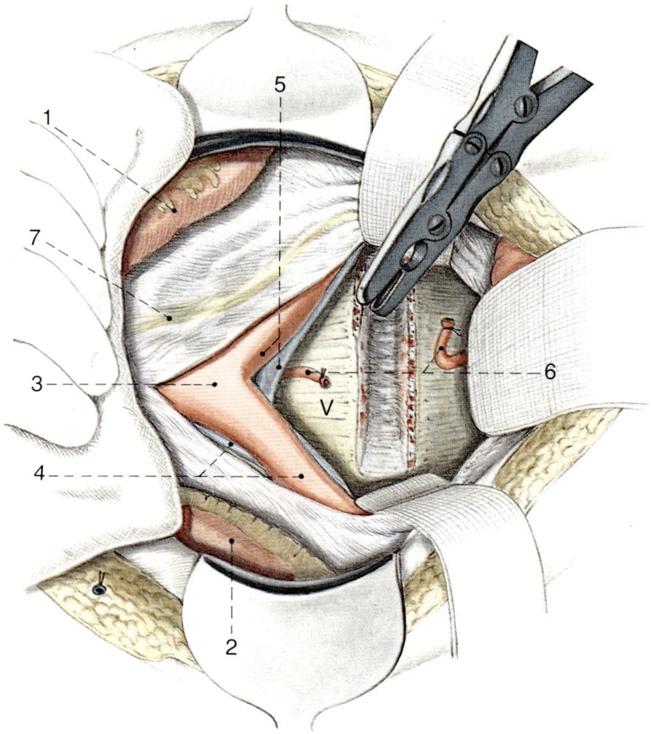

Fig. 6.**4** Removal of the remnants of the annulus fibrosus at the vertebral borders, using a rongeur.

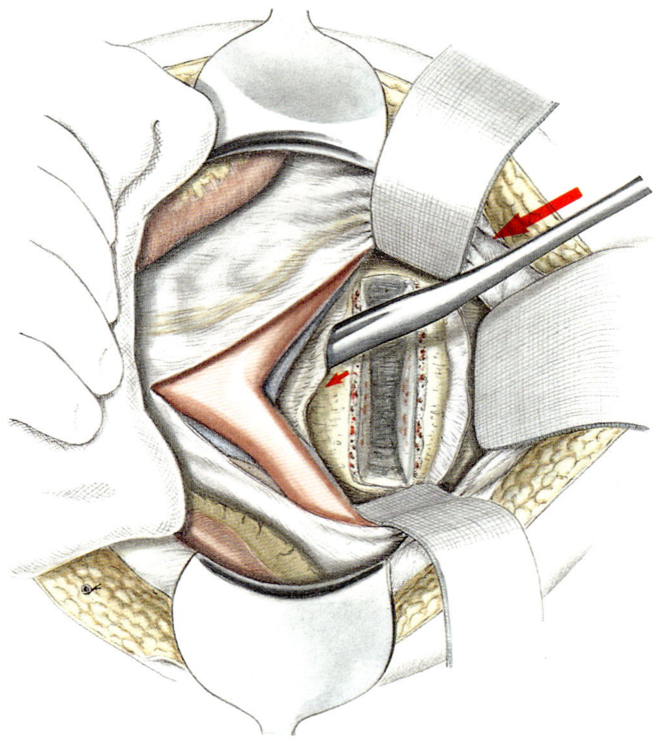

Fig. 6.**5** Debridement of the adjoining anterior wall portions of L5 and S1 by stripping the periosteum.

1 Sigmoid colon
2 Ascending colon
3 Aortic bifurcation
4 Right common iliac vessels
5 Left common iliac vessels
6 Median sacral artery
7 Superior hypogastric plexus
V Lumbar vertebral body

Graft

The following are required:

- A strong cortical or corticocancellous graft for expansion of the intervertebral space, either in the form of a homologous bank chip or as a freshly harvested autologous graft. Depending on the surgeon's perference, use can also be made of a synthetic bone substitute, provided it is sufficiently strong to withstand the compression.
- Autologous, freshly harvested cancellous bone in the form of small, thin chips or bone paste (bone mill).

The pressure-resistant graft is trimmed with a saw so that its height, depth, and shape will conform to the prepared, maximally distracted intervertebral space, and is rammed into the middle of the intervertebral space (Fig. 6.**6**). Once the spreader has been removed, the graft should be firmly wedged in with no possibility of tilting or moving; if it does not fit, its shape has to be adjusted. The free space remaining on both sides is packed with the autologous cancellous bone graft, which is compressed with a punch. The tight posterior annulus fibrosus prevents posterior penetration (Fig. 6.**7**). Finally, a layer of fine cancellous bone chips, 3–5 mm thick, is deposited anteriorly over the dissected parts of the anterior surfaces of L5 and S1, the graft, and the intervertebral space (Fig. 6.**8**). Fixation is not required; the peritoneum is closed with a running suture. After closure of the abdominal wall, the abdominal pressure holds the bone graft in place (Fig. 6.**9**).

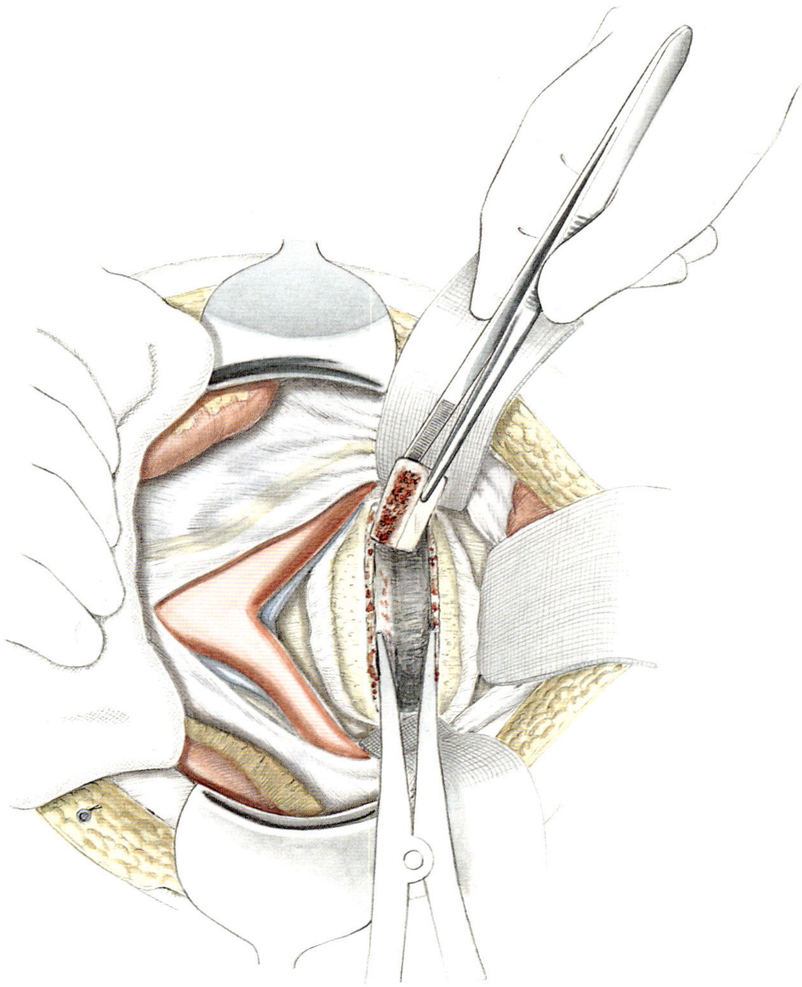

Fig. 6.**6** The trimmed, pressure-resistant graft is driven into the maximally expanded space.

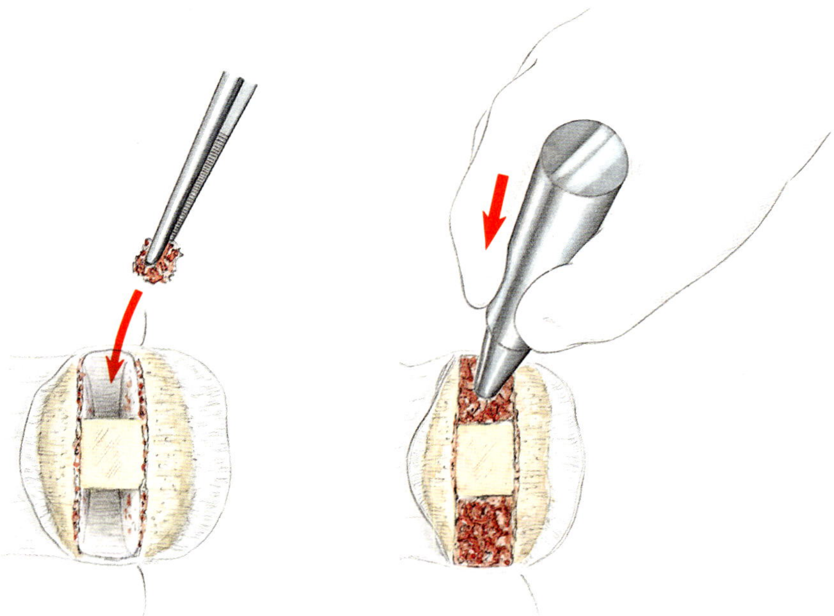

Fig. 6.**7** The remaining space is packed with autologous cancellous bone. The annulus fibrosus prevents excessive posterior penetration.

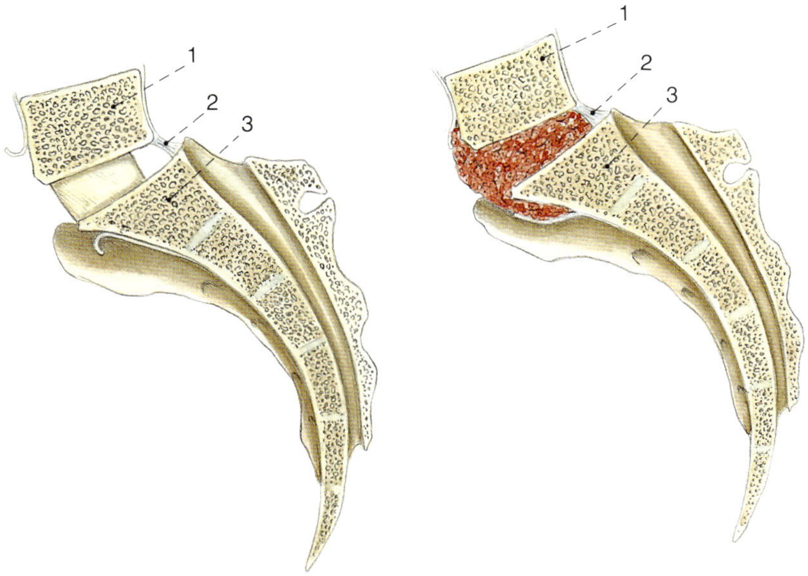

Fig. 6.**8** The debrided surface of the anterior walls of L5 and S1 are included in the fusion by application of small autologous chips or "bone paste."

1 Body of the fifth lumbar vertebra
2 Annulus fibrosus
3 Sacrum (first sacral vertebra)

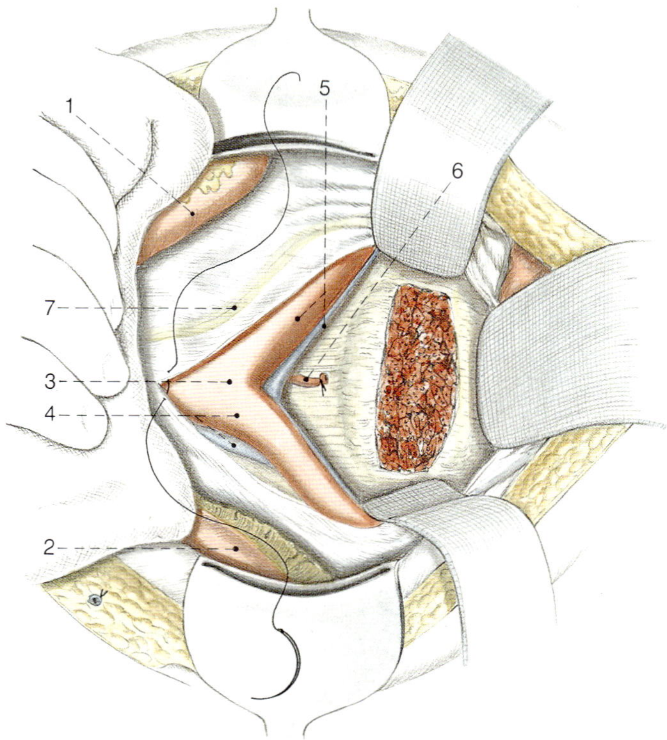

Fig. 6.**9** Completed spondylodesis. The next step is continuous suture of the peritoneum over the spondylodesis mass.

1 Sigmoid colon
2 Ascending colon
3 Aortic bifurcation
4 Right common iliac vessels
5 Left common iliac vessels
6 Median sacral artery
7 Superior hypogastric plexus

Postoperative Treatment

The patient is generally kept in bed rest without external supports, with the knees slightly supported. Only intravenous fluid substitution is advisable during the first few days, until intestinal motility is restored. The patient may be turned from side to side for nursing care. The patient is mobilized from bed with a reinforced lumbar support brace, usually after six weeks.

Pitfalls and Complications

After opening the parietal peritoneal layer, dissection of the aorta and the common right and left iliac arteries may lead to injury to the superior hypogastric plexus, particularly if the peritoneum is opened in the midline rather than on the right side as suggested. This injury may result in retrograde ejaculation in men. Another danger is ureteral injury if the dissection is extended too far laterally, as well as injury to the inferior vena cava or the common iliac veins.

Alternative Approach

The lumbosacral intervertebral disk can also be reached *retroperitoneally* from a left-sided oblique incision in the lower abdomen, as used in vascular surgery.

Anterior Monosegmental Fusion of the Other Lumbar Segments

Principal Indications

- Osteochondrosis
- Spondylodiscitis
- Spondylolisthesis

Approach

See retroperitoneal approach (caudal half) in Chapter 1, pp. 42–45.

Exposure of Vertebrae

The retroperitoneal tissue over the lumbar spine is divided in the longitudinal direction, with the sympathetic trunk being left in place laterally. Following the mandatory radiographic identification of the intervertebral disk being approached, the segmental vessels of the two corresponding vertebrae are exposed in the usual way, and are ligated and transected as far medially as possible, but not directly at the large vessels (Fig. 6.**10**). The anterior longitudinal ligament is now divided longitudinally on the side of the approach from one adjacent intervertebral disk to the other, without the latter being touched, and is then sharply lifted off the anterior surfaces of the vertebral bodies or the intervertebral disk to be resected, toward the middle of the circumference, using a knife and a dissector, so that it can be undermined and retracted with Hohmann retractors (Fig. 6.**11**). The retroperitoneal organs are protected by placing bowel towels behind the Hohmann retractors. The greater psoas muscle is freed from the intervertebral disk and retracted posterolaterally, so that the disk can be exposed as far as the intervertebral foramen (Fig. 6.**12**).

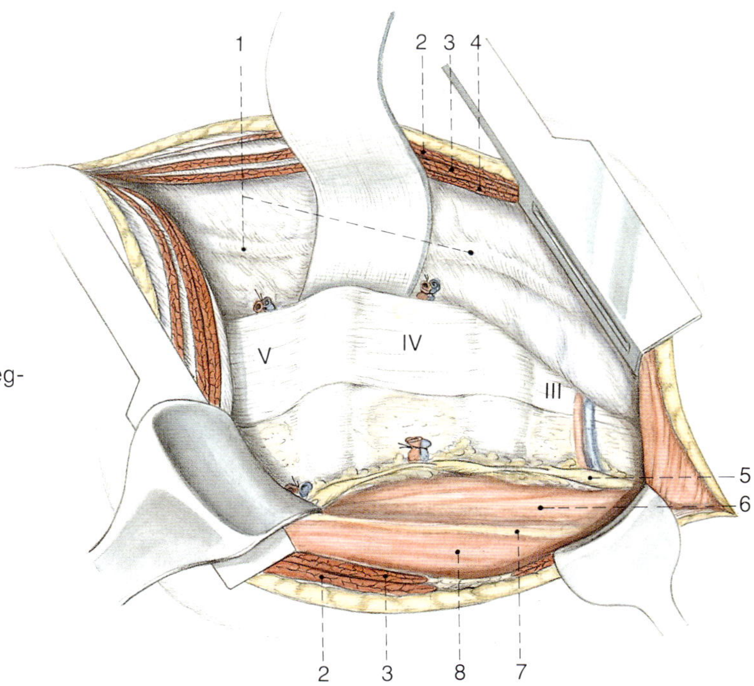

Fig. 6.**10** Exposure of the target disk (here L4–L5). The segmental vessels of both vertebrae are ligated.

1 Ureter
2 External oblique muscle of abdomen
3 Internal oblique muscle of abdomen
4 Transverse muscle of abdomen
5 Sympathetic trunk
6 Greater psoas muscle
7 Ilioinguinal nerve
8 Quadratus lumborum muscle
III–V Lumbar vertebrae

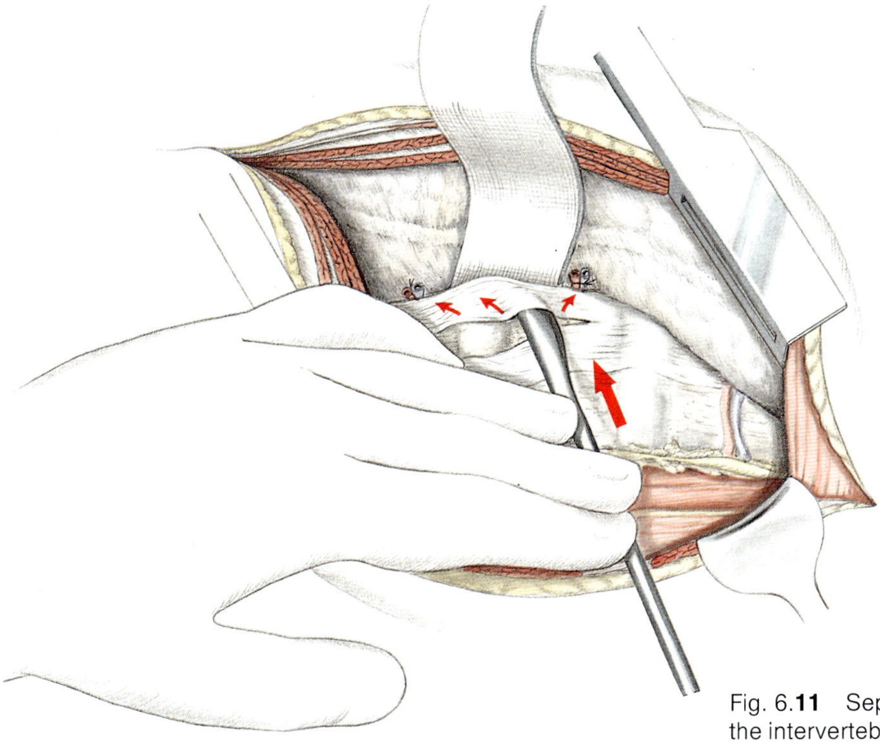

Fig. 6.**11** Separation of the anterior longitudinal ligament from the intervertebral disk and adjacent vertebral bodies. The adjacent disks must never be damaged.

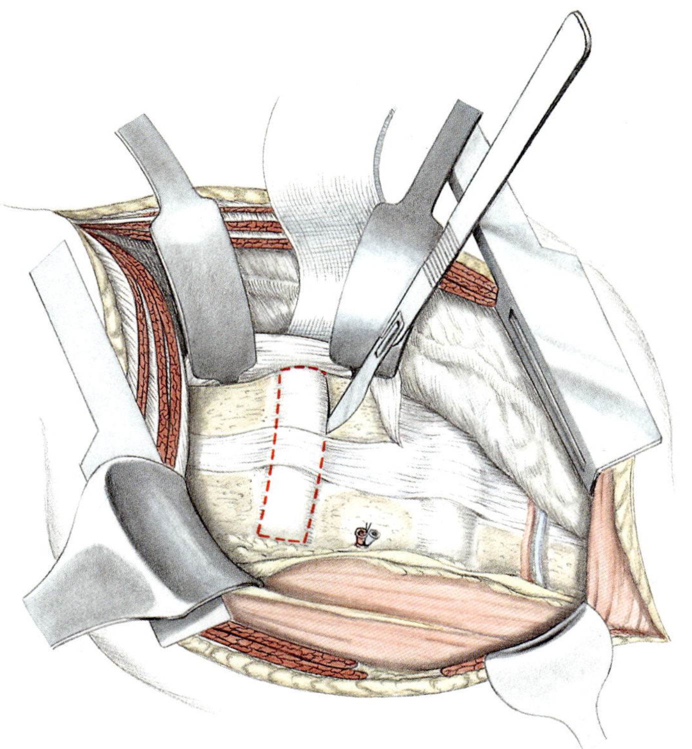

Fig. 6.**12** Lateroposterior retraction of the greater psoas muscle now exposes the entire left lateral surface and the midportion of the intervertebral disk. The annulus fibrosus in this area is resected. This is followed by dechondrification of the end plates, as shown in Fig. 6.**2**.

Objective of the Operation

The same as in lumbosacral fusion.

Operative Technique

Preparation of Graft Bed

The intervertebral disk is exposed from the left-sided intervertebral foramen to a point beyond the middle of the circumference. In this segment, the annulus fibrosus is resected with a knife (Fig. 6.**12**). The intervertebral disk is removed, and the end plates are debrided as described for the lumbosacral junction. The annulus fibrosus is left intact posterior to the spinal canal and laterally on the side opposite the dissection. In the lumbar segments, the end plates are more sharply invaginated toward the middle than they are in the lumbosacral area. It is therefore necessary to cut a groove from the side at both margins of the end plates, down to their lowest point (Fig. 6.**13**). As in the lumbosacral segment, a strong graft shaped to the maximum width of the intervertebral space is inserted, with care being taken that it extends at least to the center of the vertebra to avoid a scoliotic tilt. After removal of the spreader and straightening of the table, the graft should be solidly wedged in. The remaining fibers of the annulus fibrosus that enter at the vertebral edges are removed with the rongeur, and one-half of the left lateral surfaces of the two vertebral bodies is stripped of periosteum and debrided (Fig. 6.**14**). The free intervertebral space remaining alongside the graft can now be densely packed with finely morselized autologous cancellous bone (Fig. 6.**15**). The intrinsic cancellous bone is also inserted beneath the lifted-off anterior longitudinal ligament on the anterior side, and

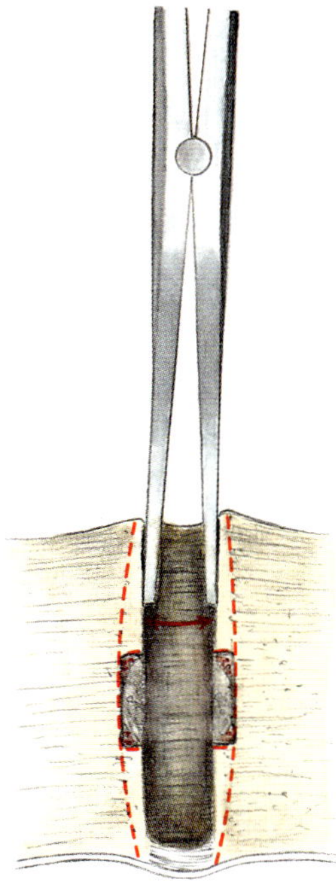

Fig. 6.**13** The sharp invagination of the end plates makes it necessary to chisel out a groove, from the side, down to the lowest point, to allow insertion of a sufficiently high graft.

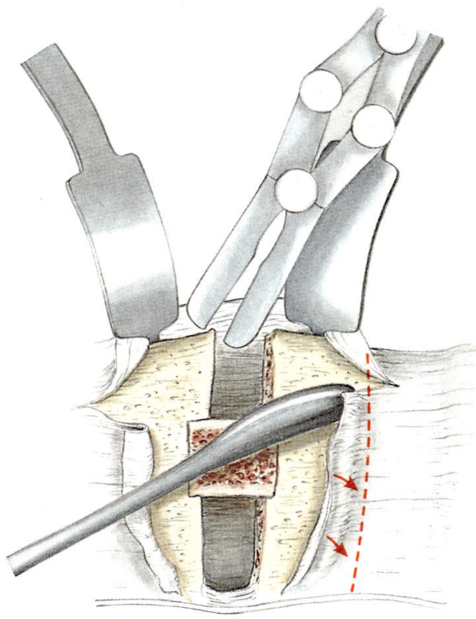

Fig. 6.**14** The trimmed, noncompressible graft, which should extend beyond the center of the vertebra, is driven in, causing expansion and lordosation. The remaining fibers at the vertebral edges are removed, and the lateral wall of the two vertebrae is debrided by denuding it of periosteum as far as the middle.

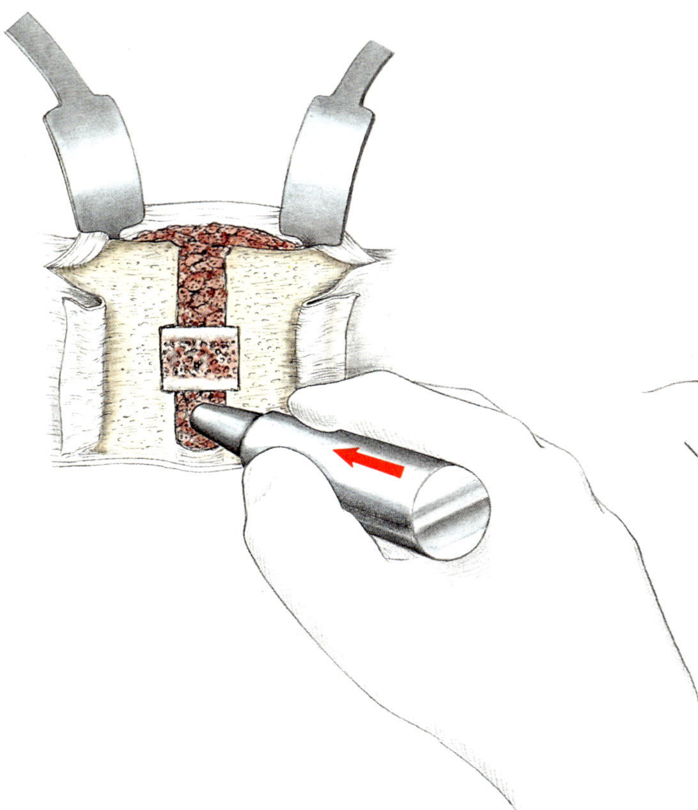

Fig. 6.**15** The remaining spaces are closely packed with small autologous bone chips. The annulus fibrosus prevents excessive penetration, in a posterior direction and toward the controlateral side.

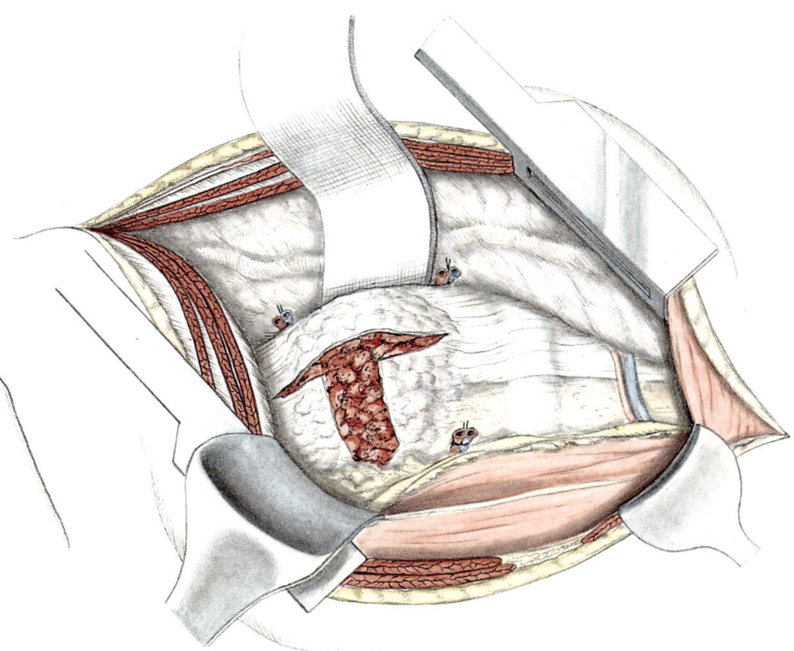

Fig. 6.**16** Completed spondylodesis. Beneath the anterior longitudinal ligament, and laterally, too, the debrided external surfaces are included in the fusion by application of small autologous bone chips (or "bone paste").

pushed laterally to the vertebral walls. Fixation is not necessary, since the relapsing peritoneal sac and the abdominal pressure will hold the graft in place (Fig. 6.**16**).

Wound Closure

Following introduction of a suction drain, the abdominal musculature, as well as the inferior posterior serratus and latissimus dorsi muscles, are closed in layers.

Pitfalls and Complications

At L5, the segmental vessels must be dissected with special care, since the venous and arterial vessels there can run a highly divergent course. Otherwise there is a danger of avulsion of the vein from its trunk. There may be epidural bleeding when the posterior portion of the annulus fibrosus is resected.

Posterior Transpedicular Stabilization Techniques

Principal Indications

- Instabilities (posttraumatic, postoperative)
- Polysegmental osteochondrosis
- Tumors and metastases
- Spondylolisthesis
- Kyphosis

Approach

See Chapter 1, pp. 68–69.

Objective of the Operation

The various procedures share the common goal of anchoring the implant so firmly—using screws are inserted from the posterior side into the vertebral bodies inside the pedicles—that sufficient stability is achieved and maintained for mobilization until consolidation of the concurrently performed bone fusion.

Operative Technique

Localization of Arch Roots

The screw entry points and alignments for the following implant systems are identical, and can be discussed together. On the lumbar vertebrae, the entry site is at the level of the center of the transverse processes of the vertebra in question, and is as lateral as the border of the cranial articular process of this vertebra (Fig. 6.**17**). The point will therefore usually lie in the sloping, oblique extensions of this articular process, so that this site should be leveled with the rongeur (Fig. 6.**18**). From this entry point, the screw should be aligned parallel to the end plate and have a 10–15 degree convergence toward the midline (Fig. 6.**17**). From the entry site, a 2-mm Kirschner wire is first drilled in at this angle to a depth of 3 cm, care being taken to ensure constant bone contact (Fig. 6.**19**).

In addition to the usual anteroposterior and lateral radiographs for determination of the segmental level, the follow-

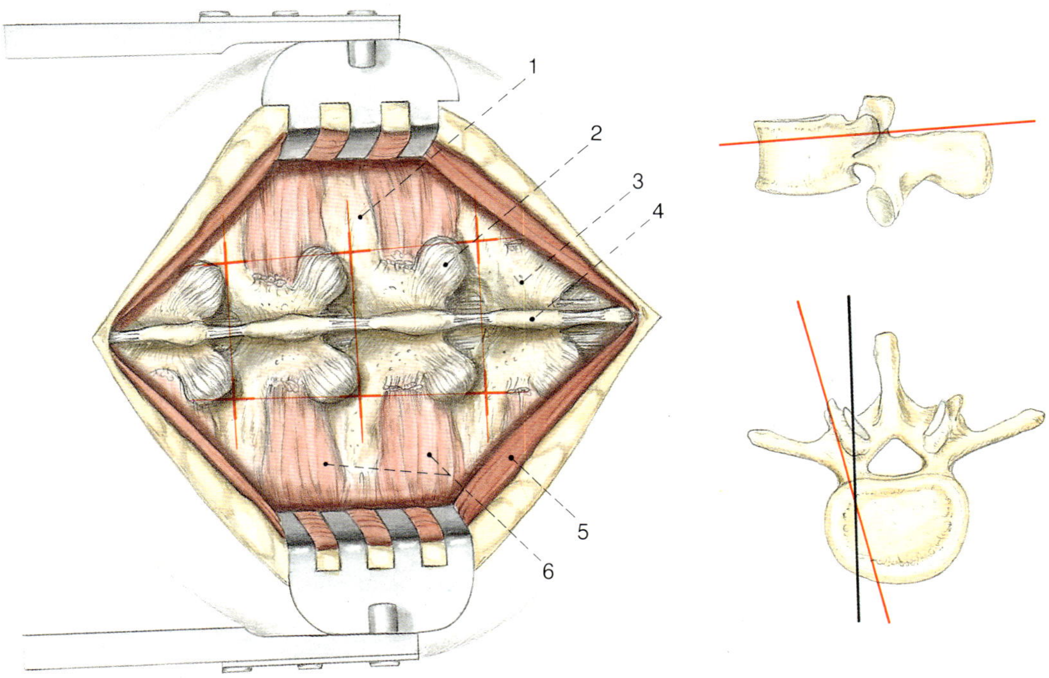

Fig. 6.**17** The entry site and drilling direction for pedicular screws at the lumbar spine in the Magerl technique.

1 Costal process
2 Zygapophyseal articulation
3 Lamina of vertebral arch
4 Spinous process
5 Longissimus muscle of the thorax
6 Multifidus muscles

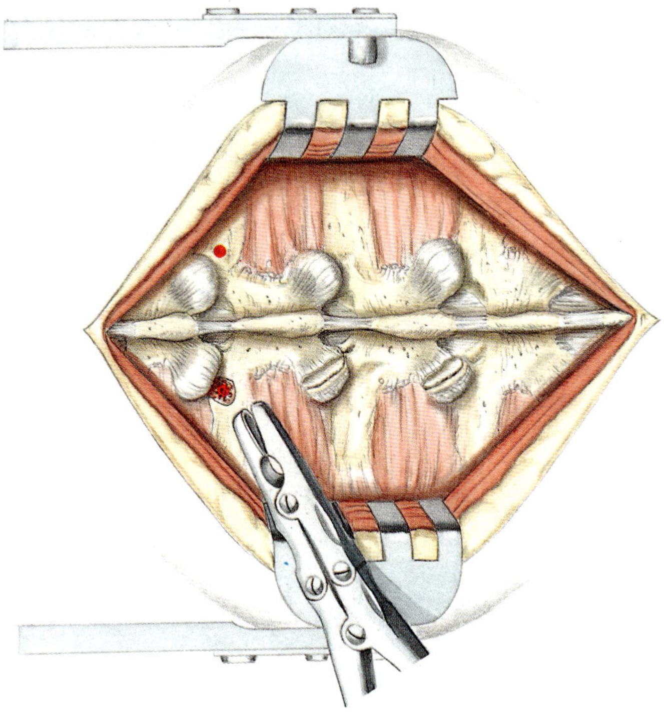

Fig. 6.**18** To prevent the Kirschner wire or the drill from sliding off the oblique surface of the base of the superior articular process, this area is leveled with a rongeur.

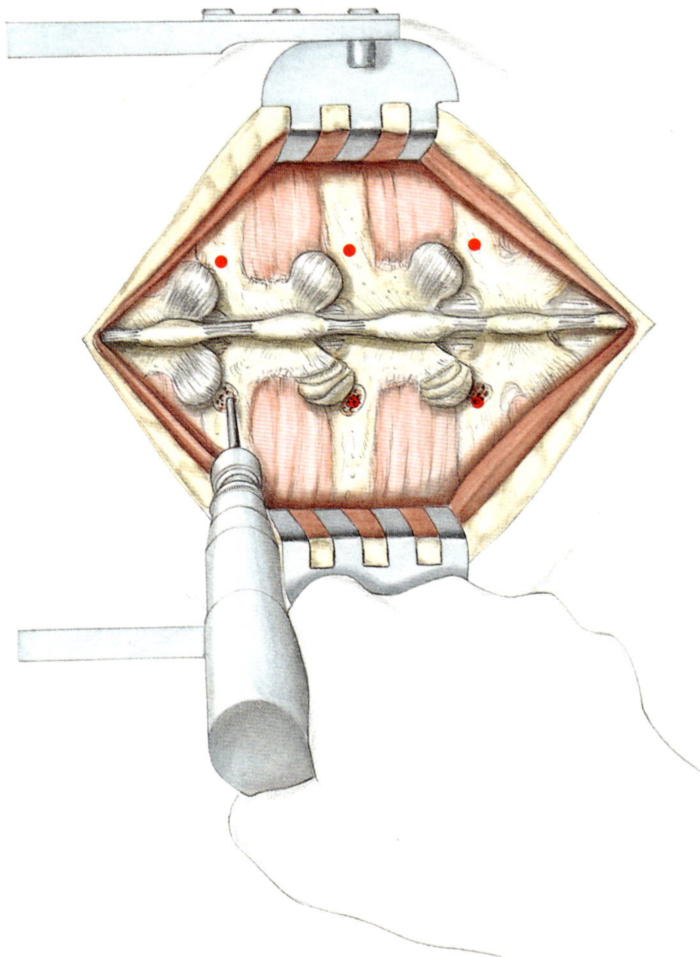

Fig. 6.**19** A 2-mm Kirschner wire is drilled in to a depth of 3 cm for image-intensifier examination.

ing method can be used to verify that the Kirschner wire is correctly positioned inside the pedicle: by slight pivoting of the tube corresponding to the convergence of the Kirschner wire, the image intensifier is brought into an exact orthograde alignment with the Kirschner wire, so that this appears as a dot in the by now readily visible oval of the arch root, if it is in the right position (Fig. 6.**20**). Later, when the drill channel has been fashioned, it is palpated for further verification with a small probe, to make certain that a bony wall is retained on all sides (Fig. 6.**25**).

Sacrum

Screws can be anchored in two directions, either converging toward the center of the promotory as above, with the depth diameter markedly smaller than in the lumbar vertebrae, or diverging laterally into the sacral alae, as shown in Figure 6.**21**.

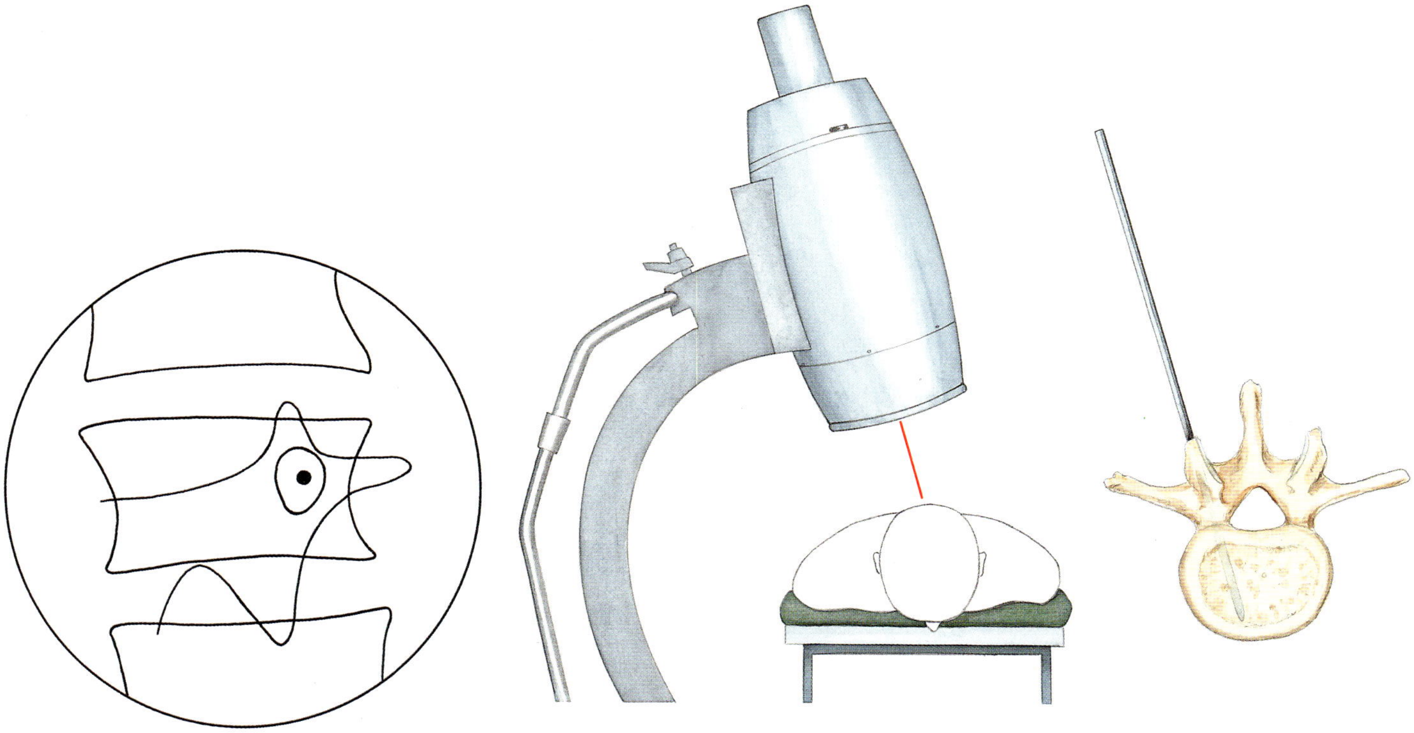

Fig. 6.**20** After exact orthograde alignment of the image intensifier with the Kirschner wire, consistent with its convergence, its position in the interior of the pedicle can be verified.

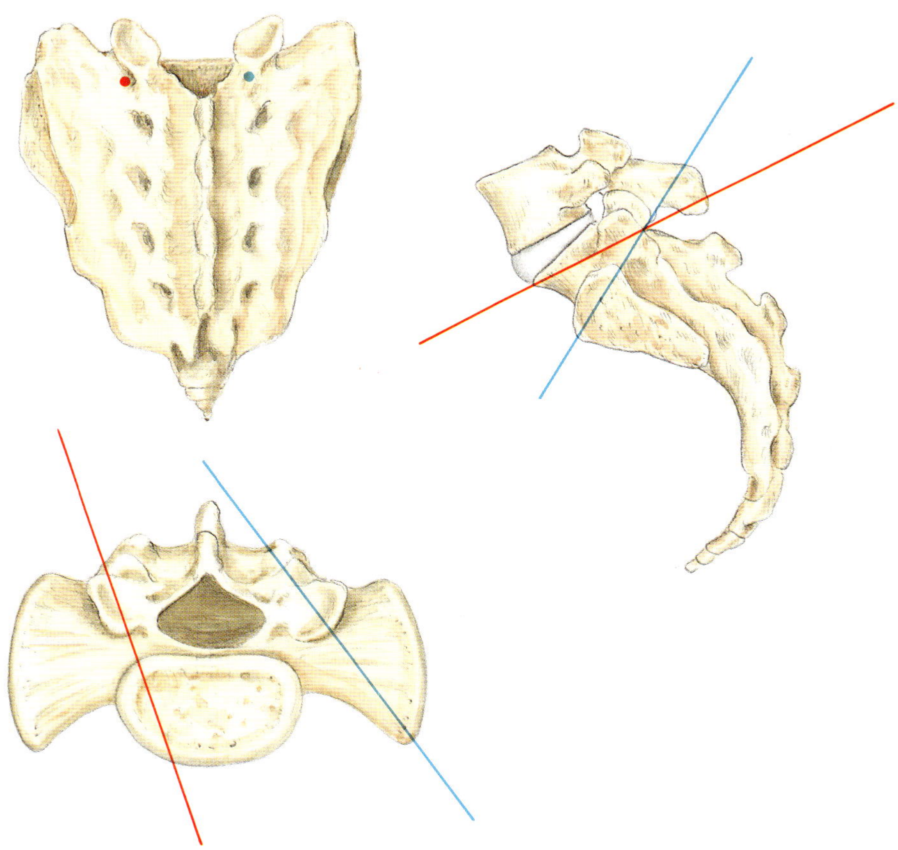

Fig. 6.**21** Possible screw fixations in the sacrum. Red line: converging toward the middle, as in the other lumbar segments. Blue line: diverging into the sacral alae.

Decortication

When the Kirschner wires are correctly positioned in all the arch roots to be instrumented, bony fusion is prepared in all the areas that will later be covered by the implant, that is, primarily at the small vertebral joints and adjacent parts of the arches. The joint capsules are resected, and the sagittally located cartilaginous joint surfaces are chiseled out and replaced by autologous bone chips. It should be borne in mind that the pair of joints directly adjoining the topmost Kirschner wires cranially belongs to the next higher motor segment, and should be preserved (Fig. 6.**22**). Decortication of the remaining parts of the arches and spinous processes, and of the transverse processes, can be delayed until after insertion of the implant in order to minimize blood loss.

If the transpedicular stabilization is necessary after a laminectomy due to stenosis of the vertebral canal, an interbody fusion can be attempted via the same approach in addition to fusion of the transverse processes. Following the usual removal of the respective intervertebral disk from

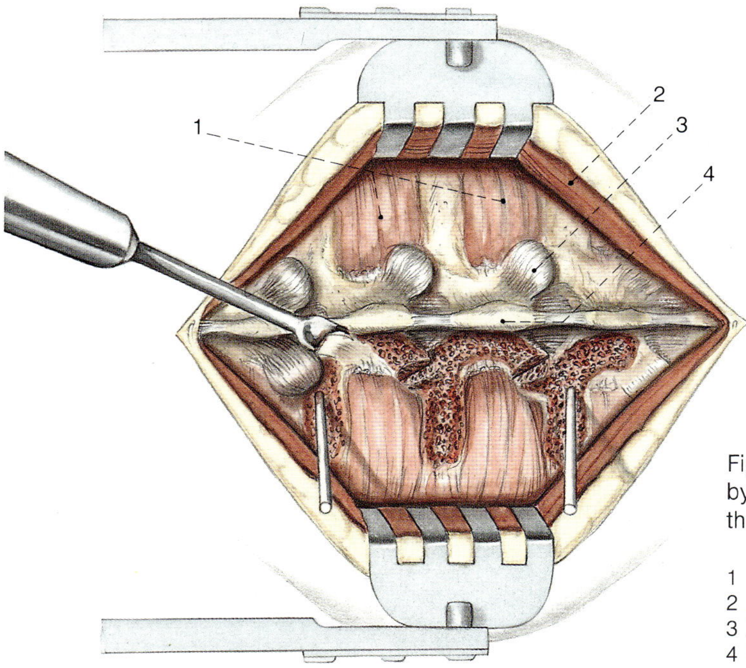

Fig. 6.**22** Preparation for fusion in segments later covered over by the implant. Resection of the joint surfaces and debridement of the adjacent arch segments.

1 Multifidus muscles
2 Longissimus muscle of the thorax
3 Zygapophyseal articulation
4 Spinous process

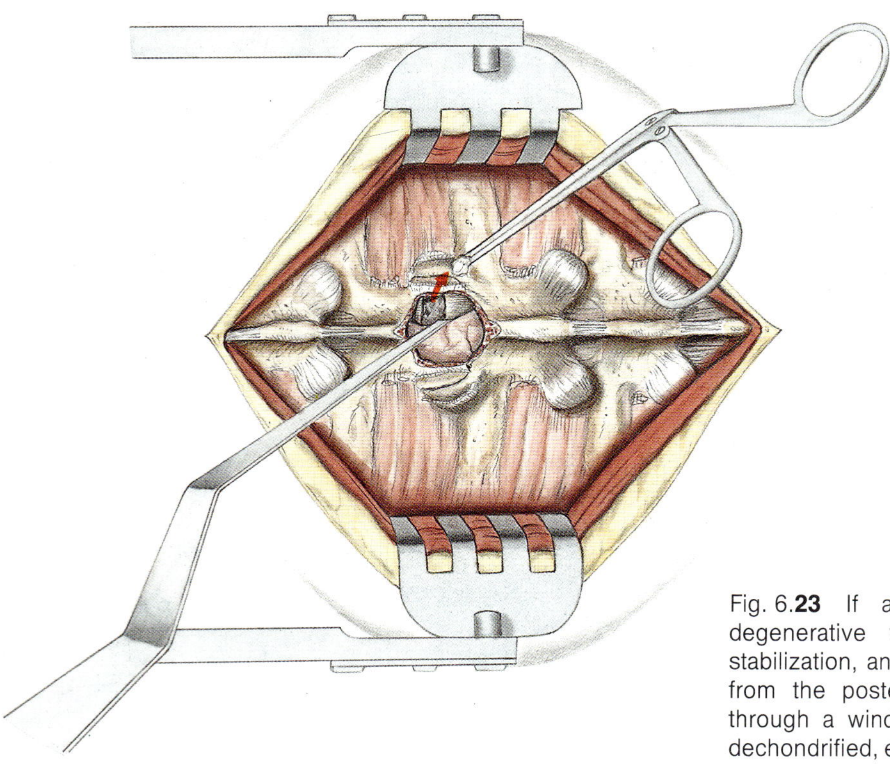

Fig. 6.**23** If an extensive decompressive laminectomy in degenerative vertebral-canal stenosis requires subsequent stabilization, an interbody spondylodesis can also be carried out from the posterior side. The intervertebral disk is removed through a window (Chapter 8). After this, the end plates are dechondrified, e.g., with an arthroscopy shaver or a sharp curet.

both sides (Chapter 8), the end plates are debrided down to bleeding bone, using a sharp curet, narrow chisel, or arthroscopy shaver (Fig. 6.**23**). Through the window in the annulus fibrosus, finely comminuted autologous bone can now be introduced from both sides into the intervertebral space and compressed with a punch (Fig. 6.**24**).

DCS Instrumentarium

Zielke's "dorsal compression spondylodesis system" (part of the universal spinal instrumentation system—Chapter 2, p. 178, Chapter 3, p. 212, and Chapter 4, pp. 230–235) consists of threaded rods and pedicular screws of various lengths, with heads that are split on top to receive the threaded rod. Cylindrical portions of the corresponding nuts on the threaded rod enter the screw head as the screw is tightened, and retain the rod firmly inside the screw head.

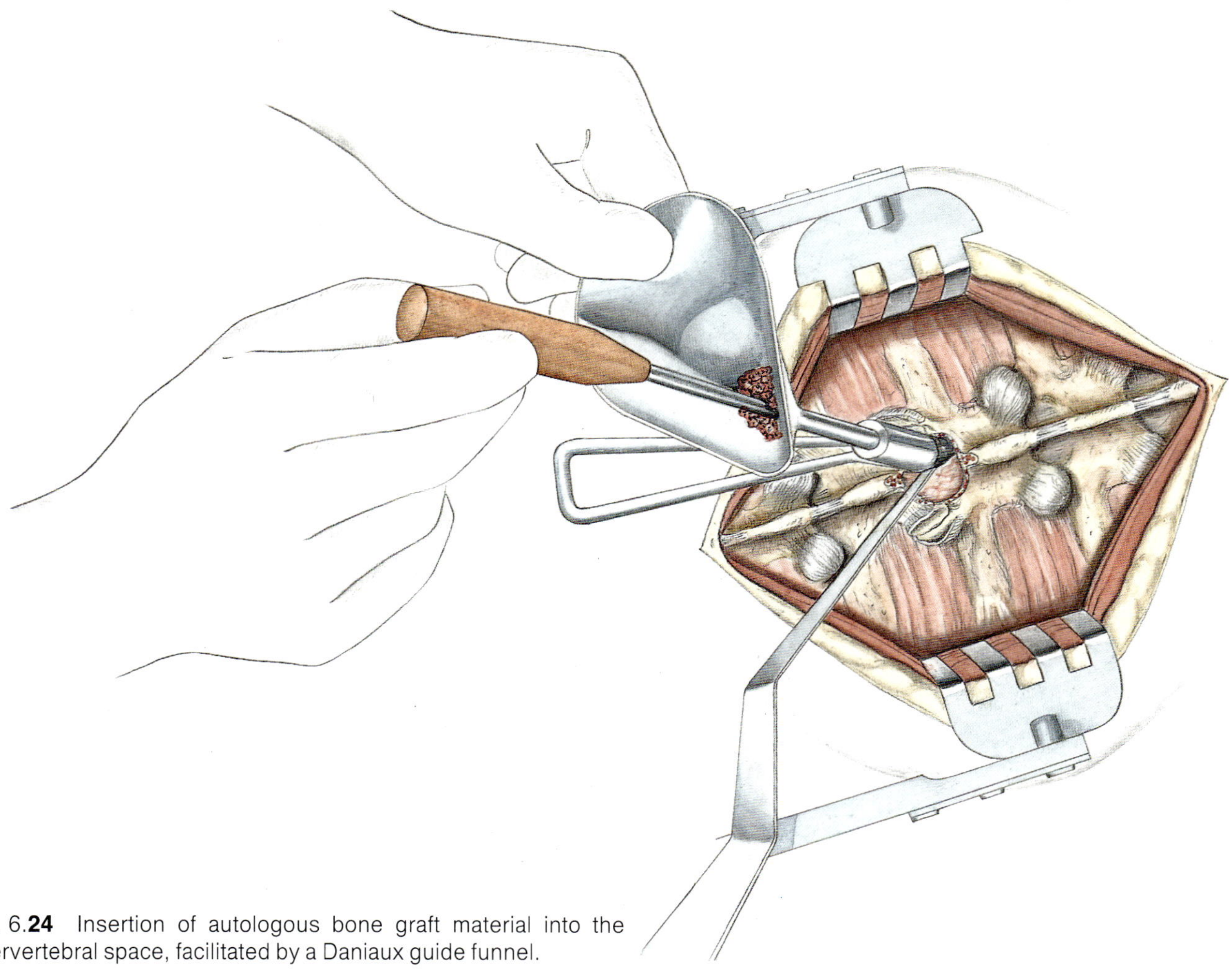

Fig. 6.**24** Insertion of autologous bone graft material into the intervertebral space, facilitated by a Daniaux guide funnel.

Mode of Action

Use is made of a tension-band implant, which in case of an instability can take the place of the lost function of the posterior articular column. A strong lordosation force can be applied around the fulcrum of the intact posterior borders of vertebral bodies (Chapter 3 and 4). In osteochondrosis, it is also possible to produce a distracting effect, but only at the price of delordosation. There is no intrinsic angular stability between the screws. The implant is preferably of a low volume.

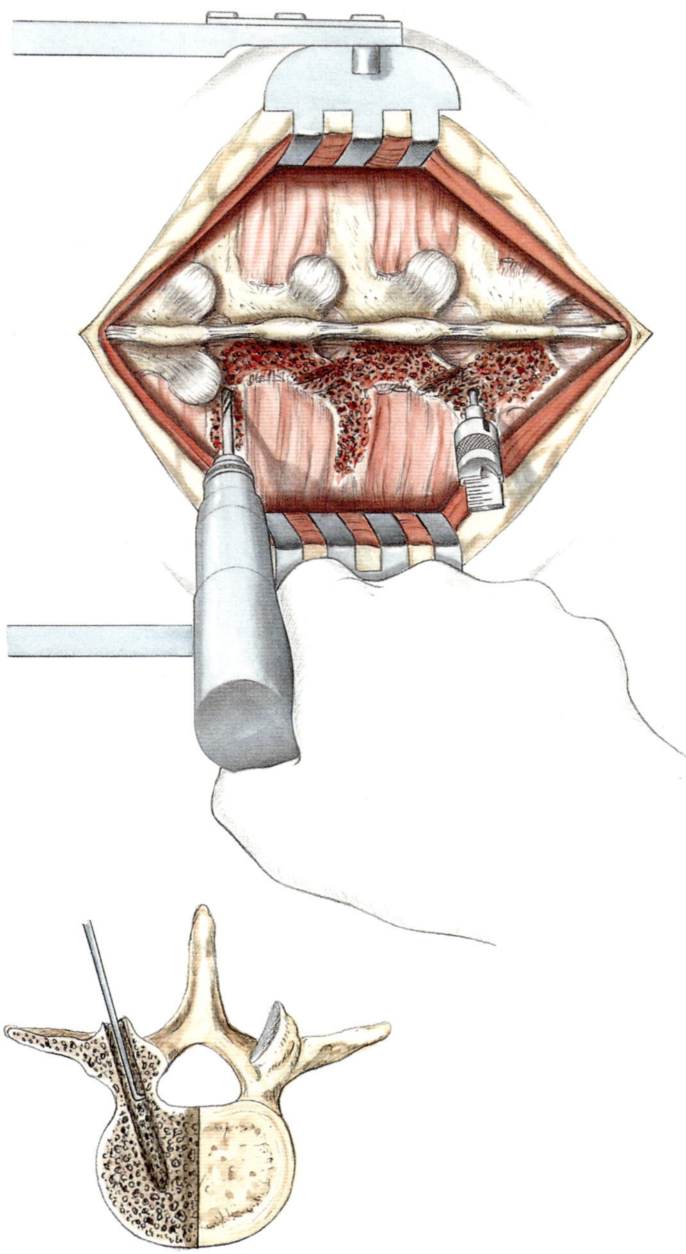

Fig. 6.**25** Drilling a screw channel in the direction of the removed Kirschner wire (Fig. 6.**27**). Using an oscillating drill proves advantageous. For safety reasons, the drill canal should be palpated with the hook of the depth gauge. If the wall shows no perforation, the position is correct; if it is not, it has to be adjusted.

Technique

The correctly placed Kirschner wires, which should be as precisely aligned in the craniocaudal direction as possible, are successively replaced by the pedicular screws, the entry sites being widened with an awl or a 3.5-mm drill. The drill channel is palpated with the hook of the depth gauge, to ascertain whether its wall is closed on all sides, meaning that its position is correct (Fig. 6.**25**). The screw can then be inserted with the special screwdriver without any pre-tapping. The screw length can be estimated by reference to the Kirschner wire during checking with the image intensifier, or by using the depth gauge in the drill canal. In the average adult patient, it is between 5 and 6 cm for the lumbar spine, and between 3 and 4 cm in the sacrum with the screw in convergent position. The threaded rod fitted with the necessary number of nut pairs is then inserted into the screw heads, and secured in the slot by approximating the nuts. In polysegmental constructs, the nuts are compressed from the middle as desired, and tightened. For this purpose, a double key which moves both nuts next to the screw head in the same direction for compression or distraction is very useful. The right and left sides are alternately, uniformly, pre-tensioned. Finally, the protruding parts of the threaded rods are clipped with rod cutters (Fig. 6.**26**).

Fixateur Interne

The fixateur interne consists of pedicular screws with a long lever, which is detached at the end of the operation and serves as a tool for reduction maneuvers. It also has longitudinal supports with an initially freely movable device for holding the pedicular screws, which can be locked after the reduction. Technical solutions for the pedicular screw–longitudinal support connection, and for separating the long lever arms, vary; Figure 6.**27** presents the model of the Swiss Osteosynthesis Association as an example.

Fig. 6.**27** Fixateur interne instrumentarium. The model of the Swiss Osteosynthesis Association is presented as example. ▸

a Mounted fixateur interne rod with universal locking plates for attachment to the pedicular screws.
b Fixateur interne rod with tension-locking plates, which can be tightened from the posterior side.
c 7-mm threaded rods of various lengths.
d 5-mm Schanz screws for transpedicular fixation.
e Universal handle for inserting Schanz screws.
f Grasping forceps for threaded tods.
h Metal-removing forceps for clipped-off Schanz screws.
i Socket wrench for tension-forceps jaw.
j Wrench.
k Bolt clipper for detachment of Schanz screw ends.

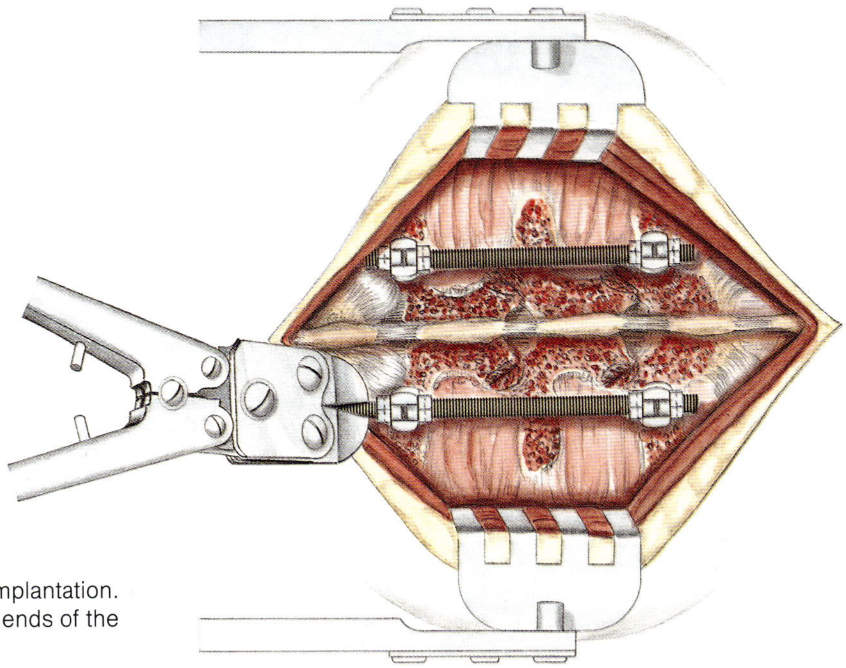

Fig. 6.**26** DCS instrumentarium (Zielke) after implantation. When all the nuts have been tightened, the protruding ends of the threaded rods are cut off.

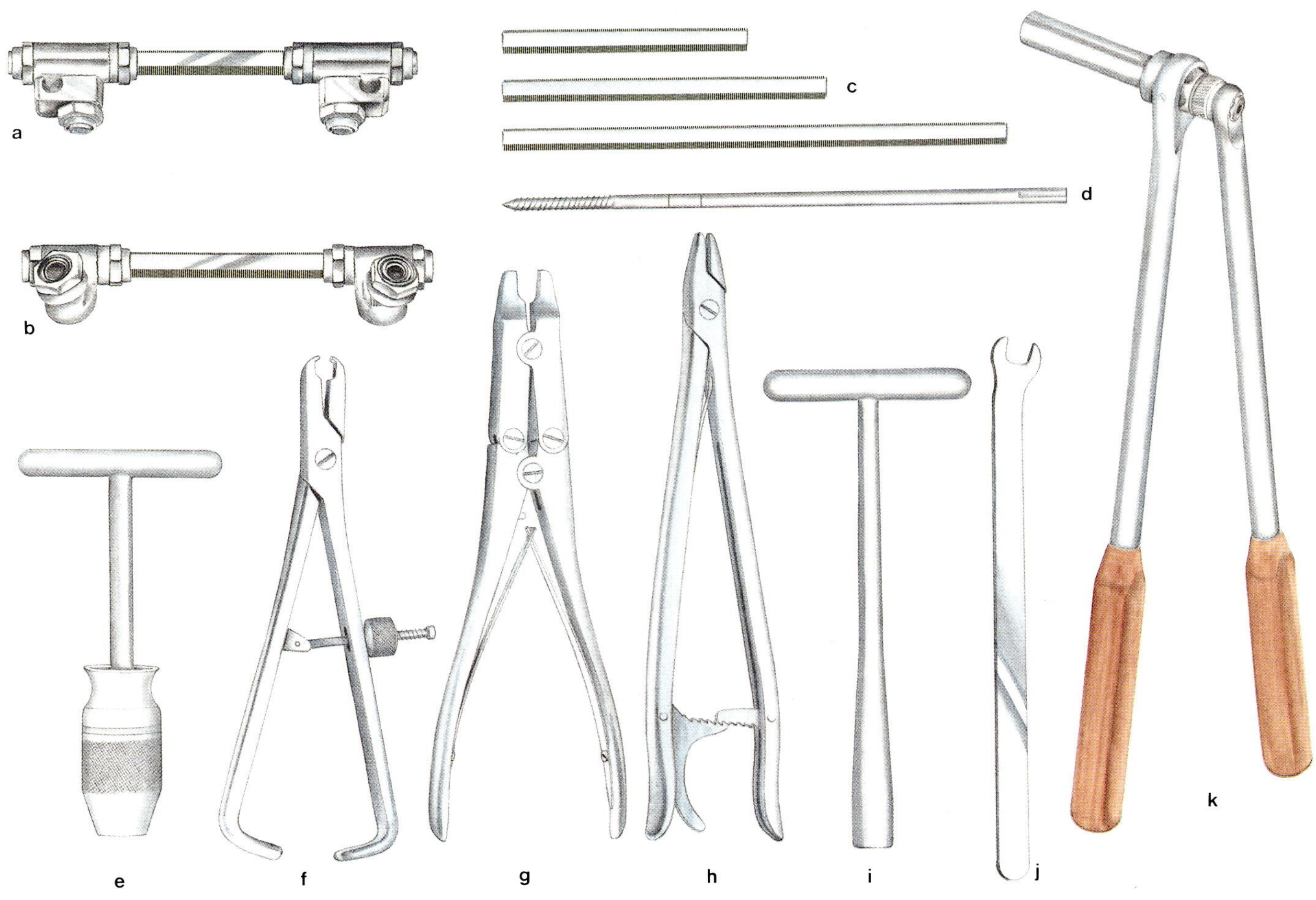

Mode of Action

Locking the holding device of the fixateur interne provides angular and rotational stability. A cross-link between the right and left longitudinal supports allows even the last degree of freedom, lateral parallel displacement, to be blocked. Apart from the screw seat, no other osseous strut points are required. Owing to the long lever arms on the pedicular screws, the fixateur interne is not only a stabilizing system, but also a reduction system. Compression, distraction, lordosation, and kyphosation can be freely combined. Monosegmental, bisegmental, or longer instrumentations, with two or more pedicular screws on each side, are possible. The implants are fairly large, depending on the design, and are, without exception, rather difficult to handle.

Assembly

The correctly placed Kirschner wires are individually replaced, in identical direction, by the pedicular screws of the fixateur, the entry points being drilled and palpated as described (Fig. 6.**25**). No pre-tapping and no further pre-drilling is needed; the screws are inserted manually with the handle. In a normal adult patient, the screw can be inserted in the lumbar spine up to a point close to the first marker (5 cm); it should not be inserted further than that without prior radiography. The longitudinal support, provided with universal locks, is then mounted on the pedicular screws in such a way that the threaded rod will lie at the spinous processes. The ensuing reduction maneuver depends entirely on the existing pathology. A general rule to be followed is that a distraction or compression should only be carried out with tightened angle locks, that is, at a fixed angle between the pedicular screws and longitudinal supports. This means that, if this is what is required, the lordosating (or kyphosating) force should always first be applied by pushing the posterior lever arms together or apart, and should then be secured by tightening of the rod locks (Fig. 6.**28**). Only then is the desired distraction (e.g., for restoration of the original height of fused intervertebral spaces) produced with the distraction nuts (Fig. 6.**29**). Finally, the counternuts are tightened on the rod. Since the angular stability depends on permanently firm seating of the nuts, these are protected against spontaneous loosening by pressing the nut rim into a depression on the threaded bolts and threaded rods. The depression on the longitudi-

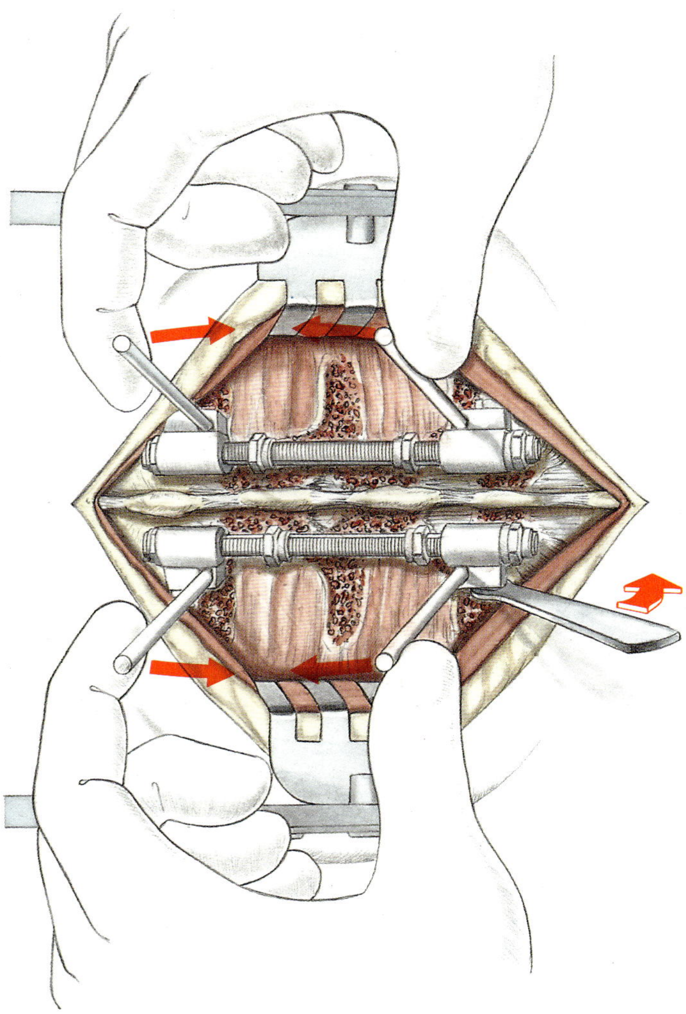

Fig. 6.**28** Adjustment for the desired lordosis by compressing the ends of the Schanz screws. This position is maintained by tightening the lateral nuts on the clamp-lock elements.

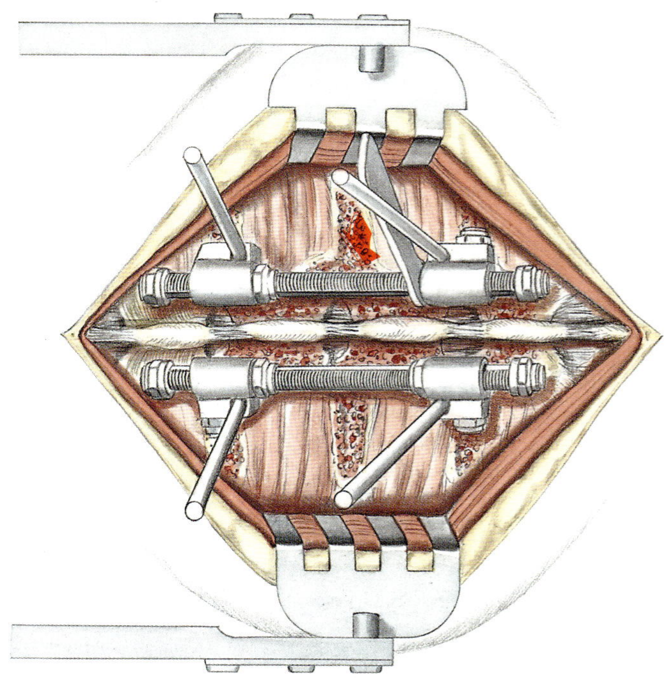

Fig. 6.**29** Parallel distraction with the aid of distraction nuts at a fixed angle between the Schanz screws and the longitudinal rod. The depression in the threaded rod first has to be aligned sagittally.

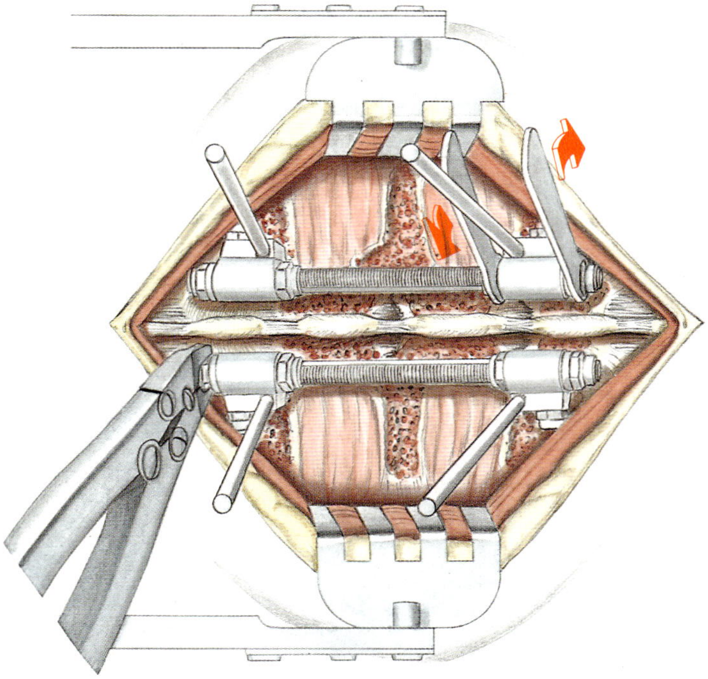

Fig. 6.**30** At the conclusion of the assembly, the counternuts are tightened and secured against spontaneous loosening by compressing the nut rim.

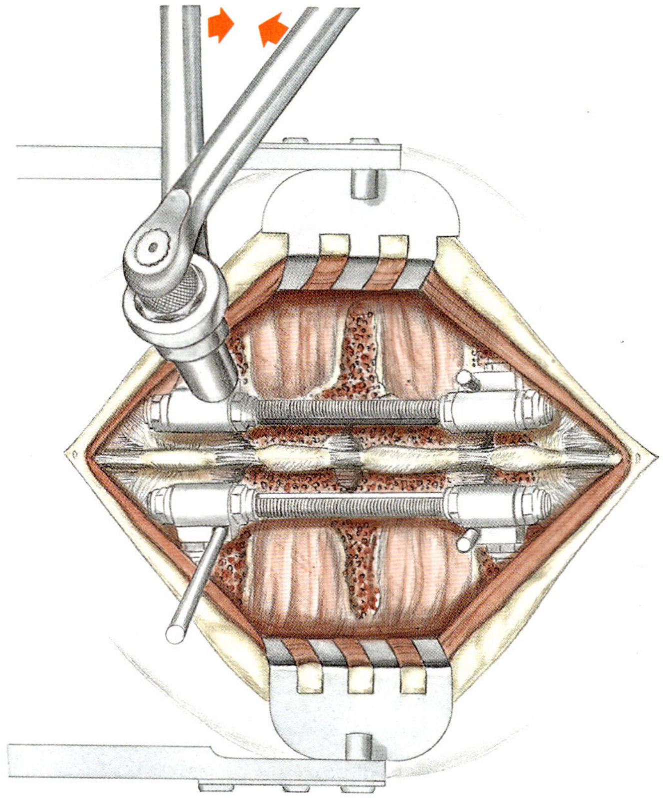

Fig. 6.**31** The protruding Schanz screws are cut off with the bolt clipper.

nal supports should be produced first in the sagittal direction; on the threaded bolts of the angle locks, it automatically runs perpendicularly (Fig. 6.**30**). The protruding lever arms of the pedicular screws are then cut off with a special bolt clipper (Fig. 6.**31**).

Posterior Spinal Plate

Spinal plates for transpedicular fixation take account of the average pedicle distance through the intervals between holes. Every other hole receives a pedicular screw, while the intermediate holes can be used, if warranted, for screw fixation of the articular masses. As a rule, therefore, plates with an uneven number of holes are used (Fig. 6.**32**).

Mode of Action

Biomechanically, the plate represents a three-point fixation system in which an anteriorly-directed pressure is exerted on the arch through the middle of the plate, while at the ends, the screws move the arches close to the plate by posterior traction. Thus, the extent of lordosis can be freely chosen for the fusion by appropriate pre-bending of the plates. Plate osteosyntheses should therefore be performed over at least three, but generally five, vertebrae. This form of stabilization has shown the greatest rigidity in experiments. The plates are not very voluminous, but they do limit the room available for osseous fusion to some extent.

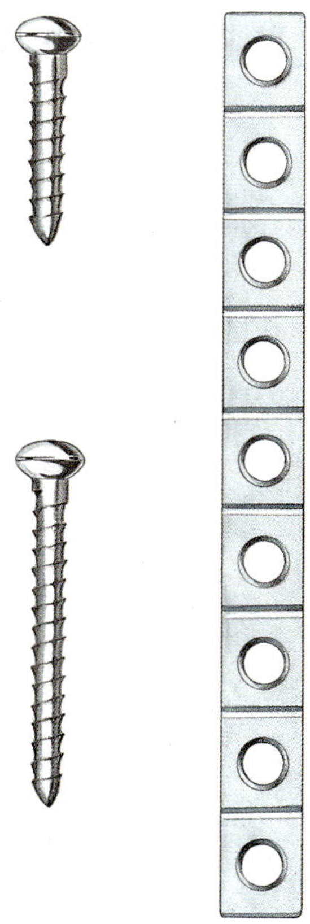

Fig. 6.**32** Posterior spinal plates for fixation to the pedicles.

Assembly

For plate osteosyntheses, only Kirschner wires are initially applied to the two end vertebrae, and then evaluated. When the posterior joints are being prepared for fusion, the highly prominent articular processes on the lumbar spine have to be considerably reduced in height with a chisel or heavy rongeur to give the plate better support (Fig. 6.**33**). The Kirschner wires are individually removed, and the screw holes are drilled in identical direction with a 3.2-mm drill. The drill canal is tested by palpation (Fig. 6.**25**). A screw length of 5 cm can be expected for the lumbar spine of an adult. Only the contex is tapped at the screw entry; after this, the pre-bent plate (Fig. 6.**34**) is fixed at its terminal holes with one screw each, but is not as yet maximally tightened (Fig. 6.**35**). Using the drill guide to center the drill point in the hole after the next, screw holes are now made in the adjacent pedicles (Fig. 6.**36**). The screwdriver applied to the end screws shows the direction in terms of convergence. When all the screws have been placed, they are alternately tightened step by step (Fig. 6.**37**).

Note
In cases of severe osteoporosis, cancellous screws, which have a wider thread, can be used instead of cortical screws.

Decortication

After completion of the construction, the remaining portions of the arches, spinous processes, and transverse processes are decorticated and packed with autologous cancellous bone chips, just as in any scoliosis operation.

Wound Closure

The laterally retracted intrinsic musculature of the back is folded back in place over the implant and the spondylodesis bone grafts. Deep suction drains are applied bilaterally. The fascia is sutured and reattached to the spinous processes.

Postoperative Treatment

The patient is positioned in bed without external supports. A neurological assessment is made immediately after the operation, followed by regular monitoring later. The patient is mobilized 3–7 days later, with or without a lumbar spine orthosis, depending on the underlying disease, the stability of the construct, and the patient's reliability.

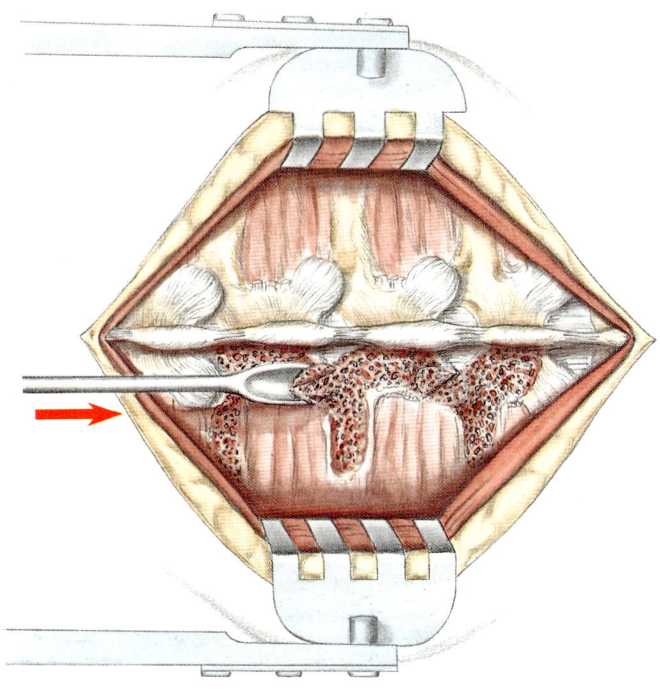

Fig. 6.**33** The highly prominent articular processes in the lumbar region are partly chiseled off to achieve a better plate seat.

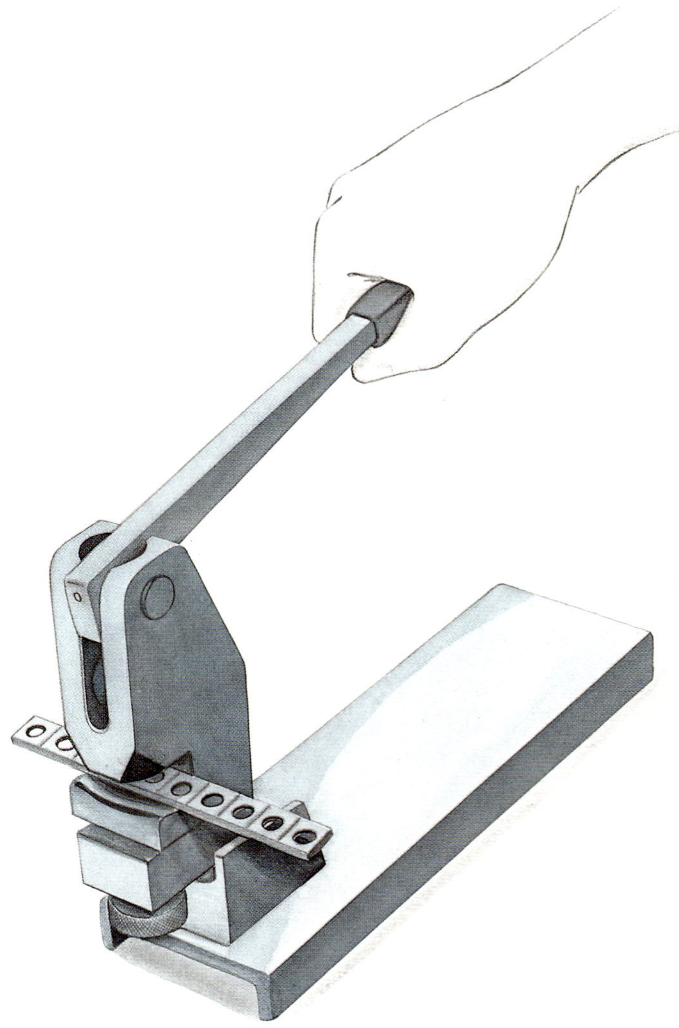

Fig. 6.**34** The plate is pre-bent in accordance with the desired lordosis.

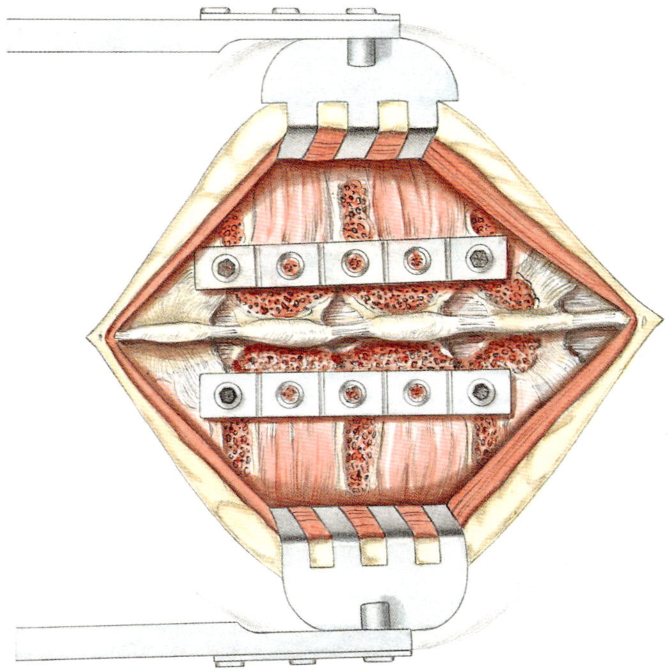

Fig. 6.**35** The plate is first fixed with the end screws, which are not tightened too much.

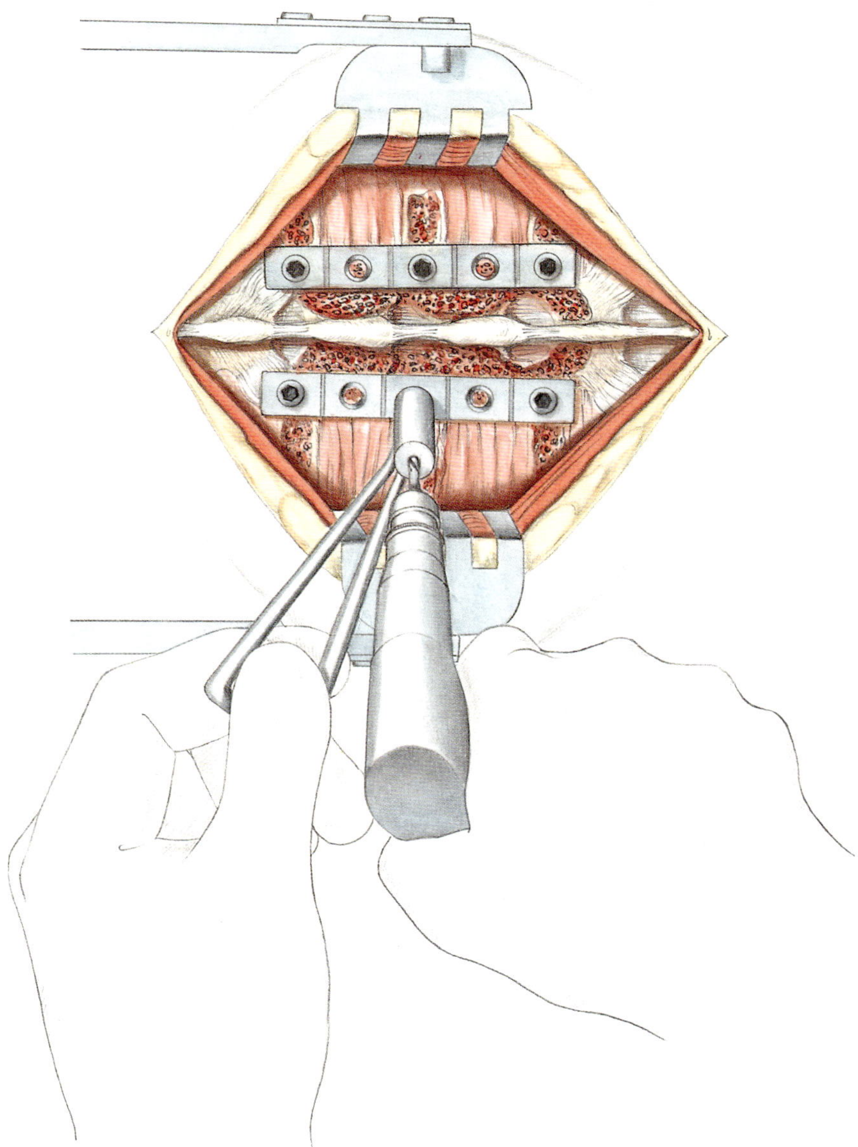

Fig. 6.**36** Using a securely mounted drill guide which centers the drill, screw holes are produced in the intermediate vertebrae through the corresponding plate hole.

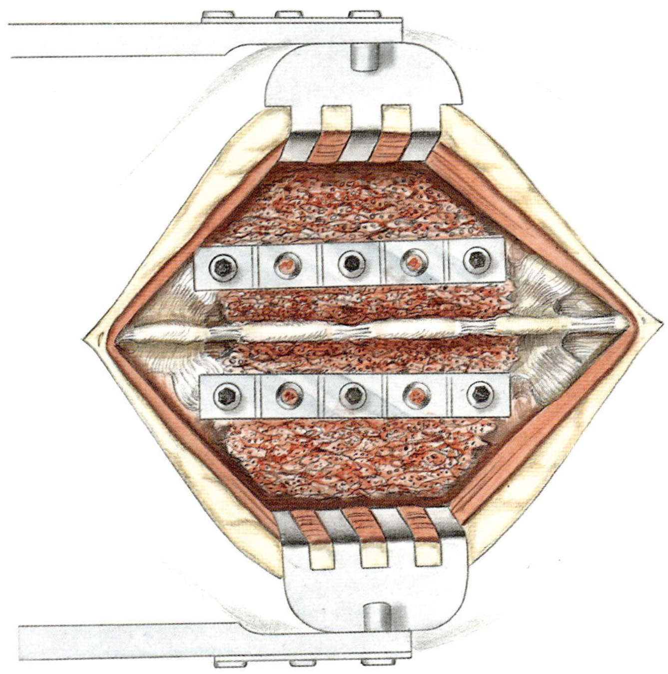

Fig. 6.**37** Completed plate osteosynthesis. At the end, the remaining portions of the arches and the spinous and transverse processes are decorticated and overlaid with autologous bone chips.

Pitfalls and Complications

The risk specific to this operation is misplacement of the pedicular screws, which can lead to root injury in the lumbar region if the screw is wrongly placed caudally to the pedicle, or medially. An excessively lateral or inadequately convergent screw position results in a reduction of stability (screw exit lateral to the vertebral body). Experience has shown that the position is rarely unduly cranial. No statistical data are as yet available about root lesions due to pedicular screws in the lumbar region. Slippage of the drill or awl, and deep penetration lateral to the vertebral body, can cause injury to the anterior vessels.

In all systems, the screw length has to be selected and verified radiographically. Perforation of the anterior vertebral wall by a long screw is not necessarily felt by the surgeon; an anterior vascular injury due to protruding screw tips is conceivable, but has not been reported thus far (1990).

Note
The above description is not sufficient for the treatment of *fractures*. The literature should be consulted on this topic.

Posterolateral Fusion of the Lumbosacral Junction (Wiltse)

Indications

- Spondylolisthesis
- Degenerative segmental instability

Approach

See Chapter 1, p. 70..

If a midline scar from previous operations is present, it can be used instead of the two paramedian skin incisions. Subcutaneously, the thoracolumbar fascia is then exposed on both sides, and its outer third divided longitudinally.

Even in patients who have not had a previous operation, Wiltse has recommended the midline skin incision for the posterolateral approach since 1988.

Operative Technique

The transverse process of L5 is debrided on its posterior surface by retracting the periosteum, and at its cranial and caudal edges by sharp dissection of the soft tissues. The capsule of the L4–L5 vertebral joint is retained, but the lateral surface of the cranial articular process of L5 can readily be included in the fusion by debridement (Fig. 6.**38**). At the sacral ala, a cranially-based lid can be lifted off with a chisel and reflected upward, so that it will rest on the transverse process of L5 and thus protect the anteriorly coursing root of L5.

Beside this graft, the thick cranial surface of the ala in particular is decorticated. The lamina of L5 and the sacral base are likewise debrided.

The iliac crest is visible at the lower edge of the approach, and can serve for harvesting of bone chips. The stripping of soft tissues for subperiosteal exposure of the external surface should not be extended more than four fingerbreadths lateral to the posterior superior iliac spine, so as to avoid injury to the sensitive cutaneous branches L1–L3 (Fig. 6.**39**). Corticocancellous and cancellous graft material can now be harvested. The quantity collected from one side is usually sufficient for bilateral fusion.

The resection gap between the L5–S1 articular processes is packed with bone graft; lengths of graft are placed from the transverse process and from the outside of the cranial articular process of L5 to the sacral ala, and from the lamina of L5 to the arch of S1 (Fig. 6.**40**).

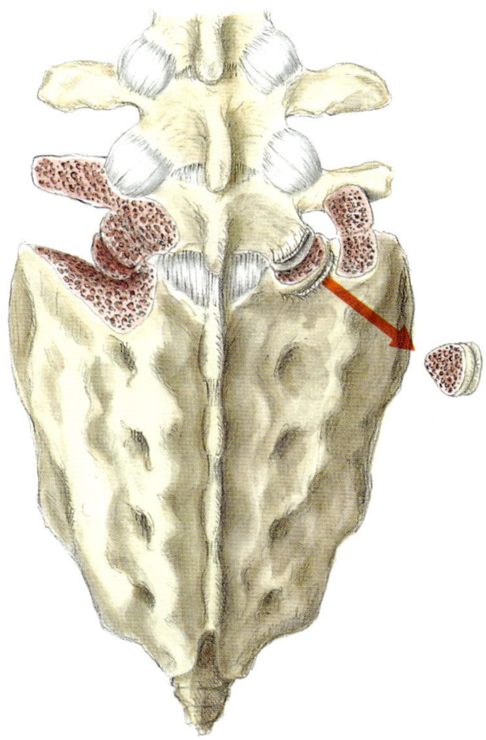

Fig. 6.**38** The marked areas of L5 and S1 in the left part of the figure are decorticated in preparation for fusion, and the L5 S1 joint surfaces are resected. Proceeding from the sacrum, a flat, based lid can also be lifted off and reflected upward onto the L5 transverse process (on the right).

Wound Closure

Following insertion of a suction drain, wound closure is effected by suture of the erector muscle of the spine and the overlying fascia.

Postoperative Treatment

The patient is positioned in bed without external support. A neurologic assessment is made immediately after the operation, followed by the usual monitoring later on. After 3–5 days, the patient can be mobilized with a lumbar cloth orthosis jacket, which can be taken off after eight weeks.

Pitfalls and Complications

Too deep a dissection between the sacral ala and the costal process of L5 can lead to injury to the fifth lumbar spinal nerve.

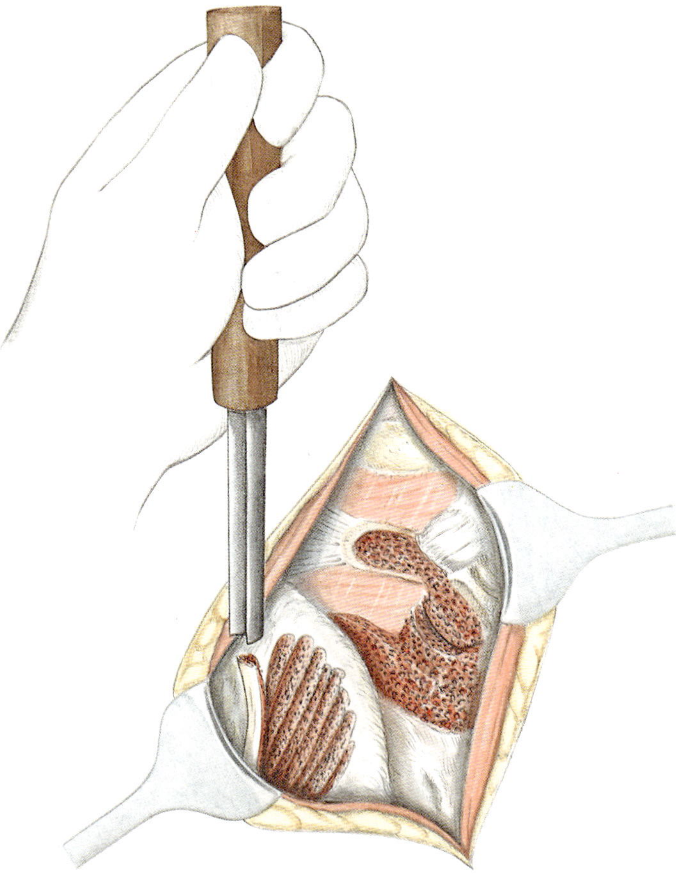

Fig. 6.**39** Bone graft is harvested from the iliac crest via the same approach. Soft tissue is stripped from the posterior superior iliac spine no farther than four fingerbreadths laterally.

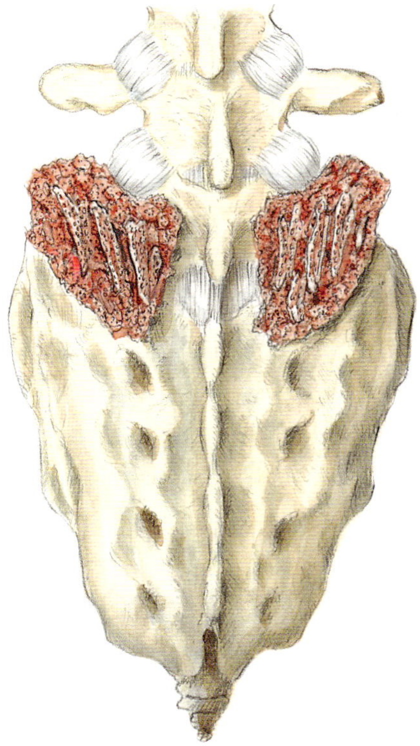

Fig. 6.**40** The completed Wiltse posterolateral lumbosacral spondylodesis.

Alternative Methods

Anterior interbody spondylodesis; posterior implant fixation using pedicular fixation systems (plate, fixateur interne).

Further Reading

Daniaux H. Transpedikuläre Reposition und Spongiosaplastik bei Wirbelkörperbrüchen der unteren Brust- und Lendenwirbelsäule. Unfallchirurgie 1986;89:197.

Dick W. Innere Fixation von Brust- und Lendenwirbelfrakturen. 2nd ed. Berne: Huber, 1987.

Dick W. Interkorporelle Spondylodese L4/L5 und L5/S1. Operat Orthop Traumatol 1989;1:43.

Freebody D, Bendall R, Taylor D. Anterior transperitoneal lumbar fusion. J Bone Jt Surg 1971;53-B:17.

Harmon PH. Anterior extraperitoneal lumbar disk excision and vertebral body fusion. Clin Orthop 1960;18:169.

Kluger P. Das Fixateurprinzip an der Rumpfwirbelsäule. In: Stuhler T, ed. Fixateur externe – Fixateur interne. Berlin: Springer, 1989.

Louis R. Chirurgie du rachis. Anatomie chirurgicale et voies d'abord. Berlin: Springer, 1982.

Magerl F. Der Wirbel-Fixateur externe. In: Weber BG, Magerl F, eds. Fixateur externe. Berlin: Springer, 1985.

Rathke FW, Schlegel KF. Wirbelsäule und Becken. In: Hackenbruch M, Witt AN, eds. Orthopädisch-chirurgischer Operationsatlas, Vol. 3. Stuttgart: Thieme, 1974.

Roy-Camille R, Saillant G, Berteaux D, Salgado V. Osteosynthesis of thoracolumbar spine fractures with metal plates screwed through the vertebral pedicles. Reconstr Surg Traumatol 1976;15:2.

Wiltse LL. The paraspinal sacrospinalis-splitting approach to the lumbar spine. Clin Orthop 1973;91:48.

Wiltse LL, Spencer CW. New uses and refinements of the paraspinal approach to the lumbar spine. Spine 1988;13:696.

Zielke K. Ventrale Derotationsspondylodese. Behandlungsergebnisse bei idiopathischen Lumbalskoliosen. Z Orthop 1982;120:320.

7 Spondylolisthesis

R. Louis

Reconstruction of the Isthmus (Pars Interarticularis)

Principle

The defect is bridged like a pseudarthrosis, with micromovements blocked by internal fixation.

Indication

Patients who are in pain despite conservative therapy, and who wish to continue their occupational and sports activities. The subjacent disk should be intact; that is, there should be no spondylolisthesis of more than 5 mm, and the disk height should not be reduced by more than one-third. The operation is performed mainly in young patients between the ages of 10 and 45. Systematic diskography is unnecessary.

Operative Technique

The technique consists of two operations:

- Grafting and osteosynthesis
- Removal of metal and verification of repair

First Stage (L5 Spondylolysis)

Positioning and Incision

Endotracheal anesthesia, prone position, support of thorax and iliac crests, with the abdomen left free. With the table extension turned down, the legs assume a 30 degree flexion relative to the torso. The skin incision runs in the midline from spinous process L3 to the sacral crest. The L5–S1 level is defined by a transvere line between the posterior superior iliac spines (Fig. 7.**1**).

The lumbar aponeurosis is freed from the spinous processes, and the muscles are retracted to the side of the joints. Hemostasis is effected by means of wet and hot compresses, followed by electrocoagulation. The laminae need to be carefully stripped of fibromuscular material (Fig. 7.**2**).

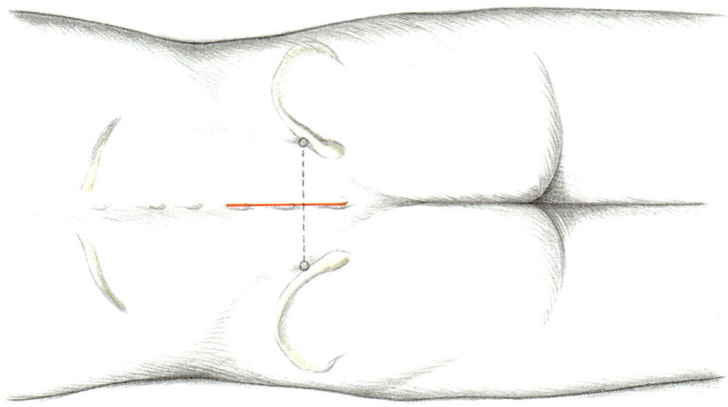

Fig. 7.**1** Median skin incision from L3 to S2. The L5–S1 segment lies at the level of a line connecting the two posterior iliac spines.

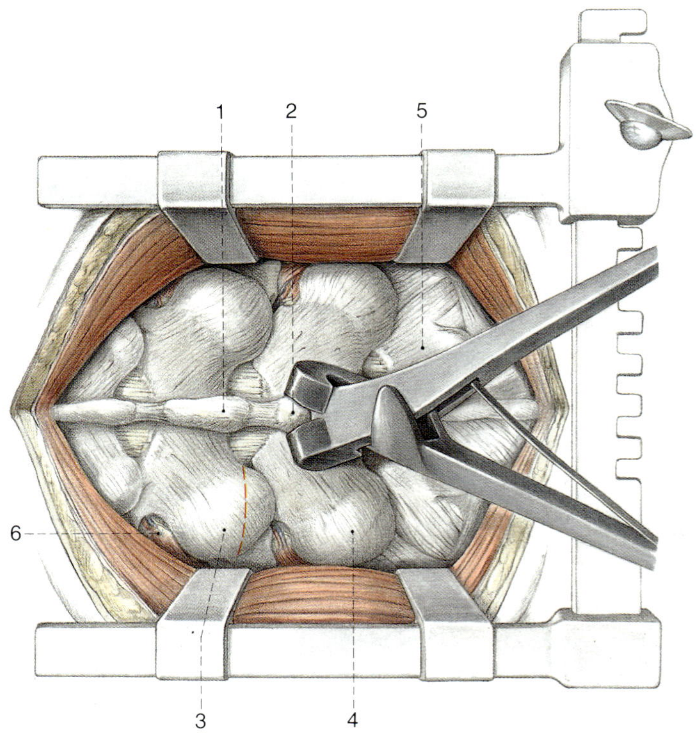

Fig. 7.**2** Exposure of arches L4–L5 and S1. Resection of the L4 and L5 spinous processes for grafting. Resection of the caudal third of the L4–L5 joints (dashed line).

1 Spinous process of the fourth lumbar vertebra
2 Spinous process of the fifth lumbar vertebra
3 L4–L5 joint capsule
4 L5–S1 joint capsule
5 Sacrum
6 Posterior branches

Harvesting of Bone Graft

The L4–L5 spinous processes are resected as far as the laminae, split in the middle, and cut into horizontal slices. Fibrous and cartilaginous matter is removed (Fig. 7.3).

Dissection of the Pars Interarticularis

Occasionally, a small Cloward retractor can be inserted into the L4–L5 interlaminar space. Fibrous and partly fatty material is removed from the lytic zone with fine forceps and rongeurs. The posterior neurovascular bundle has to be observed. The caudal third of the L4–L5 joints is then resected.

This is done for two reasons: first, to remove the main cause of the spondylolysis, namely, the tip of the lower articular process of L4; and secondly, to insert a pedicular screw into L5. At the same time, the mamillary process is removed, after which the transverse process lateral to it is exposed over a length of 4 mm. The bony portions are now debrided with curets and chisels (Fig. 7.4).

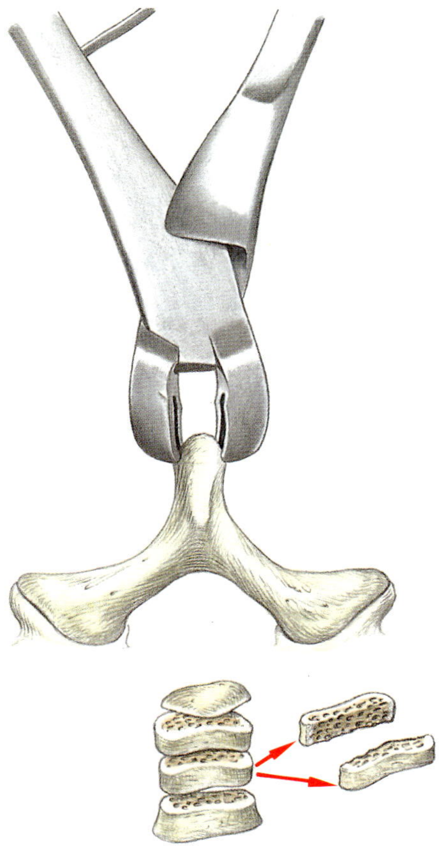

Fig. 7.**3** Removal of bone chips from the spinous processes and the vertebral arches.

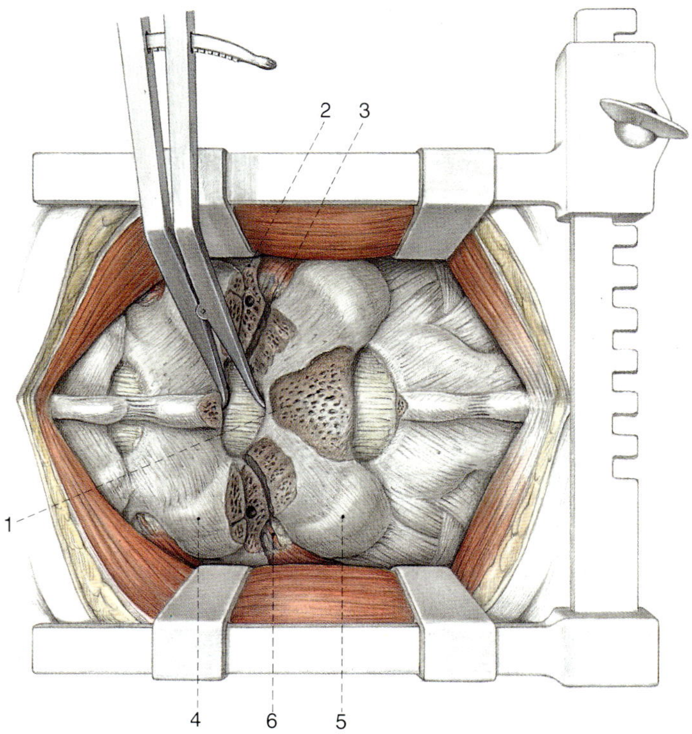

Fig. 7.**4** Exposure of the pars interarticularis and the base of transverse process. Decortication of bone. Drilling of a pedicular hole in L5.

1 Lamina of the arch of the fifth lumbar vertebra
2 Transverse process of the fifth lumbar vertebra
3 Pars interarticularis, with defect
4 L4–L5 joint capsule
5 L5–S1 joint capsule
6 Posterior branches

Preparation of Pedicular Holes

Three auxiliary lines can be used. The first runs vertically along the outer edge of the joint L4–L5 with the joint in a sagittal position, or along the middle portion of the lower articular process of L4 with the joint in a frontal position. The second is a horizontal line running 1 mm cranial to the inferior border of the joint. The third line is round, and runs cranially, outside the isthmic defect. The hole is drilled with a 3.2 mm drill; 5.5 mm screws without a tap are used, so that the drills need to penetrate to a depth of a maximum 25 mm. The drilling direction is strictly sagittal, at a slight caudal inclination of 5–10 degrees. In cases of doubt, a Kirschner wire can be provisionally introduced under image-intensifier guidance. A mandrin is placed in the drill holes (Fig. 7.**5**).

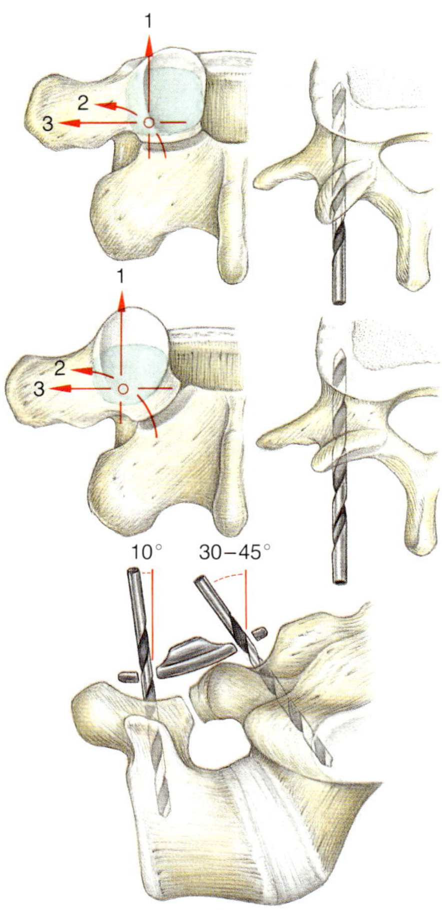

Fig. 7.**5** Anatomical markers for the pedicular screws. The position of the pedicular screw L5 is determined with the aid of three lines. The vertical line 1 depends on the position of the joint (see text).

Insertion of Bone Chips

The bone graft is introduced parallel to the isthmus, that is, obliquely from cranial–lateral to caudal–medial (Fig. 7.**6**).

Positioning of the Plate

The L5–S1 osteosynthesis is carried out with a butterfly plate, which is available in three sizes. Which size is selected depends on the interpedicular distance. While an assistant holds the plate in a sacral hole, the mandrins are removed, and are each replaced by a screw. Correct positioning of the screws has to be verified. After this, the contact between the posterior surface of the plate and the laminae is checked. For ideal apposition of the plate, it is often necessary to remove parts of the lamina. The holes in the ilium should be slanted caudally and laterally at an angle of 30–45 degrees. Screw fixation of the iliosacral joints should be avoided. The screw length in adults averages 40–45 mm for pedicular screws and 45–50 mm for sacral screws.

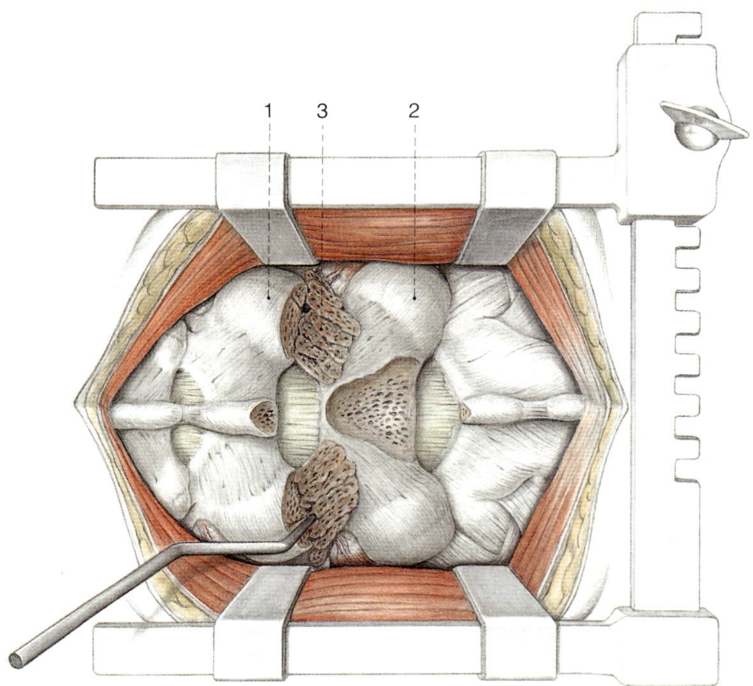

Fig. 7.**6** The pedicular holes are temporarily taken up by a mandrin which permits the application of bone graft, while at the same time securing the screw entry site.

1 L4–L5 joint capsule
2 L5–S1 joint capsule
3 Pars interarticularis

The screws are tightened diagonally. Verification by image intensifier is necessary. Muscular twitching in the gluteal region indicates that the screw is malpositioned (Fig. 7.7).

Wound Closure

The wound is closed in four layers: three deep layers with absorbable material, and a superficial layer with nonabsorbable sutures.

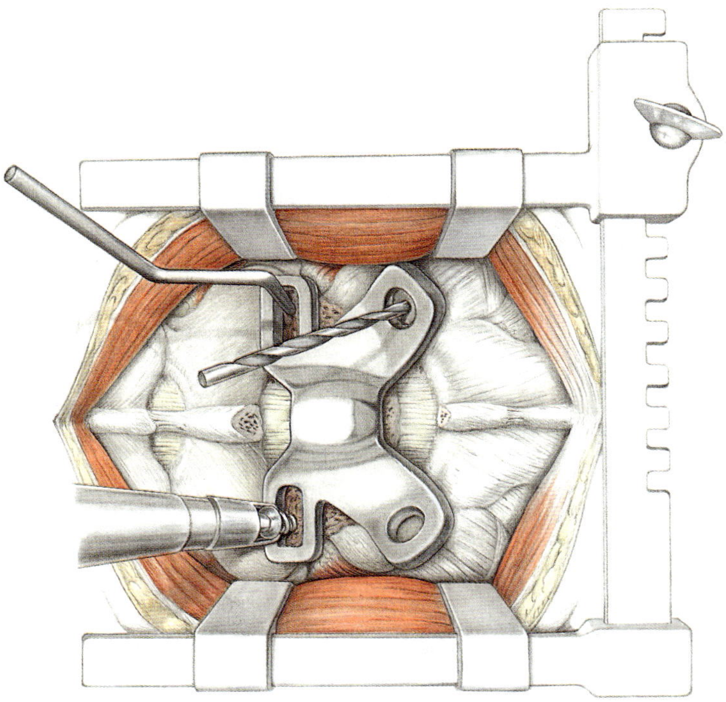

Fig. 7.**7** Application of the L5–S1 lumbosacral plate. The L5 pedicular mandrins are removed and replaced by 5.5 mm screws. The holes for the sacral screws are drilled doubly oblique through the mounted plate at an angle of 30–40 degrees to the sagittal and horizontal planes.

Postoperative Treatment

The patient is mobilized on the first postoperative day, wearing a sacroiliac brace. This is designed not for external fixation, but to remind the patient that he should avoid excessive movement during the first six months. During the first three months, sitting in the normal position is not permitted; instead, the thigh should be aligned with the longitudinal axis of the torso and the knee flexed 90 degrees.

Second Stage

At the end of the third month, radiographs and, occasionally, tomograms are taken. In patients under 18 years of age, we remove the plate at the end of the fourth month, and in patients over 18 at the end of the sixth month. At the same time, consolidation of the pars interarticularis is verified, and joint mobility is tested.

On occasion, partial bone bridging of the joints of L4–L5 or L5–S1 is observed. This should be removed until the joints have become mobile.

Technical Modifications

- Spondylolysis of L4 or L3. In these cases, the butterfly plate cannot be used. Use of two plates, fixed with pedicular screws, is then recommended (Fig. 7.**8**).
- Polysegmental spondylolyses: bilateral plates are applied over the entire spondylolysis zone.
- Spondylolysis with spina bifida: in this case, bone graft has to be harvested from the iliac crest.

Pitfalls and Complications

Pseudarthroses.

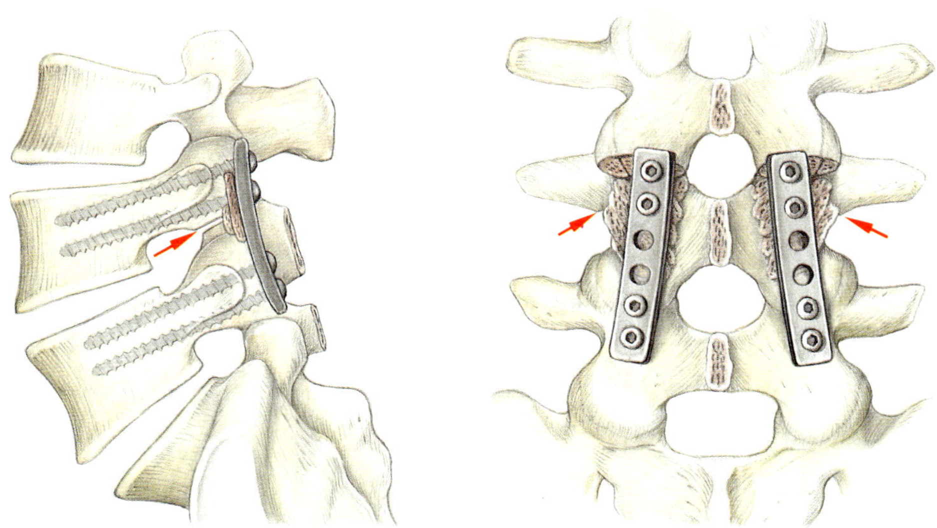

Fig. 7.**8** Osteosynthesis of the interarticular reconstruction in spondylolysis of L4 with a mobile L5–S1 segment. Following insertion of a bone graft into the defect, the osteosynthesis is effected by two plates that have been transpedicularly fixed in L4 and L5.

Reduction with Combined Fusion

This technique has two parts: an anterior approach with reduction and reconstruction of the anterior column, and a posterior approach, usually eight days later, for reconstruction of the posterior columns.

Principle

Rupture of the three columns at the lumbosacral junction leads to vertebral instability. This consists of an interruption of the two posterior columns and formation of a cleft in the area of the intervertebral disk. For a certain period, the musculature is able to compensate for this instability. However, as soon as pain develops, the instability is decompensated. Stabilization of the three columns becomes necessary. There should be combined anterior and posterior fusion; it should be confined to the lytic zone and secured by an internal osteosynthesis. A severe spondylolisthesis can lead to vertebral stenosis, which in later years can give rise to conus symptoms, as we have observed in two cases 20 years after a fusion operation without reduction.

Indications

The operation is indicated for spondylolisthesis with a slip of more than 5 mm and signs of intervertebral disk degeneration. Refractory complaints should also be present.

This applies especially to younger patients who do not want to have their physical activities restricted. The operations are contraindicated in patients over 45, obese patients, and in the presence of larger osteophytes that extend into the vertebral canal.

Anterior Approach

Normally, the anterior approach is used in the first session and the posterior one in a second session. For the anterior approach, there are two technical variants, depending on the perioperative or preoperative possibilities of reduction.

Positioning and Incision

Under endotracheal anesthesia, with the patient in a supine position, the feet are attached to the table with shoes, while at the same time traction is exerted on the skull with the aid of a leather cuff and a dynamometer. The bone graft is harvested (fibula). This is followed by slow reduction under image-intersifier control. For this purpose, the operating table is flexed under the sacrum at an angle of 30–40 degrees, and a lumbar hyperlordosis is produced. The traction on the spine is slowly increased to 15–25 kg within 5–10 minutes. In patients with moderate spondylolistheses of 10–40%, it is nearly always possible to achieve a reduction by this method (Fig. 7.**9**).

Transperitoneal Approach

See Chapter 1, pp. 52–55.

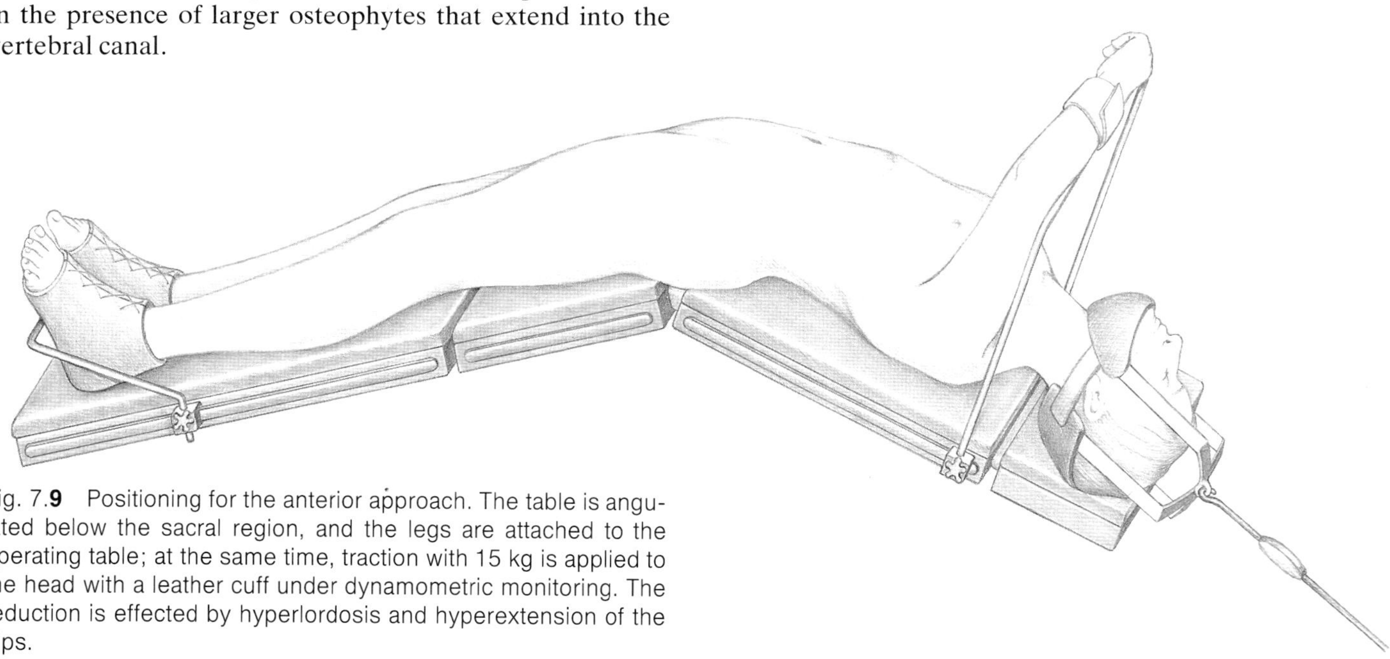

Fig. 7.**9** Positioning for the anterior approach. The table is angulated below the sacral region, and the legs are attached to the operating table; at the same time, traction with 15 kg is applied to the head with a leather cuff under dynamometric monitoring. The reduction is effected by hyperlordosis and hyperextension of the hips.

Exposure of the Last Lumbar Intervertebral Disks

Figure 7.**10** presents the anatomical site in front of the fifth lumbar vertebra and the promontory.

First option: interiliac approach, after mobilization of the large vessels with peanut swab sticks. Exposure of intervertebral disks after insertion of pins into the fifth lumbar vertebra. Hemostasis of the median sacral artery and vein. In half of the cases, this approach is suitable for exposure of the L5–S1 intervertebral disk and of the middle third of L4–L5 intervertebral disk (Fig. 1.**94**).

Second option: The left iliac vein is temporarily ligated. This vein occasionally crosses the fifth lumbar vertebra; it is therefore dissected free of the artery with cotton swab sticks and secured with a vessel loop. The vessel loops are pulled through a Redon drain 10 cm long, and are then fixed with a clamp, as a result of which the vein completely collapses (Fig. 7.**11**).

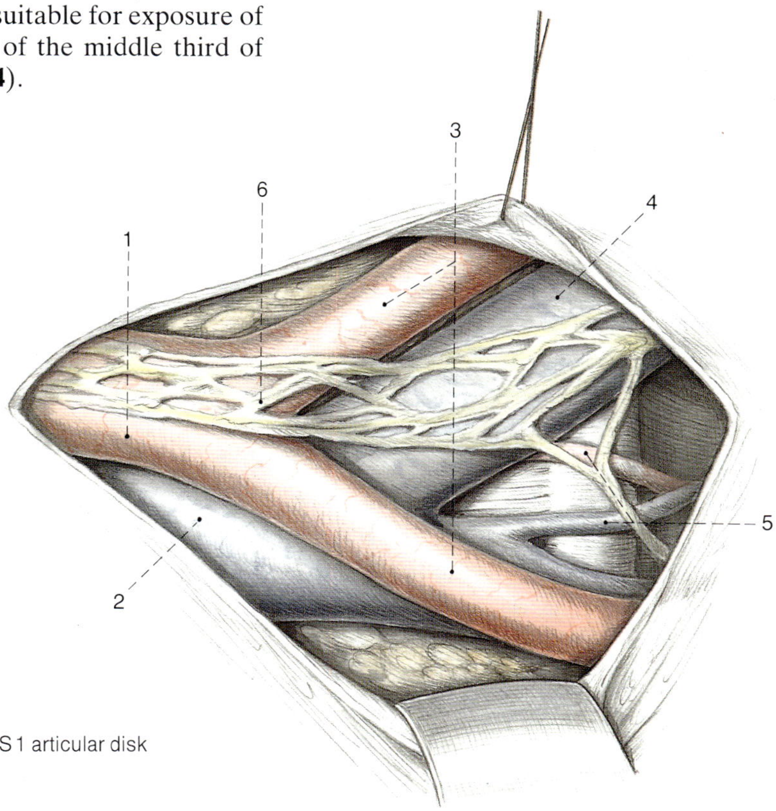

Fig. 7.**10** Anatomical site.

1 Abdominal aorta
2 Inferior vena cava
3 Common iliac arteries
4 Left common iliac vein concealing the L5–S1 articular disk
5 Median sacral vessels
6 Superior hypogastric plexus

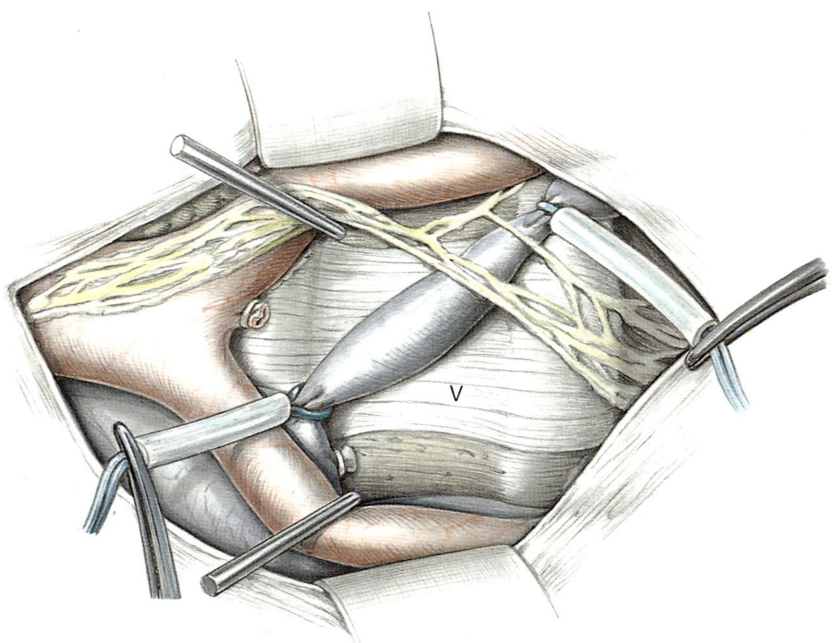

Fig. 7.**11** Temporary ligation of the left common iliac vein allows exposure of the L4–L5 and L5–S1 intervertebral disks.

V Lumbar vertebra

Third option: Mobilization of the aorta toward the right. This is necessary if the L4–L5 intervertebral disk is concealed by the aortic bifurcation. In such cases, both lumbar arteries have to be mobilized, beginning on the left, and ligated to permit displacement of the aorta to the right (Fig. 7.**12**).

Fourth option: In an aortocaval approach with exposure of the L3–L4 intervertebral disk, the midline between the inferior vena cava and the aorta has to be exposed, which requires ligation of two segmental lumbar vessels at the level of the L3 and L4 vertebrae.

The intervertebral disk is exposed after insertion of four Steinmann nails (Fig. 7.**13**).

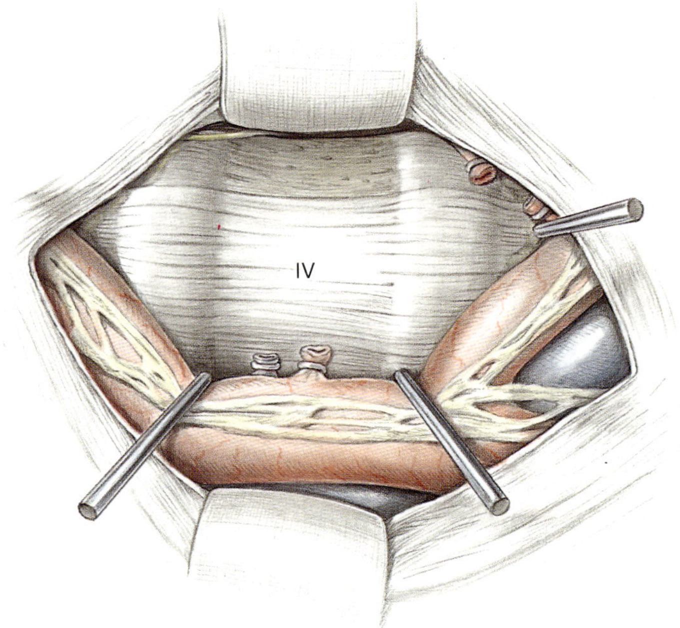

Fig. 7.**12** Exposure of L3–L4 and L4–L5 intervertebral disks by dissection of the aorta to the right. The left lumbar collateral vessels have been divided.

IV Lumbar vertebra

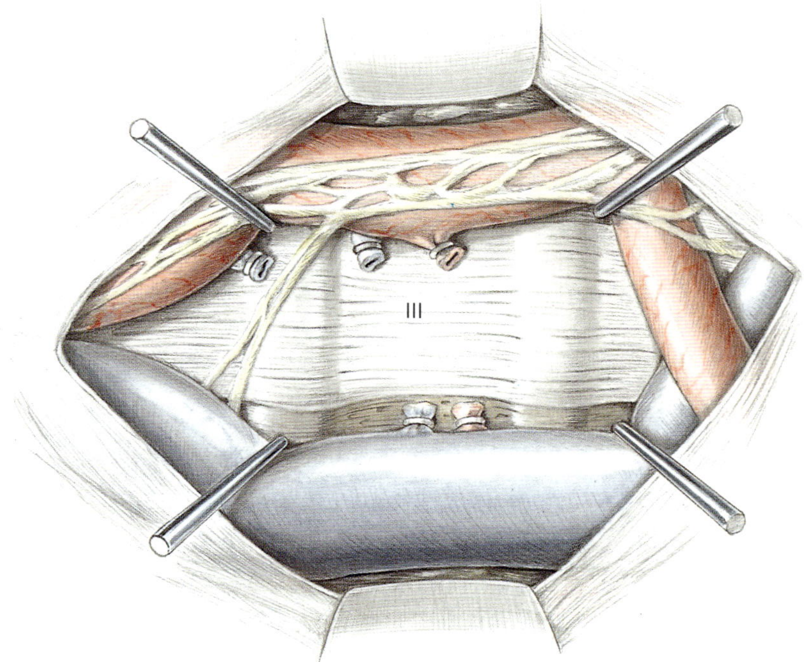

Fig. 7.**13** Interaortocaval approach following ligation of one to two lumbar vessels for exposure of the L2–L3 and L3–L4 intervertebral disks.

III Lumbar vertebra

Operative Technique

Transbody Fixation

If reduction of the spondylolisthesis during surgery can be adequately performed by the reduction procedure mentioned above, the reduction is maintained by transbody insertion of a fibular graft. A 5-cm fibular graft is required for monosegmental fusion, and a 7-cm graft for two segments. The graft is harvested by a lateral incision in the medial area of the fibular shaft. A Kirschner wire is introduced from the upper plate of L5 at an angle of 45 degrees with the anterior surface of L4 and is drilled in, under image-intensifier guidance, in the middle of the first sacral vertebra. The tip of the wire should lie 4 cm below the L5–S1 intervertebral disk (Figs. 7.**14**, 7.**15**). A cannulated 8-mm drill is now entered above the Kirschner wire. The drill point should lie 3 cm below the L5–S1 intervertebral disk (image-intensifier guidance) (Fig. 7.**16**).

The fibular graft is tapered distally, and is driven in after removal of the drill and the Kirschner wire. The walls of the fibula must not be removed (Fig. 7.**17**). A Gelfoam is placed, and the partial peritoneum is then closed by continuous suture without drainage.

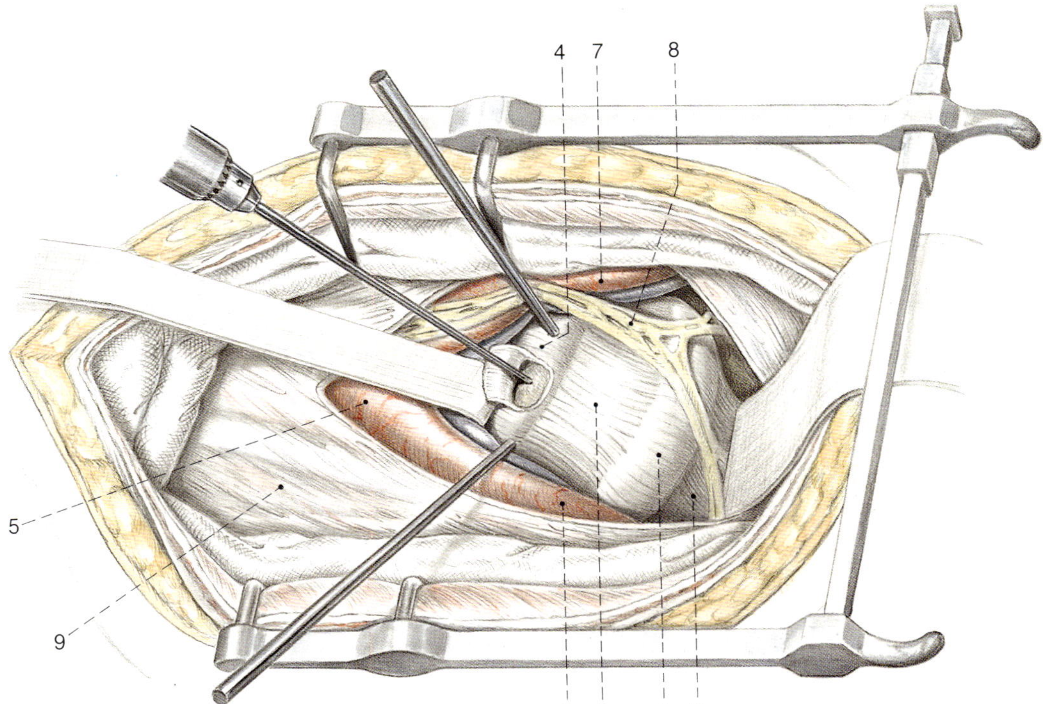

Fig. 7.**14** Anterior stabilization technique. A Kirschner wire is drilled through the vertebral bodies of L5 and S1.

1 Body of the fifth lumbar vertebra
2 L5–S1 intervertebral disk
3 Sacrum
4 L4–L5 intervertebral disk
5 Abdominal aorta
6 Right common iliac artery
7 Left common iliac artery
8 Superior hypogastric plexus
9 Parietal peritoneum

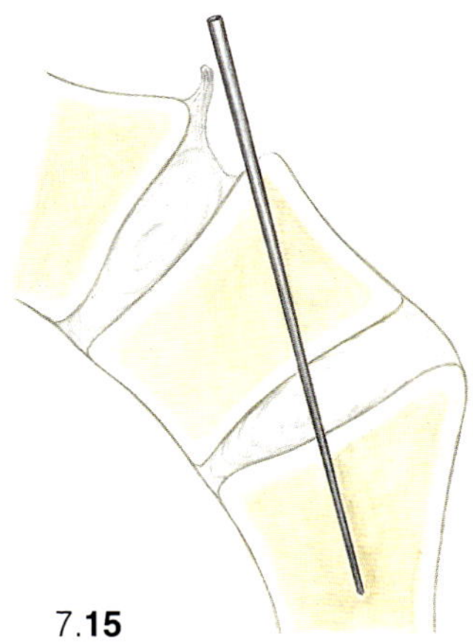

7.**15**

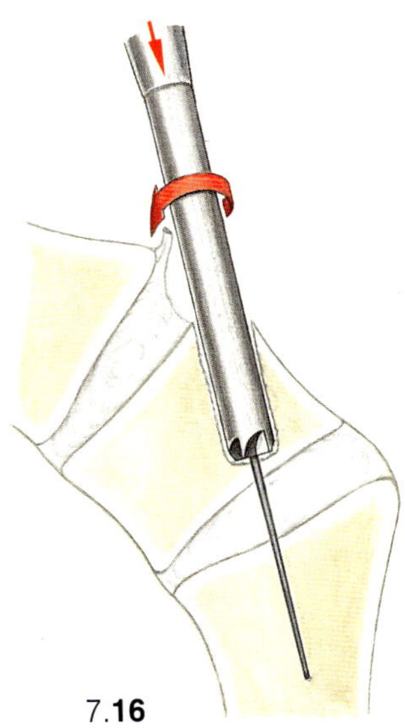

7.**16**

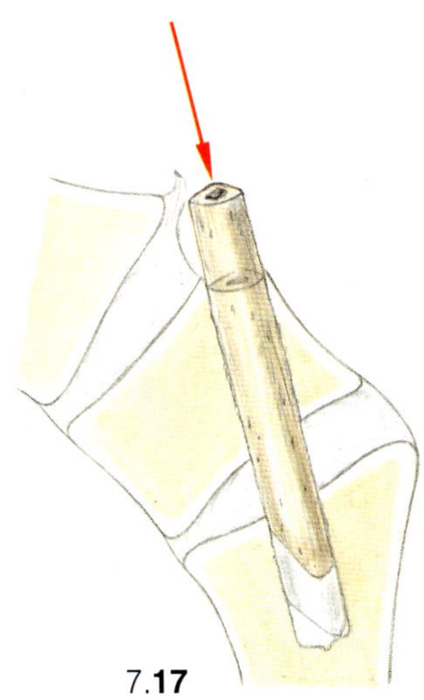

7.**17**

Fig. 7.**15** The position of the Kirschner wire from the L5 end plate into the vertebral body S1. To be verified by image identifier.

Fig. 7.**16** The cannulated drill that is placed above the Kirschner wire.

Fig. 7.**17** Insertion of a fibular segment 5 cm in length. The caudal portion of the fibula is beveled to prevent the tip from sliding off posteriorly.

Instrumental Reduction with Transbody Screw Fixation

If a closed reduction is not accomplished perioperatively, instrumental reduction is necessary. This involves an axial elevation of L5 and posterior translation of this vertebra as well as of the spine. The elevation is made possible by complete excision of the L5–S1 intervertebral disk. To protect the roots and the venous plexus, two posterolateral lamellae of the disks are left in plate (Fig. 7.**18**). Following excision of the intervertebral disk with a chisel and a curved curet, four elevators (of 90, 120, and 150 degrees, and a flat elevator) are introduced successively. Each elevator is propped on the end plate of the sacral plateau with the aid of a hook and raised, stretching the L5–S1 intervertebral disk space (Figs. 7.**19** and 7.**20**). By opening the disk space, it is now possible to remove the disk and the middle third of the posterior annulus fibrosus. This should visualize the dura, so that the spinal canal can be inspected. As soon as the last (flat) elevator can be inserted and the intervertebral space can be opened 18–20 mm anteriorly and 8–10 mm posteriorly (Figs. 7.**21** and 7.**22**), the reduction is secured with two Kirschner wires that are drilled through L5 and S1. For posterior reduction of the fifth lumbar vertebra, a special instrument is applied, consisting of a hook supported by the posterior edge of S1 and a cylinder coaxially screwed in above it, which moves the L5 vertebral body in a posterior direction in the midline. Before starting the posterior reduction, the Kirschner wires have to be removed. After image-intensifier examination and completion of the reduction, the Kirschner wires are reinserted so as to keep the reduction provisional (Figs. 7.**23**, 7.**24**). The end plates of L5 and S1 should not be damaged during excision of the intervertebral disk, since this would hamper the reduction. Guided by the image converter, a 7.5-mm Judet screw is now entered from the end plate of L5 in the median line, up to 4 cm below the L5–S1 intervertebral space.

Next, a fibular graft is cut into two pieces, 8–10mm and 18–20 mm in length, the shorter fragments being applied posterior to the screw and the longer fragments anterior to the screw. The screw is then turned tight, bringing the grafts under compression (Figs. 7.**25**, 7.**26**).

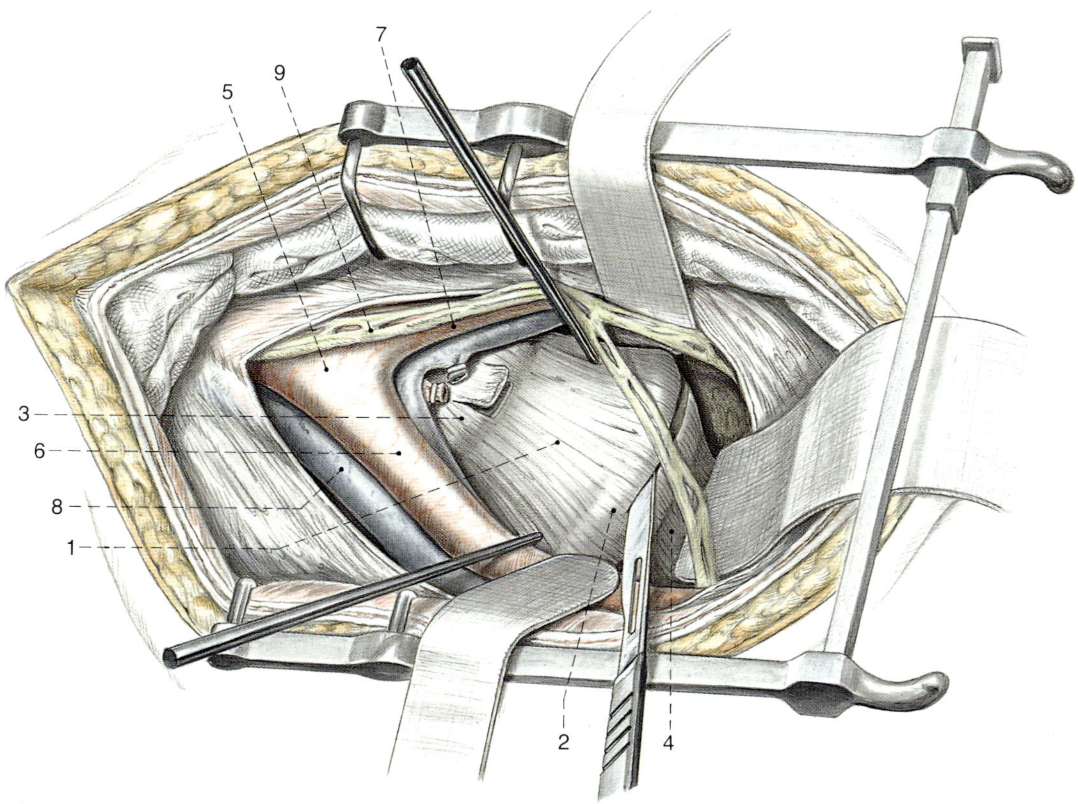

Fig. 7.**18** Technique of reduction and anterior fusion. Excision of the L5–S1 intervertebral disk.

1 Body of the fifth lumbar vertebra
2 L5–S1 articular disk
3 L4–L5 articular disk
4 Sacrum
5 Abdominal aorta
6 Right common iliac artery
7 Left common iliac artery
8 Right common iliac vein
9 Superior hypogastric plexus

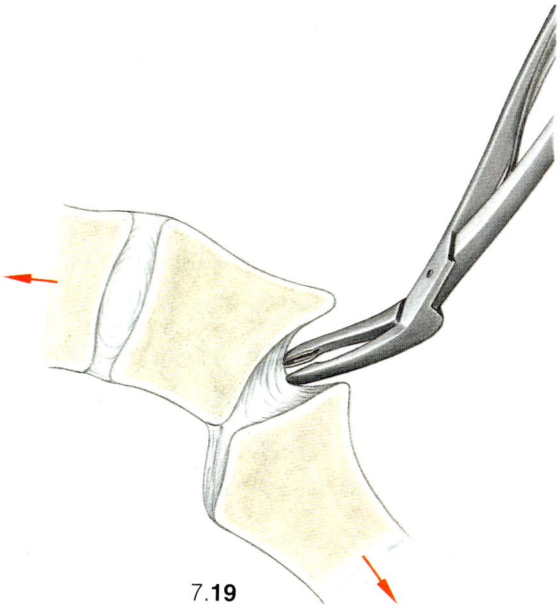

7.19

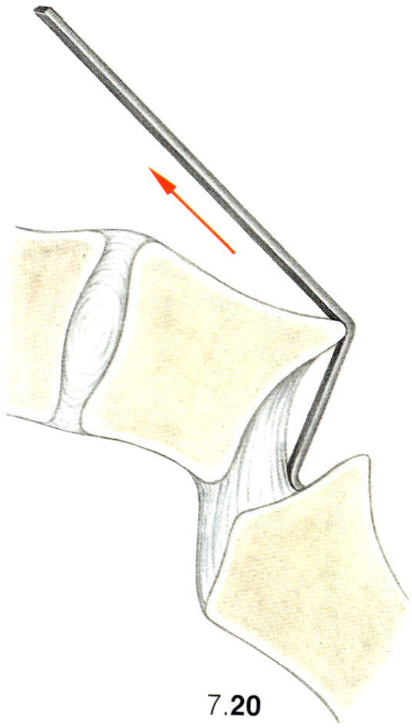

7.20

Fig. 7.**19** Excision of the L5–S1 intervertebral disk, except for the posterolateral parts.

Fig. 7.**20** Progressive elevation of the L5 vertebral body with special elevators propped on the sacrum.

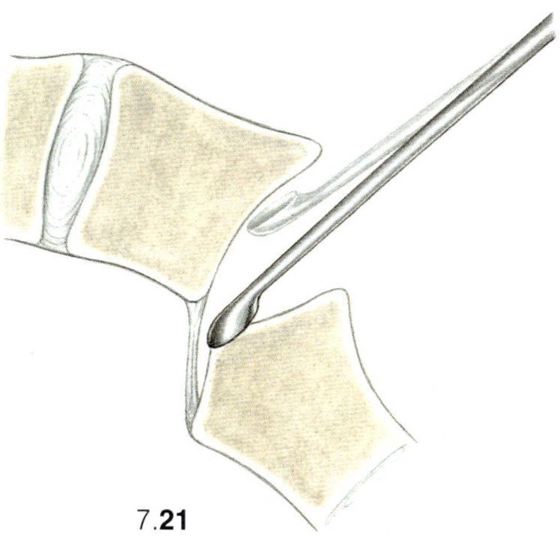

7.21

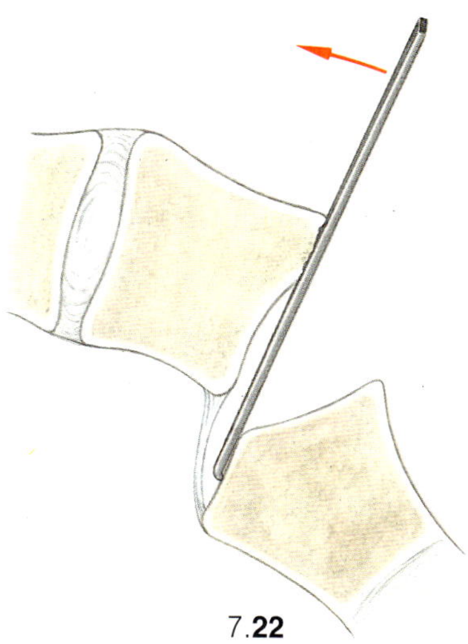

7.22

Fig. 7.**21** Excision of the remnants of the L5–S1 intervertebral disk with a sharp curet.

Fig. 7.**22** Final elevation of the L5 vertebral body with a flat elevator.

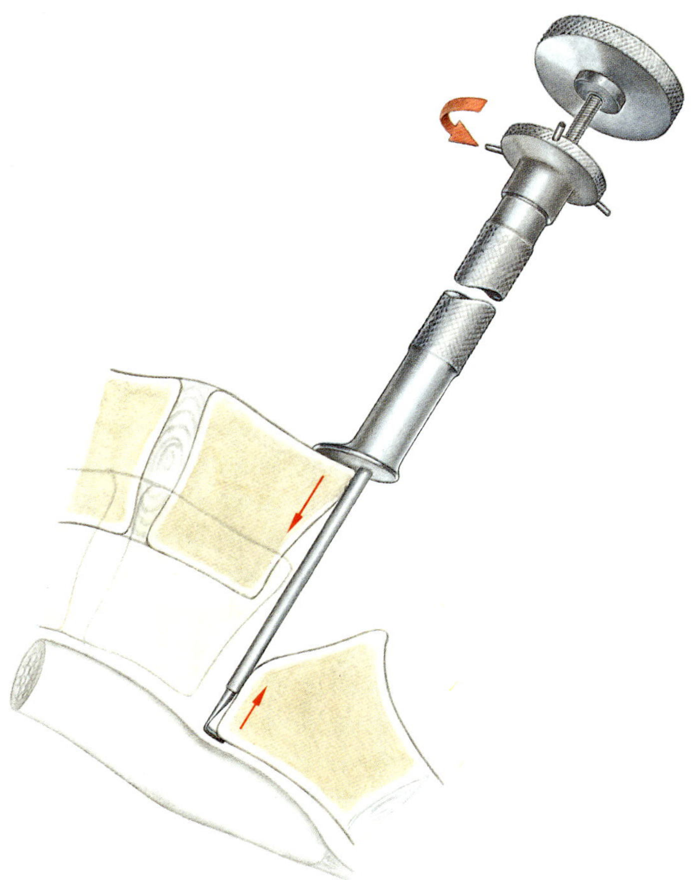

Fig. 7.**23** Insertion of a reduction tool and posterior transposition of L5 guided by the image intensifier.

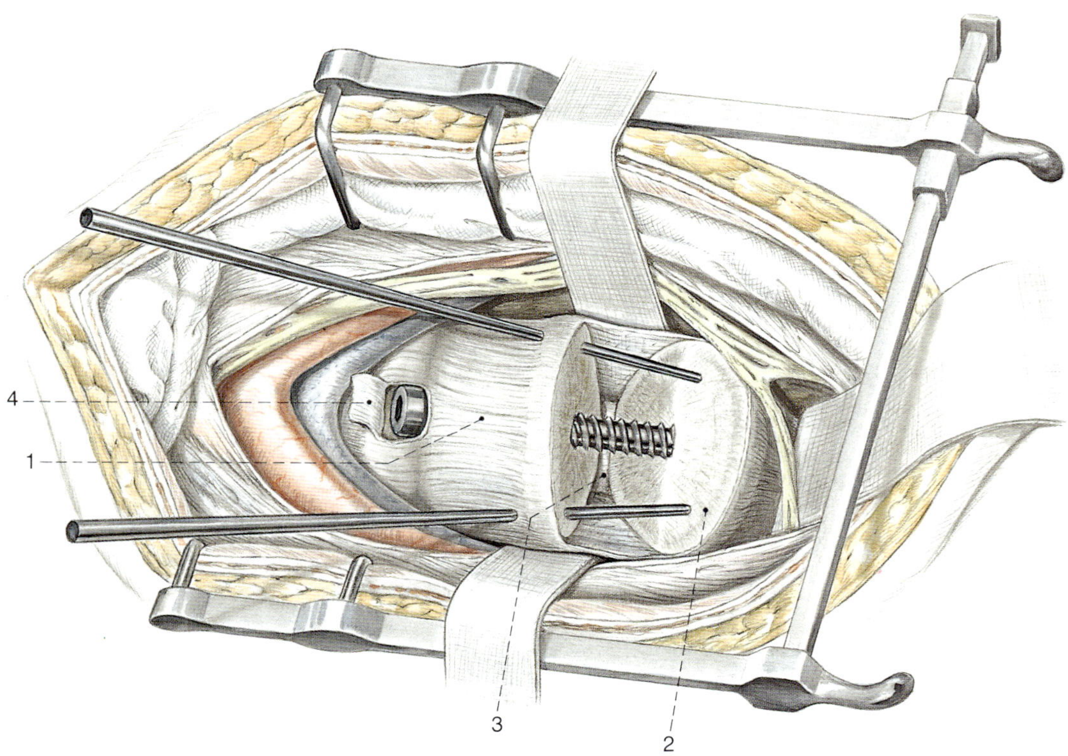

Fig. 7.**24** Temporary fixation of the reduction with two Steinmann nails. Insertion of the median Judet screw (7.5 mm diameter), to be monitored by image intensifier.

1 Body of the fifth lumbar vertebra
2 Base of the sacrum
3 Spinal dura mater
4 Annulus fibrosus

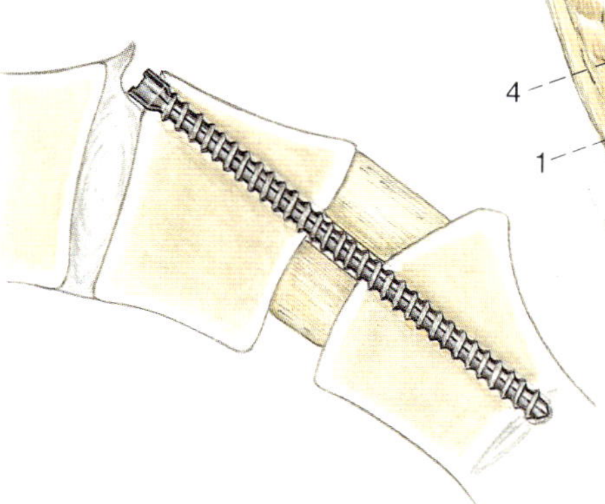

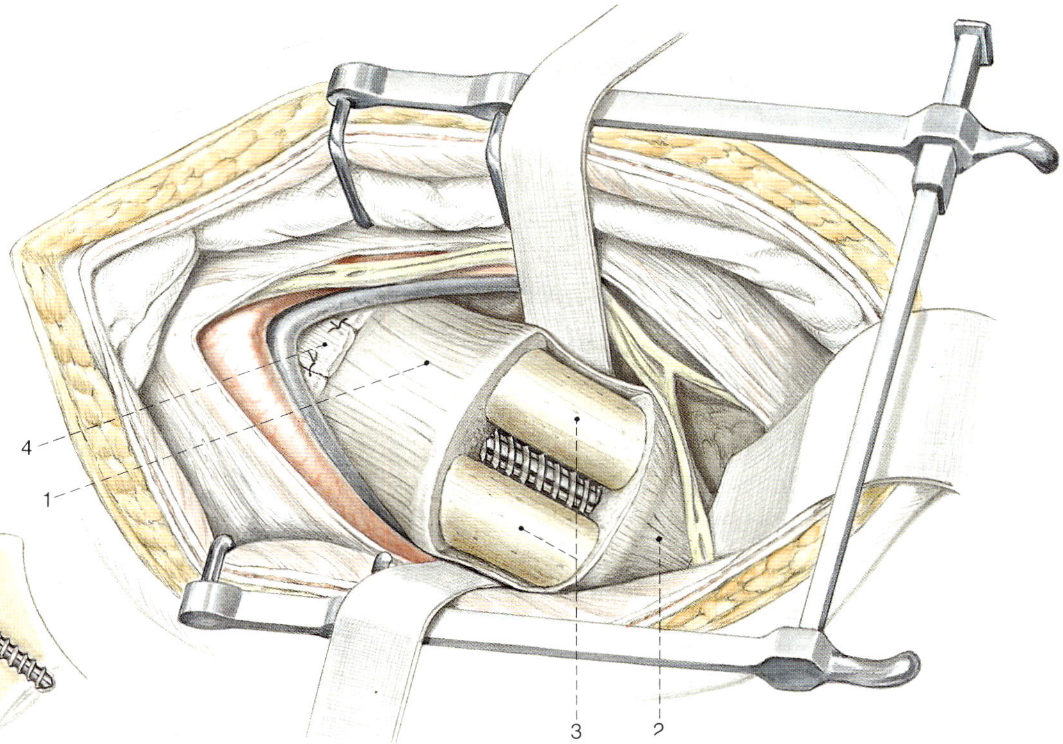

Fig. 7.**25** The screw position and the vertical fibular graft in the sagittal plane.

Fig. 7.**26** Status after anterior arthrodesis. Transbody screw, four fibular chips, and closure of the L4–L5 disk in front of the screw head.

1 Body of the fifth lumbar vertebra
2 Sacrum
3 L5–S1 intervertebral space with fibular graft
4 Closure of the annulus fibrosus in front of the screw head

Wound Closure

A Gelfoam is inserted, and the parietal peritoneum is closed by continuous suture without drainage (Fig. 7.**27**). The abdominal wall is closed with interrupted sutures for the peritoneum and the rectal aponeurosis. Suture of the subcutis and the skin follows.

Postoperative Treatment

Parenteral alimentation is advisable until the intestine is functioning normally again (flatus, defecation) on the second or third postoperative day. Postoperative preventive antibiotic and anticoagulant therapy is indicated. The patient should rest in bed until the eighth day after the operation.

Pitfalls and Complications

- Cauda equina syndrome due to entry of the fibula into the spinal canal, or due to incomplete removal of the intervertebral disk.
- L5 root lesion after reduction, due to isthmic ossification.
- Ejaculation disorders.
- Screw fracture.

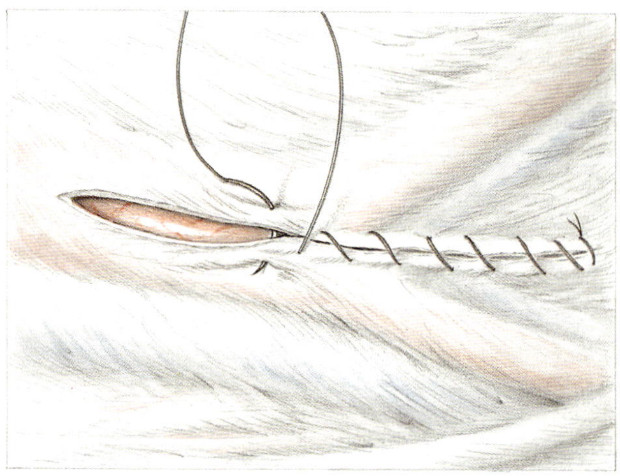

Fig. 7.**27** Closure of the parietal peritoneum by continuous suture without drainage.

Posterior Approach

Operative Technique

If there is no neurologic lesion, exploration of the spinal canal is not necessary. Reconstruction of the pars interarticularis (isthmus) and fusion of joints L5–S1 are required. The space between the sacrum and the inferior facets of L5 is also debrided and packed with corticocancellous chips, as is the pars interarticularis (Fig. 7.**28**). The butterfly plate is then fixed, and its position checked with the image intensifier (Fig. 7.**29**).

Postoperative Treatment

A patient who has undergone instrumented reduction can get out of bed with a lumbar support or body cast on the first postoperative day. If a body cast is used, the cutaneous sutures should be made with absorbable material. The body cast should be windowed in the umbilical region and well contoured over the iliac crest. It is worn for four months, and replaced for another two months, by a removable orthosis. During the first three months after the operation, the patient should sit with the thigh extended.

Technical Modifications

If there have been previous operations, removal of the internal fixation and a transverse osteotomy at the level of the L5–S1 foramen are occasionally required before the first session in order to mobilize the segment. In the presence of radiographically demonstrable supernumerary ossification centers in the area of the isthmic lesions, a posterior approach to remove these ossification centers is necessary before making the anterior approach, so that root lesions can be avoided. In cases of spina bifida, the added use of iliac bone graft is required. In reductions for severe spondylolisthesis, the course of the anterior root has to be followed after reduction. If the L5 root is unduly stressed after the reduction, a gutter should be formed in the sacral alae in order to relax the roots. Additionally, the thighs should remain in a flexed position during the first few days.

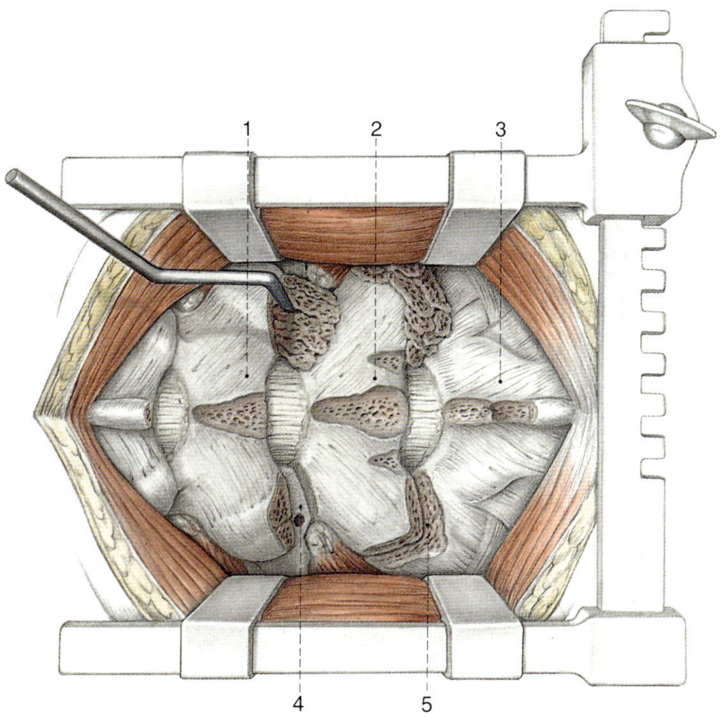

Fig. 7.**28** Second, posterior approach with anterior and posterior arthrodesis. Left: Dissection of the bone portions to be fused, placement of the L5 pedicular screw, and debridement of the L5–S1 vertebral joints. Right: Insertion of a mandrin into the pedicle of L5 and application of corticocancellous chips from the resected spinous processes.

1 Arch of the fourth lumbar vertebra
2 Arch of the fifth lumbar vertebra
3 Sacrum
4 L4–L5 joint space
5 L4–S1 joint space

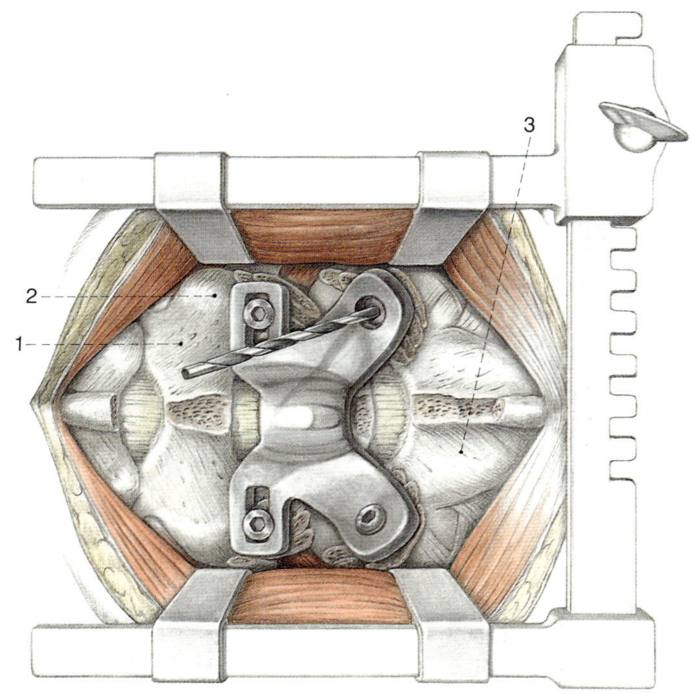

Fig. 7.**29** Insertion of the lumbosacral plate.

1 Arch of the fourth lumbar vertebra
2 L4–L5 joint capsule
3 Sacrum

Posterior Decompression With or Without Arthrodesis

Indication

In elderly patients, or patients who do not engage in any sports, the posterior approach alone may suffice. If there is neurologic damage, decompression is required in addition.

Operative Technique

A median longitudinal incision and exposure are followed by laminectomy with removal of the posterior, mobile arch. If necessary, the laminectomy has to be extended in a cranial or caudal direction. The dural sac is inspected and, if necessary, further decompression is carried out in the area of the vertebral joints or the disk. After this, a graft arthrodesis of the posterior column is performed, the resected arch serving as graft material. For fixation, use is made either of two plates or, if only the segment L5–S1 is being fused, the butterfly plate. In older patients with a rigid spine, decompression alone, without arthrodesis, is enough.

Further Reading

Louis R. Fusion of the lumbar and sacral spine by internal fixation with screw plates. Clin Orthop 1986;203:18.

Louis R, Maresca C. Les arthrodèses stables de la charnière lombosacrée (70 cas). Rev Chir Orthop 1976;62(suppl 2):70.

Louis R, Maresca C. Stabilisation chirurgicale avec réduction des spondylolyses et des spondylolisthésis. Int Orthop 1977;1:215.

8 Neurosurgical Operations

H.-J. Reulen

Transoral Approach in Dens Elevation

The transoral approach provides a very good overview of the clivus, the anterior arch of the atlas, the body of C2, and the intervertebral disk C2–C3. if necessary, the body of C3 can be reached as well. Laterally, the occipital condyle and the lateral parts of C1 and C2, with the respective joints, can be exposed (Fig. 8.**1**).

Indications

Elevation of the dens due to congenital or acquired basilar impression (Paget's disease, rheumatoid arthritis); os odontoideum; tumors of the clivus (chordoma, etc.).

Diagnosis

The diagnosis is made by computed tomography (CT) or magnetic resonance imaging (MRI). With the latter, sagittal sections such as those shown in Figure 8.**1** can be obtained. This makes a detailed visualization of bony structures and soft tissues, and precise planning of the operation possible. Radiographic tomograms can be used for specific problems.

Approach

See Chapter 1, pp. 2–3.

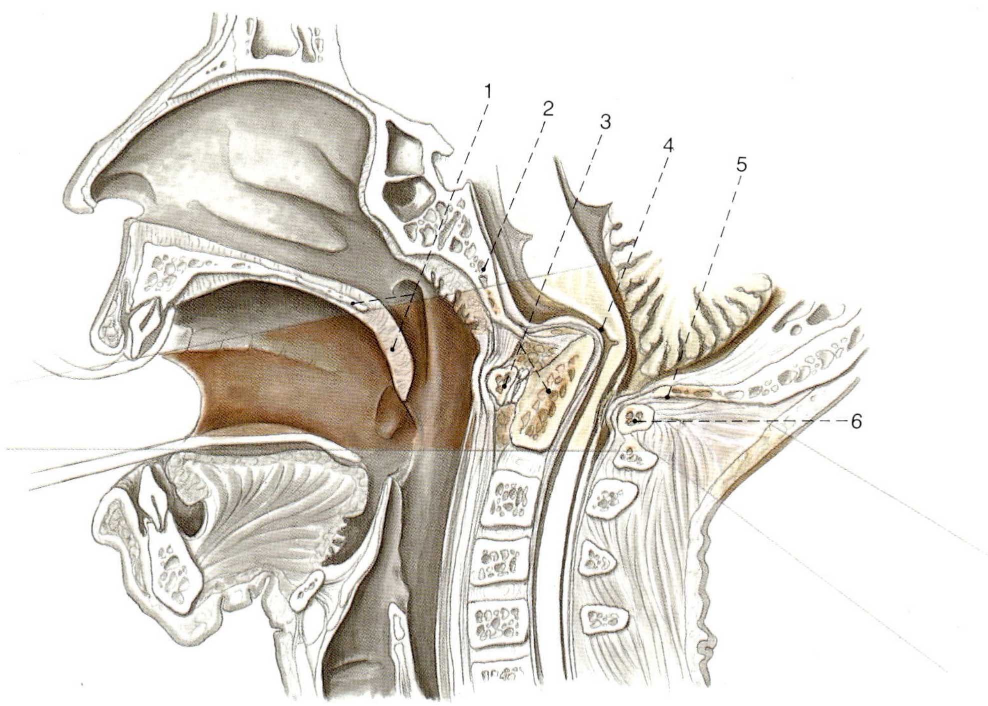

Fig. 8.**1** The transoral approach in basilar impression with elevation of the dens (rheumatoid arthritis). The medulla oblongata is massively compressed by the dens. Also shown is the possibility of posterior decompression, with removal of the posterior arch of the atlas and enlargement of the great occipital foramen

1 Hard palate and soft palate
2 Clivus
3 Anterior arch of the atlas and dens axis
4 Medulla oblongata, compressed
5 Great foramen
6 Posterior arch of the atlas

Preoperative Preparation, Positioning, and Incision

After a nasopharyngeal smear has been taken and sensitivity tested, an antibiotic is given prophylactically via a parenteral route. The patient is in the supine position, with the chest slightly raised; the cervical spine is hyperextended and the head slightly lowered, to prevent aspiration of blood (Fig. 8.**2**). Using a mouth gag, such as the Crowe–Davis, for example, the mouth is opened wide and the tongue depressed (Fig. 8.**3**). The tube is affixed to the mouth gag. The hypopharynx is packed with sterile gauze, and the oral and pharyngeal mucosa and the skin around the mouth are disinfected.

If access to the body of the second cervical vertebra is required, it is sufficient to retract the soft palate and the uvula upward by means of two rubber catheters that are brought out through the nose (Fig. 8.**3**). On the other hand, if the atlas and the clivus are to be exposed, the uvula and the soft palate have to be split in the middle, and the mucosa of the hard palate has to be retracted laterally and fixed with stay sutures (Fig. 8.**4**). If necessary, about 1–2 cm of the posterior portion of the hard palate can then be resected with a rongeur or chisel. A preoperative sagittal MRI in the midline facilitates planning of the resection, since the topmost structure to be accessed is readily recognizable when compared with the hard palate (Fig. 8.**1**). A lateral radiograph intensifier may occasionally be necessary and helpful.

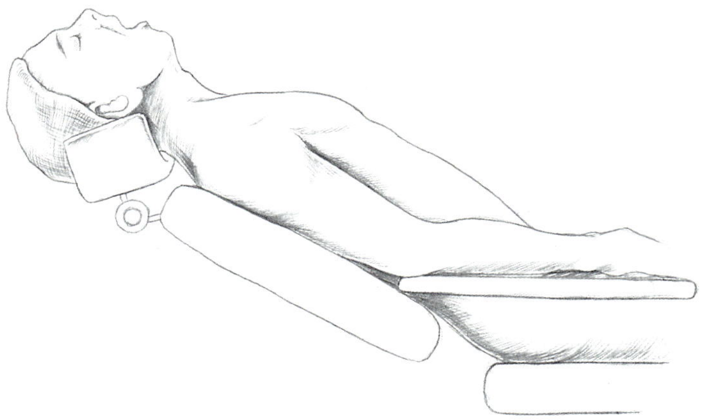

Fig. 8.**2** Positioning for the transoral approach.

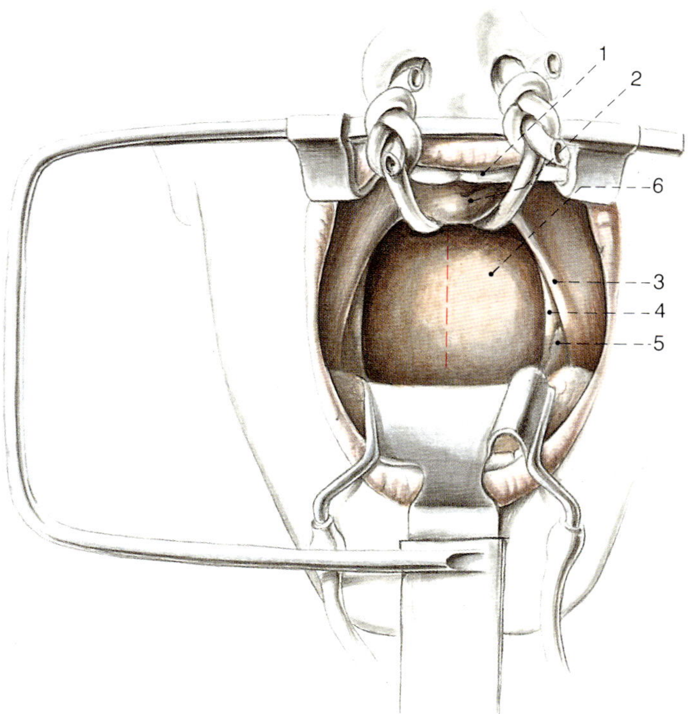

Fig. 8.**3** Inserted mouth gag with lateral groove for the tube. The upper stirrup is placed over the row of teeth, while the lower blade is placed over the tongue and the base of the tongue. Shown here is a method of superiorly retracting the soft palate and the uvula using two rubber catheters.

1 Superior dental arch
2 Uvula and soft palate
3 Palatoglossal arch
4 Palatopharyngeal arch
5 Palatine tonsil
6 Posterior wall of the pharynx

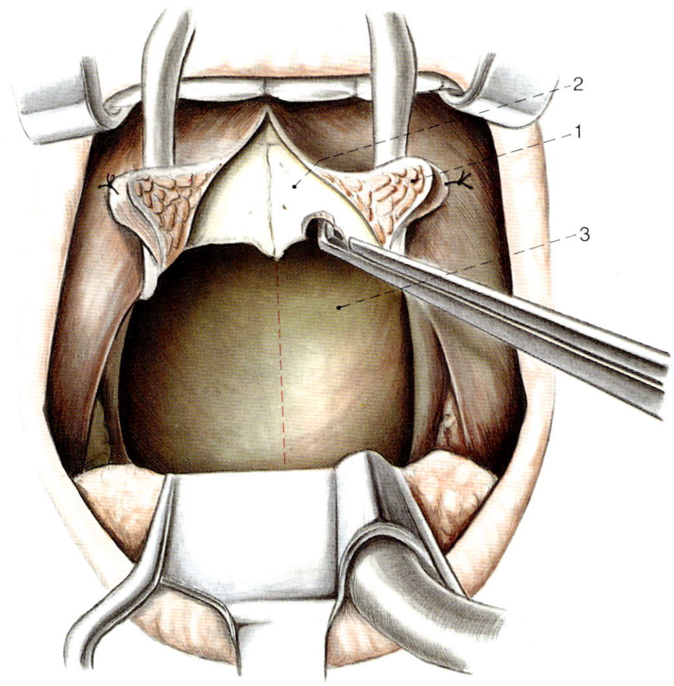

Fig. 8.**4** The uvula and the soft palate are split in the middle, and the mucous membrane has been retracted over the hard palate. The hard palate can be resected with a rongeur or chisel (optical magnification).

1 Uvula
2 Hard palate
3 Posterior wall of the pharynx

Operative Technique

Exposure of the Clivus and Arch of the Atlas

By palpating the posterior wall of the pharynx, the anatomy can be identified. The anterior arch of the atlas is readily palpable, and shows a hump (anterior tubercle) in the midline; the disk between C2 and C3 protrudes slightly.

The posterior wall of the pharynx is longitudinally incised in the midline (Fig. 8.**5**). The pharyngeal mucosa, the muscular layer of the superior constrictor, and the pharyngobasilar fascia, are successively divided. These layers, together with the longus colli muscle arising from the arch of the atlas, are laterally retracted subperiosteally on both sides (Fig. 8.**6**). The mucosa and the muscular layer are retracted with stay sutures or special gags. The anterior arch of the atlas, the body of the axis, and the inferior margin of the clivus are now defined. The approach can be expanded upward or downward, depending on the pathology. Generally speaking, it is even possible to reach the third cervical vertebra, but this requires exerting considerable pressure on the base of the tongue. Also, the layer of soft tissue over the third cervical vertebra is much thinner, so that later closure may prove difficult.

The present example describes resection of the dens axis in a case of marked elevation associated with acquired basilar impression following rheumatoid arthritis. To reach the odontoid process and the body of the axis, the anterior arch of the atlas has to be removed with a microdrill (Fig. 8.**7**). If, as in the present case, the dens has migrated far upward into the intracranial space, the caudal portion of the clivus has to be removed as well (Fig. 8.**8**).

In such cases, a reactive–degenerative, partly calcified tissue several millimeters thick is usually found between the arch of the atlas and the dens. After removal of this tissue, the odontoid is increasingly reamed out, using optical magnification and a microdrill (diamond drill), until only a thin shell remains. This can be cautiously detached and removed without exerting any pressure on the spinal cord posteriorly. Because of the danger of infection, the dura behind the dens must not be injured. If this should exceptionally occur nonetheless, the dura defect is closed with fascia lata and fibrin glue.

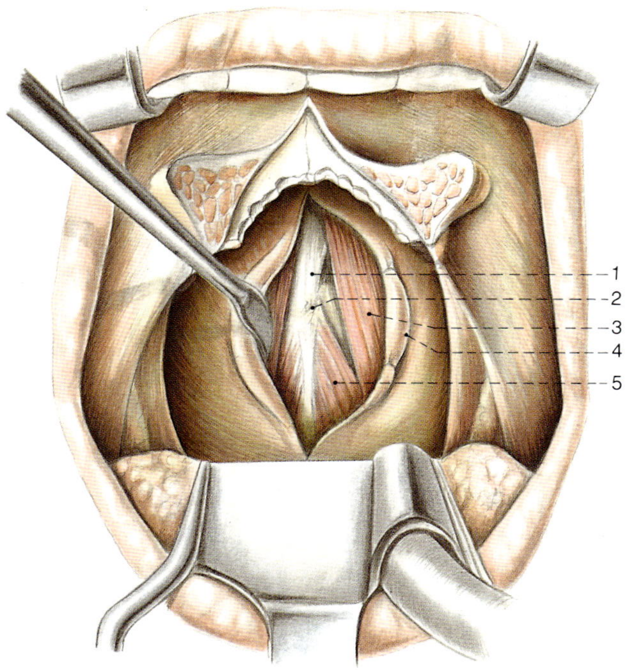

Fig. 8.**5** The posterior wall of the pharynx is split in the midline; the arch of the atlas with the anterior tubercle, the longus colli, and the longus capitis muscle are visualized.

1 Anterior longitudinal ligament
2 Anterior tubercle of atlas
3 Longus capitis muscle
4 Posterior wall of the pharynx
5 Longus colli muscle

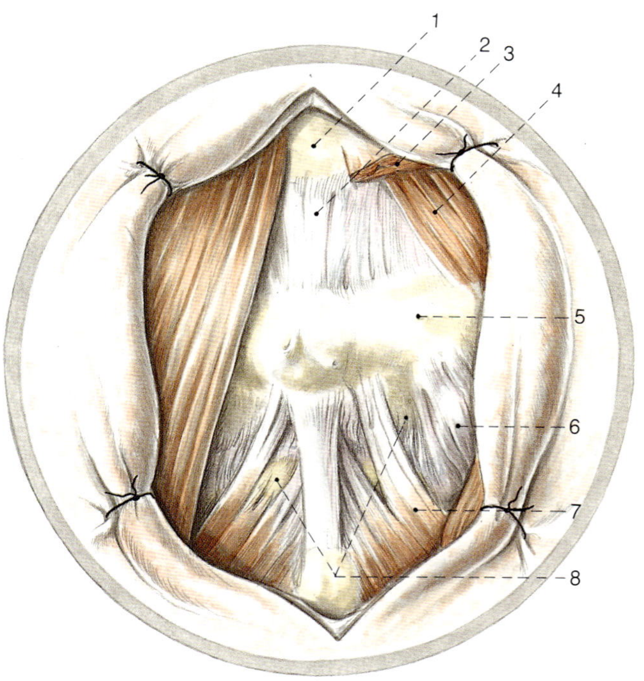

Fig. 8.**6** The longus colli and longus capitis muscles are subperiosteally retracted laterally, possibly after partial division at the insertion. A small soft-tissue retractor is then introduced to keep these muscles in lateral retraction (optical magnification).

1 Clivus
2 Anterior atlanto-occipital membrane
3 Longus capitis muscle
4 Rectus capitis anterior muscle
5 Anterior arch of atlas
6 Joint capsule of the lateral atlantoaxial articulation
7 Longus colli muscle
8 Body of the axis

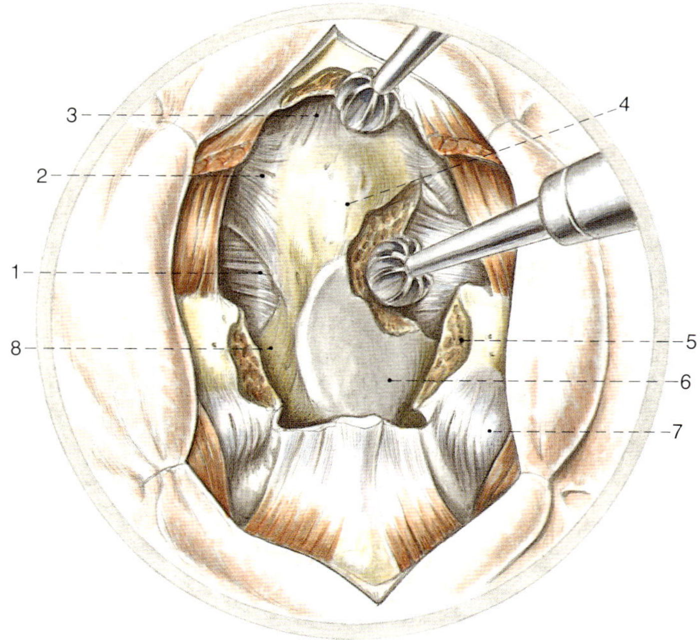

Fig. 8.7 The anterior arch of the atlas and part of the clivus have been removed with a drill. The dens is hollowed out and removed down to its base (optical magnification).

1 Transverse ligament of the atlas
2 Alar ligaments
3 Apical dental ligament
4 Dens axis
5 Anterior arch of the atlas
6 Anterior articular facet
7 Capsule of the lateral atlantoaxial articulation
8 Body of the axis

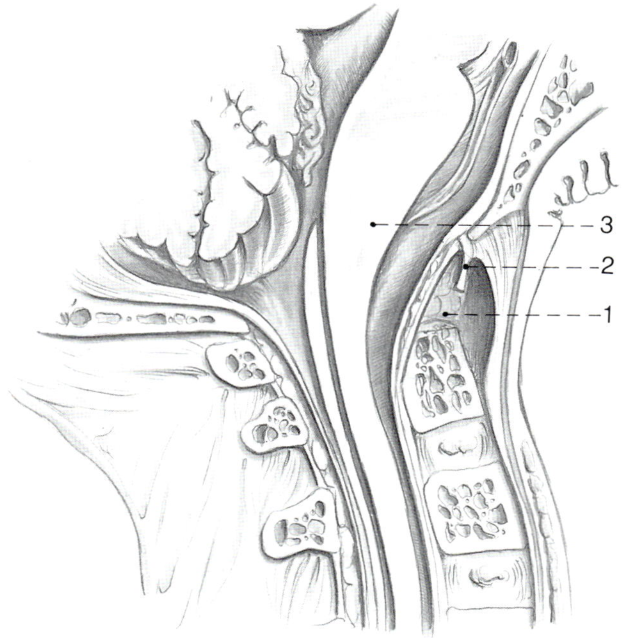

Fig. 8.8 Decompression of the medulla oblongata after resection of the dens.

1 Cavity following resection of the dens axis
2 Apical dental ligament
3 Decompressed medulla oblongata

Wound Closure

Special care should be taken when closing the posterior wall of the pharynx. First the muscle layer and then the mucosa are tightly closed with absorbable sutures. The uvula and the soft palate are approximated with loose absorbable sutures. The packing is removed after drainage, and the pharynx is examined to verify removal of all the material. If fusion and stabilization are desired, possible anchoring points for a plate osteosynthesis are the clivus or the occipital condyle at the base of the skull, the lateral mass at C1, and the body area at C2 (Harms and Schmelzle 1987).

Postoperative Treament

Parenteral antibiotic therapy is continued prophylactically for at least three days. If no stabilization was required, the patient is mobilized on the first day after the operation. The wound at the oropharynx is inspected daily, and the patient is instructed to rinse with antiseptic solution. A soft collar is worn around the neck for two or three weeks.

Complications

Infection can be prevented for the most part by determining the presence of causative organisms and their sensitivity preoperatively, and giving antibiotics prophylactically. In the event of injury to the dura, watertight closure of the dura is imperative; the patient should be monitored for possible signs of meningitis postoperatively. The importance of careful closure of the posterior wall of the pharynx should be borne in mind.

Cervical Myelopathy in Spondylosis

Posterior spondylophytic osteophytes can narrow the spinal canal considerably at one or more levels. Hypertrophy of the ligamentum flavum is usually associated with this condition, so that the spinal cord, too, may be compressed anteriorly and posteriorly. This compression, as well as the constant, movement-dependent microtrauma of the spinal cord, compromising its local blood supply, leads to a slowly progressive instability of gait, atactic disturbances, and paraspasticity of the legs. If more than one level, e.g., two adjacent segments, is affected in cervical myelopathy, both levels can be treated by the Smith–Robinson operative technique; alternatively, a corpectomy and interbody fusion (pp. 256–263) may be considered.

Diagnosis

Medial spondylophytes (Fig. 8.**9**) lead to chronic cord damage (see above); if lateral osteophytes are present in the area of the uncus at the same time, a monoradicular syndrome of the affected root, with pain, paresthesias, and sensorimotor deficits, may supervene. Most commonly involved are the levels C4–C5, C5–C6, and C6–C7. Radiographs of the cervical spine in four planes are needed, as are myelograms or CT myelograms. Motion films of the cervical spine in anteflexion and retroflexion may reveal additional instability in a motion segment, which is not uncommon. MRI with sagittal cuts is best suited to demonstrate the spondylotic osteophytes and the level of compression of the cervical cord; in axial cuts, this technique is still surpassed by computed tomography. Narrowing of the sagittal diameter of the spinal canal to less than 13 mm is considered pathological.

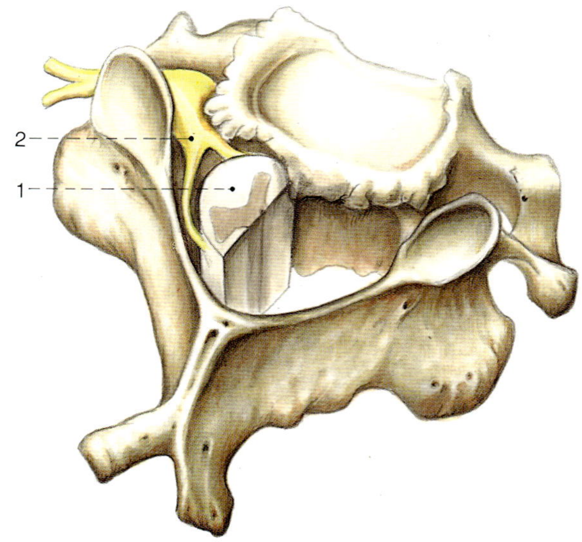

a

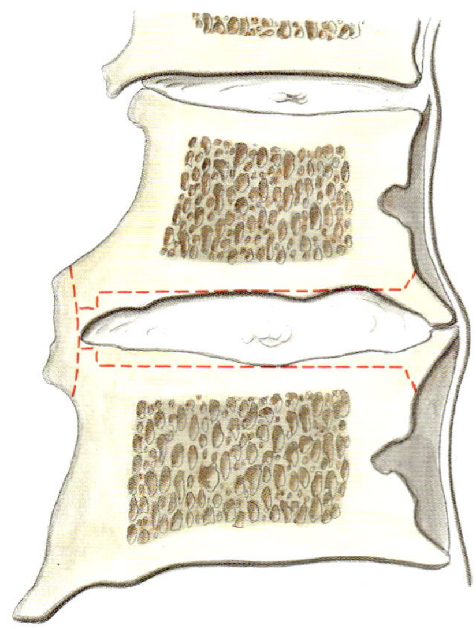

b

Fig. 8.**9a** Medial and lateral spondylotic jagged edges in a posterior semilateral view. Compression of the left spinal cord and left nerve root.
b In the saggital section, the necessary resection of the spondylophytes is shown in the midline (red dashed line).

1 Spinal medulla, cervical segment
2 Spinal nerve

Approach

See Chapter 1, pp. 4–12.

Exposure of the anterior side of the cervical spine is followed by identification of the appropriate level. For this purpose, a needle is inserted into the putative intervertebral space and monitored with the aid of a lateral radiograph image intensifier. If pronounced anterior osteophytes are present, they are removed with a rongeur or a drill, so that the intervertebral space can be exposed (Fig. 8.**10**).

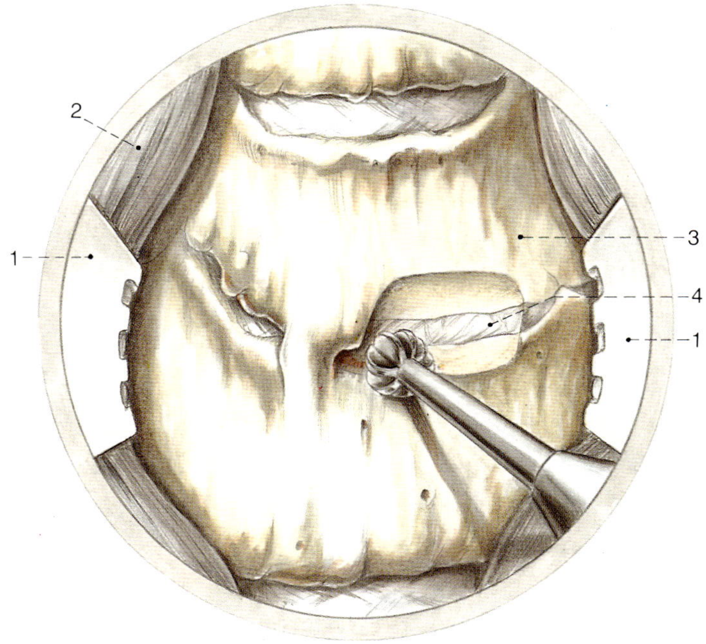

Fig. 8.**10** Resection of the anterior spondylotic osteophytes with a drill or rongeur (optical magnification). For the sake of clarity, the anterior longitudinal ligament is not shown.

1 Spreader blade
2 Longus colli muscle
3 Body of the fifth cervical vertebra
4 Intervertebral disk

Operative Technique

Removal of the Intervertebral Disk

The anterior longitudinal ligament and the annulus fibrosus are excised with a knife over their entire width. The annulus fibrosus, like the intervertebral disk, is removed with a rongeur 2–3 mm wide. Remnants of the intervertebral disk, especially in the lateral area of the intervertebral space, can be removed with a small, curved curet until the annulus fibrosus or the posterior longitudinal ligament comes into view posteriorly. The further course of the operation can be facilitated by expanding the intervertebral space (Fig. 8.**11**).

The Cloward vertebral body spreader should be placed as far laterally in the intervertebral space as possible (Fig. 8.**11**). If there is not enough room to insert the spreader, a larger opening can be cut with the microdrill. The superior and inferior end plates of the adjacent vertebrae are then carefully dechondrified with a small curet, but the subchondral bone is left intact.

Removal of Posterior Osteophytes

In preparation for grafting, the sclerosed end plate is slightly roughened and opened with a ball-tipped reamer. The posterior osteophytes are thinned, and removed up to the posterior longitudinal ligament, using a microdrill and a diamond drill (2 mm diameter). Optical magnification with a magnifier or surgical microscope greatly facilitates this operative step (Fig. 8.**11**).

The posterior longitudinal ligaments is freed from the osteophytes with a fine rectangular dissector. The remaining osteophytes can now be resected piece by piece with a fine angulated curet or a fine 40-degree angle punch (jaw width 2 mm) (Fig. 8.**12**). The curet is cautiously inserted behind the osteophyte; a piece is then broken off and displaced into the intervertebral space. This procedure is repeated until the osteophyte has been completely removed. As a rule, portions of the posterior longitudinal ligament are resected as well; absence of the protective longitudinal ligament partly or completely exposes the dura. It is therefore advisable to proceed with great caution in this phase, and to handle the instruments well supported. Resection of posterior osteophytes with a chisel is inadvisable, since this may lead to very severe damage, additional to the already existing compression of the spinal cord.

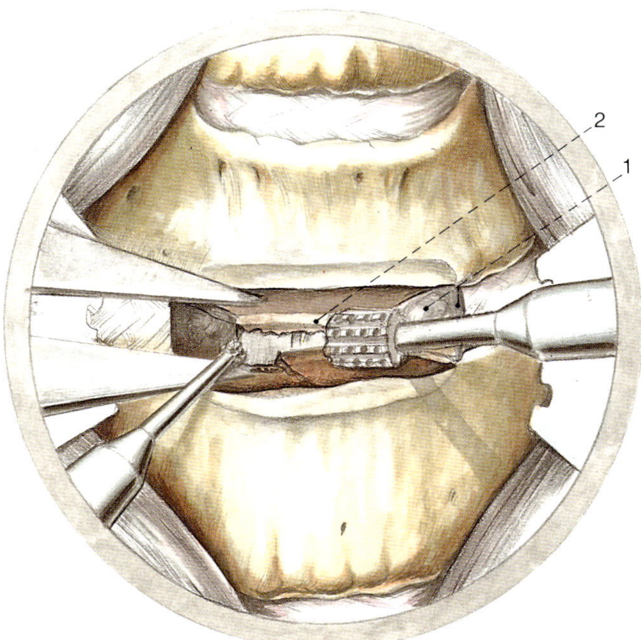

Fig. 8.**11** After expansion of the intervertebral space, the osteochondrotic end plates are debrided, and the graft bed is prepared. The posterior spondylotic osteophytes are resected with a diamond drill, rongeur, or curet.

1 Intervertebral disk
2 Posterior spondylotic osteophytes

Lateral osteophytes are removed with the rongeur until the nerve root is completely decompressed. This can be verified at the end by passing a fine probe along the edge of the bone. If resection of lateral osteophytes should lead to venous bleeding, this can easily be controlled by cautious packing with Gelfoam or the like.

The depth of the graft bed is now measured (Fig. 8.**13**). Harvesting, preparation, and implantation of the bone graft are carried out as described in Chapter 5 (pp. 252–255).

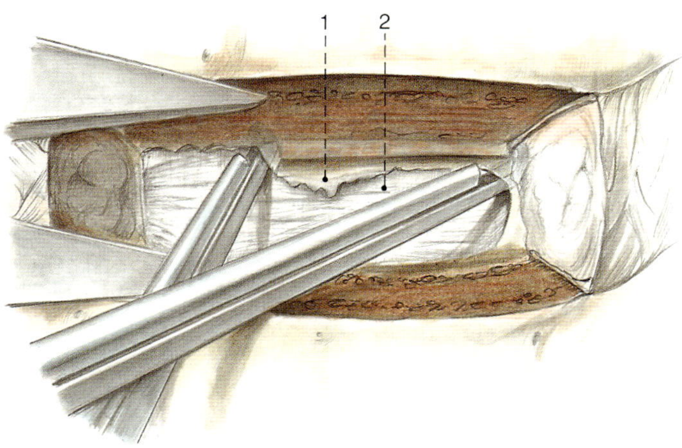

Fig. 8.**12** Resection of a medial spondylotic osteophyte, using a fine rongeur.

1 Medial spondylotic osteophyte
2 Posterior longitudinal ligament

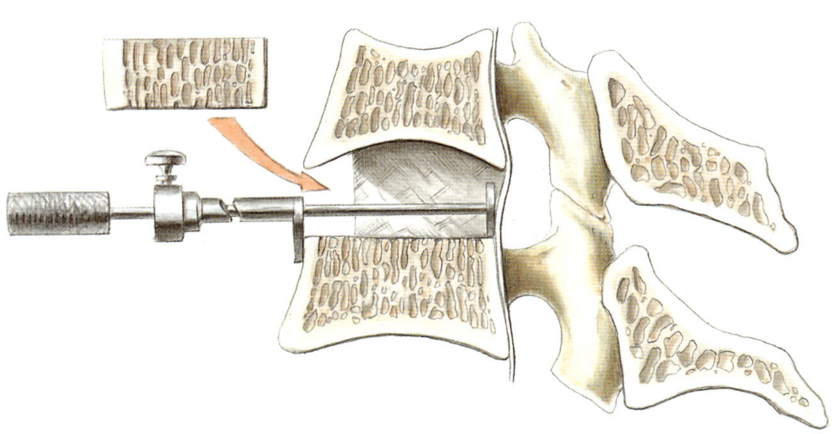

Fig. 8.**13** Depth measurement of the graft bed.

Postoperative Treatment

Immediately after the operation, the head is placed flat between two firm pillows. Starting on the first postoperative day, the patient is mobilized with an orthoplast collar (Camp collar, for example), which has to be worn for 6–8 weeks. If the lateral radiograph shows good consolidation after this time, the collar can be taken off. Physical therapy for the cervical and nuchal musculature should follow.

Complications

Excessive retractor pressure on the trachea causes sore throat and hoarseness. The patient can be led to inhalation therapy for 2–3 days after the operation, in addition to analgesic–anti-inflammatory drugs. If hoarseness does not subside within 4–7 days, a lesion of the recurrent or superior laryngeal nerve must be suspected. In rare cases, Horner's syndrome is observed when the ipsilateral sympathetic trunk over the longus colli muscle has been injured. Care should therefore be taken to detach this muscle with caution and to apply the retractors appropriately. Injury to the esophagus is avoidable if the dissection is performed properly.

Thoracic Disk Herniation

Incidence and Localization

Thoracic disk herniation is extremely rare (approx. 0.2–0.8% of all herniated disks), and is found preferentially between T8 and T12, and most commonly at T11–T12. Acute, soft herniations (approx. 30%) are usually located mediolaterally, in contrast to calcified older herniations, which are almost invariably in a medial location (approx. 70%) (Arce and Dohrmann 1985).

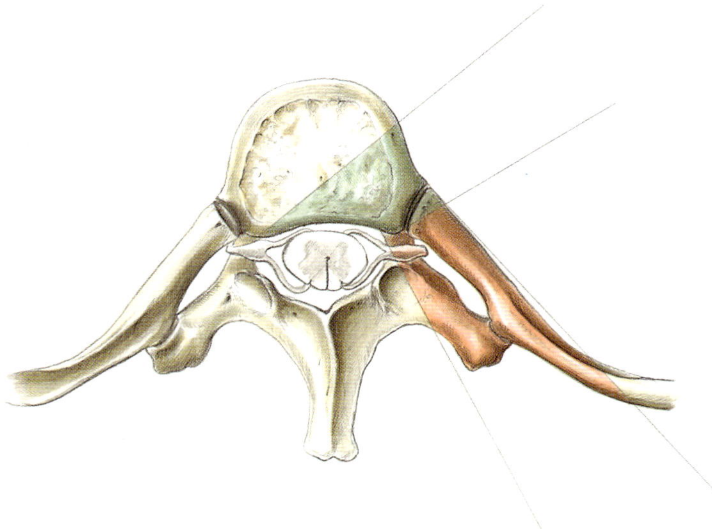

Fig. 8.**14** The posterolateral approach via costotransversectomy (red), and the anterolateral approach following thoracotomy (green).

Indications and Diagnosis

Back pain in the midline is frequently the initial symptom. About 70% of patients then develop motor and sensory disturbances such as the Brown–Séquard syndrome, while the remainder only experience radicular symptoms, that is, pain and sensory deficits. The diagnosis is nowadays made by computed tomography—preferably after intrathecal administration of contrast agents—or by magnetic resonance imaging.

Approaches

Owing to the high risk of spinal cord injury, the approach by conventional laminectomy has been completely discarded, and ought not to be used any longer today. At the present time, several variants of the *posterolateral approach* by costotransversectomy and an *anterolateral approach* following thoracotomy are recommended. The two approaches, and the structures to which they give access, are indicated in Fig. 8.**14**.

In our opinion, the *anterolateral transthoracic approach* affords the widest range of options. The approach to lateral and medial herniations is clear and simple; the dura is in full view at all times, and the risk of a cord lesion or damage to the neurovascular structures is minimal. Resection of bones and ligamentous structures is reduced to a minimum, and there is no danger of postoperative instability. This approach is also suitable for larger tumors (e.g., hourglass neurinoma) or for vertebral resection with ensuing stabilization. The necessity of opening the pleura and retracting the lung, risking a possible postoperative respiratory dysfunction, is a *disadvantage*. For older patients, therefore, preoperative evaluation of respiratory function and, if necessary, appropriate preparation are recommended.

The *posterolateral approach* via costotransversectomy offers advantages in lateral herniations, but it is of very limited value when a larger process extends into the thorax, and particularly for medially located processes. A herniated disk near the midline is hardly accessible without compression of the dural sac and its contents. Another *drawback* is the extensive division of the back musculature. Additionally, there is a risk of injury to the anterior radicular artery and, at the level between D8 and D12, of the Adamkiewicz artery. According to Lazorthes et al. (1973), the Adamkiewicz artery runs between T7 and T8 in 15% of cases, between T9 und T12 in 75% of cases, and between L1 and L2, usually on the left side, in 10%. This should always be taken into account, particularly with a posterior approach.

As we see it, costotransversectomy is indicated when a thoracotomy is out of the question for medial or technical reasons, or when processes in the spinal canal with little extraspinal extension are to be removed in one and the same session.

Anterolateral Transthoracic Approach

Positioning and Incision

See Chapter 1, pp. 13–16, regarding the positioning and incision in the transthoracic approach to the thoracic spine T4–T11.

In case of a lateral herniation, the thoracotomy will be performed on the same side; for medial herniations, right-sided thoracotomy is more advantageous, because of the vascular situation (left-sided course of the aorta). For exposure of only two or three vertebrae, an intercostal posterolateral thoracotomy is adequate, so that rib resection is unnecessary. It is important to note that because of the descending course of the ribs, the approach should generally be made two ribs above the level corresponding to the center of the lesion. Following thoracotomy and application of the chest spreader, the lung is retracted anteriorly; this affords a good overview of the anterolateral surface of the thoracic spine.

Anatomical Site

The anatomy of the anterolateral aspect of the thoracic spine and the posterior mediastinum is presented in Chapter 1, pp. 16–21, and in Figure 8.**15**.

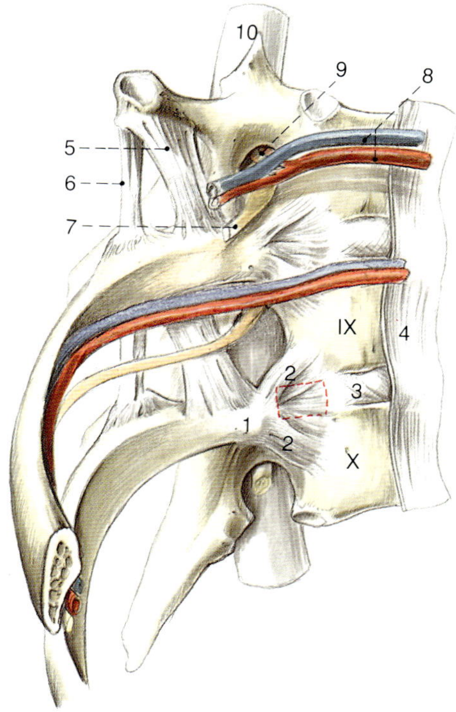

Fig. 8.**15** Anatomical site of the right lateral surface of thoracic spine. The sympathetic trunk and the greater splanchnic nerve have been removed.

1 Rib head
2 Radiate ligament of the head of the rib
3 Intervertebral disk
4 Anterior longitudinal ligament
5 Superior costotransverse ligament
6 Lateral costotransverse ligament
7 Intercostal nerve
8 Intercostal vessels
9 Anterior radicular artery
10 Dural sac
IX–X Thoracic vertebrae

Operative Technique

Instrumentarium

Thoracotomy via the anterolateral approach requires the usual instruments; particularly long instruments are needed for removal of the intervertebral disk (Fig. 8.**16**).

Level identification is accomplished by counting the vertebrae from the caudal side in the lateral beam of an image converter, using a needle inserted into the intervertebral space, or by counting the ribs along the medial side of the thorax from above. When counting the ribs, it should be borne in mind that a given rib shares its articular surface with the thoracic vertebra at the same level, and may also have a small articular surface at the next higher vertebra. (The disk space T8–T9, for example, may lie at the superior margin of the ninth rib, but the rib may also overlie it to some extent.)

After this, the parietal pleura is incised rectangularly and dissected free laterally, attention being paid to the subjacent intercostal neurovascular structures, the sympathetic trunk, and the various branches to the greater splanchnic nerve. The two pleural ends are fixed with stay sutures (Fig. 8.**17**). The sympathetic trunk and, if necessary, the branches to the greater splanchnic nerve as well, are mobilized with the dissector and retracted with the aid of a vessel loop. The intercostal artery and vein are retracted, so that the lateral aspect of the disk is exposed.

After identification of the intervertebral disk, the radiate ligament of the rib head and the lateral portion of the annulus fibrosus are incised (area enclosed by dashed line in Fig. 8.**15**) and removed with a rongeur. The inferior portion of the radiate ligament of the rib head is left intact, so as to protect the intercostal nerve and the anterior radicular artery and vein (neurovascular structures) that run through the intervertebral foramen (Fig. 8.**18**). Using a curet, the disk can now cautiously be freed from the vertebral end plate and removed. Using a microdrill (initially a rose-head burr, later a diamond burr) and continuous lavage, the space thus produced is rectangularly expanded (approximately 10 × 15 mm) by trimming bone from the upper and lower vertebral body (Fig. 8.**18**). Another part of the disk can be removed by curet from the resultant cavity, and the space can again be cautiously expanded until the posterior border of the vertebral body and the posterior longitudinal ligament are reached (Fig. 8.**19**). Occasionally, it may be of advantage to rotate the patient about 10 degrees toward the contralateral side, so that the drill can be applied relatively parallel to the posterior aspect of the vertebra, avoiding injury to the posterior longitudinal ligament and, above all, to the dura. A mediolateral herniation is now readily visualized and

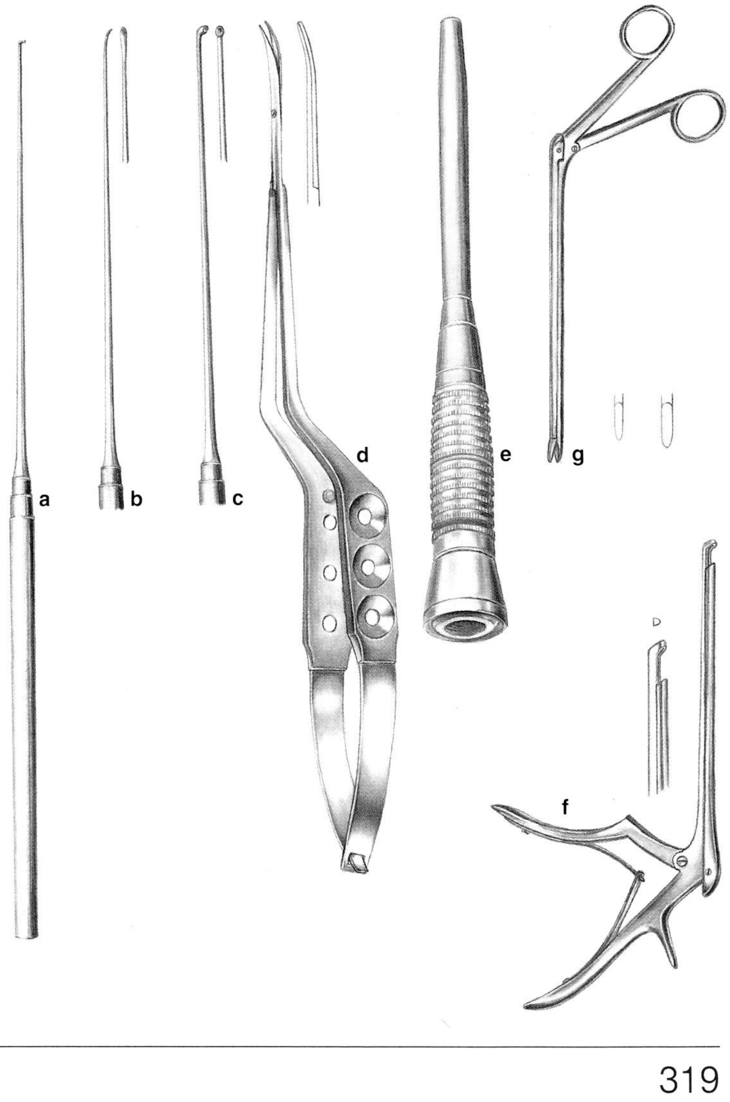

Fig. 8.**16** Special instruments for discectomy by the anterolateral approach.
a Blunt probe, 23–25 cm long.
b Narrow microdissector, 23–25 cm long.
c Sharp microcuret, 23–25 cm long.
d Curved microdissecting scissors, 22.5–23.0 cm long.
e Long holder for microdrill.
f Kerrison rongeur (2–3 mm wide), 20–23 cm long.
g Love rongeur (3 mm wide), 20–23 cm long.

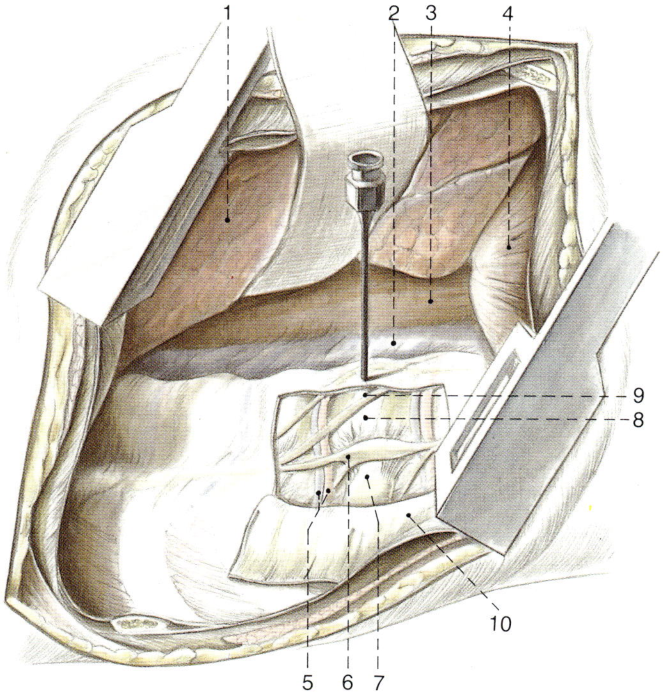

Fig. 8.**17** Radiologic level determination by insertion of a needle into the intervertebral space. Incision of the parietal pleura. Fixation of the pleural ends with stay sutures.

1 Right lung
2 Azygos vein
3 Esophagus
4 Thoracic diaphragm
5 Intercostal vessels
6 Sympathetic trunk with ganglion and communicating branch
7 Head of rib
8 Intervertebral disk
9 Greater splanchnic nerve
10 Parietal pleura

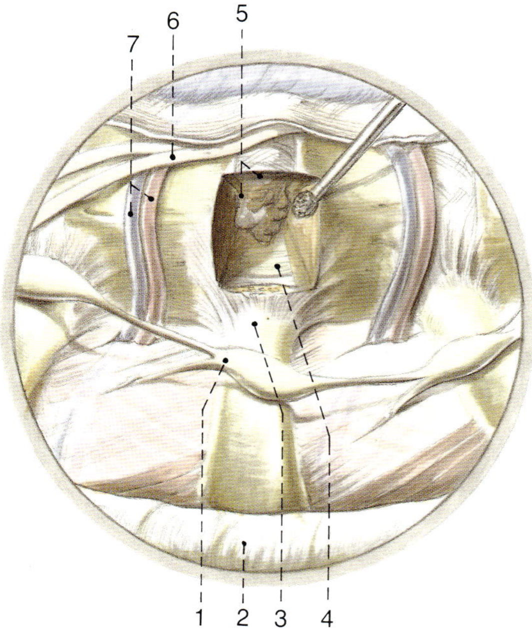

Fig. 8.**18** After incision of the annulus fibrosus and freeing of the intervertebral disk with a rongeur, the intervertebral space is enlarged with a microdrill, and the posterior wall of the vertebral bodies and the posterior longitudinal ligament are exposed. Optical magnification.

1 Sympathetic trunk
2 Parietal pleura, reflected
3 Head of rib
4 Posterior longitudinal ligament
5 Annulus fibrosus and pulpy nucleus
6 Greater splanchnic nerve
7 Intercostal vessels

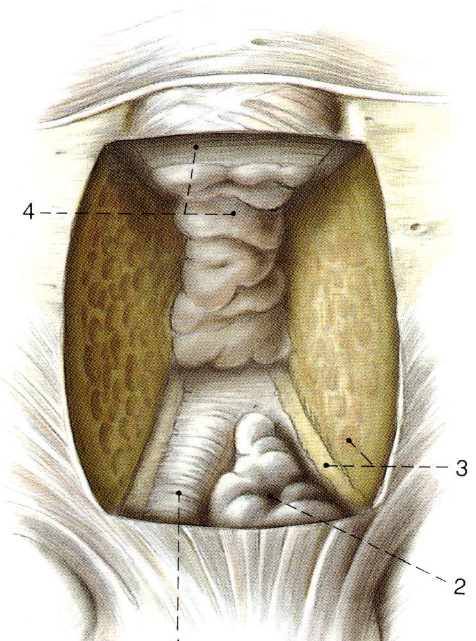

removable with a rongeur (Fig. 8.**19**). If the protrusion lies very far laterally, that is, near or in the intervertebral foramen, the cavity is expanded laterally, preserving the posterior longitudinal ligament, until the disk fragments can be removed. In the presence of a medial, calcified herniation, on the other hand, the osteophytic masses are now cautiously removed—using a surgical microscope or magnifying glasse—with a diamond burr and continuous irrigation (Fig. 8.**20**).

Fig. 8.**19** Exposure of a mediolateral soft disk herniation. Optical magnification.

1 Posterior longitudinal ligament
2 Intervertebral disk sequestrum
3 Intervertebral space enlarged by means of a microdrill
4 Annulus fibrosus and pulpy nucleus

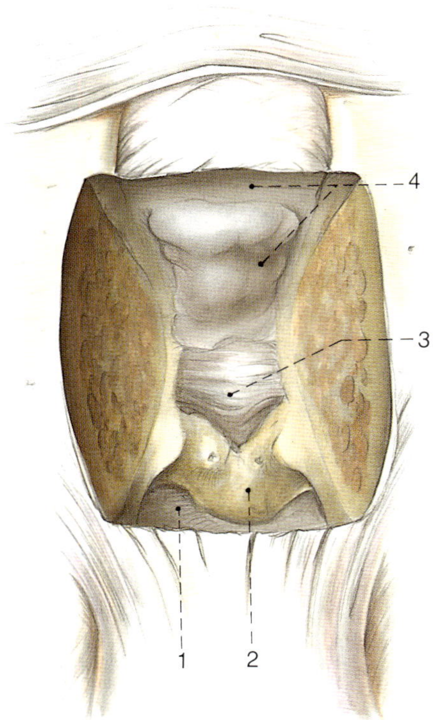

Fig. 8.**20** Exposure of medial exophyte with compression of the dura and the thoracic spinal cord.

1 Dural sac
2 Calcified medial disk herniation
3 Posterior longitudinal ligament
4 Annulus fibrosus and pulpy nucleus

Wound Closure

Subsequently, the previously fashioned pleural flap is closed with interrupted sutures. After removal of the retractors, application of a chest tube and inflation of the lung, wound closure is effected as described on pp. 22–23.

Posterolateral Approach After Costotransversectomy

A laterally situated disk hernia can be accessed via a modified costotransversectomy (Seeger 1982). This only requires removal of half the width of the rib and the transverse process (Fig. 8.**22**). A better view is obtained by complete removal of a rib and a transverse process. In the presence of a tumor, such as a spinal metastasis or an hourglass neurinoma, a hemilaminectomy preserving the vertebral joint can be performed afterwards. When larger paravertebral processes, or a whole vertebra, are involved, the anterolateral approach offers far better visualization, and is less risky.

Positioning

The approach can be made from either side, depending on the site of the lesion. The operation is carried out with the patient in prone position, the side to be operated on being slightly raised by placing pads under the thorax and the pelvis, so that a tangential view can be obtained. For approaches to the upper thoracic spine, we place both arms forward, so as to turn the scapula away from the midline as far as possible (Fig. 8.**21**).

Localization

If the spinous processes are used to identify the level, it should be borne in mind that the tip of the spinous process of T1 lies about 1 cm lower than the inferior margin of this vertebra; in the case of T5 and T6, it is even lower by a whole vertebral breadth, while at T12 it again lies at the lower border of the vertebra. Localization with reference to the ribs is difficult, too, since they are not consistently palpable. Precise localization of the intervertebral space is therefore best accomplished by paramedian insertion of a needle and lateral image-intensifier control.

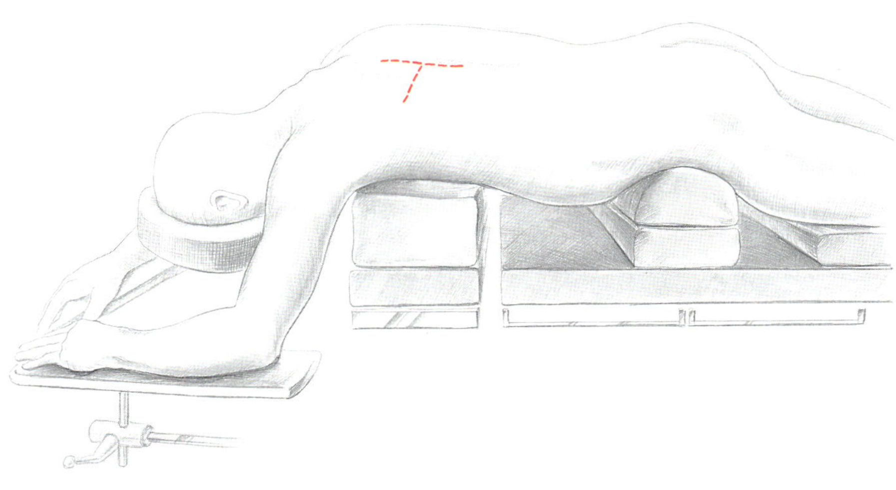

Fig. 8.**21** Positioning for a posterolateral approach to the thoracic spine with outstretched arms. Skin incision.

Anatomical Site

Figure 8.**22** shows the bony and ligamentous structures of the posterolateral approach to the thoracic spine from the surgeon's point of view. The dashed red line indicates the resection lines on the rib and the transverse process. The rib head with its articular surface (facies articularis capitis costae), which is separated into a cranial and a caudal part by a transverse ledge on the second to tenth ribs, is in apposition to the superior and inferior costal fovea of the vertebral bodies; the ninth rib, for example, adjoins vertebral bodies T9 and T8.

Incision

We used a T-shaped incision (Fig. 8.**21**; see also Chapter 1, pp. 60–63). The transverse limb of the skin incision is at the level of the intervertebral space or the vertebra to be exposed (about 12 cm), while the longitudinal incision runs over the spinous processes (about 8 cm). The two skin flaps are sufficiently mobilized in cranial and caudal directions.

After transverse division of the superficial muscle layer (trapezius muscle), the deep musculature of the back (erector muscle of the spine), with its tendinous insertions, is first separated from the spinous processes and retracted from the vertebral arches and the joints with an elevator, and is then transected about 5–7 cm laterally with the electrocautery (Fig. 8.**23**). The rib that leads to the vertebral body or intervertebral space in question is now identified. Since ribs 3–11 attach by about two-thirds to the same vertebra, and by about one-third to the next higher

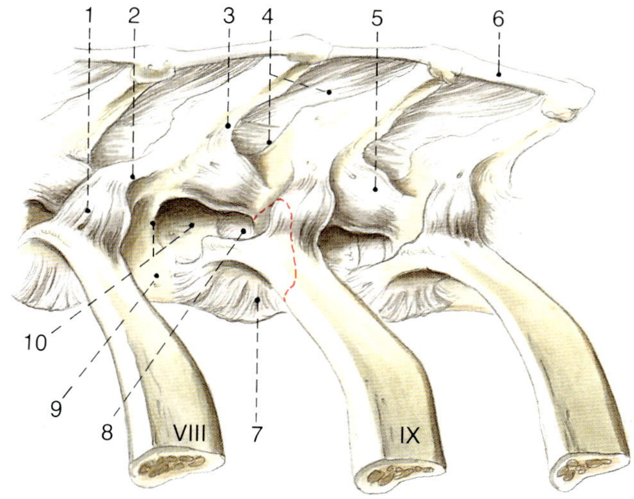

Fig. 8.**22** Surgical anatomy of the bony and ligamentous structures in the posterolateral approach to the thoracic spine.

1 Costotransverse articulation
2 Transverse process of the eighth thoracic vertebra
3 Spinous process of the eighth thoracic vertebra
4 Interspinal ligament and ligamentum flavum
5 Joint capsule
6 Supraspinal ligament
7 Radiate ligament of the head of the rib
8 T8–T9 intervertebral disk
9 Eighth thoracic vertebra
10 Pedicle of vertebral arch and intervertebral foramen
VIII–IX Ribs

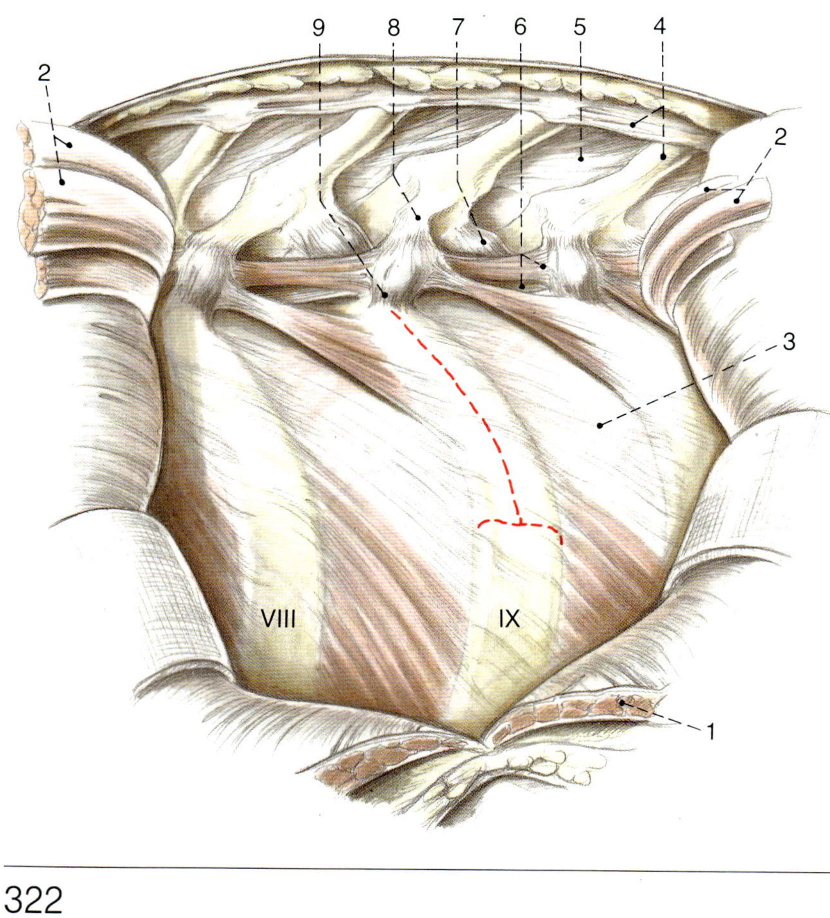

Fig. 8.**23** Operative site after cranial and caudal dissection of muscle flaps. Division of rib periosteum and subperiosteal detachment of the rib over a length of about 8 cm (dashed red line). After opening of the costotransverse joint capsule and removal of the transverse process at the base, the rib is laterally divided with rib cutters, and exarticulated after careful detachment of the costovertebral joint capsule.

1 Trapezius muscle
2 Erector muscle of the spine
3 External intercostal muscles
4 Spinous process and supraspinal ligament
5 Interspinal ligament
6 Intertransverse muscle and intertransverse ligament
7 Zygapophyseal articulation
8 Transverse process
9 Costotransverse ligament and costotransverse articulation
VIII–IX Ribs

vertebra, it is sufficient for a small access to the intervertebral disk to remove only the upper half of the corresponding rib or transverse process. For larger processes, resection of the rib and transverse process provides a better overview.

Operative Technique

Costotransversectomy

The rib and the corresponding transverse process are freed and removed as described in Chapter 1 (pp. 60–63). During detachment of the rib from the costotransverse articulation, there is a danger of injury to the anterior radicular artery (Adamkiewicz artery), which arises here from the intercostal artery. The parietal pleura below the rib periosteum is bluntly retracted from the vertebral bodies and the intervertebral disk, using small cotton-tipped sponge sticks.

Exposure and Removal of Herniated Disk

The course of the intercostal nerve, the intercostal artery coming from the anterior side, with the origin of the anterior radicular artery, and—for larger processes—the sympathetic trunk, are now exposed (Fig. 8.**24**). The neurovascular bundle can be carefully retracted to provide an overview of the intervertebral disk and the herniation. If ligation of the intercostal artery is required, this should be done at the T9–T12 level, because the Adamkiewicz artery (anterior radicular artery) may arise from it not anterior to the vertebral body but laterally, below the rib.

The intervertebral disk can now be incised (Fig. 8.**25**, red dashed line) and removed with small rongeurs (Fig. 8.**26**). A rectangular probe is used to verify complete decompression of the dural sac and the nerve root.

Wound Closure

Before wound closure, positive-pressure breathing should be performed to make certain that the parietal pleura has not been injured. Injury to it would require insertion of a chest tube. The wound is closed by reapproximation of the divided musculature layer by layer. See also Chapter 1, p. 62.

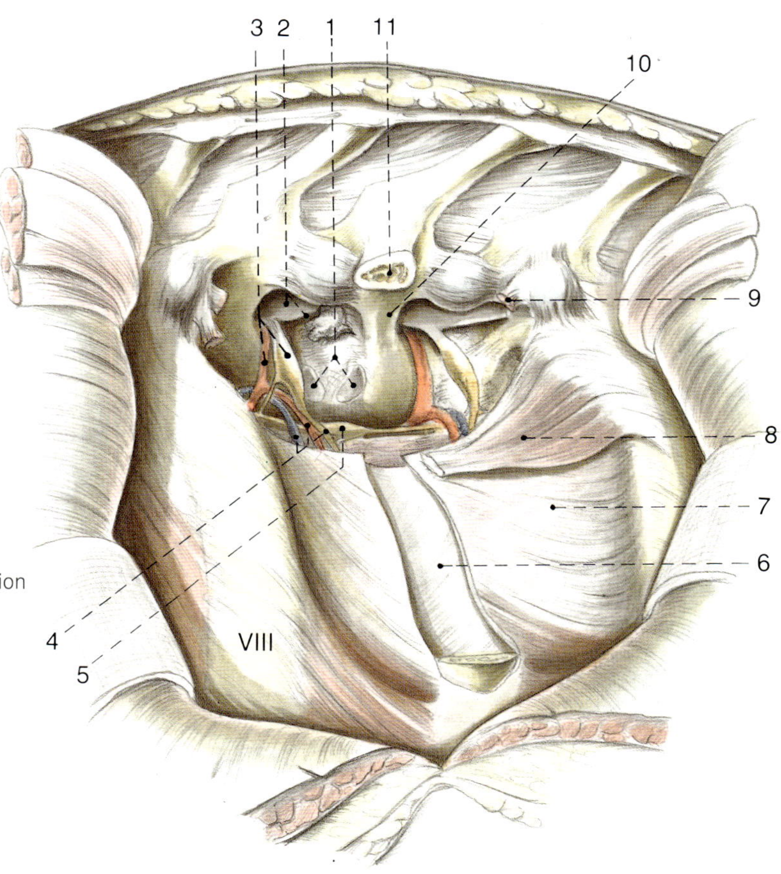

Fig. 8.**24** After freeing the rib and resecting the transverse process, the intervertebral disk being sought is visualized and, above it, the intervertebral foramen with the structures passing through it; the dural sac can be seen in the spinal canal.

1 T8–T9 intervertebral disk and superior and inferior costal fovea
2 Dural sac, indented by disk hernia
3 Radiculomedullary artery and intercostal nerve, with spinal ganglion
4 Intercostal artery, vein and nerve
5 Sympathetic trunk
6 Parietal pleura and periosteum
7 External intercostal muscles
8 Semispinalis thoracis muscle
9 Intertransverse muscle (separated)
10 Pedicle of the vertebral arch
11 T9 transverse process
VIII Rib

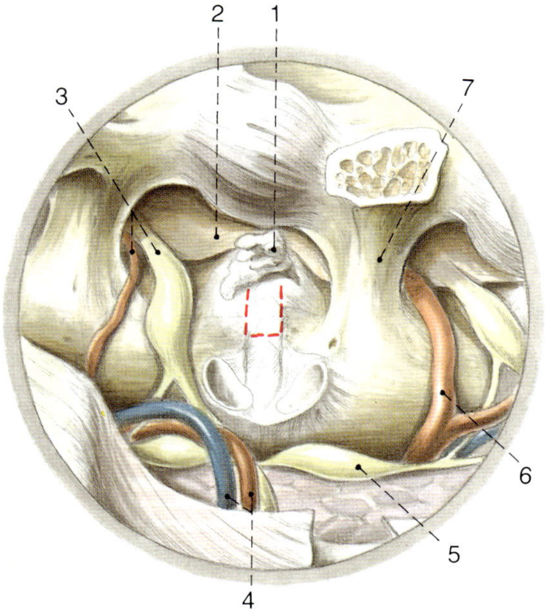

Fig. 8.**25** The structures are more easily discernible after optical magnification. The emerging mediolateral disk hernia compressing the dural sac and the nerve root is visible.

1 Disk hernia and intervertebral disk
2 Dural sac
3 T8 spinal nerve and anterior radicular artery
4 Intercostal artery, vein and nerve
5 Sympathetic trunk
6 Radiculomedullary (Adamkiewicz) artery
7 Pedicle of the ninth thoracic vertebra

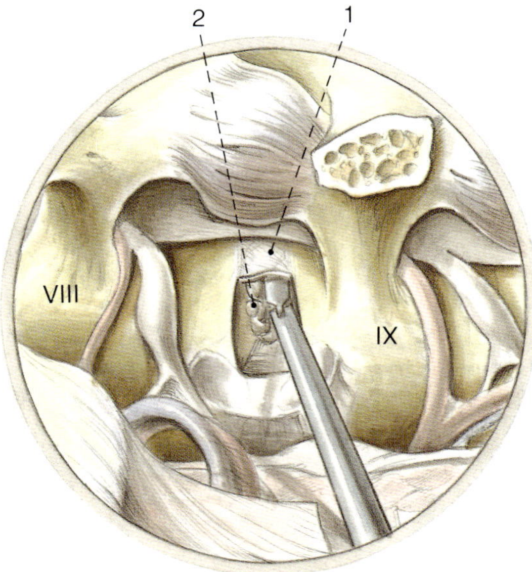

Fig. 8.**26** After incision of the intervertebral disk, the hernia and a portion of the intervertebral disk (so far as accessible) are removed with a rongeur.

1 Annulus fibrosus with perforation site
2 Intervertebral disk
VIII–X Vertebrae

Lumbar Disk Herniation

Indications and Diagnosis

Absolute indications (requiring emergency operation):

- Cauda equina compression syndrome.
- Acute severe paresis of functionally important muscles.

Relative indications (operation performed only after unsuccessful conservative therapy with at least 14 days of bed rest):

- Severely painful, refractory radicular syndrome.
- Chronic and recurrent radicular pain syndrome, with mild neurologic deficits, or none.

Besides the clinical, neurological examination, plain anteroposterior and lateral radiographs of the lumbar spine (information about abnormalities at the lumbosacral junction) should be obtained and myelography or—preferably today—computed tomography performed. The latter, possibly in conjunction with reconstructions, is at present superior to MRI.

A negative myelogram calls for added CT scanning, so that a so-called extracanalicular herniation or another rare pathological condition in the intervertebral canal may not be overlooked. In the event of inadequate visualization, a thin-layer CT (1.5 mm) with reconstructions may provide better information.

Clarification of the following questions is critical:

- At what level is the clinically affected nerve root compressed?
- What is the cause of the compression?
  - Disk herniation
  - Stenosis of the lateral recess
  - A pathological process in the intervertebral canal
  - A far-out syndrome

The most common cause is disk herniation. It should be remembered, however, that there also is "sciatica without disk herniation."

Symptomatic herniated disks are present at two levels at the same time in only about 2–4% of cases. The precise level should therefore be determined preoperatively on the basis of the clinical picture and the neuroradiological findings. A polysegmental exploration, or actual removal, of two adjacent intervertebral disks is associated with a higher rate of poor results. We aim for a *monosegmental* approach.

We also seek to avoid hemilaminectomy, that is, complete resection of a hemiarch. This imposes a unilateral stress on the motor column, and creates the danger of a new disease, that is, of a facet syndrome, or instability with persistent lumbago or pseudoradicular complaints, or both.

Positioning

Various positions are employed; examples are the genufacial and the knee–chest positions (Chapter 1, Fig. 1.**123**). They have in common the purpose of kyphosing the lumbar spine and widening the interlaminar spaces. We have adopted modified genupectoral positioning (Fig. 8.**27**). This has advantages over the genufacial position in elderly patients, obese patients, and patients with hip prostheses. Patients with stiff hip or knee joints are placed in a flat prone position, with padding under the thorax and pelvis. The abdomen should always be free, so that venous reflux and increased venous bleeding during the operation can be avoided.

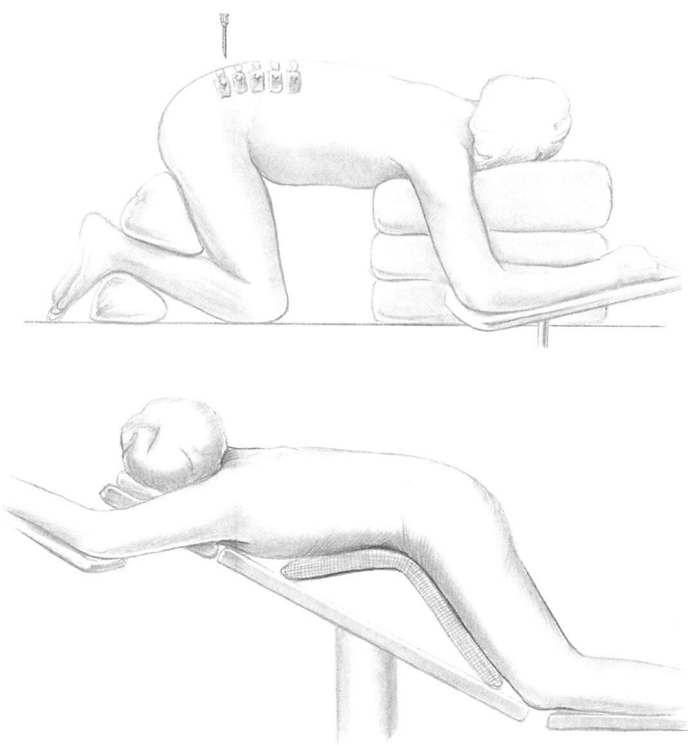

a

b

Fig. 8.**27** Positioning. a Genufacial position; b modified genupectoral position.

Locating the Level for Surgery

We recommend that the level of the segment to be operated on should be verified using the image intensifier prior to the start of the operation. To do this, a needle is inserted alongside the next higher spinous process (that is, alongside the L4 spinous process in operations on L4–L5) until it makes contact with the L4 arch. The arch may, in addition, be marked with a small amount of dye.

Incision and Exposure of the Surgical Field

The incision, detachment of the musculature from the spinous processes and the laminae, and exposure of the surgical field by the conventional technique are described on p. 71 above.

Additionally, we will discuss the Caspar approach here, using a special instrumentarium (Fig. 8.**28**). With the use of this instrument, a median skin incision about 3 cm long, from the middle of one spinous process to the other, is sufficient. At L3–L4 and L2–L3, the skin incision is made a little higher, as the intervertebral space here lies farther below the upper arch than at L4–L5 and L5–S1.

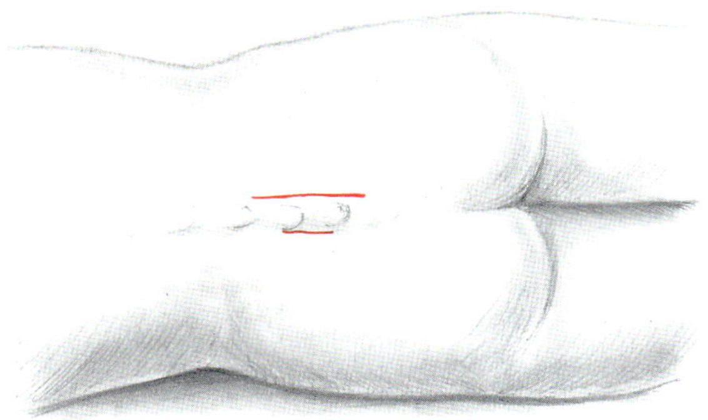

Fig. 8.**28** Incision—on the right for conventional technique (about 6–8 cm); on the left for the Caspar technique (3 cm). Either incision is placed in the midline.

The subcutaneous tissues are divided as far as the thoracolumbar fascia, and a retractor is applied. A curved opening is made in the fascia about 1 cm from the midline; the fascia is separated from the musculature and retracted with the aid of two stay sutures (Fig. 8.**29**). The semispinalis and multifidus muscles are bluntly retracted from the interspinous ligament from caudal to cranial. The tendinous insertions are sharply divided at the inferior border and the lateral surface of the spinous processes (Fig. 8.**30**). As a rule, detachment of the tendinous insertions from a single spinous process, the next higher one, is sufficient.

Using an elevator and a folded-out sponge, the paraspinal musculature is retracted over the vertebral joints (Fig. 8.**31**). The superior and the inferior hemiarch and the ligamentum flavum are now freed of soft tissue. The muscle retractor (Caspar speculum) is then inserted over a grooved Langenbeck retractor and turned 90 degrees with the handle toward the assistant (Fig. 8.**32**). The speculum is then opened until it is solidly anchored in the musculature cranially and caudally. The opened speculum should expose the entire ligamentum flavum, a portion of the inferior hemiarch, and about one-third of the width of the superior hemiarch (Fig. 8.**33**). A second retractor may be used for lateral retraction of the musculature. From this point on, use is made of optical magnification (operating microscope; focal length 300–350 mm, eyepiece 12×, or loupe 2.5–3.5×).

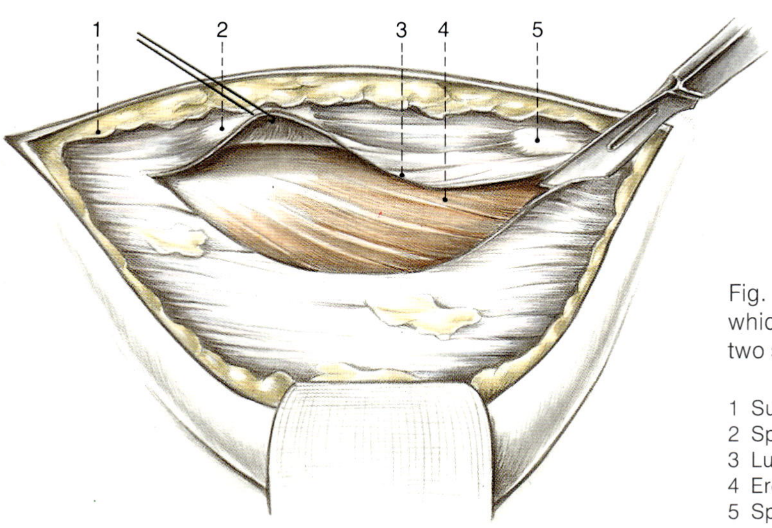

Fig. 8.**29** A curved opening is made in the lumbosacral fascia, which is then separated from the musculature and retracted with two stay sutures (right side).

1 Subcutis
2 Spinous process of the fifth lumbar vertebra
3 Lumboposterior fascia, open
4 Erector muscle of the spine
5 Spinous process of the fourth lumbar vertebra

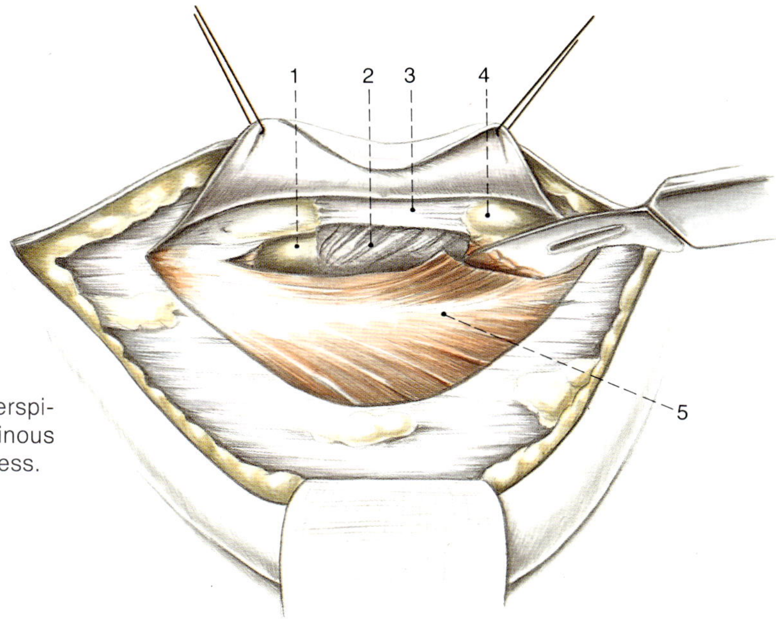

Fig. 8.**30** The musculature is bluntly retracted from the interspinal ligament from caudal to cranial, after which the tendinous insertions are sharply separated at the superior spinous process.

1 Spinous process of the fifth lumbar vertebra
2 Interspinal ligament
3 Supraspinal ligament
4 Spinous process of the fourth lumbar vertebra
5 Multifidus and semispinalis lumbalis muscles

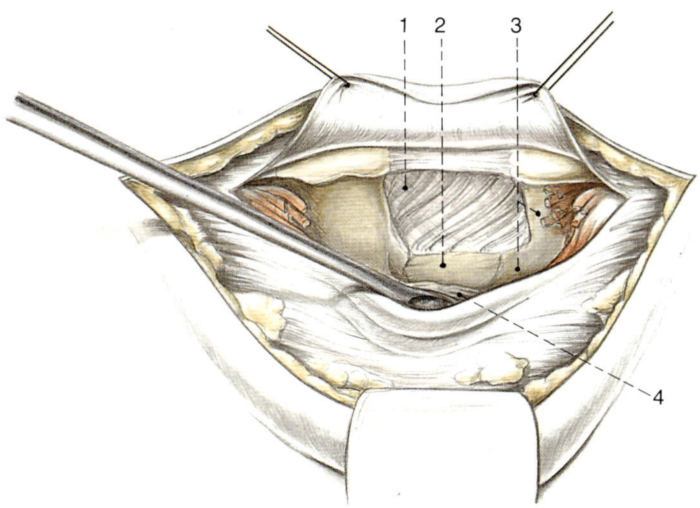

Fig. 8.**31** Lateral detachment of the musculature, using a raspatory, over the two vertebral arches and the intervertebral joint. The upper and lower vertebral arches, the articulation, ligamentum flavum, and interlaminar space serve as orientation aids.

1 Interspinal ligament
2 Ligamentum flavum
3 Spinous process and arch of the fourth lumbar vertebra
4 L4–L5 zygapophyseal articulation

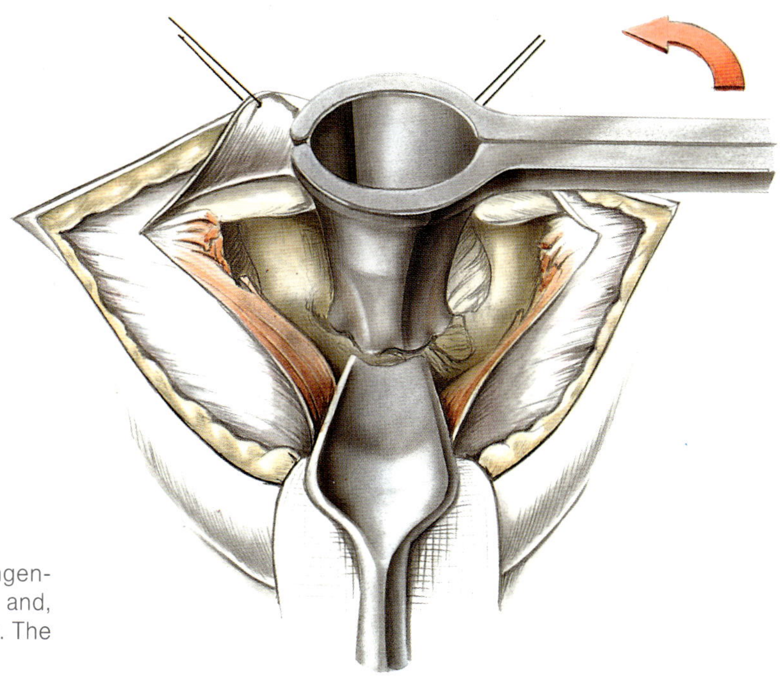

Fig. 8.**32** Retraction of the musculature with grooved Langenbeck probes. The muscle retractor (speculum) is inserted and, with the handle, given a 90-degree turn toward the assistant. The retractor is then opened.

Opening the Ligamentum Flavum and Laminotomy

(Fig. 8.**33**)

(The terms interlaminar fenestration and laminotomy are used synonymously.) The ligamentum flavum is incised cruciformly and removed with punches of varying size (2 mm, 3 mm, 5 mm). It is normally 2–3 mm thick, but may range up to 8 mm in elderly patients.

Note: In the presence of large hernias, the nerve root and the dural sac can be posteriorly displaced by high pressure, so that lack of caution during opening entails a risk of injury.

The laminotomy (interlaminar fenestration) is enlarged as required by resection of portions of the superior and inferior hemiarches, and possibly of the medial third of the facet joint, using variously sized rongeurs or a microdrill. This enlargement is based on the articular distance from the spinous process and on the location of the intervertebral space and the herniation. In view of the importance of this operative step, some anatomical details will be discussed here.

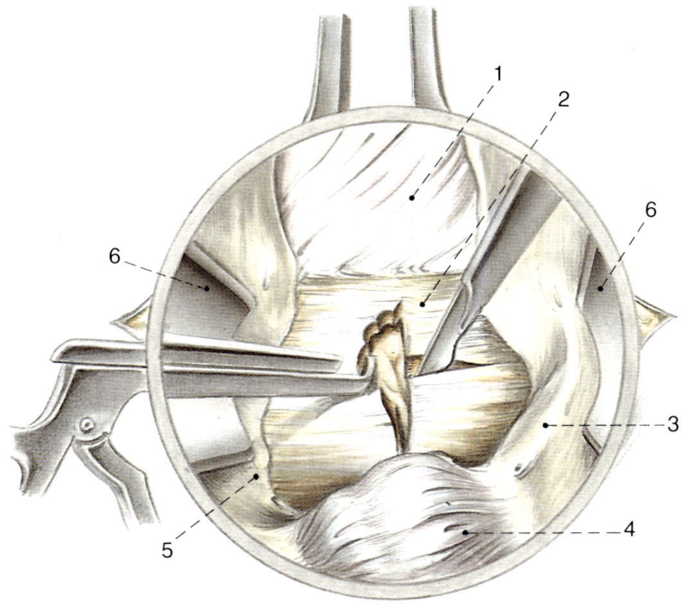

Fig. 8.**33** View through the speculum. Optical magnification. The ligamentum flavum is opened with a scalpel and subsequently resected with punches.

1 Interspinal ligament
2 Ligamentum flavum
3 L4 hemiarch
4 Zygapophyseal articulation
5 L5 hemiarch
6 Blades of the speculum

Surgical Anatomy

The normal dimensions of the interlaminar windows L3–L4, L4–L5, and L5–S1, including their maximal and minimal values, are shown in Figure 8.**34**. The intervertebral disk is drawn in relation to them. It can be seen that the intervertebral disk can be reached without removing part of the upper hemilamina only at L5–S1. At L4–L5, it is usually necessary, and at L3–L4 always necessary, to remove about 4–6 mm from the upper arch in order to gain access to the intervertebral disk. By the same token, the articular distance from the midline is sufficiently wide only at L5–S1; at L4–L5 and particularly L3–L4, the inferior articular process and the joint conceal the course of the nerve root, which normally arises at the level of the intervertebral disk (lateral recess, p. 340). In this case, resection of the medial border of the joint can hardly be avoided if the nerve root is to be accessed without damaging traction. For this reason, it is necessary to be certain about the location of the hernia in relation to the intervertebral space: at the same level, above, or below it. Accordingly, an attempt may be made to preserve the joint and to remove bone from the upper or lower hemiarch in order to reach the herniation. The laminotomy, therefore, is not always performed in the same way, but is adapted to the individual circumstances (Fig. 8.**34**).

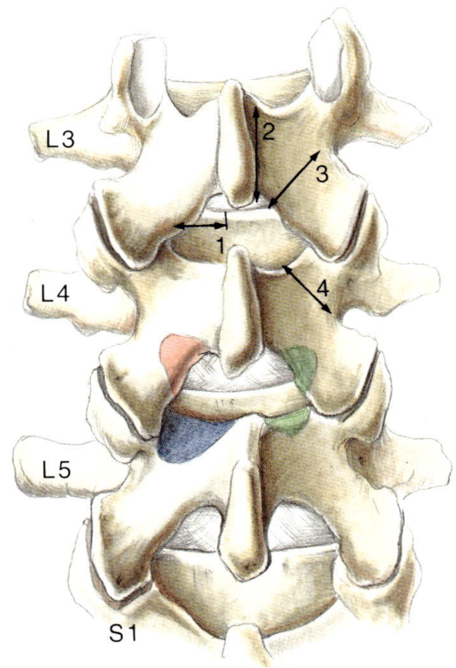

Fig. 8.**34** The most important dimensions of the interlaminar windows L3–L4, L4–L5 and L5–S1.

	Level	Variations (mm)	Mean (mm)
1 Articular distance from the midline	L3–L4	3– 7	5
	L4–L5	3–10	6
	L5–S1	7–13	9
2 Height of the vertebral arch	L3	20–32	23
	L4	16–29	21
	L5	14–22	17
3 Width of the inferior articular process	L3	12–19	16
	L4	12–22	17
	L5	13–24	18
4 Width of the superior articular process	L3	12–22	16
	L4	12–21	16
	L5	13–20	16

Green: Laminotomy in mediolateral disk herniation at the level of the intervertebral space.

Red: Laminotomy in cranially slipped herniation, the joint being largely preserved.

Blue: Laminotomy in caudally slipped herniation. The joint is not opened.

Operative Technique

Dissection to the Nerve Root (Spinal Nerve)
(Fig. 8.**35**)

In recent herniations, the epidural fat pad surrounding the dural sac and the nerve root, and serving as a gliding layer, is retained; after chronic compression, it is usually considerably thinned out. This gliding layer should be transected only at its lateral attachment, and should be retracted medially with the root (Fig. 8.**35**). It protects the root against subsequent adhesions. A venous chain with horizontal connections runs like a rope-ladder over the posterior longitudinal ligament. These connecting vessels are coagulated with *bipolar* forceps. If they were pulled from lateral to medial, they would lacerate far laterally at the trunk, and severe venous hemorrhages might result, usually requiring nonselective, gross coagulation. The venous system is often initially congested, and is always decongested after removal of the hernia.

Exposure and Removal of the Hernia
(Figs. 8.**36**–8.**40**)

In the next step, the relation of the hernia to the dural sac and the nerve root is clarified with the aid of a fine dissector or probe. Using a fine suction tip (2.5 mm diameter), the root is retracted medially and explored with a 90-degree probe between the longitudinal ligament and the neural structures; any loose fragment that may be found is mobilized and removed (Fig. 8.**36**).

As mentioned above, the operating surgeon should be aware of the location of the herniation preoperatively, having determined it by CT, and should plan his approach through appropriate bone resection. Even today, this simple rule is the one probably disregarded most frequently, despite the good diagnostic techniques that are available, so that overlooked fragments, neurologic deficits, and unnecessary bone resections result. The most common locations of disk herniations are shown in Figure 8.**37**.

Mediolateral Disk Herniations

So-called mediolateral herniations are by far the most common (around 88%). They may lie at the level of the intervertebral space, but more often they have slipped off caudally, and less often cranially. The former are usually subligamentous sequestra; the two latter types tend to be loosely dislocated hernias.

When the herniation is at the level of the intervertebral space, or slightly above it, the gliding layer, the root, and the dural sac are cautiously retracted medially and held and protected with a curved nerve-root retractor (Fig. 8.**38**).

A loose fragment is now removed, or, in the case of subligamentous hernias, the longitudinal ligament is ovally incised over the hernia (Figs. 8.**36**, 8.**38**), and the fragment is cautiously teased out with a small pituitary forceps. We have found that the Williams (Codmann) forceps is best suited for this operative step.

An oval window is now cut into the annulus fibrosus, and the intervertebral disk is removed as nearly completely as

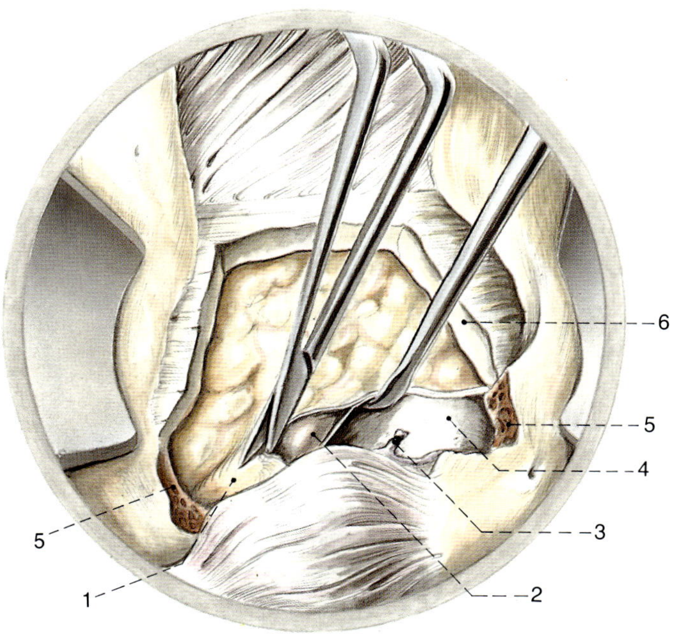

Fig. 8.**35** Division of the gliding layer lateral to the nerve root. Using a dissector, the nerve root with the gliding layer is medially retracted over the disk herniation.

1 Epidural gliding layer
2 Spinal nerve
3 Coagulated horizontal veins
4 Subligamentous disk herniation
5 Resected hemiarch
6 Resected ligamentum flavum

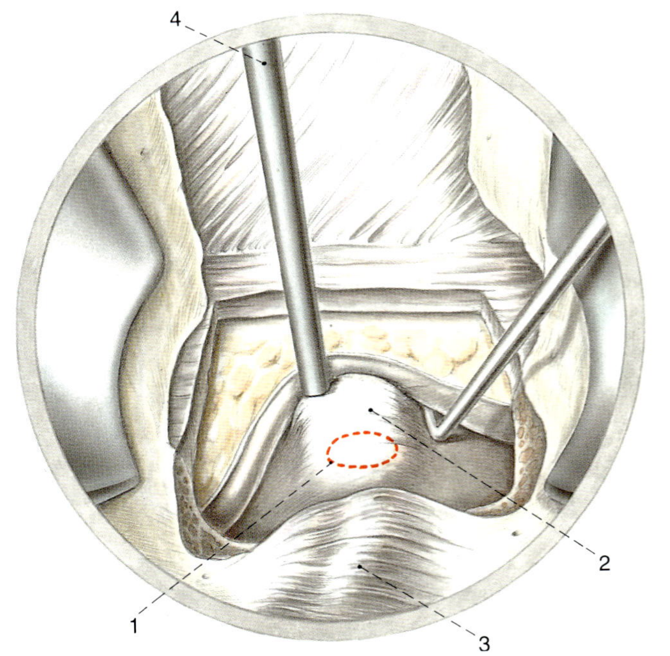

Fig. 8.**36** The location of the hernia is explored with a probe. The root is medially retracted with a fine suction tip. Line of incision for fenestration of the longitudinal ligament and the annulus fibrosus.

1 Incision line
2 Subligamentous disk herniation
3 Zygapophyseal articulation
4 Suction tip

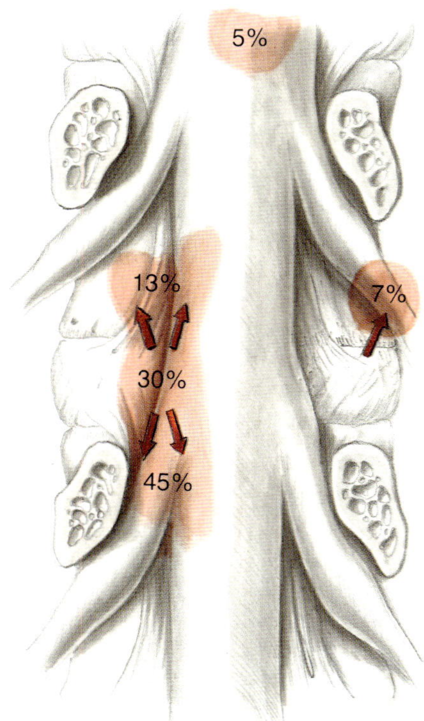

Fig. 8.**37** Possible disk herniations and their frequency distribution.

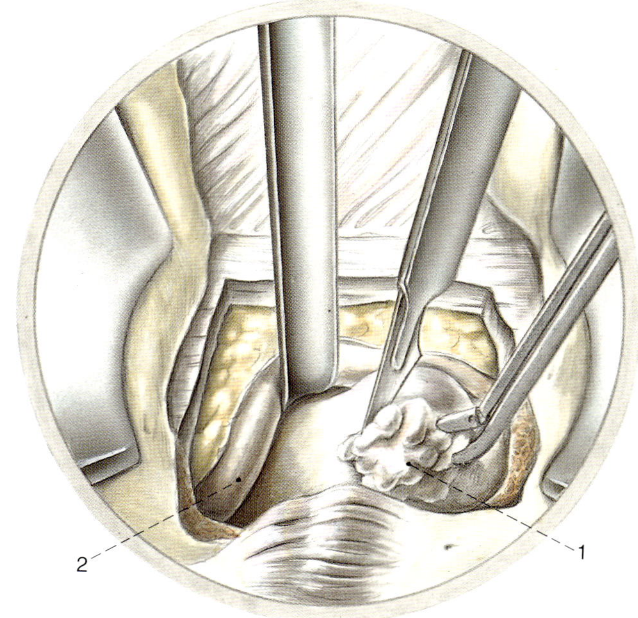

Fig. 8.**38** Insertion of a root retractor over the hernia. Incision of the posterior longitudinal ligament and the annulus fibrosus. The subligamentous sequestrum juts out.

1 Intervertebral disk sequestrum
2 Spinal nerve

possible first using straight pituitary forceps (3 mm, 4 mm, 5 mm wide), and then, medial and lateral, angulated pituitary forceps (3 mm, 4 mm) (Fig. 8.**39**). The cartilaginous end plates are retained. In conclusion, the probe can be used for medial, lateral, and possibly subligamentous exploration, to ensure that no part of a sequestrum has been overlooked (Fig. 8.**40**).

Caution: Tilting of the root hook can cause additional neurologic deficits. Many authors therefore shun root retractors, and instead use two nerve paddies, which are advanced cranially and caudally lateral to the nerve root.

If there is a caudally-displaced mediolateral herniation at the shoulder of the root origin (Fig. 8.**41**), the above procedure for exposure and removal of the hernia is equally applicable, provided the herniation is not too large. If it is very large, on the other hand, possibly accompanied by a loose fragment of sequestrum, it is advisable first to remove the loose sequestrum from the shoulder and only then to retract the root medially, without pressure, and to open and clear out the intervertebral space as described above.

Mediolateral disk hernias may slip off caudally alongside the nerve root, and then compress the latter in the lateral recess or at the entry to the intervertebral canal (Fig. 8.**42**). The position of the pedicle is important, since the nerve courses along its oblique internal surface. The pedicle begins 2–3 mm below the superior edge of the corresponding vertebral body; its inferior border lies approximately 8 mm above the lower edge of the vertebral body (Figs. 8.**34**,

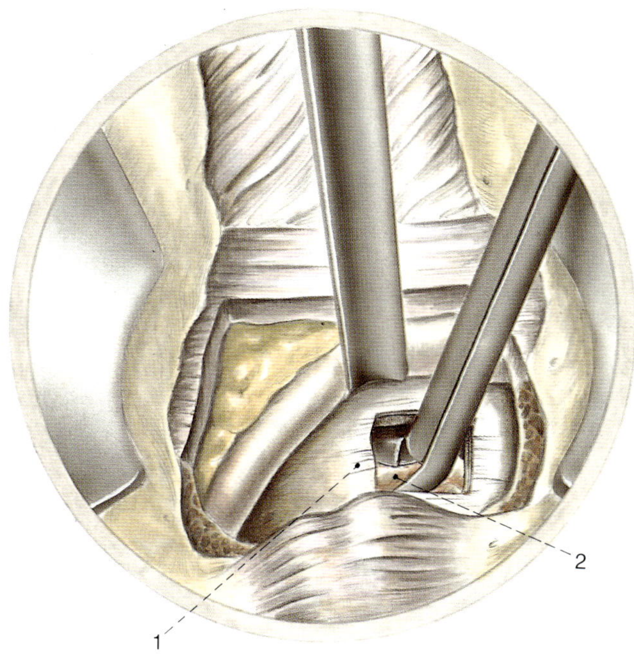

Fig. 8.**39** Removal of degenerated pulpy nucleus from the intervertebral space with different types of grasping forceps.

1 Posterior longitudinal ligament and annulus fibrosus
2 Intervertebral disk

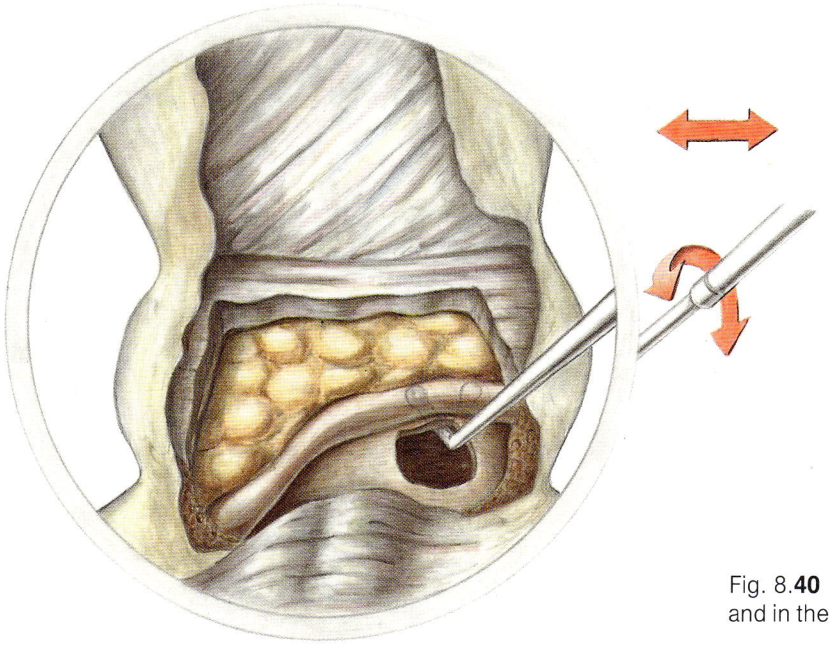

Fig. 8.**40** Follow-up probing with the probe below the ligament and in the intervertebral space.

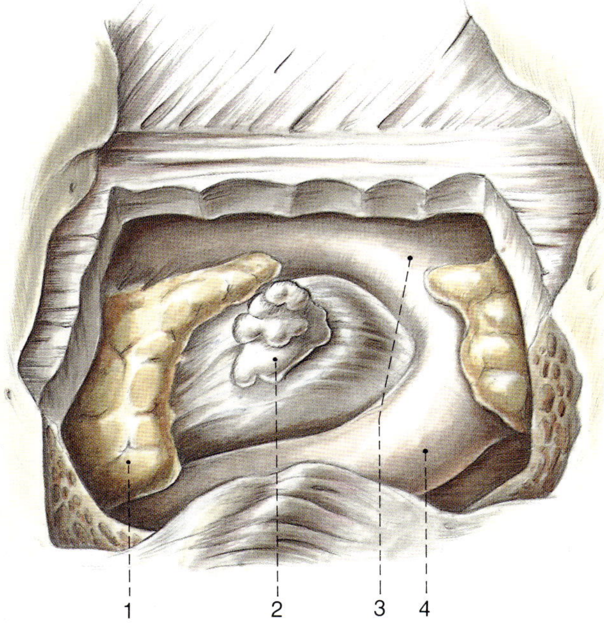

Fig. 8.**41** Partly perforated hernia in the shoulder of the root origin. At the lower hemiarch, the resection has been slightly enlarged.

1 Peridural fatty tissue (interrupted for better visualization)
2 Perforated hernia
3 Spinal dura mater
4 Spinal nerve

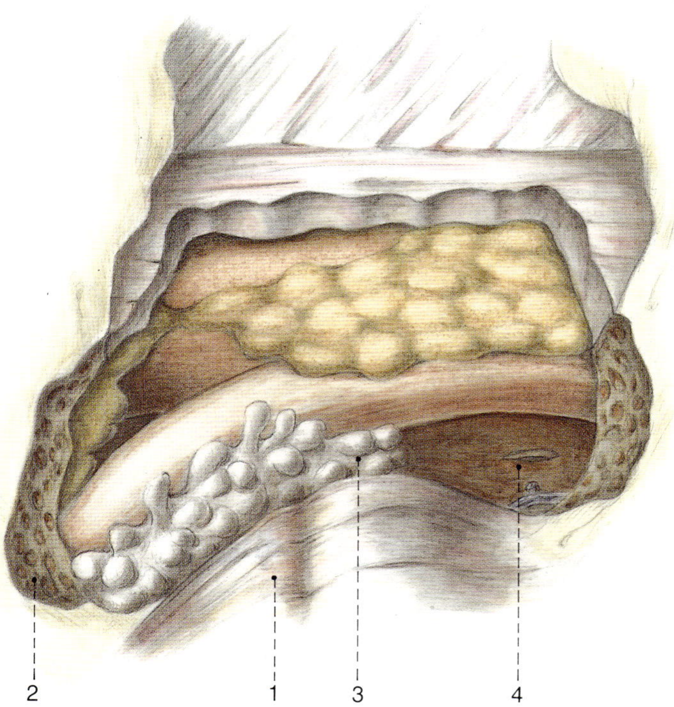

Fig. 8.**42** A sequestrum that has slipped down laterally alongside the pedicle. Note the bone resection (see also Fig. 8.**34**).

1 Zygapophyseal articulation
2 Resection extended caudally and laterally
3 Loose intervertebral disk sequestrum
4 Perforation site and height of the intervertebral space

8.**37**). The sequestrum may lie between the inner side of the pedicle and the nerve root (Fig. 8.**42**); the site of perforation is not always discernible. The intervertebral disk may be completely level. If the sequestrum has been detected preoperatively, 5 mm to at most 10 mm of the lamina and the base of the superior articular process are removed along the nerve root, without touching the joint if possible. The caudal enlargement, with the anatomical dimensions, is presented in Figure 8.**34**. If the longitudinal ligament is intact and the intervertebral disk is not protruding, we are inclined not to remove it.

Access is also difficult to sequestra that have slipped laterally upward; they often lie hidden in a pocket formed by the waist of the posterior wall of the vertebral body and the posterior longitudinal ligament, and may compress the next higher root in the intervertebral canal. A herniation concealed in such a pocket is not infrequently overlooked, and may cause persistent symptoms postoperatively. As shown in Fig. 8.**43** enough bone has to be removed from the superior lamina and the inferior articular process (Fig. 8.**43**), care being taken that the base of the pars interarticularis is not thinned out excessively.

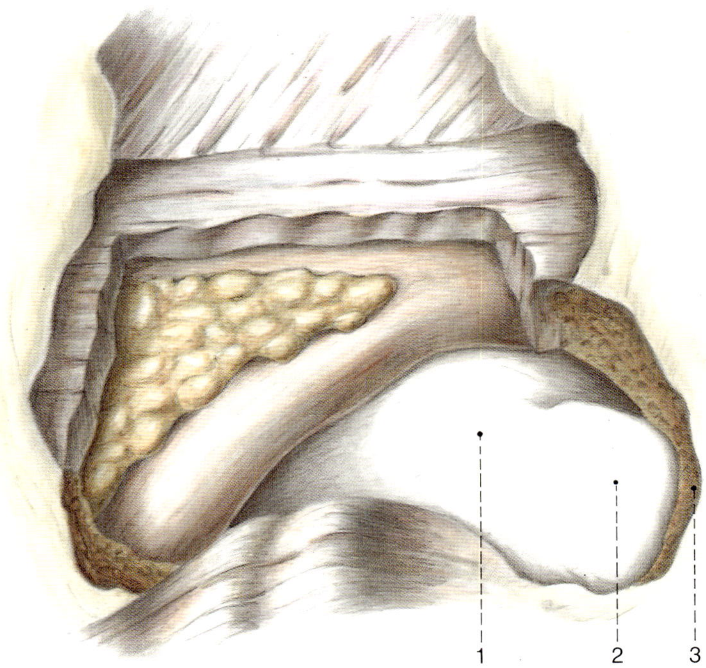

Fig. 8.**43** A subligamentous sequestrum that has slipped upward laterally and which can compress the root arising at the level of this intervertebral disk, as well as the root lying above it.

1 Level of the intervertebral disk
2 Subligamentous hernia that has slipped upward laterally
3 Cranially and (above the joint) laterally enlarged resection

Medial Disk Herniations

(Fig. 8.**44**)

Smaller medial disk hernias are usually positioned subligamentously, while larger ones are loosely sequestered and strongly compress the dural sac in the middle, so that the root is practically immovable. Removing them is technically very difficult under these circumstances. If a portion of the sequestrum can be grasped, it is carefully teased out, reduced *piece by piece,* and removed. Another method consists in first carrying out a fenestration of the longitudinal ligament and the annulus lateral to the root, and removing as much intervertebral disk material as possible from the intervertebral space. Once this has been done, it is easier to tease out the median sequestrum and to morcellate and remove it. Removing a large sequestrum in one piece is extremely dangerous, and can lead to severe neurologic deficits or even complete rectovesical paralysis, so that such a procedure would be extremely ill-advised. A number of experienced surgeons actually prefer a complete laminectomy under these special circumstances.

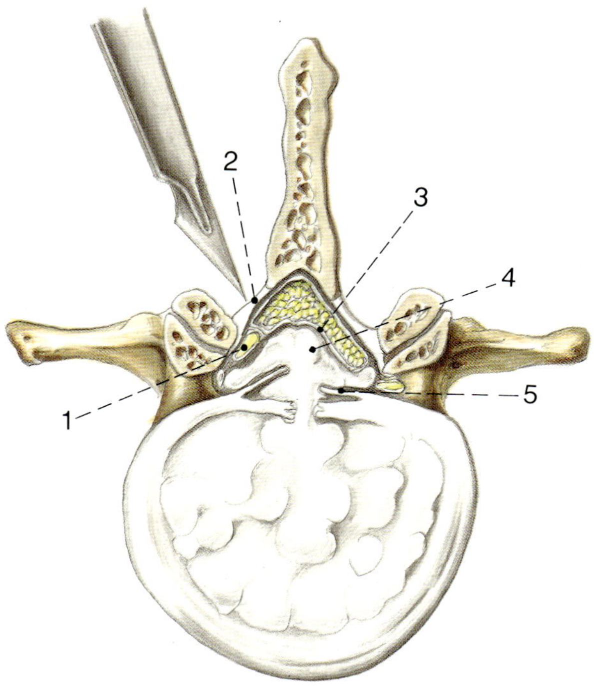

Fig. 8.**44** A large medial hernia with a subligamentous and freely dislocated portion. The dura and the spinal nerve are severely compressed. Guard against damage to the dura or the root during opening of the ligamentum flavum.

1 Posteriorly displaced spinal nerve
2 Ligamentum flavum
3 Compressed dural sac
4 Intervertebral disk sequestrum
5 Posterior longitudinal ligament and annulus fibrosus

Fundamentals

The question of whether the intervertebral disk should be entirely removed in all cases has not been conclusively answered. Like most authors, we generally clear the intervertebral space as much as possible, using various pituitary forceps. Because of the danger of injury to the end plates, no follow-up curettage with sharp curets is carried out. Studies of cadaver preparations have shown that about 25% of the pulpy nucleus is not reached by this technique. An exception to this rule is an isolated free sequestrum with a well-preserved annulus fibrosus in younger patients, only the dislocated portion being removed. A few authors have recommended that only the rupture site should be bluntly enlarged, and loose intervertebral disk material should be removed with fine grasping forceps (Williams 1983). This may offer the advantage of little biomechanic disturbance, but it also has the drawback of a higher relapse rate.

Root-sheath fibrosis. Unduly vigorous manipulation of the nerve root by pressure, traction, or coagulation leads to injury to the investing structures and fibers, to swelling, hyperemia, and intradural fibrotic alterations (root-sheath fibrosis), which may later cause persistent pain. In case of doubt, we are inclined to remove slightly more bone, rather than to retract the root or the dural sac too far.

Epidural fibrosis. The extent of epidural scar formation with consequent traction neuropathy is determined by a variety of factors. These are rules to be followed in order to avoid it:

- Avoidance of extensive lesions of the longitudinal ligament, coagulation, destruction of venous plexus, etc.
- Preservation of the fatty tissue and gliding layer around the root.
- Careful hemostasis and insertion of a Hemovac suction drain for 24–48 hours. With proper technique, only about 20 to 50 mL of blood should be lost in this operation. Collection of blood in the laminotomy window leads to ingrowth of capillaries, fibroblast formation, collagen deposits, etc.
- The laminotomy window can be packed with a free subcutaneous fat graft; this should always be done in recurrent herniations.

Injury of vertebral joint. Under which conditions persistent or new back pain or pseudoradicular symptoms develop after injury to a vertebral joint as the result of an instability or a facet syndrome is not known at present. We therefore avoid injuring the joint capsule and the articular surfaces whenever this is possible without added traction on the nerve root.

Surgically Relevant Anatomical Variations

In the so-called *conjoined root,* there is a common origin of two nerve roots from the dural sac. They may run through the intervertebral foramen jointly or separately. Owing to the limited possibilities of evasion or operative mobilization, this root is more susceptible to compression (Fig. 8.**45**).

In case of a *rectangular origin of the root,* it arises at a lower level than usual, that is, below the level of the intervertebral disk, and it then runs nearly horizontally toward the intervertebral foramen (Fig. 8.**45**).

If the *origin is extremely high,* the root arises above the disk. A herniation is then more likely to occur at the shoulder between the dural sac and the nerve root (Fig. 8.**45**).

Postoperative Treatment

A neurologic assessment is made immediately after the operation. The patient is placed in a completely flat position; older patients are mobilized on the first postoperative day, and younger ones on days 2–3. Treatment with low-dose heparin is started at the beginning of the operation and terminated at the time of mobilization. For several days after the operation, analgesics with sedative and muscle-relaxant action are prescribed. A very conservative program of physiotherapy (a few isometric exercises) is initiated, and the patient is usually discharged after removal of the sutures on day eight. Apart from the restriction of physical activity for six weeks, the patient is advised not to sit down during the first two postoperative weeks. Swimming is permitted by the second week.

Sciatica will be largely absent after the operation, but may occur once again between days four and seven. If it is still present on the eighth day, a follow-up CT is recommended, so that an overlooked fragment, a recess stenosis, or early recurrence can be ruled out.

Complications

Besides general complications, such as wound infection, thrombophlebitis, and pulmonary embolism, three specific complications may develop:

Anterior perforation of the annulus fibrosus. This may lead to injuries to the great abdominal vessels or the visceral organs, or both (Fig. 8.**46**). The incidence of this complication may amount to 1 in 1000 to 1 in 6000. Perforation with bleeding requires immediate laparotomy and closure of the affected vessel. Anterior perforation without visible bleeding necessitates intensive surveillance with monitoring of hemoglobin, abdominal symptoms, and possibly computed tomography to rule out a retroperitoneal hematoma.

Spondylodiskitis. The incidence of this reported in the literature is 0.3–1.5%; under rigorous aseptic precautions, it should be below 1%. It manifests itself in a secondary temperature rise, very severe lumbar and usually bilateral radicular pain, and an increase in the erythrocyte sedimentation rate. A skeletal bone scan will show a nonspecific concentration after two weeks; a radiographic tomogram

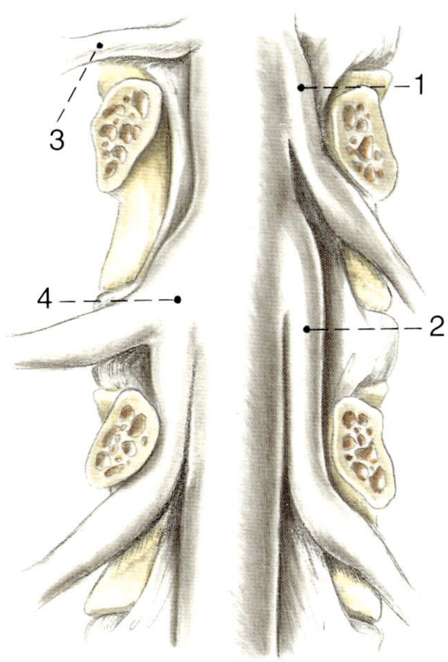

Fig. 8.**45** Conjoined root, rectangular root origin, high root origin.

1 Normal root origin
2 High root origin
3 Rectangular root origin
4 Conjoined root

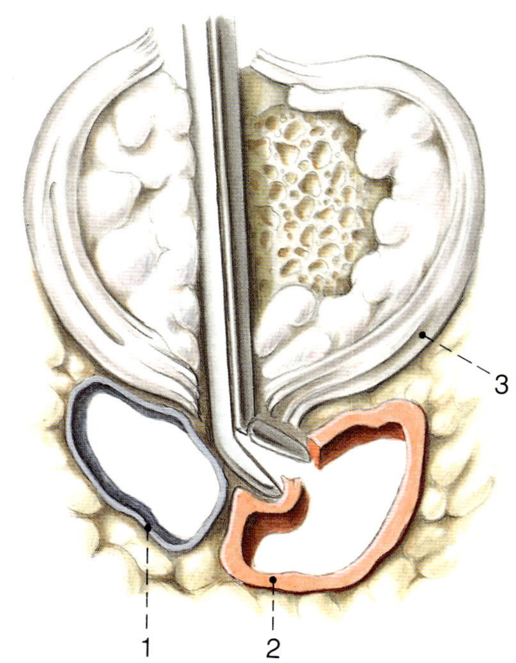

Fig. 8.**46** Anterior perforation of the intervertebral space with injury to the abdominal aorta (top view).

1 Inferior vena cava
2 Abdominal aorta
3 Annulus fibrosus

will disclose dissolution of end-plate structures after 3–4 weeks at the earliest. The pathogenic micro-organisms involved are usually staphylococci. The initial treatment should comprise strict bed rest and antibiotics, at least until the erythrocyte sedimentation rate begins to decrease.

Additional neurologic deficits. In large herniations, the dural sac and the root may be displaced far posteriorly, so that careless resection of the ligamentum flavum may result in injury to the nerve root or the dural sac. In addition, an undetected conjoined root may be stretched out over a hernia and hardly recognizable as a root (Fig. 8.**45**). During the operation, care should be taken not to manipulate the root unnecessarily, and not to tilt the root retractor. Finally, there is a possibility of severe dura and root lesions from rongeurs with jaws opening wider than 90 degrees (Figs. 8.**47**, 8.**48**). Use of such rongeurs ought to be avoided. A dural lesion has to be closed to avert a pseudomeningocele.

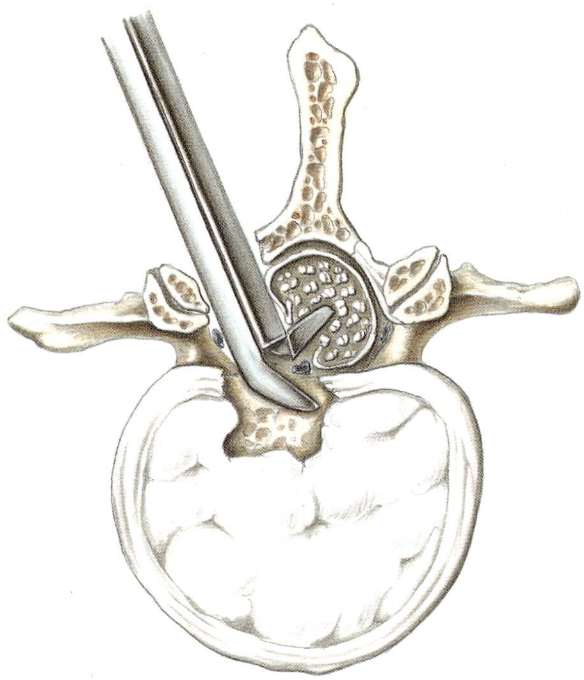

Fig. 8.**47** Injury to the dural sac and nerve fibers due to use of the wrong or faulty instrumentation, or both.

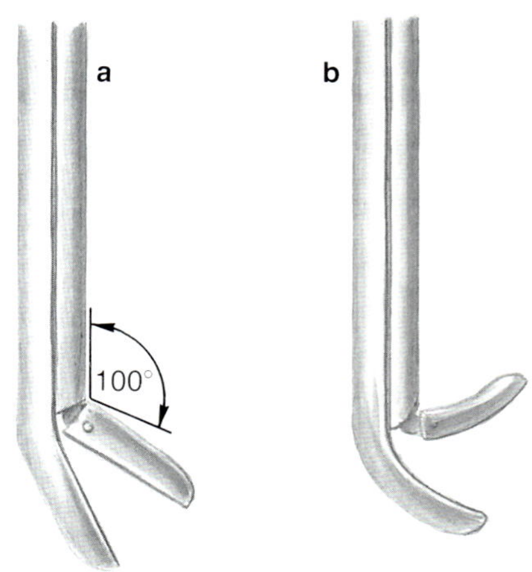

Fig. 8.**48** Rongeurs with an opening angle to the operating axis of more than 90 degrees should be avoided. **a** Correct, **b** wrong.

Extracanalicular Disk Herniation

Synonyms: Extraforaminal herniation, extreme lateral herniation.

The incidence of extracanalicular disk herniation is reportedly 4–12% of all lumbar disk herniations. The herniation lies within and outside the intervertebral canal; it is freely perforating in more than 80% of cases, and has slipped cranially into the waist of the vertebral body. The nerve root is displaced in cranial and posterior directions (Fig. 8.**49**). Because of the great distance from the midline, ranging up to 35–40 mm, it cannot be removed through interlaminar fenestration without resection of the inferior articular process. Unilateral destruction of the joint, however, may lead to instability in conjunction with debridement of the intervertebral space, and may become the cause of persistent lumbago or pseudoradicular symptoms. For this reason, a lateral, extraspinal approach has been developed (Reulen et al. 1987).

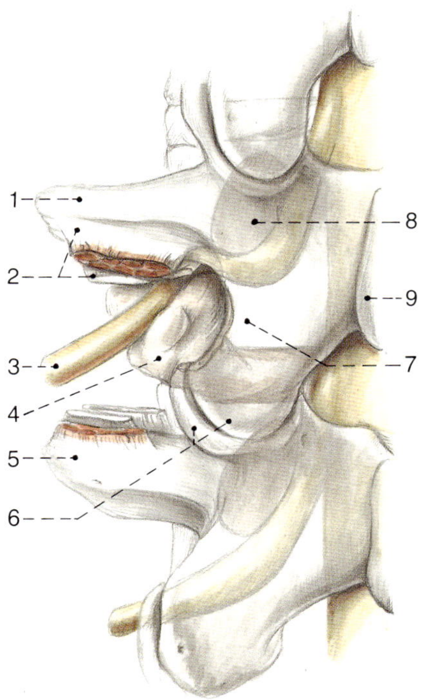

Fig. 8.**49** An extracanalicular disk hernia (left side). Shown here are the origin of the L4 nerve root at the L3–L4 level and its course along the pedicle as the upper boundary of the intervertebral canal. As a result of the herniation, the root is displaced upward and posteriorly. Note the relation of the hernia and the root to the L4–L5 intervertebral disk.

1 Transverse process of the fourth lumbar vertebra
2 Intertransverse muscle and intertransverse ligament
3 L4 spinal nerve
4 Disk herniation
5 Transverse process of the fifth lumbar vertebra
6 L4–L5 zygapophyseal articulation
7 L4 pars interarticularis
8 Pedicle of arch of the fourth lumbar vertebra
9 Spinous process of the fourth lumbar vertebra

Diagnosis

An extracanalicular herniation affects the root that arises at the level of the suprajacent intervertebral disk (example: root L4 arises at the level of the intervertebral space L3–L4, and is compressed in the intervertebral canal L4–L5). The myelogram will not show an extracanalicular disk herniation; it is detected by axial CT using narrow sections.

Operative Technique

The positioning is the same as that in lumbar disk herniation. The level is verified by means of a lateral radiographic image intensifier.

The superior spinous process of the affected level is used for orientation, that is, the spinous process L4 in the example of L4–L5. The skin incision is made about 1.5 cm off the midline; it extends 4 cm each superiorly and inferiorly from the L4 spinous process. The posterior fascia is split about 1.5 cm off the midline, retracted medially with two stay sutures, and then the tendinous insertions of the longissimus muscle and the multifidus muscles are dissected free of the L4 spinous process and the spinous processes above and below. The musculature is laterally retracted far enough to expose the joint of the affected level completely, as well as the suprajacent joint with the attachment of the transverse process (Fig. 8.**50**). The following landmarks are now used for another orientation: the L4 spinous process, L4 arch, L4 interarticular portion, L4–L5 vertebral joint, and L4 transverse process. A heavy muscle retractor (Aesculap BV 349) is then inserted, with the mandril being anchored medially in a notch of the spinous process that has been cut with the microdrill, while the blade laterally retracts the musculature between the two transverse processes L4 and L5 (Fig. 8.**50**). From the vantage point of the operating surgeon, the L4–L5 intervertebral disk now lies beneath the L4 pars interarticularis and the upper margin of the L4–L5 joint. Using the microdrill, several millimeters are removed from the lateral border of the pars interarticularis, and possibly also from the upper margin of the joint (Fig. 8.**51**). In order to spare the nerve root, the intertransverse ligament and the intertransverse muscle have been left in place up to this point, and are only now removed with a punch. This usually results in bleeding from the branch of the lumbar artery (posterior branch), which passes through here together with the posterior branch of the spinal nerve. The bleeding is controlled by *bipolar* coagulation. The lateral branches of the ligamentum flavum are carefully removed with the rongeur (Fig. 8.**52**). The lateral opening of the intervertebral canal and the cranial portion of the intervertebral disk are now brought into view. From this time on, use should be made of a loupe or an operating microscope. The nerve root is dissected free from the surrounding fatty tissue; it is usually displaced cranially and posteriorly. Accordingly, the free sequestrum is found most frequently medial and caudal to the nerve root (Fig. 8.**52**). The nerve root can be cranially retracted with a suction tip and the sequestrum or sequestra removed. If it is a loose sequestrum and no hole can be found in the annulus fibrosus, we dispense with debridement of the intervertebral space (Fig. 8.**53**). Following careful hemostasis, a Hemovac drain is inserted and the wound is closed in layers. Postoperative care is the same as in mediolateral disk herniation.

At the L5–S1 level, the pars interarticularis is extremely short, the sacrum may ascend steeply in a cranial direction, and the L5 transverse process may be positioned very low, so that the approach is extremely difficult and should be used only by experienced surgeons.

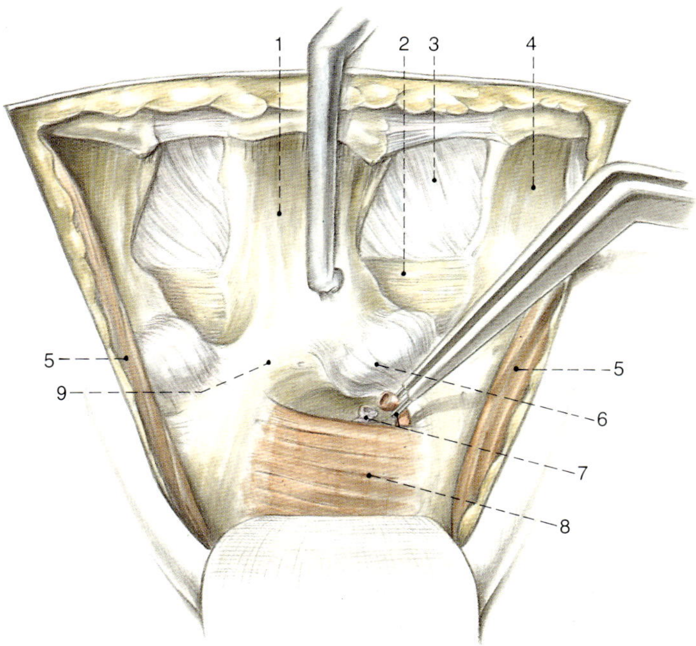

Fig. 8.**50** Operative site (left side) following retraction of the musculature of the back and insertion of retractor. The intertransverse muscle, L4–L5 vertebral joint, and the pars interarticularis are shown.

1 Spinous process of the fourth lumbar vertebra
2 Ligamentum flavum
3 Interspinal ligament
4 Spinous process of the fifth lumbar vertebra
5 Multifidus and semispinalis lumbalis muscles
6 L4–L5 zygapophyseal articulation
7 Lumbar artery and vein (posterior branch)
8 Intertransverse muscle
9 L4 pars interarticularis

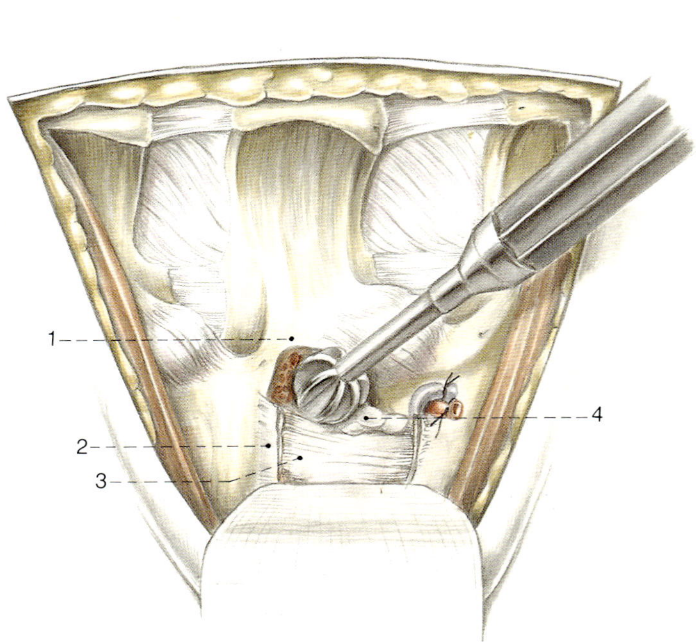

Fig. 8.**51** Reaming-out of the pars interarticularis and superior joint boundary. The intertransverse muscle has been separated at the insertions; the intertransverse ligament is preserved.

1 Pars interarticularis
2 Intertransverse muscle, divided
3 Intertransverse ligament
4 Perineural fatty tissue

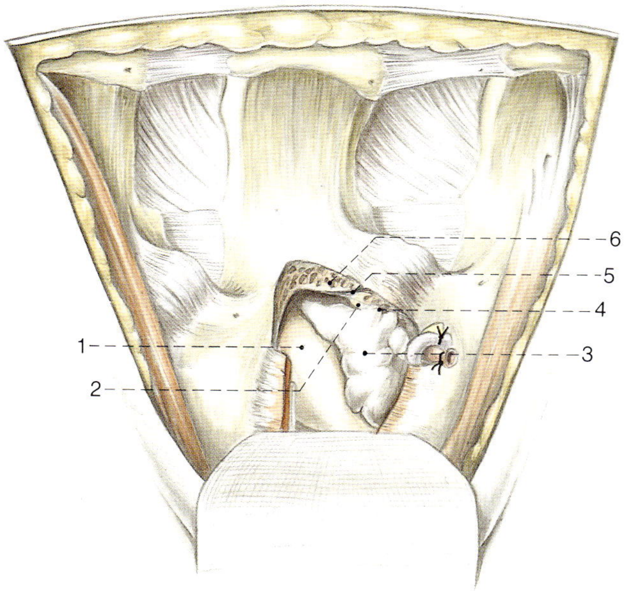

Fig. 8.**52** After retraction of the fatty tissue, the nerve root or the spinal ganglion and the loose sequestrum are visualized. The intervertebral disk is concealed.

1 L4 spinal nerve
2 Ligamentum flavum
3 Disk herniation
4 Superior articular process of the fifth lumbar vertebra
5 L4–L5 zygapophyseal articulation
6 Inferior articular process of the fourth lumbar vertebra

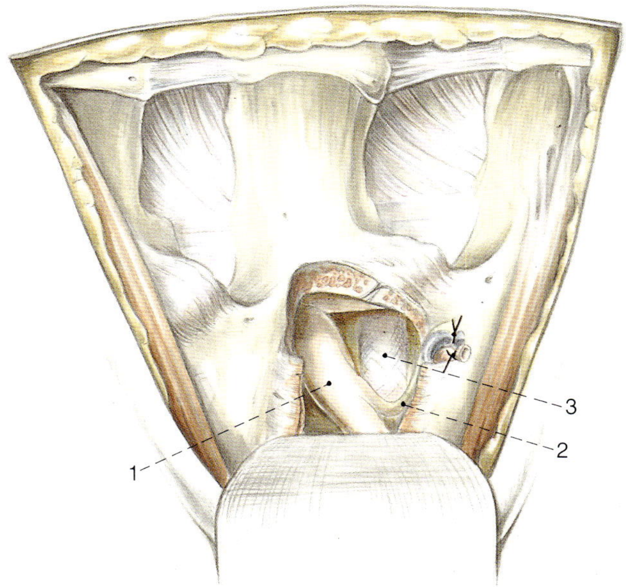

Fig. 8.**53** Status after removal of the loose sequestrum. The disk can now be seen; it is outwardly intact.

1 Spinal nerve
2 Posterior branch of the L4 spinal nerve
3 Intervertebral disk

Stenoses in the Lumbar Spinal Canal

A chronic degeneration of the intervertebral disk with *narrowing of the intervertebral space* sets in motion a series of other degenerative processes which, individually or in combination, may be responsible for compression of the neural elements in the spinal canal, in the recessus lateralis, or in the intervertebral foramen: bulging of the tendinous ring and the ligamentum flavum, scalloping of the vertebral body, loosening of the ligamentous apparatus and the joint capsules, superior subluxation of the superior articular process with narrowing of the anteroposterior diameter of the upper portion of the intervertebral foramen, posterior displacement of the next higher vertebra, overloading of the facet joints with hypertrophic alterations of the superior articular process (Fig. 8.**54**) ("superior facet syndrome"), and hypertrophy of the inferior articular process with resulting spinal stenosis (Fig. 8.**55**).

The two most common stenotic syndromes are discussed below.

Stenosis of the Lateral Recess (Superior Facet Syndrome)

The nerve root coursing in the lateral recess can be increasingly compressed by degenerative changes in the superior articular process (Fig. 8.**55**). The L4–L5 and L5–S1 joints are affected most frequently. An overlooked stenosis of the lateral recess is the most common cause of an unsatisfactory outcome of an intervertebral disk operation.

Symptoms

A narrow lateral recess is associated with monoradicular, generally unilateral pain, which increases under stress. Paresthesias may supervene; sensory or motor radicular deficits are rather unusual.

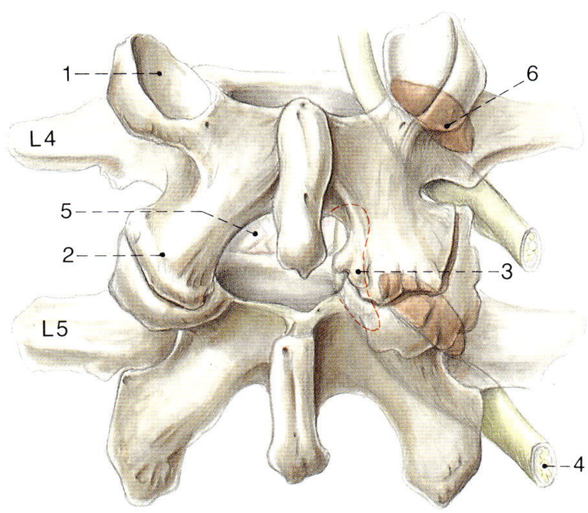

Fig. 8.**54** Right-sided spondylotic alterations of the L4–L5 vertebral joint. Posterior view. Resection for decompression of the nerve root (dashed red line).

1 Superior articular process of the fourth lumbar vertebra
2 Inferior articular process of the fourth lumbar vertebra
3 Spondylotic changes in the L4–L5 zygapophyseal articulation
4 L5 spinal nerve
5 Intervertebral disk
6 Pedicle of the arch of the fourth lumbar vertebra, traced

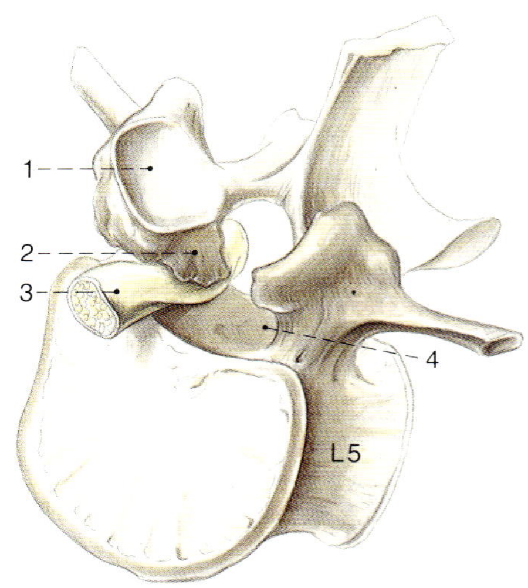

Fig. 8.**55** Stenosis of the lateral recess due to formation of medial spondylophytes on the joint surface of the L5 superior articular process. Note the compression of the L5 nerve root at the cranial end of the lateral recess.

1 Superior articular process of the fifth lumbar vertebra
2 Medial spondylotic scallops
3 L5 spinal nerve (in constricted lateral recess)
4 Normal lateral recess

Diagnosis

Axial CT sections at intervals of 3 mm or less are important, and allow visualization of the transverse anatomy of the spinal canal and the lateral recess and possibly of other pathological processes. The height of the recess should be at least 4 mm. Lower values are characterized as relative stenosis, and values under 3 mm are nearly always associated with root compression.

Surgical Anatomy

The facet of the superior articular process forms the roof of the lateral recess, while it is bounded anteriorly by the posterior surface of the vertebral body and the intervertebral disk (Figs. 8.**54**, 8.**55**). The nerve root leaves the dural sac at approximately the level of the intervertebral disk, and then enters the lateral recess, which turns into the intervertebral canal at the level of the superior margin of the pedicle (Fig. 8.**54**). Under pathological conditions—intervertebral disk degeneration, narrowing of intervertebral space, increased loading of joints—the medial border of the superior articular process develops a spondylotic scalloping (Fig. 8.**55**), and as a result of this, or added intervertebral disk protrusion, the nerve root is compressed.

At L4, L5, and S1, the superior articular process protrudes cranially 4–11 mm (average 7 mm) above the superior border of the corresponding vertebral body, that is, beyond the superior border of the adjoining intervertebral disk. This should be taken into account in decompression. Since the superior articular process has a somewhat anterior inclination at its upper end, the lateral recess is lowest at its upper entrance; it widens in a caudolateral direction toward the intervertebral canal.

Operative Technique (Recessotomy)

Exposure of the joint and the interlaminar window is accomplished as in the conventional approach to the lumbar intervertebral disk (Chapter 1, p. 71). For decompression of the affected nerve root, the hypertrophic medial portion of the superior articular process has to be removed (dashed red line in Figs. 8.**54** and 8.**56**). For this purpose, about 5–6 mm is initially removed from the superior hemiarch, followed by the medial third of the inferior articular process, down to the articular surface (Fig. 8.**57**). Finally, the superior articular process, which is now visualized, is carefully removed with its hypertrophic marginal bulges (Fig. 8.**57**), until the subjacent nerve root is completely decompressed (Fig. 8.**58**). The narrowness of the recess severely compromises the nerve root; it is best protected by using a microdrill for the resection. If angulated rongeurs are employed, resection of the medial edge of the superior articular process and the marginal bulges should be carried out with fine punches (jaw width of 2 or 3 mm). How much should be removed from the superior and inferior articular process or from the vertebral joint cannot be specified, given the highly variable anatomical dimensions. The joint may extend far medially (Fig. 8.**34**), and the dural sac far laterally. The main consideration is that the nerve root should be decompressed, and that its course should be freely visible. It may be taken as a general rule, however, that resection of the articular surfaces should be kept to a minimum. Another point to be borne in mind is that the inferior articular process should not be excessively thinned out at its isthmus, the pars interarticularis, since it may otherwise fracture under stress.

Not infrequently, a narrow lateral recess occurs in combination with a small protrusion of the intervertebral disk. The decision as to whether debridement of the disk is appropriate has to be made in each individual case.

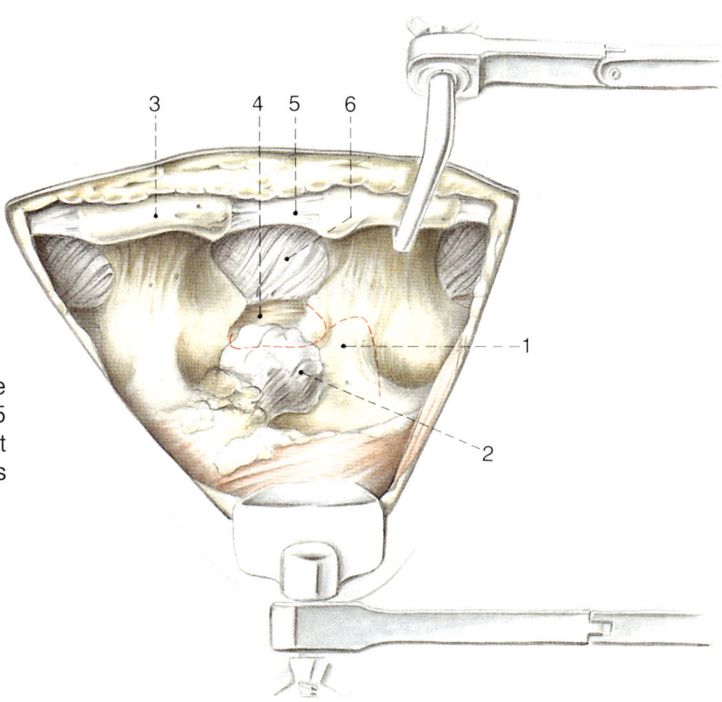

Fig. 8.**56** Operative site after freeing of the intrinsic musculature of the back and exposure of the vertebral joint and the L4–L5 interlaminar space. Right side. Decompression of the nerve root by resection of the inferior and superior articular processes (dashed red line).

1 Arch of the fourth lumbar vertebra
2 Joint capsule of the L4–L5 zygapophyseal articulation
3 Spinous process of the fifth lumbar vertebra
4 Ligamentum flavum
5 Supraspinal ligament
6 Interspinal ligament

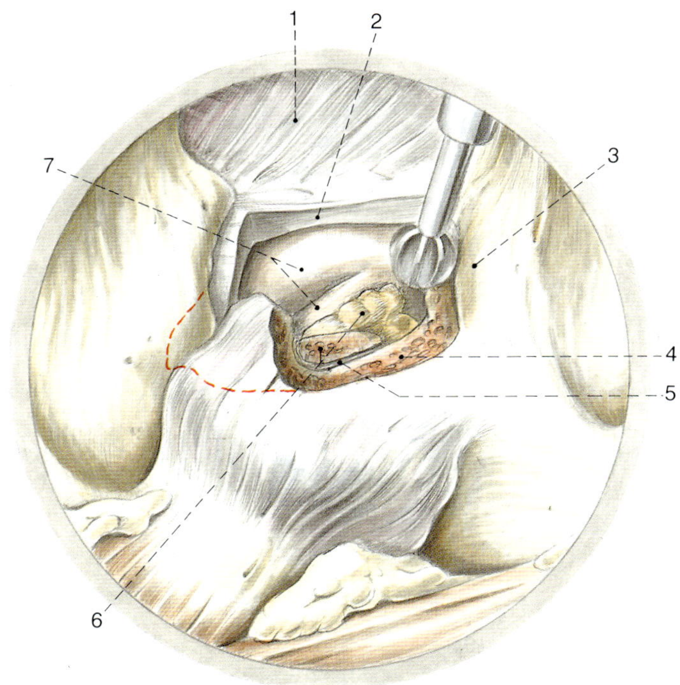

Fig. 8.**57** Resection of the inferior articular process with microdrill or rongeur. Optical magnification.

1 Interspinal ligament
2 Ligamentum flavum, partly removed
3 Arch of the fourth lumbar vertebra
4 Inferior articular process of the fourth lumbar vertebra
5 Zygapophyseal articulation
6 Superior articular process of the fourth lumbar vertebra with spondylotic scallops
7 Spinal dura mater and spinal nerve L 5

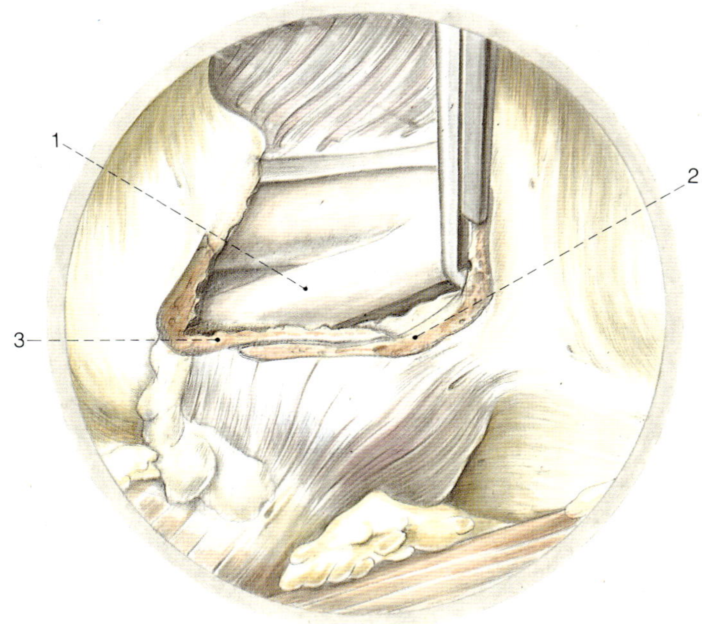

Fig. 8.**58** Status after decompression of the nerve root. Optical magnification.

1 Spinal nerve
2 Inferior articular process of the fourth lumbar vertebra
3 Superior articular process of the fourth lumbar vertebra

Stenosis of Lumbar Spinal Canal

Lumbar spinal canal stenoses may be congenital or acquired. The more common, acquired form generally appears at ages over 60. In this form, the sagittal or transverse diameters of the spinal canal, or both, are reduced at one or more levels by osteophytic appositions on the facet joints, by hypertrophy of the arches, and by thickening of the ligamentum flavum (Fig. 8.**59**). The critical area lies below the thickened vertebral arch or at the level of the vertebral joints. In most cases, the lateral recess is narrowed at the same time (see above), so that there is nerve root compression in addition to compression of the dural sac with the cauda equina.

Spondylotic marginal bulges on the posterior side of the vertebral body or intervertebral disk protrusion may be additional space-limiting factors. A sagittal diameter of the spinal canal of between 10 and 15 mm is considered a relative stenosis, and a diameter of less than 10 mm a absolute stenosis. The latter also manifests itself *clinically* without any other space-reducing factors.

Symptoms

Low back pain and bilateral sciatic-type pain is typical. This is occasionally accompanied by paresthesias and weakness of the thighs that are experienced after the patient has walked a certain distance, forcing him to sit down (intermittent claudication). Walking uphill or while leaning forward is usually less painful than walking downhill or with an erect gait.

Diagnosis

Since the clinical findings often do not permit determination of the exact level of compression of the cauda equina, evaluation of the entire lumbar spinal canal is necessary. A myelogram with the typical hourglass-shaped constriction of the dural sac at the level of the vertebral joints facilitates the decision as to whether one or more levels are involved. A CT study of all levels is far more costly. Radiographs of the lumbar spine are always needed to detect malformations or pathological conditions.

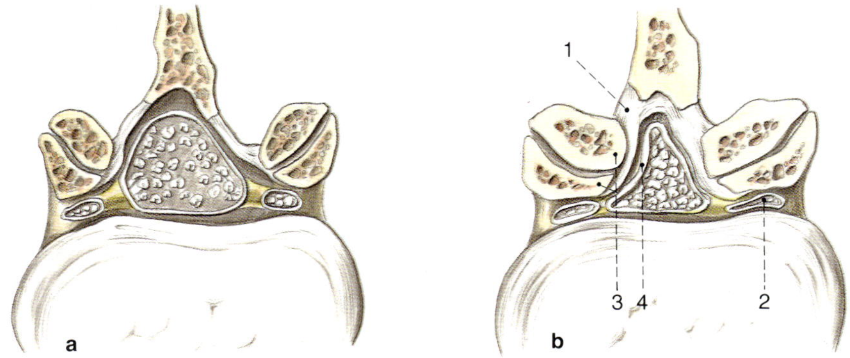

Fig. 8.**59** Acquired stenosis of the spinal canal, with concomitant stenosis of the lateral recess. **a** Normal condition, spinal canal triangular. **b** Constriction of the spinal canal on the lateral and anteroposterior diameters, with compression of the cauda equina due to thickening of the bony arch, spondylotic osteophytes, and thickening of the ligamentum flavum.

1 Thickened ligamentum flavum
2 Compressed nerve root
3 Spondylotic scallop
4 Compressed dural sac

Positioning and Incision

The positioning is the same as that for lumbar disk herniation, or the patient can be placed in prone position, with padding under the chest and the iliac crest. The skin incision depends on the number of levels involved. It should go beyond the spinous process of the affected level, extending to 1–2 spinous processes superiorly and inferiorly. The subcutis is divided down to the fascia, and a retractor is introduced.

Operative Technique

Exposure of Posterolateral Vertebral Elements

The thoracolumbar fascia is dissected free near the bone on both sides of the spinous processes (Chapter 1, Fig. 1.**113**). The tendinous insertions of the semispinalis and multifidus muscles are sharply separated with a knife, at the periosteum, from the lower edge of the spinous processes. Using an elevator, the paraspinal musculature is bilaterally retracted laterally over the vertebral joints. The thickened vertebral arches and joints are now exposed (Fig. 8.**60**) and, together with the ligamentum flavum, are debrided of tissue remnants with cotton-tipped tissue dissectors or the rongeur.

Removal of Stenosis

If only one level is involved, the vertebral arch affected, with the spinous process, is removed completely; one-fourth of the vertebral arch below it is also removed. To this end, the spinous process of the arch to be resected is first resected with a rongeur, and the vertebral arch is thinned out posteriorly (Fig. 8.**61**). Using a curved dissector, the ligamentum flavum is retracted from the lower border of the arch. This is an important step, since the dura may be adherent to the ligamentum flavum, and there is no epidural fat at the level of the compression (watch out for injury of the dura). The remainder of the arch is removed with an angulated Kerrison rongeur (4 or 5 mm wide) (Fig. 8.**62**). Using a 5-mm rongeur, the lower shoe should be moved parallel to the bone, and should not be obliquely tilted. If the spinal canal is severely constricted, there is danger of compression of the cauda equina, with resultant additional neurologic deficits.

The lateral part of the ligamentum flavum is now removed with a smaller rongeur (2 or 3 mm wide) as far as its junction with the bone or joint. At this point, the medial third of the joint may be removed with the angulated rongeur or, preferably, a microdrill (Fig. 8.**62**). It is important not to resect the joint and the inferior articular process too extensively, and to make certain that the isthmus remains sufficiently thick. The width of the isthmus (pars interarticularis) can be palpated in a lateral direction with a dissector.

This eliminates the stenosis of the dural sac, and with adequate decompression the dura will begin to pulsate

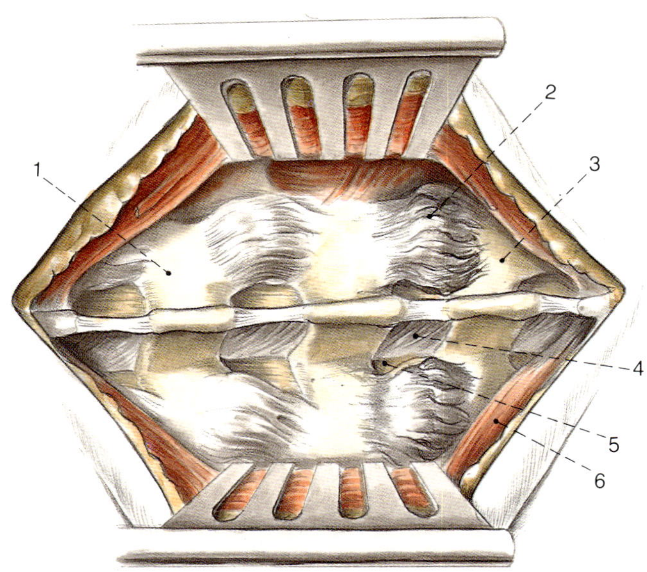

Fig. 8.**60** Operative site after detachment of the intrinsic musculature of the back. Note the severely thickened joints and the narrow interlaminar space.

1 Lamina of arch of the third lumbar vertebra
2 Joint capsule of the L4–L5 zygapophyseal articulation
3 Lamina of arch of the fifth lumbar vertebra
4 Interspinal ligament
5 Ligamentum flavum
6 Intrinsic musculature of the back, retracted

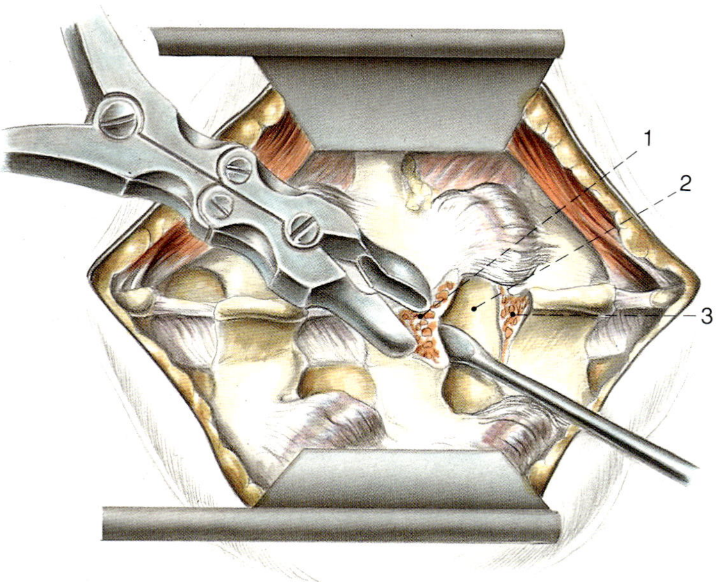

Fig. 8.**61** Resection of spinous process and thinning of the L4 arch with a rongeur. The ligamentum flavum is retracted with a dissector.

1 Spinous process of the fourth lumbar vertebra, resected
2 Ligamentum flavum
3 Spinous process and arch of the fifth lumbar vertebra, partly removed

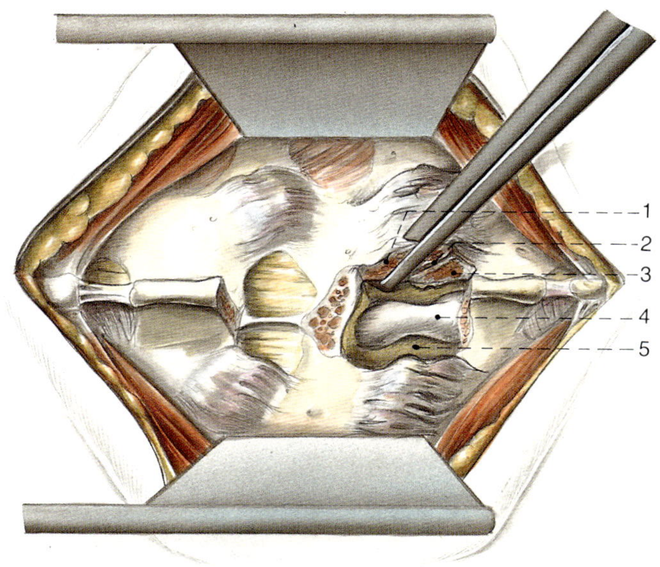

Fig. 8.**62** Removal of the remnants of the L4 arch with a rongeur. The dural sac is distinctly constricted by the thickened arch, the thickened ligamentum flavum, and osteophytes.

1 Inferior articular process of the fourth lumbar vertebra
2 L4–L5 zygapophyseal articulation
3 Superior articular process of the fifth lumbar vertebra
4 Spinal dura mater
5 Ligamentum flavum, thickened

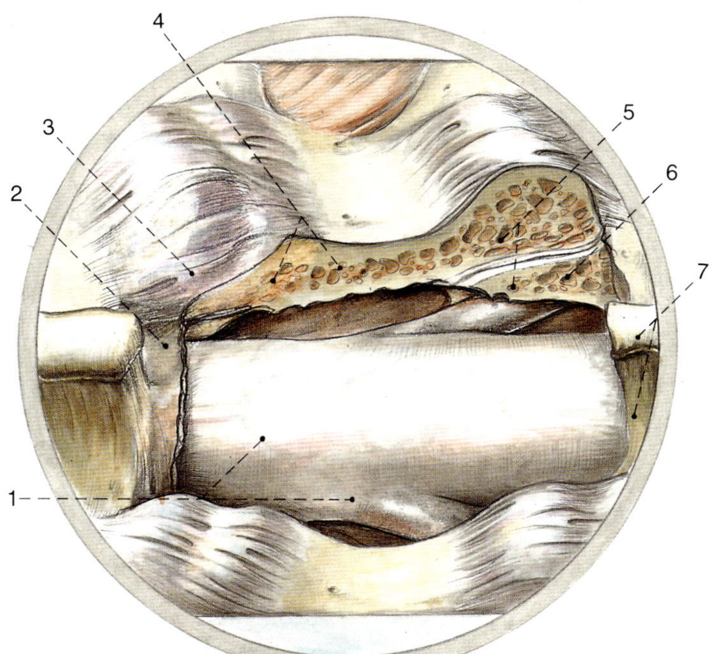

Fig. 8.**63** Operative site after completed laminectomy of L4, approximately a quarter of L5, and foraminotomy for roots L4 and L5.

1 L4 dural sac and root
2 Partly resected L3 spinous process and arch
3 L3 inferior articular process
4 L4 superior articular process and arch
5 L4–L5 zygapophyseal articulation
6 L5 superior articular process
7 Partly resected L5 spinous process and arch

normally again (Fig. 8.**63**). If the arthrectomy is confined to one-third, postoperative instability may be anticipated in 2–5% of the patients (White and Wiltse 1977). However, if a degenerative spondylolisthesis is already present, a progressive subluxation may develop, so that primary stabilization should be considered. In our estimation, a diskectomy is not necessary, even when there is some protrusion and marginal osteophytes are present; this would only aggravate the risk of postoperative instability. If two or—less commonly—more levels are affected, the decompression is extended as needed.

If a recessotomy is to follow, the procedure described on p. 341 is applicable.

Wound Closure

Owing to the danger of epidural hematoma, hemostasis should be carried out with great care. After insertion of an epidural Hemovac drain, the wound is closed by approximating suture of the musculature and, successively, the fascia, subcutis, and skin.

Postoperative Treatment

From the first day onward, the patients are increasingly mobilized, and they are discharged on days 8–10. Analgesics are usually needed during the first few postoperative days. The patients are given an exercise program, and are advised to increase their activities slowly during the first month.

Complications

The frequently present adhesions between the dura and the ligamentum flavum create the risk of dural or neural lesions. Before removal, the ligamentum flavum should therefore be bluntly separated from the dura with a dissector. A dural injury requires watertight closure, to avoid aspiration of cerebrospinal fluid via the Hemovac drain (danger of decompression syndrome, with symptoms ranging from severe headache to obtundation). Complications such as instability, epidural hematoma, and compression of the cauda equina by outsided rongeurs are referred to above.

Further Reading

Alonso WA, Black P, Connor GH, Vematsu S. Transoral, transpalatal approach for resection of clivus chordoma. Laryngoscope 1971;81:1621–31.

Arce CA, Dohrmann GJ. Thoracic disk herniation. Surg Neurol 1985;23:356–612.

Benini A. Ischias ohne Bandscheibenvorfall: Die Stenose des lumbalen Wirbelkanals. Berne: Huber, 1976.

Caspar W. Die mikrochirurgische Operationstechnik nach Caspar. Aeskulap-Sonderprospekt S-020, 1974;20.

Ebeling U, Reulen HJ. Mikrochirurgische Technik bei lumbalen Bandscheibenoperationen. Ist sie der konventionellen Methode überlegen? Jahrb Neurochir 1988;143–160.

Epstein JA, Epstein BE, Lavine L. Nerve root compression with narrowing of the lumbar spinal canal. J Neurol Neurosurg Psychiatr 1962;25:165–76.

Harms HJ, Schmelzle W. Indications and limits of the transoral entry for treatment of fractures, luxations and tumors of the vertebral column. In: Schwenzer N, Pfeifer G, eds. Fortschritte der Kiefer- und Gesichts-Chirurgie. Vol. 32. Stuttgart: Thieme, 1987:206–8.

Kirkaldy-Willis WH. Lumbar spondylosis and stenosis. In: Canthed JC, ed. Lumbar spine surgery. Baltimore: Williams and Wilkins, 1983.

Lazorthes G, Gonaze A, Djindjan R. Vascularisation et circulation de la moëlle épinière. Paris: Masson, 1973.

Loew F, Caspar W. Surgical approach to lumbar disk herniations. In: Krayenbühl H, et al., eds. Advances and technical standards in neurosurgery. Vol. 5. Berlin: Springer, 1978:153–174.

Mixter W, Barr IS. Rupture of the intervertebral disk without involvement of the spinal canal. New Engl J Med 1934;211:210–15.

Perot PL Jr, Munro DD. Transthoracic removal of midline thoracic disk protrusions causing spinal cord compression. J Neurosurg 1969;31:452–8.

Ransohoff J, Spencer F, Siew F, Gage L Jr. Transthoracic removal of the thoracic disk: report of three cases. J Neurosurg 1969;31:459–61.

Reulen HJ, Pfaundler S, Ebeling U. The lateral microsurgical approach to the "extracanalicular" lumbar disk herniation. Acta Neurochir 1987;84:64–7.

Safdari H, Baker RL II. Microsurgical anatomy and related techniques to an anterolateral transthoracic approach to thoracic disk herniation. Surg Neurol 1985;23:589–93.

Schneck CD. The anatomy of lumbar spondylosis. Clin Orthop 1985;193:20–37.

Seeger W. Microsurgery of the spinal cord and surrounding structures: anatomical and technical principles. Berlin: Springer, 1982.

Verbiest H. Neurogenic intermittent claudication with special reference to stenosis of the lumbar vertebral canal. Amsterdam: Elsevier, 1976.

White AH, Wiltse LL. Postoperative spondylolisthesis. In: Weinstein PR, Ehini F, Wilson CB, eds. Lumbar spondylosis: Diagnosis, management, and surgical treatment. Chicago: Yearbook, 1977.

Williams RW. Microlumbar discectomy: a surgical alternative for initial disk herniation. In: Canthen JC, ed. Lumbar spine surgery. Baltimore: Williams and Wilkins, 1983.

9 Rheumatoid Instability

F. Kerschbaumer

The following distinctions are made:

- Atlantoaxial anterior instability (Figs. 9.**1**–9.**3**), aggravated by insufficiency of the transverse ligament of the atlas.
- Occipitocervical vertical instability, with pseudobasilar impression (Fig. 9.**4**).
- Subaxial instability. This is treated by segmental fusion from an anterior and a posterior approach (Chapter 5, Fusion of the Cervical Spine).

Indications

- Severe pain, not improved by orthotic support.
- Neurologic defects: pareses, transverse cord lesions, myelopathy, radicular lesions, disorders of perception.

Operative Methods

- Posterior atlantoaxial fusion
- Posterior occipitocervical fusion
- Anterior transoral operations

Preoperative Preparation in Patients with Neurologic Deficits

Preoperative traction by means of Crutchfield tongs or a halo is recommended, especially in the presence of an incomplete transverse neurologic deficit. Daily lateral radiographs of the cervical spine and clinical monitoring of the neurologic deficits are indicated. After general preoperative preparations and remission of the neurological symptoms, the operation can generally be planned within 3–4 days.

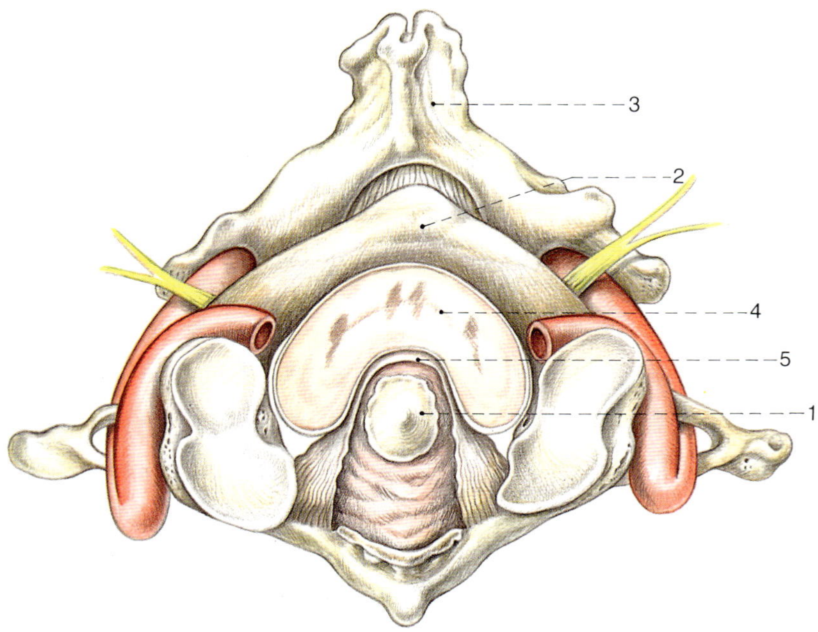

Fig. 9.**1** Insufficiency of the atlantal transverse ligament in anterior subluxation of the atlas in the transverse plane.

1 Dens of the axis
2 Posterior arch of the atlas
3 Posterior arch of the axis
4 Medulla oblongata
5 Transverse ligament of the atlas

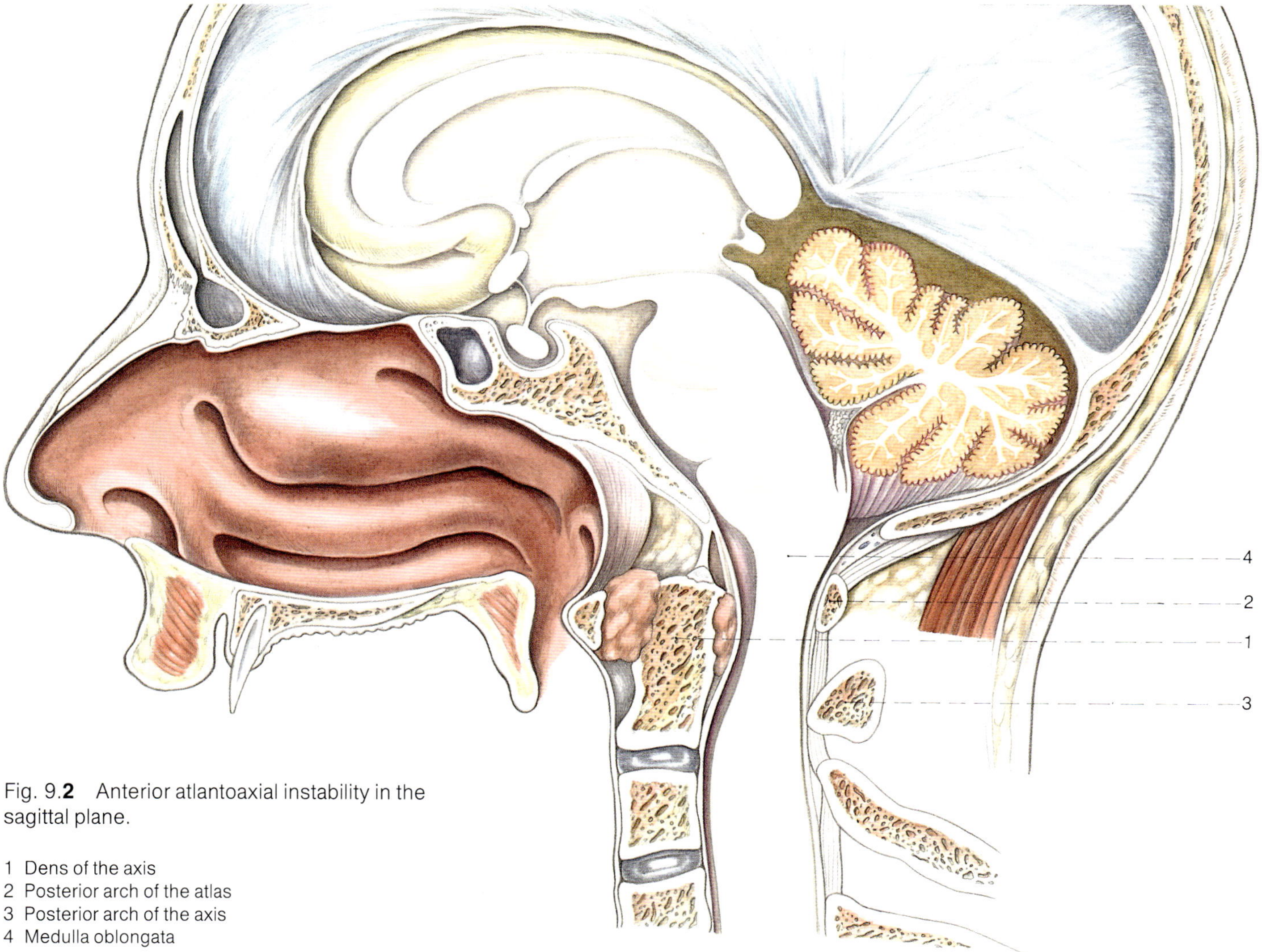

Fig. 9.**2** Anterior atlantoaxial instability in the sagittal plane.

1 Dens of the axis
2 Posterior arch of the atlas
3 Posterior arch of the axis
4 Medulla oblongata

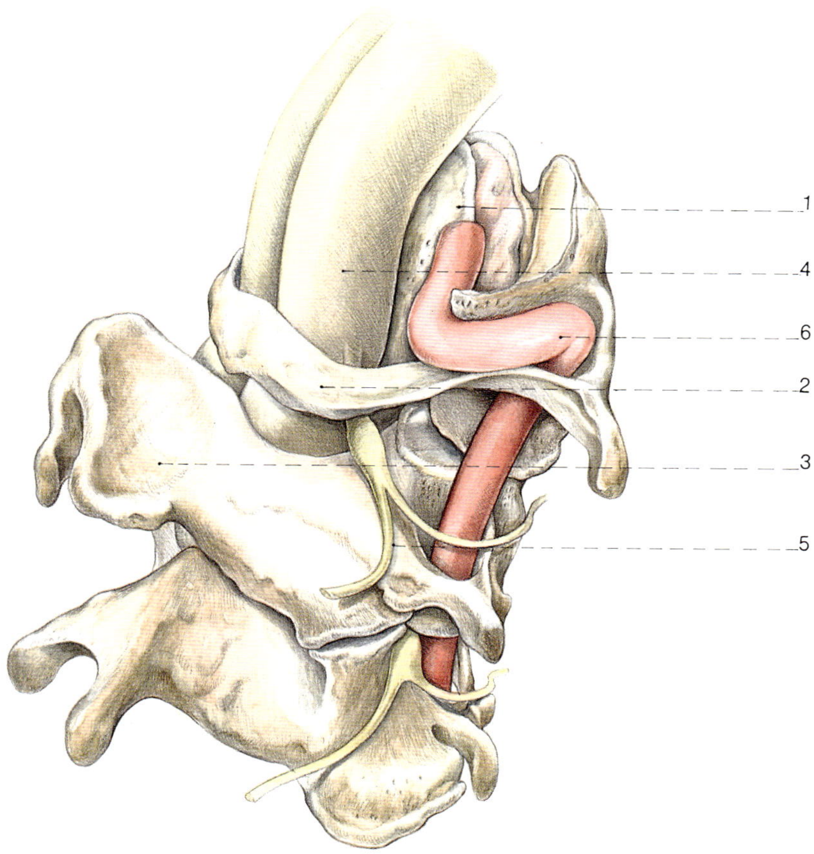

Fig. 9.**3** Cord compression in anterior atlantoaxial instability.

1 Dens of the axis
2 Posterior arch of the atlas
3 Spinous process of the axis
4 Medulla oblongata
5 Greater occipital nerve
6 Vertebral artery

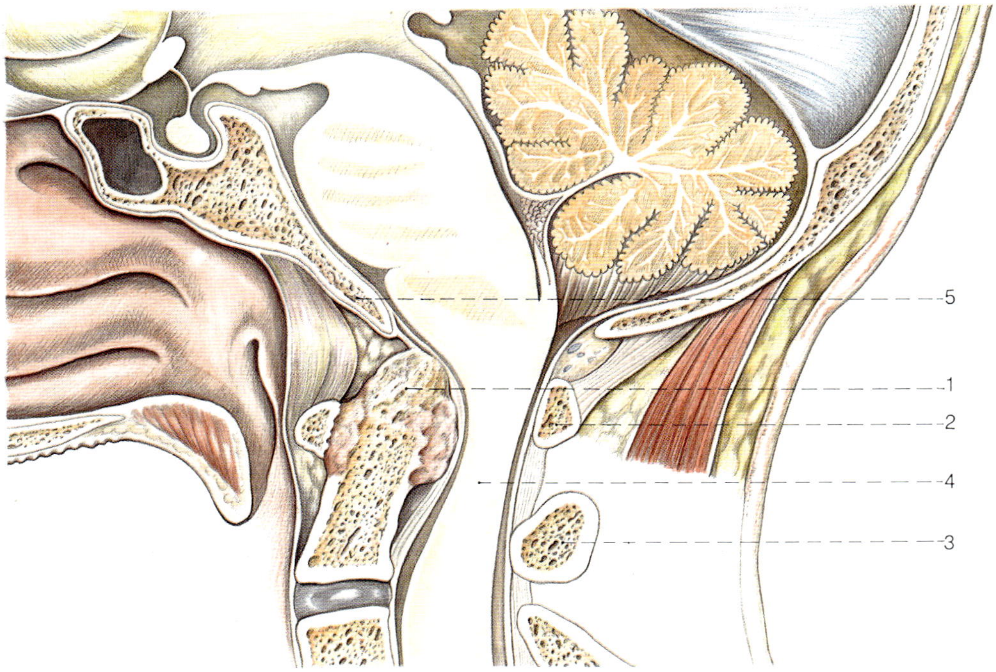

Fig. 9.**4** Secondary basilar impression with compression of the cord from the front.

1 Dens of the axis
2 Posterior arch of the atlas
3 Posterior arch of the axis
4 Medulla oblongata
5 Clivus

Posterior Operations

Positioning and Anesthesia

Surgery is generally performed under oral intubation, or, if this is not possible, with intubation by a tracheostomy. The patient is placed in the prone position, with bolsters under the thorax and the anterior superior iliac spine. The head is fixed in a slightly flexed position in a padded horseshoe head holder (Fig. 1.**97**). On the day before the operation, the back of the neck and the occiput are shaved. For clear exposure of the operative field, both shoulders are pulled distally with wide adhesive straps.

Preoperatively, the positions of the atlas and the axis are checked with the aid of a laterally-directed image intensifier. Anterior dislocation of the atlas has to be prevented by appropriate positioning. Anesthetic equipment is positioned on the side of the operating table approximately at the level of the pelvis. This leaves the upper part of the table free for the surgeon and his team.

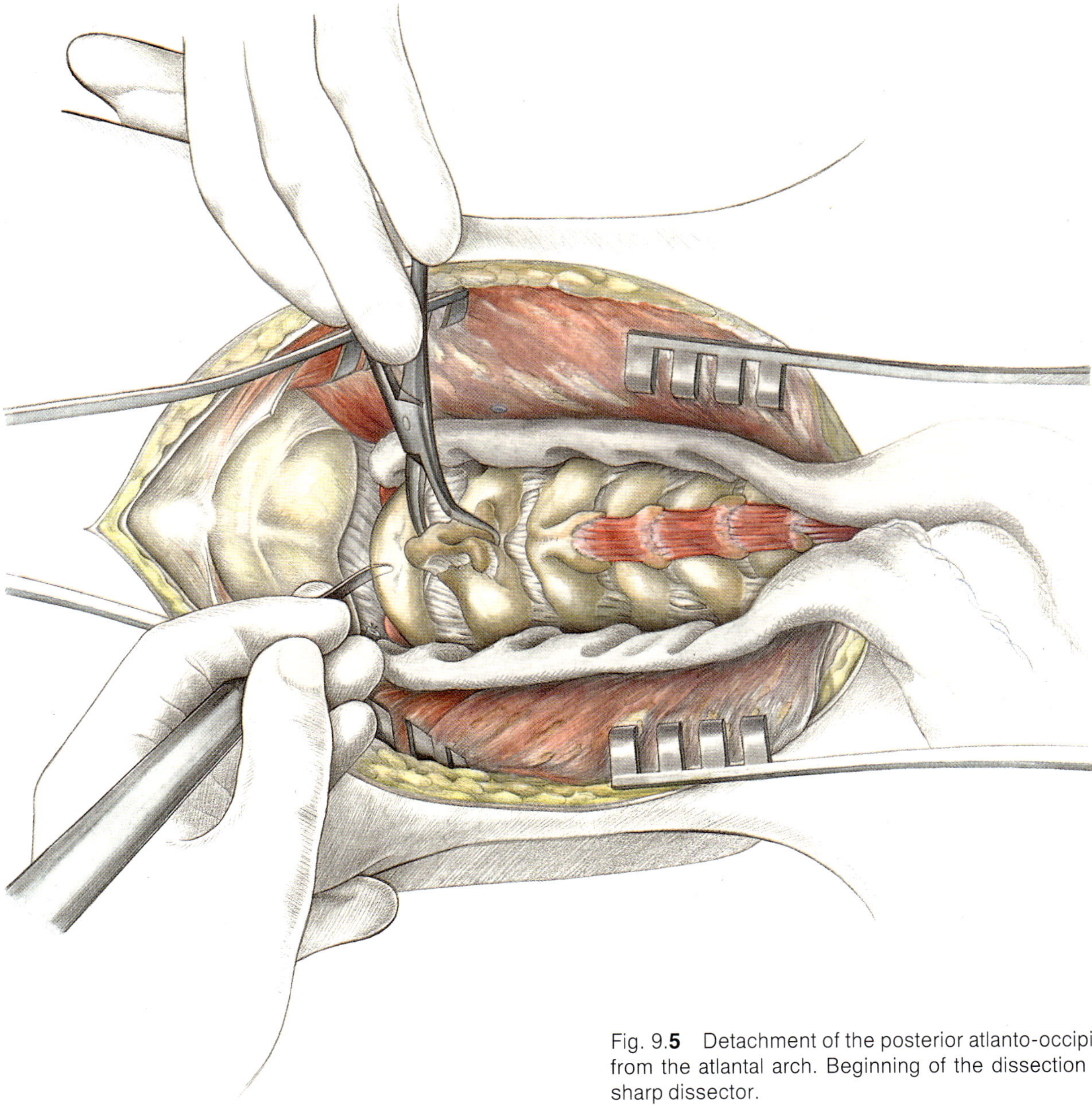

Fig. 9.**5** Detachment of the posterior atlanto-occipital membrane from the atlantal arch. Beginning of the dissection with a curved sharp dissector.

Posterior Atlantoaxial Fusion

The posterior atlantoaxial fusion (Brooks–Southwick), with the use of two interlaminar bone grafts, creates a stable rotatory fusion between C1 and C2. The Gallie technique is similar, but provides less rotatory stability. The technique according to Magerl is technically and instrumentally more demanding.

Approach

See Chapter 1, pp. 56–59.

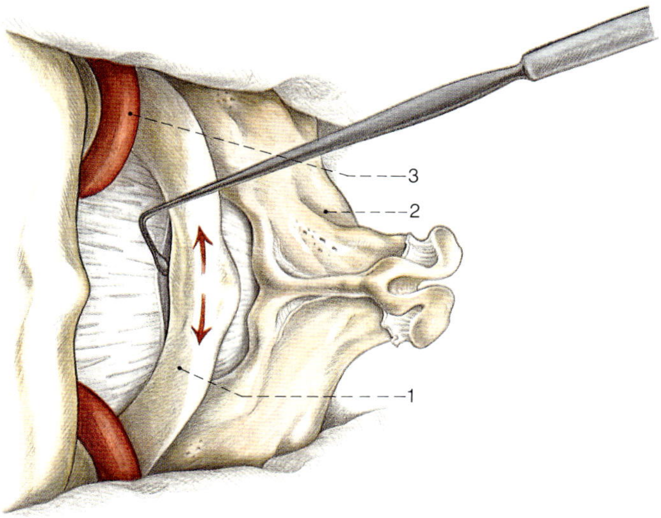

Fig. 9.**6** Further sublaminar dissection with a curved probe.

1 Posterior arch of the atlas
2 Posterior arch of the axis
3 Vertebral artery

Operative Technique

Brooks–Southwick Method

Using a narrow, sharp and curved elevator the posterior atlanto-occipital membrane is detached in the midline, beginning at the cranial border of the atlas, for a length of about 1 cm toward each side. The same procedure is followed from the caudal side (Fig. 9.**5**). The porotic, anteriorly dislocated arch of the atlas is frequently adherent to the dura. These adhesions can be carefully divided by rotary movements with a blunt probe (Fig. 9.**6**). Next, the ligamentum flavum is freed from the lamina of the axis, caudally at first and then cranially (Figs. 9.**7**, 9.**8**). Four soft wires 0.8 mm thick and about 30 cm long are looped at one end, slightly bent with pliers and armed with a suture. The suture and the wire can now be passed under the arches of C1 and C2 with a narrow wire passer (Fig. 9.**9**). The wire should be prevented from "sinking" into the spinal canal; the wire ends are therefore immediately grasped with a clamp and drawn posteriorly (Figs. 9.**10**, 9.**11**). In the same way, three additional wires are passed through below the laminae and lifted out of the operative field (Fig. 9.**12**). Using a ball-tipped reamer, the laminae of the atlas and the axis are debrided on both sides of the midline (Fig. 9.**13**).

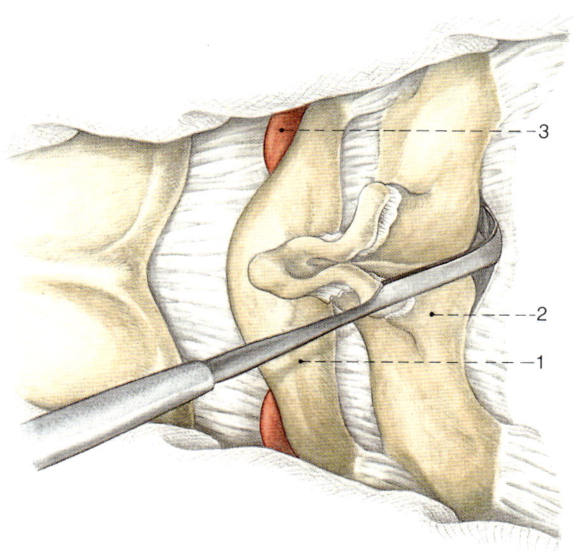

Fig. 9.**7** Detachment of the ligamentum flavum from the caudal border of the C2 arch.

1 Posterior arch of the atlas
2 Posterior arch of the axis
3 Vertebral artery

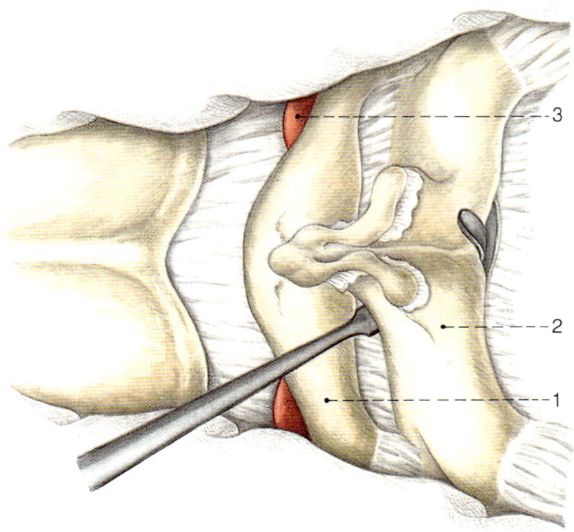

Fig. 9.**8** Sublaminar dissection of the arch of the axis from the cranial side.

1 Posterior arch of the atlas
2 Posterior arch of the axis
3 Vertebral artery

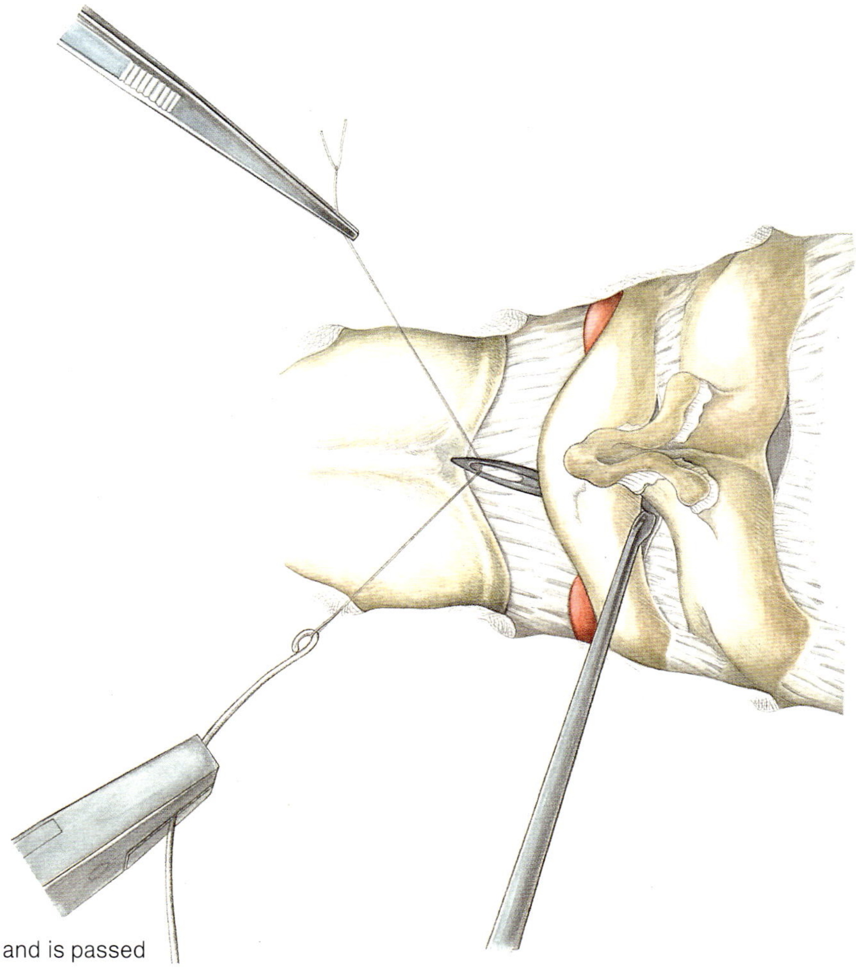

Fig. 9.**9** The steel wire has a suture attached to it, and is passed below the vertebral arch with a wire passer.

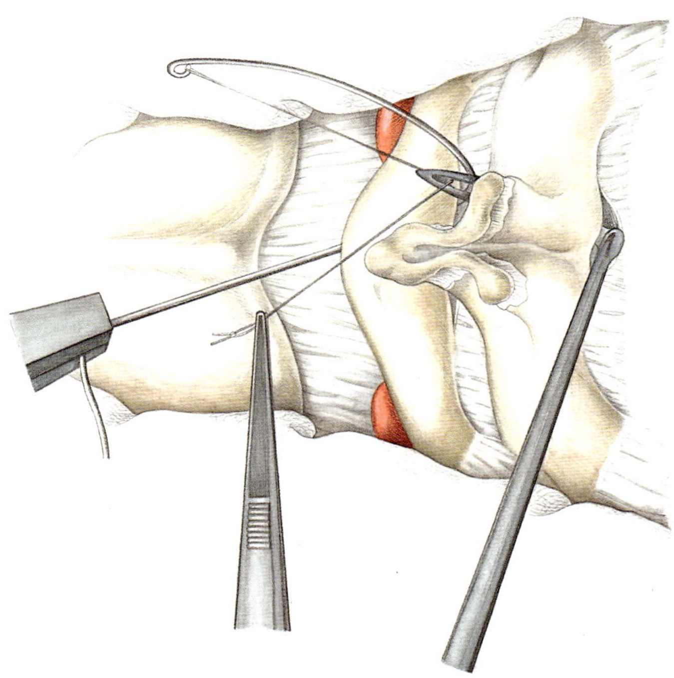

Fig. 9.**10** Passage of the wire below the arch of the axis.

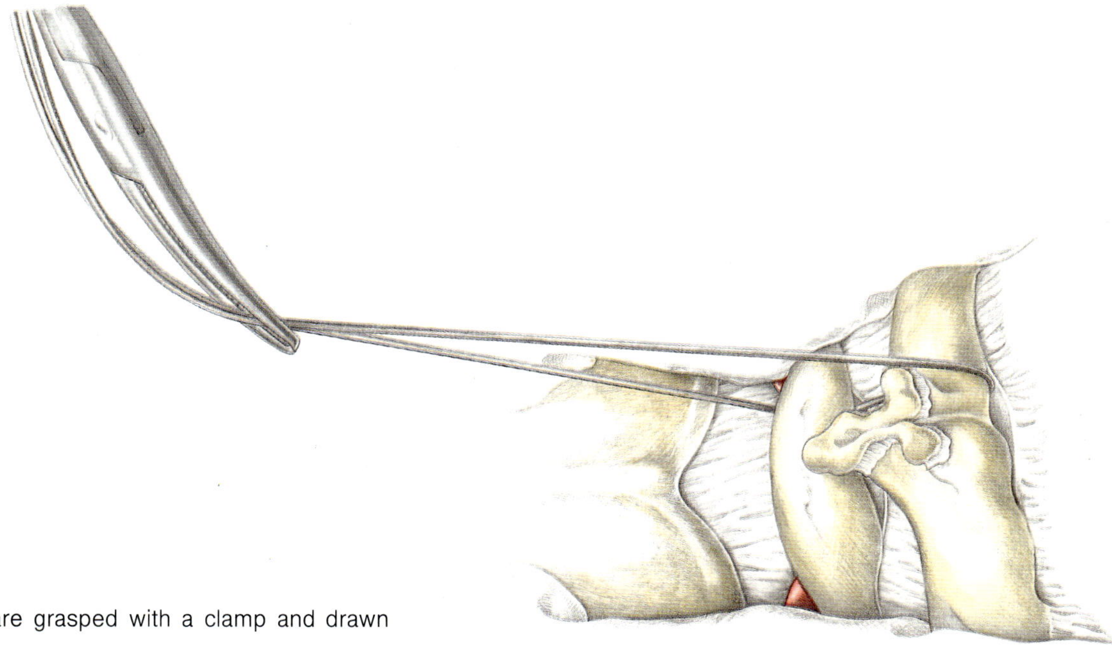

Fig. 9.**11** The wire ends are grasped with a clamp and drawn posteriorly by the assistant.

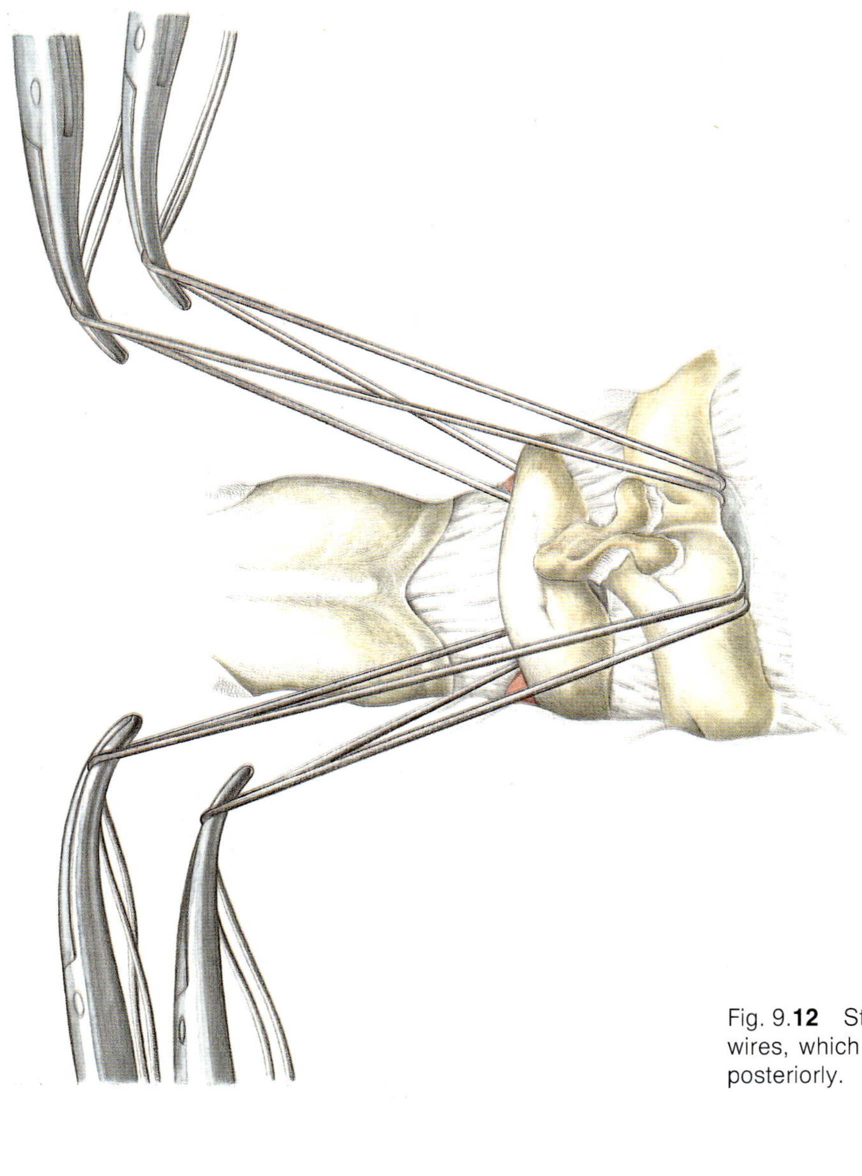

Fig. 9.**12** Status following sublaminar passage of the four steel wires, which are grasped with clamps at the ends and retracted posteriorly.

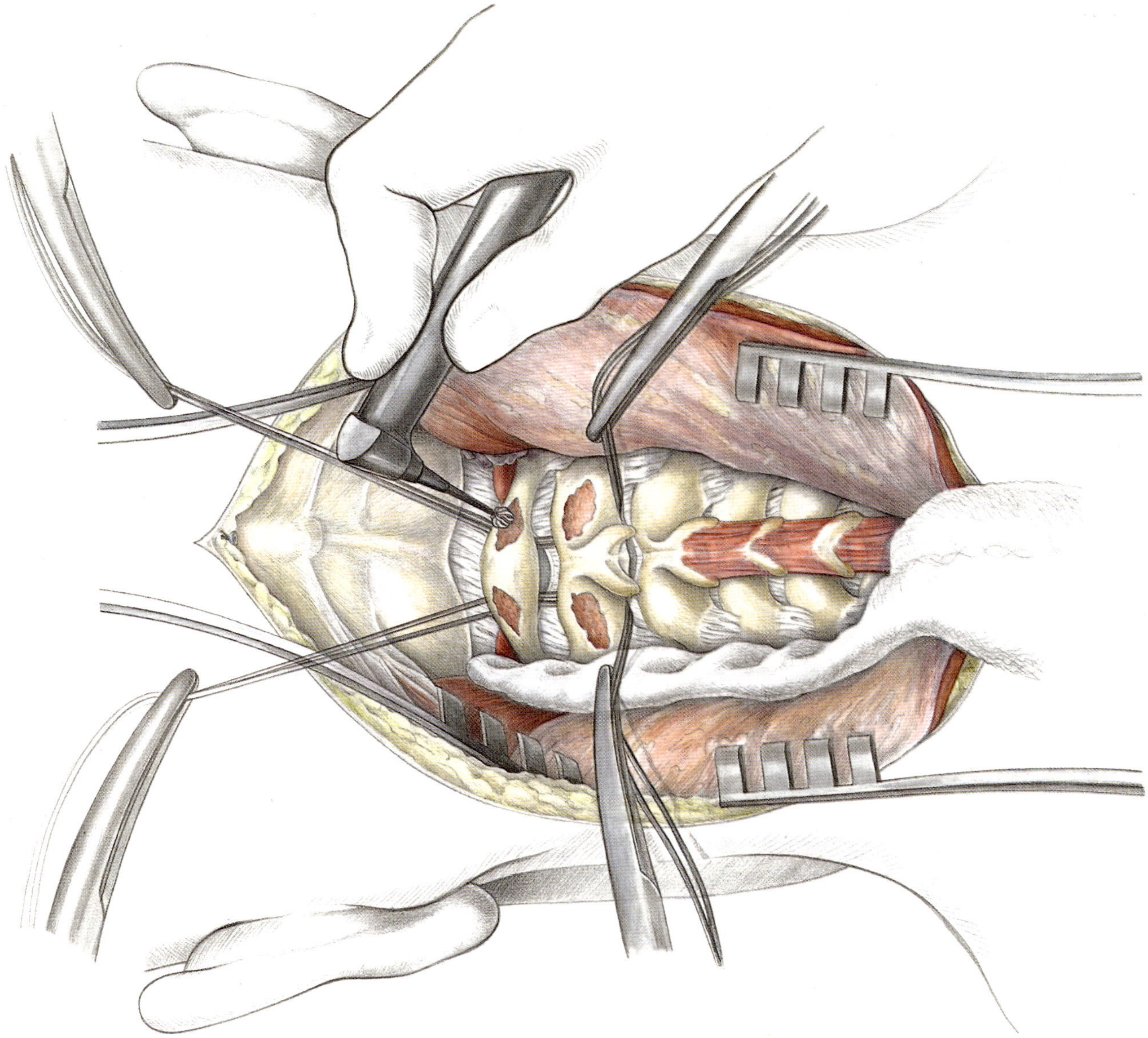

Fig. 9.**13** Debridement of the laminae of the atlas and axis with a ball-tipped reamer.

Two previously removed corticocancellous iliac-crest grafts are notched in four places and fitted flush between the laminae on both sides of the spinous process of C2. These grafts are cortically supported by the laminae; a cancellous bridge 5 mm thick remains between the laminae (Figs. 9.**14**, 9.**15**). After application of the first chip, the occiput is slightly extended under image intensifier control (lateral beam) until complete reduction of the anterior dislocation of the atlas has been achieved. Using moderate traction, the two wire ends are now grasped and twisted (Fig. 9.**16**). Reresection of the cranial portion of the graft may be required. Cancellous grafts from the pelvis are inserted in the midline, after which the second corticocancellous graft is introduced (Figs. 9.**17**, 9.**18**).

Fusion in the sagittal plane is shown in Figure 9.**19**.

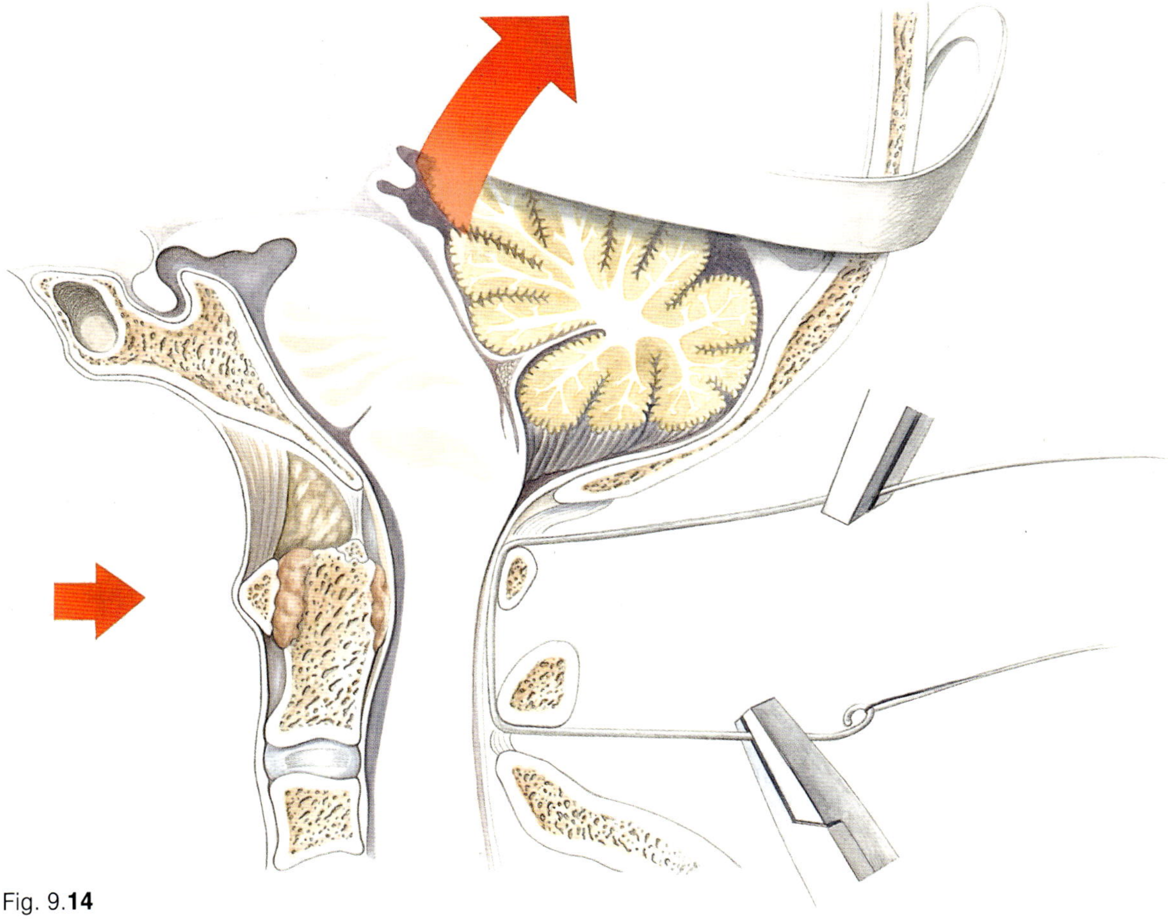

Fig. 9.**14**

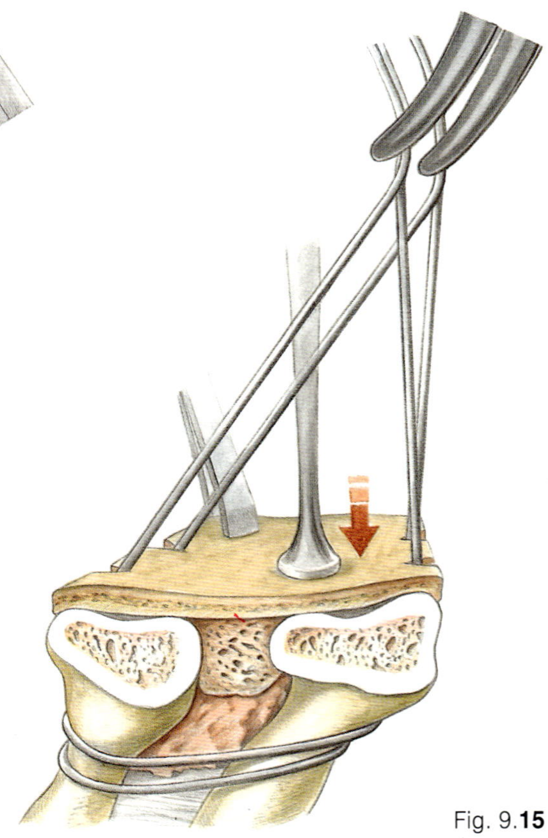

Fig. 9.**15**

Fig. 9.**14** Traction of the occiput; reduction of dislocation (image-intensifier control).

Fig. 9.**15** Insertion of an appropriately trimmed corticocancellous iliac graft between the atlas and the axis.

Fig. 9.**16** Wire fixation of a bone graft and insertion of additional cancellous grafts in the midline.

Fig. 9.**17** Insertion of the second corticocancellous graft and fixation with the laterally placed wire. After this, both of the wires in the midline are twisted.

Fig. 9.**18** Status after fixation of both grafts.

Fig. 9.**19** Checking the reduction and fusion with the image intensifier.

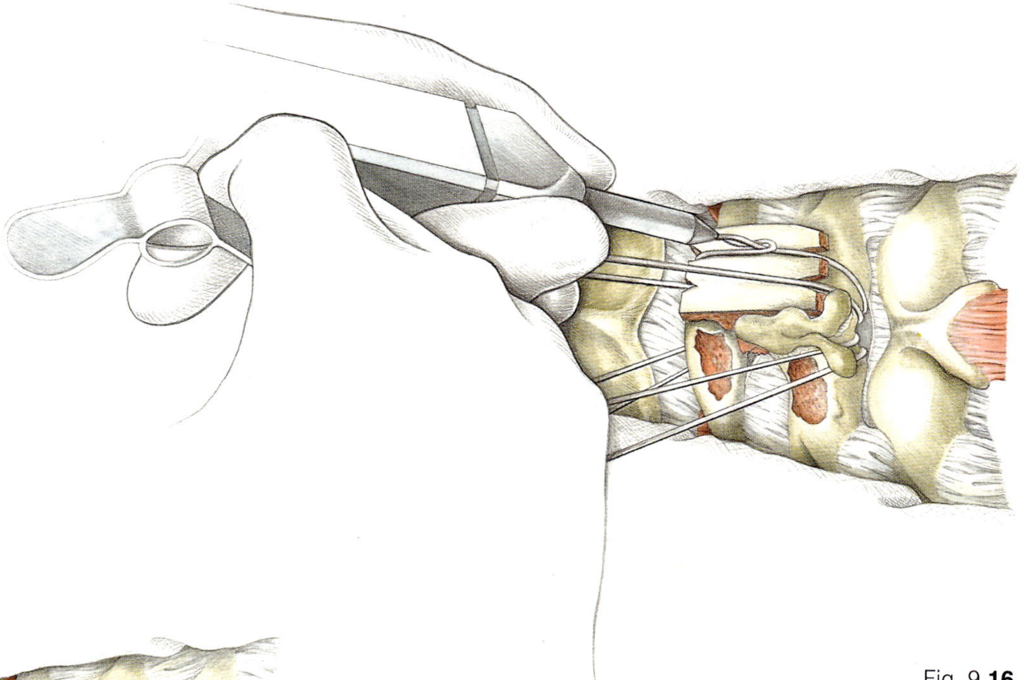

Fig. 9.**16**

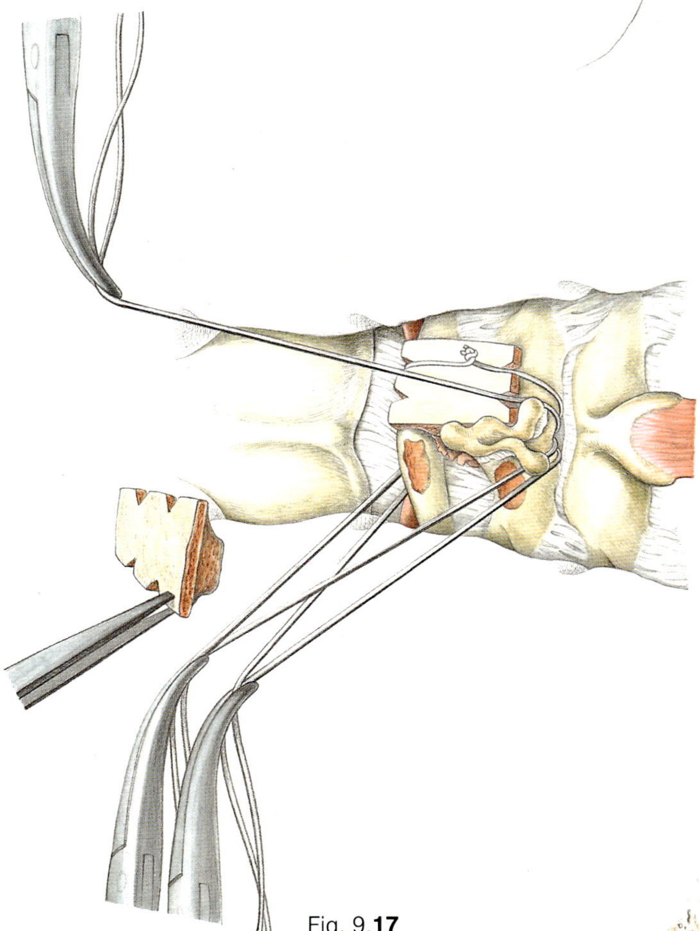

Fig. 9.**17**

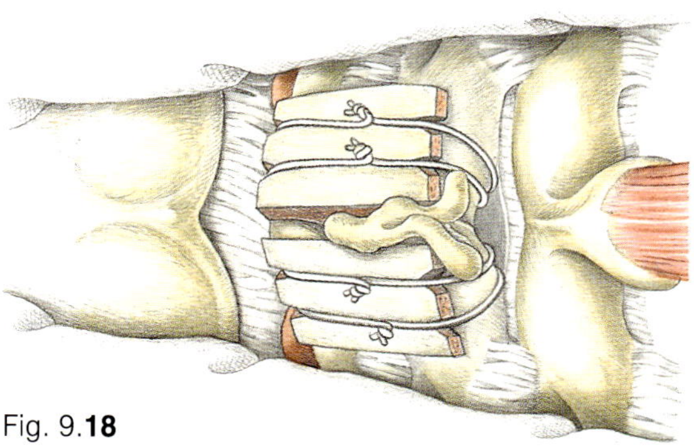

Fig. 9.**18**

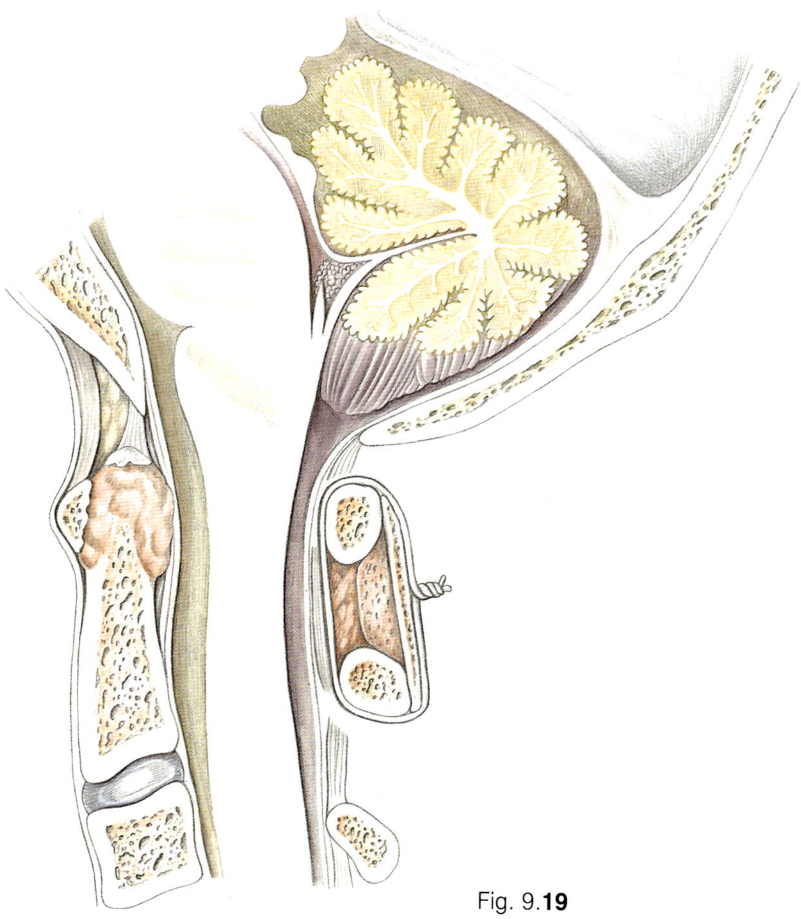

Fig. 9.**19**

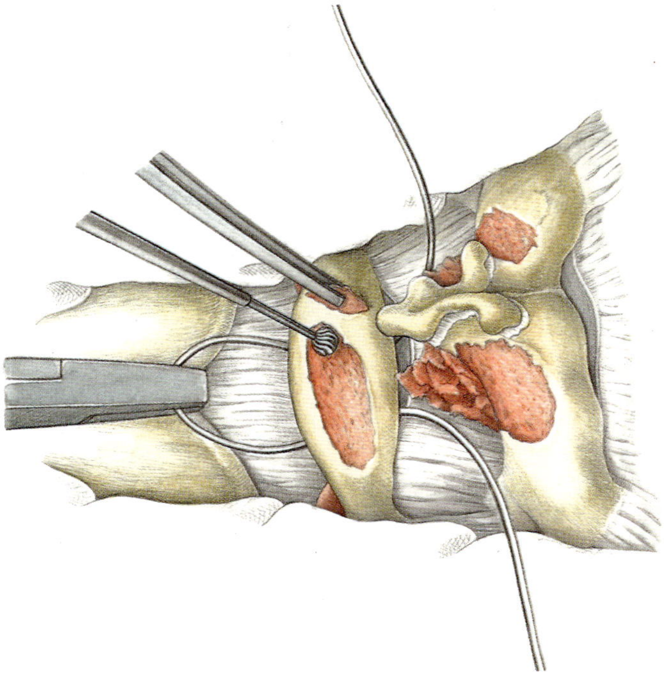

Fig. 9.**20** The arches of the atlas and the axis are decorticated, a wire loop is pulled through from caudal to cranial, and cancellous chips are packed between the atlas and the axis.

Gallie Method

In this method, a centrally positioned graft "riding" on the spinous process of the axis is used. A drawback of this technique is its lower rotatory stability compared with the Brooks method. An advantage is a less demanding operative procedure; in particular, no time-consuming sublaminar wiring of the axis is required.

A U-shaped excision is made in the caudal end of a previously harvested corticocancellous iliac graft. Channels for the wire are fashioned at both ends. Following decortication of the atlantal arch and of the spinous process and adjacent parts of the axial arch, the corticocancellous graft is provisionally inserted, and reshaped if necessary. After removal of the graft, a soft, flexible wire 0.9 mm thick and 30 cm long is bent in the middle to form a loop and is passed below the arch of the atlas from the caudal side. Cancellous-bone chips are placed on the ligamentum flavum between the atlas and the axis (Fig. 9.**20**). At the caudal end of the spinous process of the axis, two small grooves are made with the rongeur. The graft is now introduced and the wire loop is pulled from cranial to caudal over the graft and the spinous process of the axis (Fig. 9.**21**). The wire ends are tightened and twisted in a posterior direction over the graft (Fig. 9.**22**).

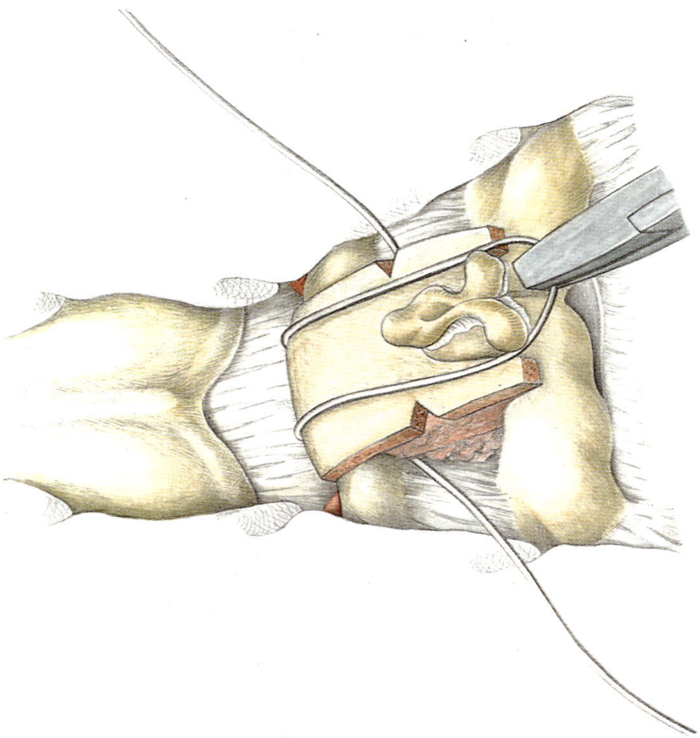

Fig. 9.**21** A previously-fashioned corticocancellous iliac graft which has received a U-shaped distal cut and two lateral grooves is inserted between the arches of the atlas and the axis. The wire loop is pulled over the spinous process of C2.

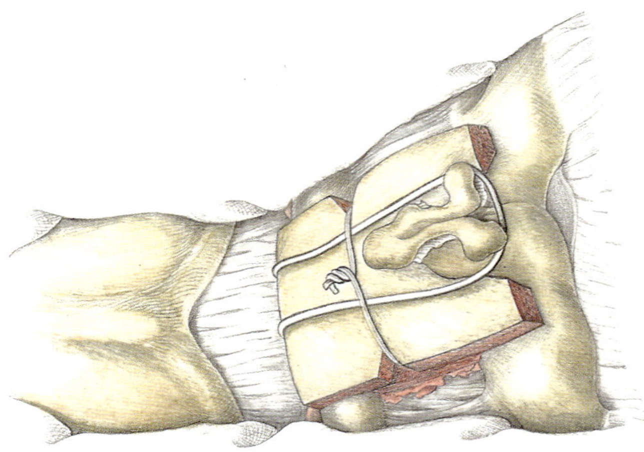

Fig. 9.**22** Status after fixation of the Gallie corticocancellous graft.

Transarticular Screw Fixation (Magerl)

Transarticular screw fixation is a technically demanding operation, but it gives greater stability than other methods of atlantoaxial fusion.

Under image-intensifier control, the cervical spine is flexed preoperatively. This is necessary to allow entry of the drill for the C1–C2 fusion at the correct angle. However, anterior dislocation of the atlas must be avoided in this position. The cervical spine is exposed caudally as far as the T2 spinous process.

After exposure of the cervical spine and the occipitocervical junction, a wire loop is passed under the arch of the atlas from cranial to caudal, the free ends of the wire being pulled under the loop. Thus, reduction of the atlas dislocation can be obtained by posterior traction. Slight traction by the assistant keeps the wire retracted posteriorly. The C1–C2 joints are now dissected from caudal to cranial along the arch of the axis. Exposure of the lower edge of the atlantal arch should be avoided in order to spare the greater occipital nerve. To spare the vertebral artery, the joint should also not be dissected laterally. The spinous process of C2 is now pushed manually in a cranial and, if possible, in an anterior direction. A drill 2.7 mm long is applied flush just medial and cranial to the C2–C3 joint after it has been marked with an awl, and is advanced, under lateral image-intensifier control, through the lamina and the C1–C2 articulation into the articular mass of the atlas (Fig. 9.**23**). When the tap hole has been cut, a cortical small-fragment screw of appropriate length (average 48 mm) is driven in (Fig. 9.**24**). The lower edge of the atlantal arch and the cranial portion of the spinous process and of the axial lamina are now decorticated with a reamer. A U-shaped corticocancellous iliac graft and cancellous-bone chips are fitted between the arch of the atlas and the spinous process of the axis (Figs. 9.**25**, 9.**26**). After engaging the C2 spinous process, the wire is tightened. The posterior parts of the C1–C2 joint can be sparingly debrided and packed with cancellous bone.

Postoperative Treatment

Postoperatively, a collar of plaster (padded) or any plastic material is applied. Use of an external support is recommended for a period of four months.

Pitfalls and Complications

Improper dissection of the C1–C2 joints may result in injury to the greater occipital nerve. The transarticular screw fixation can lead to injury to the vertebral artery if the drill is inserted laterally. The drilling should be done with the control of the image intensifier. Anterior perforation by the drill bit must be avoided because of the risk of damage to retropharyngeal structures.

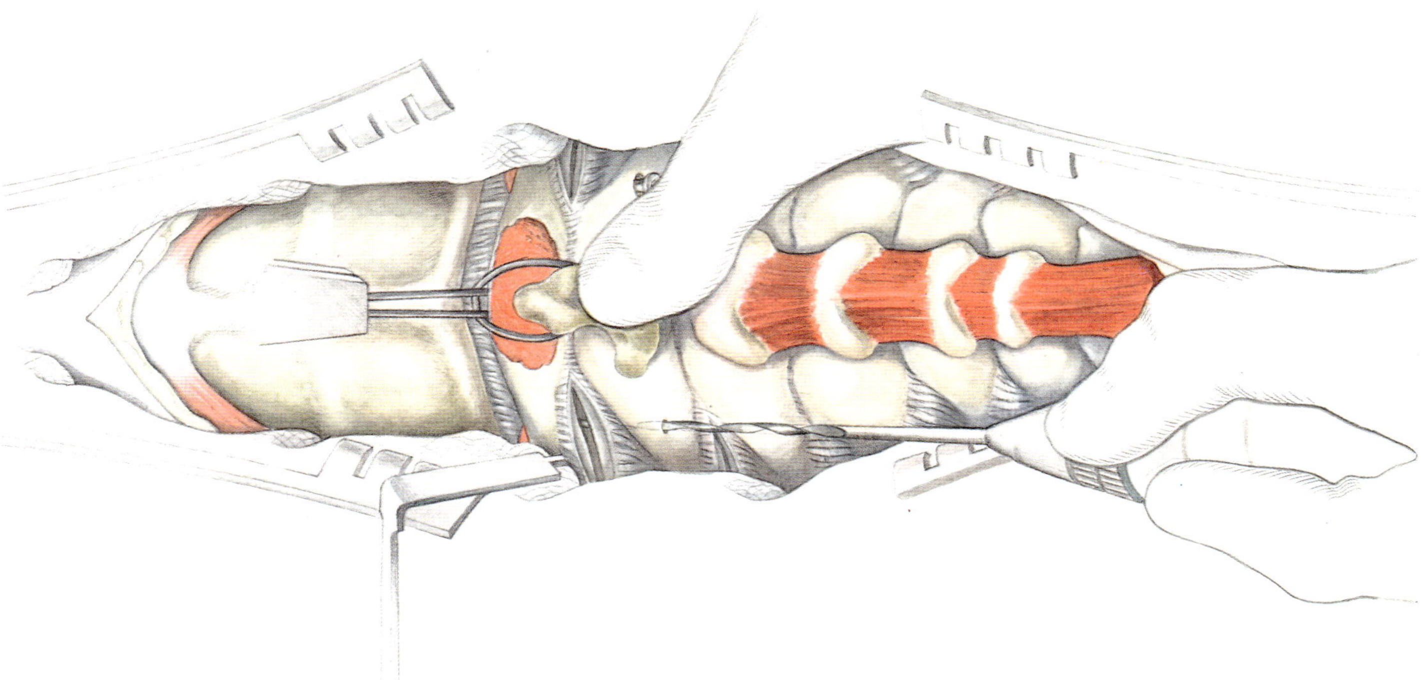

Fig. 9.**23** Following dissection of the C1–C2 joints from the caudal end and exposure of the joint space, a drill 2.7 mm wide is applied from the lower border of the axis arch and inserted under image-intensifier control in a shallow ascending line. The drilling direction should be verified by lateral radiography. An assistant pulls the arch of the atlas in a posterior direction with the aid of the wire loop, and thus corrects the anterior dislocation of the atlas. If necessary, the spinous process of the axis may be carefully tilted with the thumb to ensure safe intra-articular placement of the drill bit.

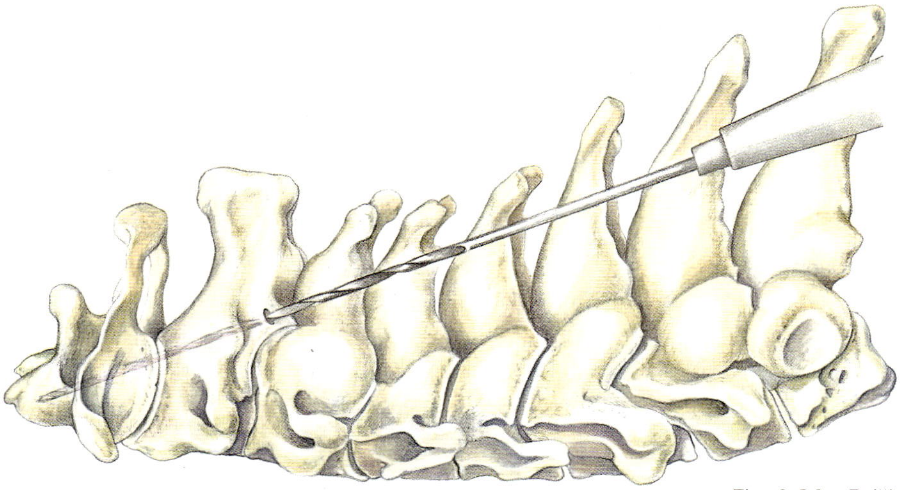

Fig. 9.**24** Drilling of hole on the left and status after fixation of the right C 1 – C 2 vertebral joint with a small-fragment screw.

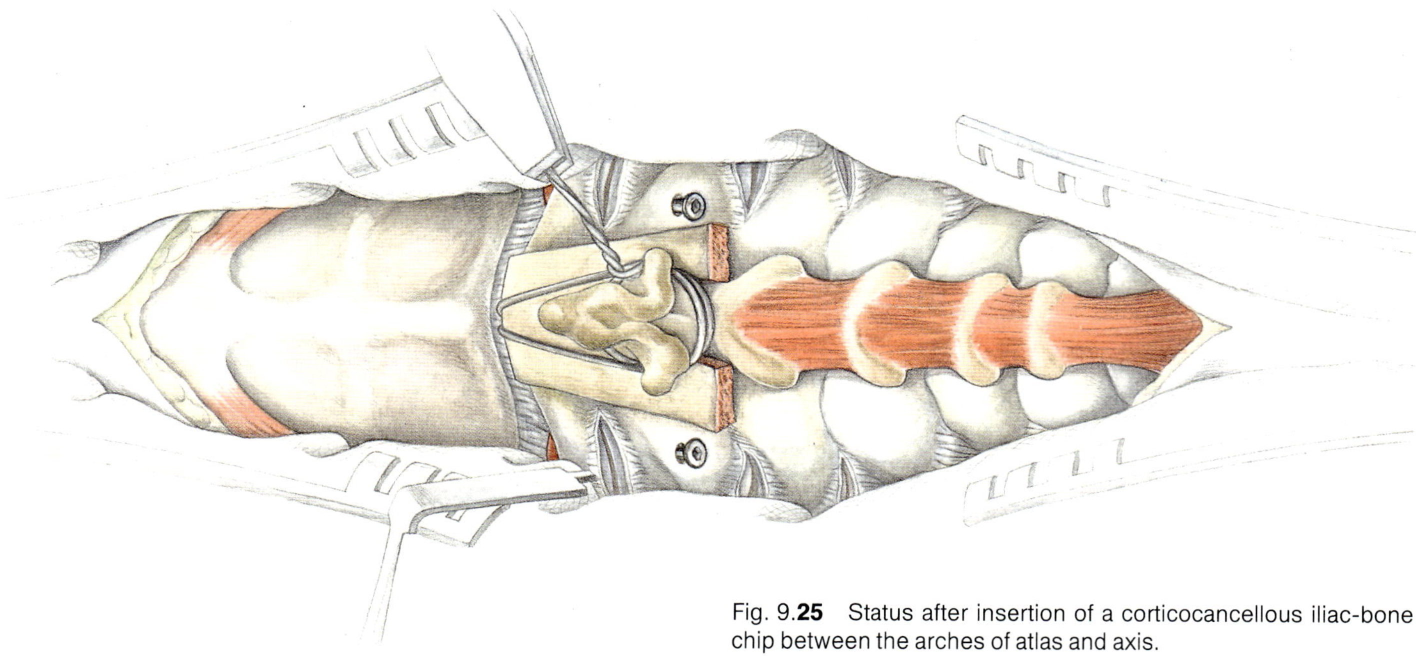

Fig. 9.**25** Status after insertion of a corticocancellous iliac-bone chip between the arches of atlas and axis.

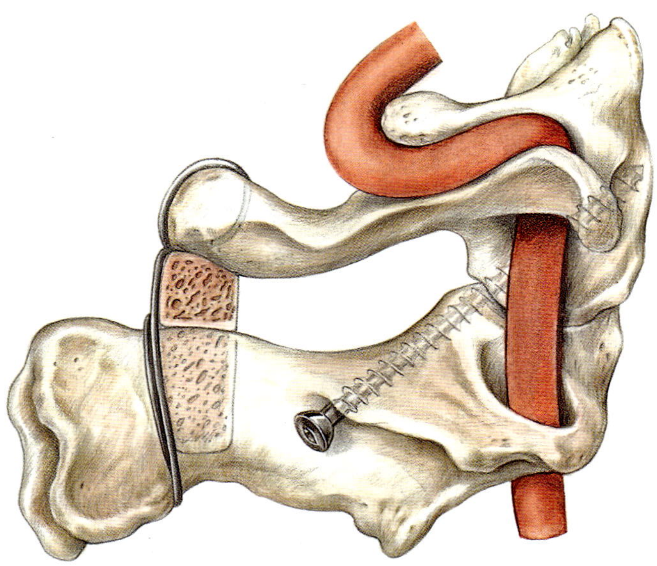

Fig. 9.**26** Status following screw fixation of the joints and fixation with a horseshoe-shaped graft.

Posterior Occipitocervical Fusion

Posterior occipitocervical fusion is indicated for destruction of the C0–C1 joint surfaces, for secondary basilar impression, and for anterior dislocation of the atlas or posterior subluxation due to pathological dens fractures.

Approach

See Chapter 1, pp. 56–59.

Positioning

All occipitocervical fusions, and specifically operations using the Gschwend and Brattström technique, are carried out, as a general rule, in traction by means of Crutchfield tongs, a Mayfield headrest, or a halo ring.

Operative Technique

Geschwend Method

About 1.5 cm lateral to the midline and caudal to the occipital protuberance, one drill hole each is made with the special drill, and two Gschwend screws are inserted (Fig. 9.**27**). This is followed by sublaminar dissection of the arches of the atlas and the axis, by removing the interspinal ligament between C2 and C3, and by sparing resection of the cranial portions of the C3 arch (Fig. 9.**28**). Two wires are then passed sublaminarly under the arches of C1 and C2, and the arches are decorticated with the ball-tip reamer (Fig. 9.**29**). Another wire is placed around both screw necks and underneath the arch of C1. A reduction of the atlantal arch can now be achieved by posterior traction (Figs. 9.**30**, 9.**31**). A transverse groove is then cut into the occipital bone with a ball-tipped reamer. A sufficiently long corticocancellous bone graft is harvested from the iliac crest; at its distal end, a U-shaped cut is made with a saw (Fig. 9.**32**), and the graft is prepared with a rongeur at its inferior border in such a way that it fits flush into the interlaminar region (Fig. 9.**33**). The graft is then punched in (Fig. 9.**34**). Next, the central graft is wired around the spinous process of C2 (Fig. 9.**35**) after radiographic control. After this, two additional small corticocancellous grafts from the iliac crest are placed between the arches of C1 and C2 and fixed by wire (Fig. 9.**36**). The appropriate positions of the atlas, the axis, and the graft are now verified by lateral radiographs (Fig. 9.**37**).

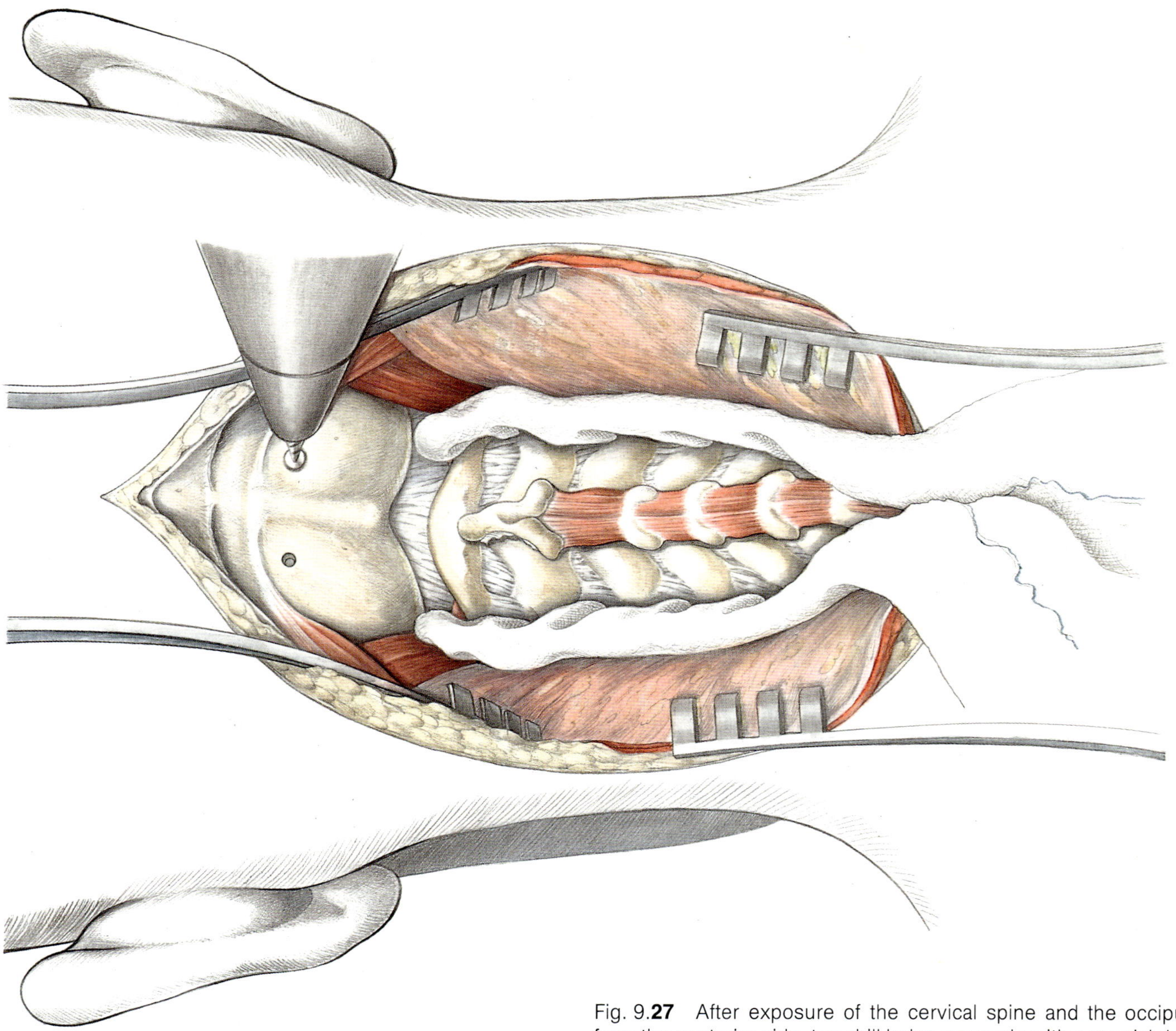

Fig. 9.**27** After exposure of the cervical spine and the occiput from the posterior side, two drill holes are made with a special drill on both sides of the midline.

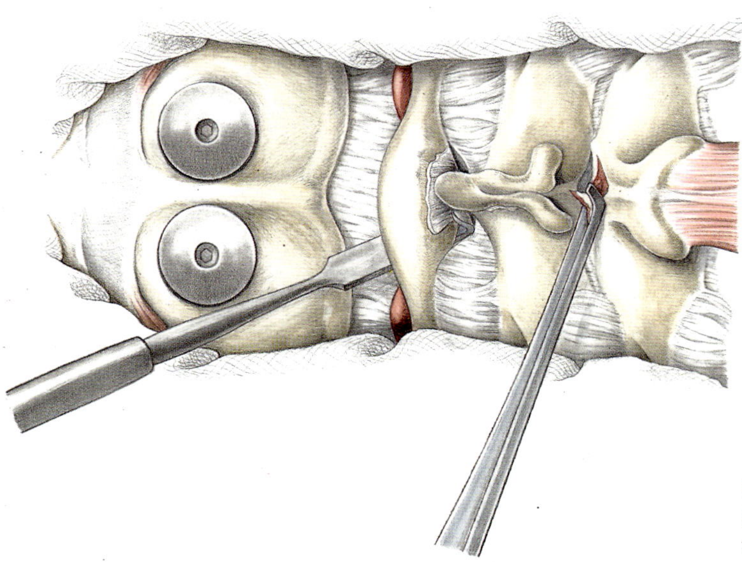

Fig. 9.**28** Sublaminar dissection of the atlantal and axial arches. Sparing resection of the cranial portions of the C3 arch. Flat and wide-headed Gschwend screws are driven into the occiput.

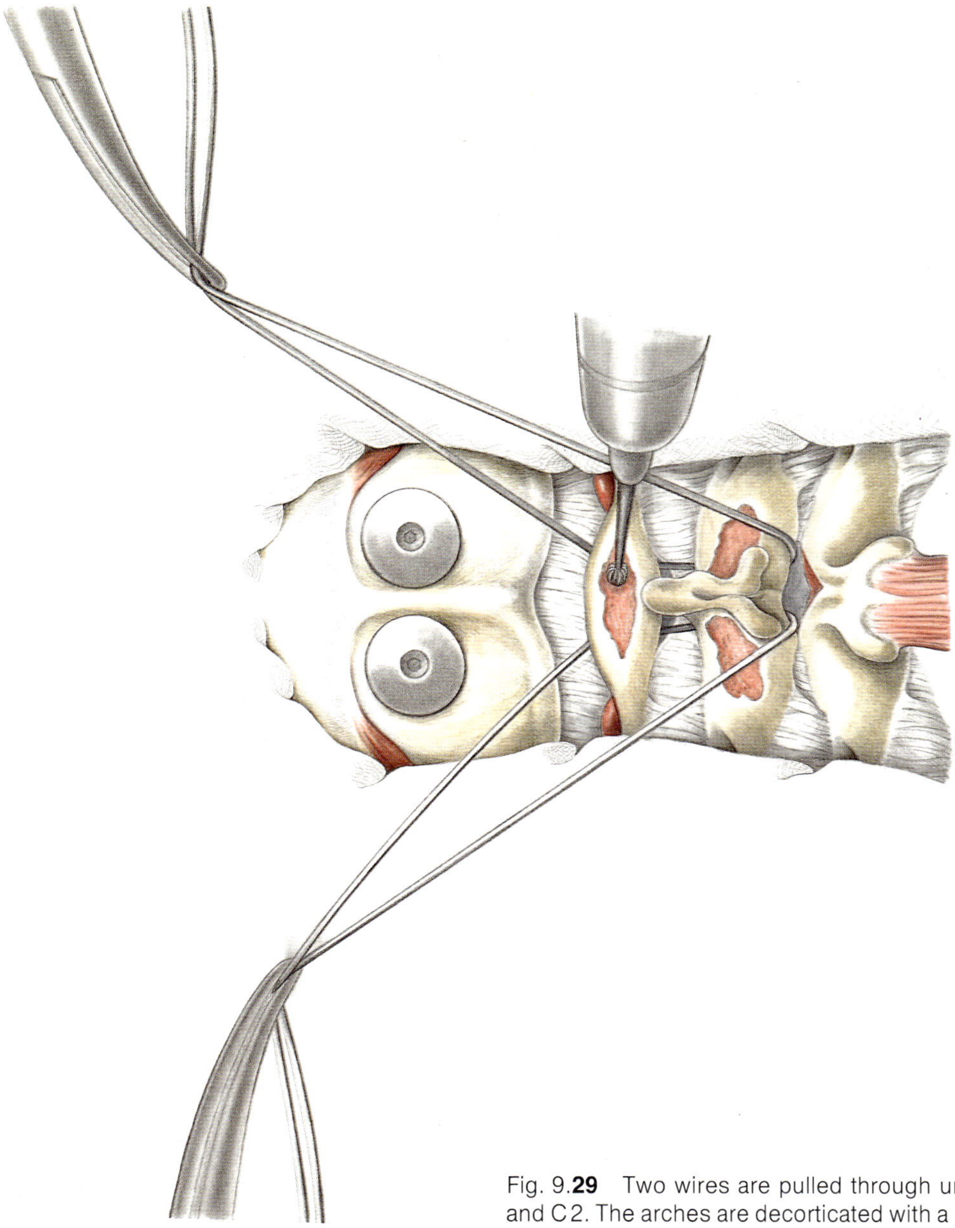

Fig. 9.**29** Two wires are pulled through under the arches of C1 and C2. The arches are decorticated with a ball-tipped reamer.

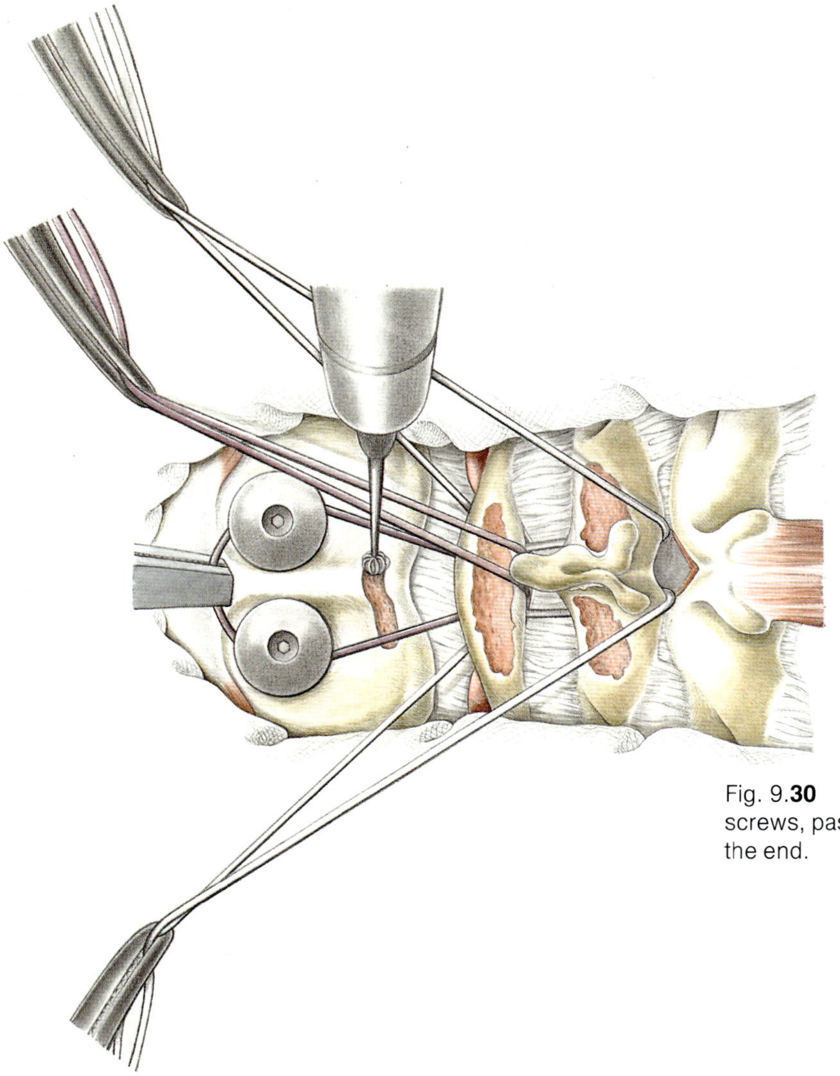

Fig. 9.**30** A central wire is placed around the necks of both screws, passed under the arch of C 1, and grasped with a clamp at the end.

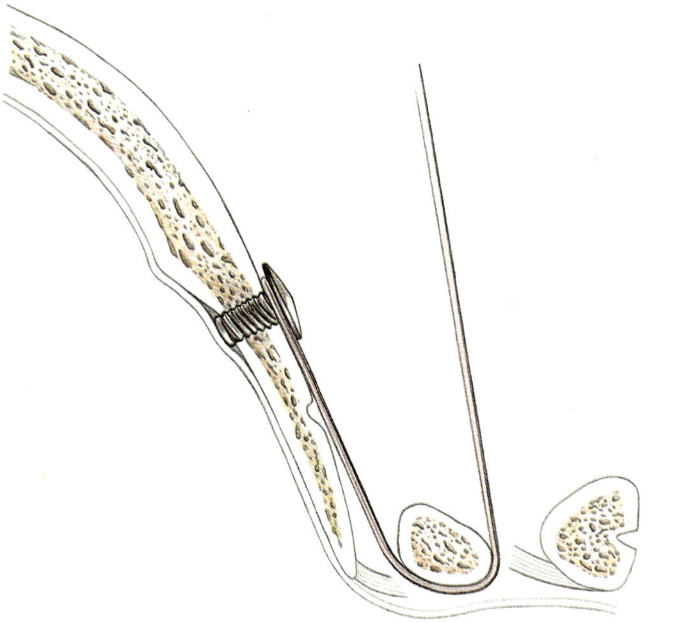

Fig. 9.**31** The malposition can be reduced by posterior traction (sagittal plane).

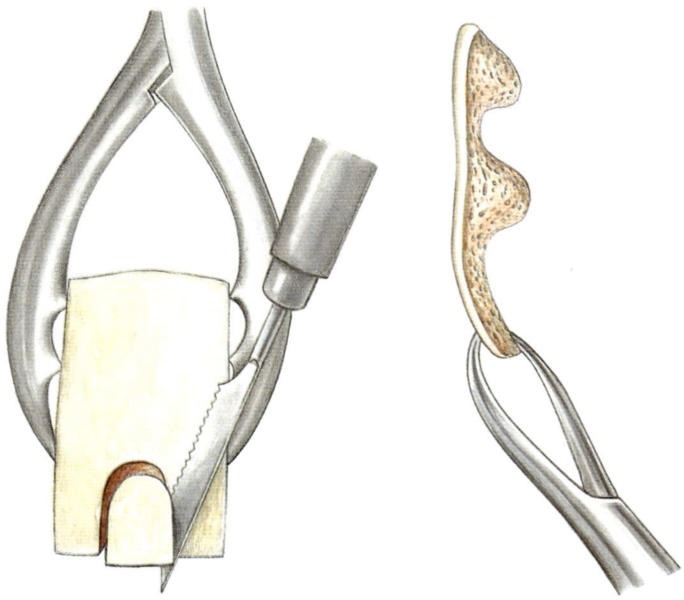

Fig. 9.**32** Harvesting of a corticocancellous graft from the iliac crest; the graft is given a horseshoe shape at the lower end.

Fig. 9.**33** The graft is fashioned so that cancellous bony bridges are obtained between the occiput and the atlas, as well as between the atlas and the axis.

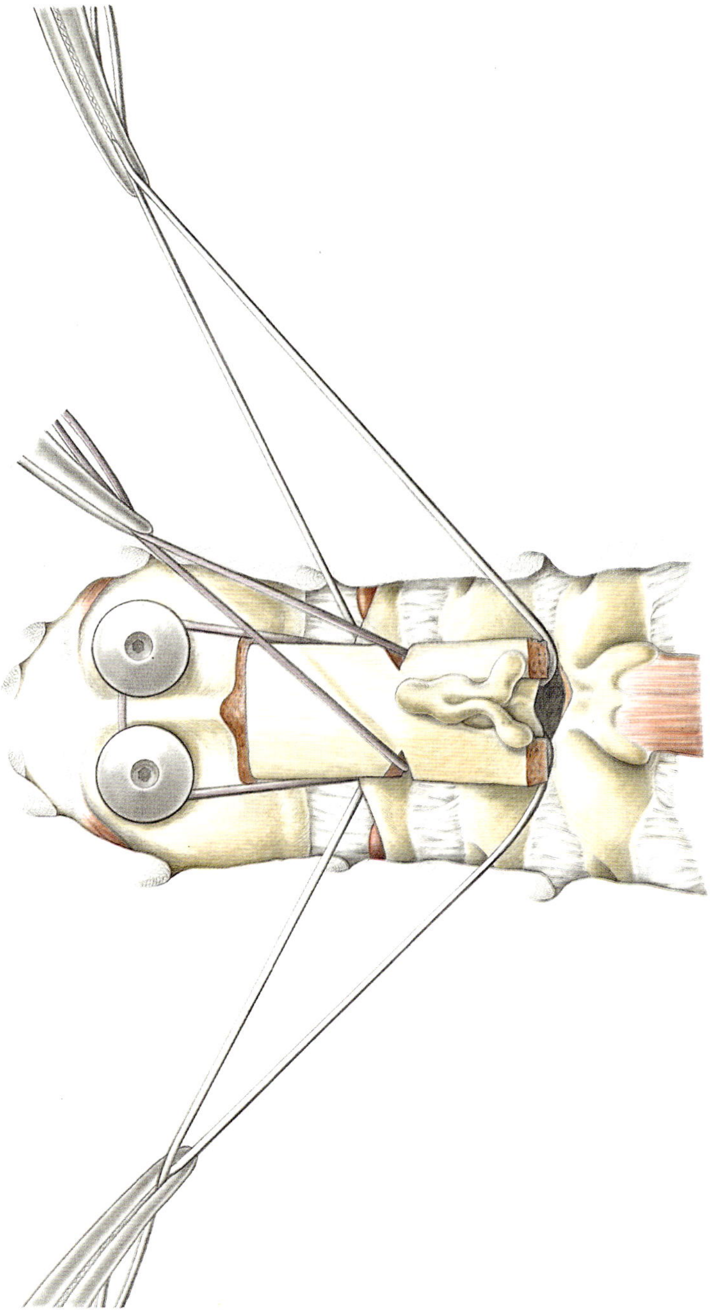

Fig. 9.**34** Status after introduction of the corticocancellous graft.

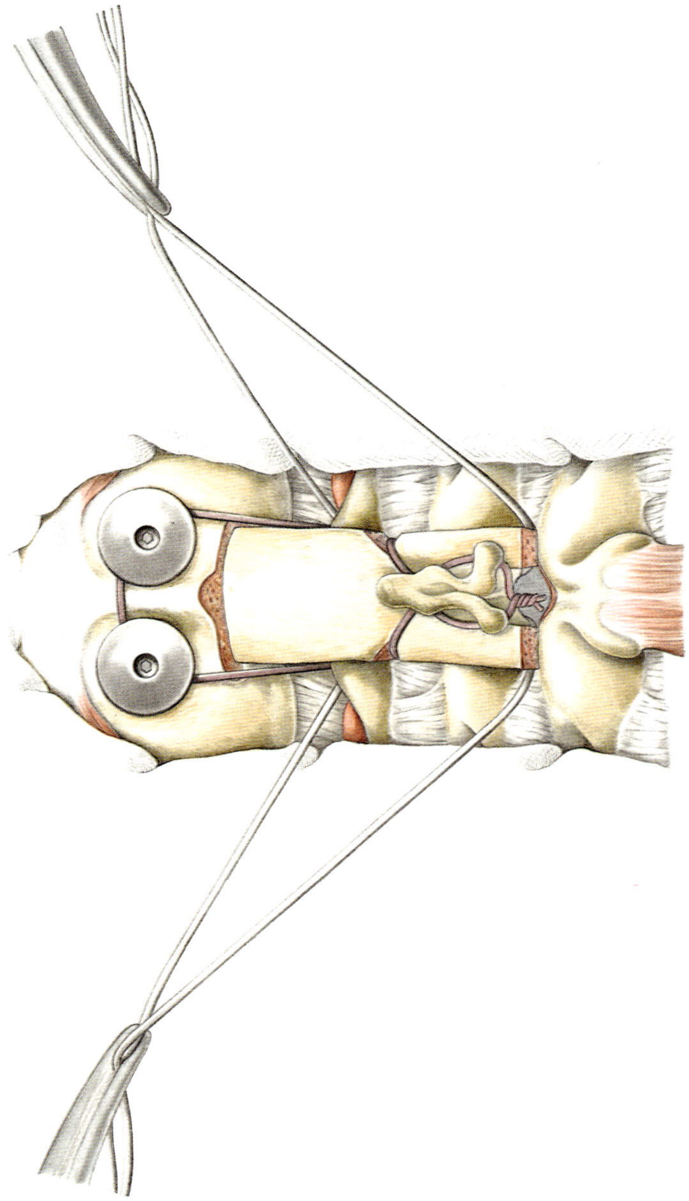

Fig. 9.**35** After reduction, the central graft is fixed under traction (lateral radiographic control) over the spinous process of the axis by wiring.

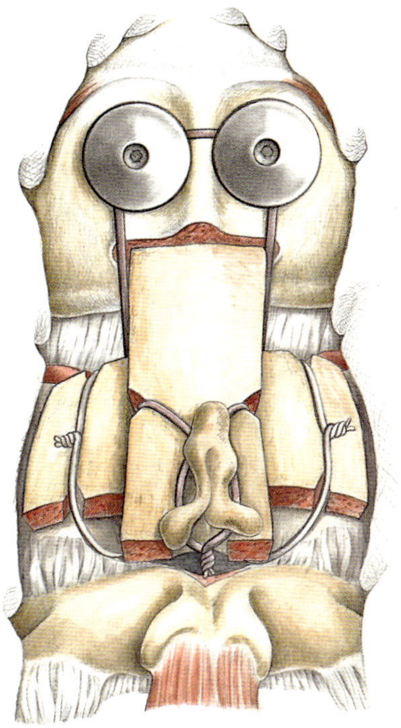

Fig. 9.**36** Status after insertion of two laterally placed corticocancellous grafts and wire fixation.

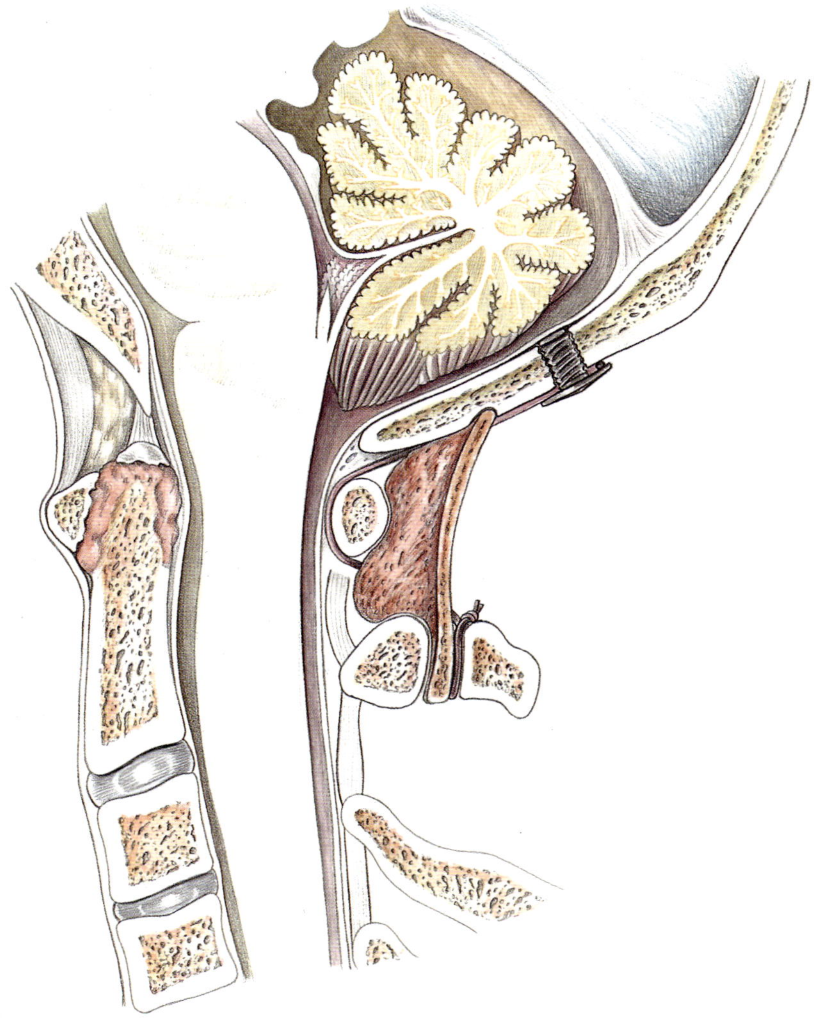

Fig. 9.**37** Status after Geschwend fusion between the occiput, C1, and C2 (sagittal plane).

Brattström Method

On both sides of the midline, four drillholes are made in the occipital squama with a calibrated neurosurgical trephine drill. Using angulated elevators or curved blunt probes, the dura is cautiously detached from the occipital squama (Fig. 9.**38**). This is followed by decortication of the occipital squama and of the atlantal and axial arches with a high-speed ball-tipped drill. A soft and flexible wire about 40 cm long and 0.9 m thick is looped at one end, pulled throuth the holes on one side of the occipital squama, and is then brought out again through the holes on the contralateral side from cranial to caudal. If the wire cannot be inserted from caudal to cranial, two wires approximately 30 cm long can be passed epidurally through one side each from cranial to caudal. The cranial part of the wires can now be twisted. After this, the caudal wire ends are pulled sublaminarly beneath the arch of the atlas (Fig. 9.**39**). Before this, the posterior atlantooccipital membrane and the ligamentum flavum were retracted for a length of about 1.0 cm on both sides of the midline. If necessary, lateral image-intensifier control is now performed, and the existing subluxation is reduced by extension of the occiput. A Kirschner wire 2 cm long and 1.5 mm thick is placed around the spinous process of C2. One side is reinforced with methylmethacrylate, and after the cement has cured, the wire is twisted over the spinous process of the atlas and the Kirschner wire. To avoid heat injuries, ample irrigation is necessary during the polymerization process. After this, the occiput, the atlas, and the axis on the contralateral side are covered with cancellous-bone chips (Figs. 9.**40** and 9.**41**).

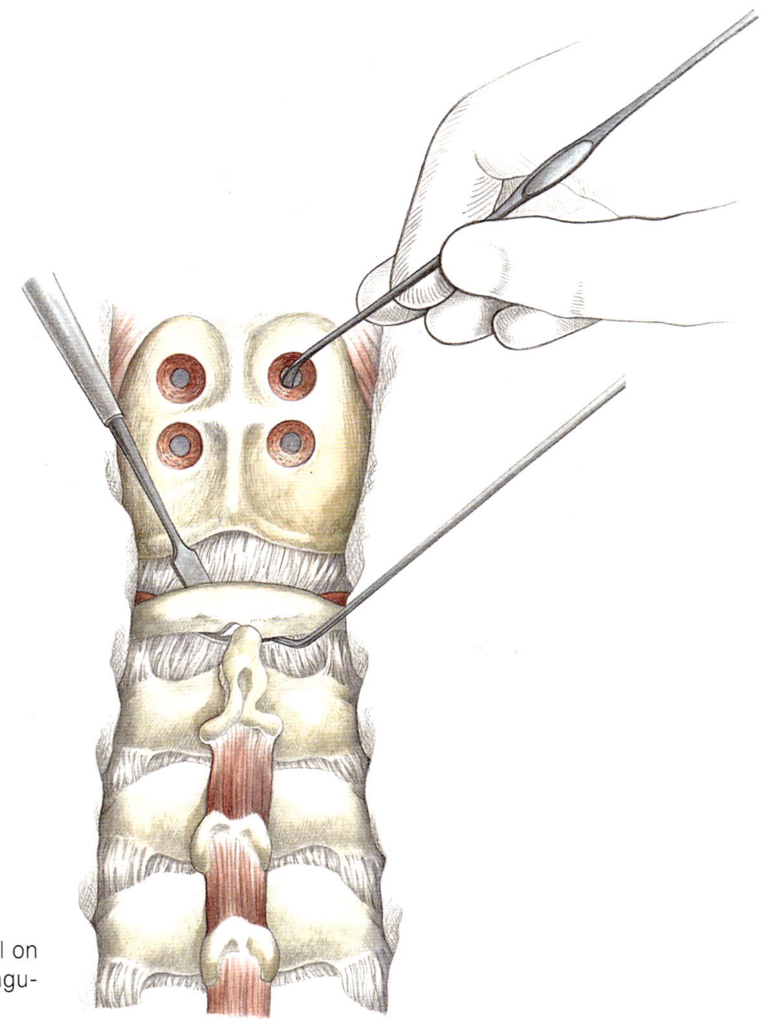

Fig. 9.**38** Two drill holes each are made with a trephine drill on both sides of the midline. The dura is carefully freed with angulated elevators.

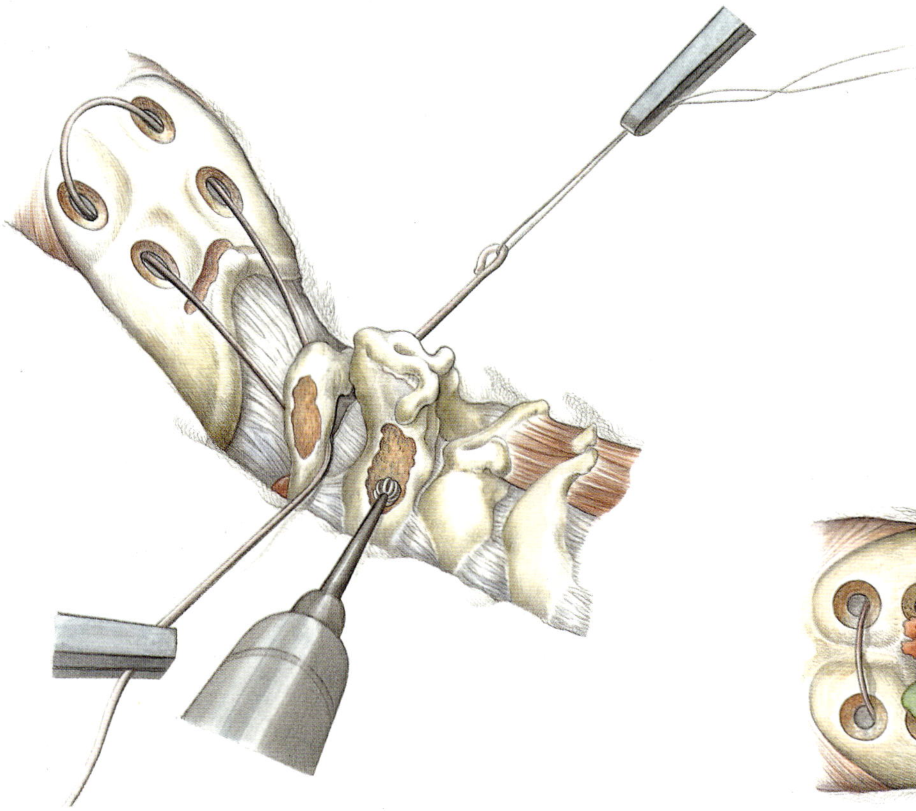

Fig. 9.**39** When the wire has been passed through the drill holes in the occiput, the wire ends are pulled under the atlantal arch, grasped with one clamp each, and retracted superiorly. The atlantal and axial arches are debrided, and a groove is cut into the occipital bone.

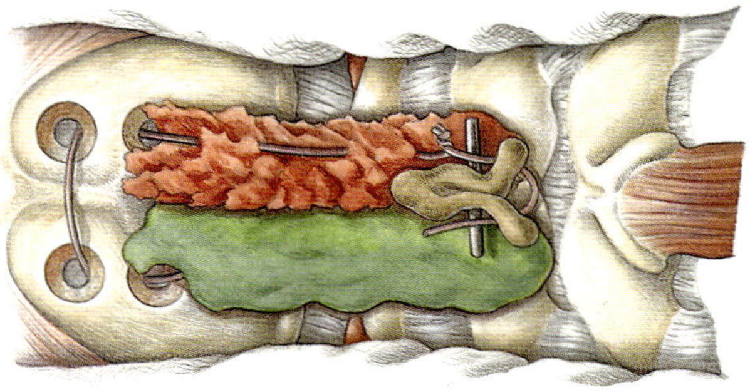

Fig. 9.**40** Following insertion of a Kirschner wire through the spinous process of the axis, the anterior dislocation of the atlas is reduced under traction (lateral radiographic control). A cement plug is now introduced from one side, and when it has cured, the wire over the spinous process of the atlas and the Kirschner wire is twisted. On the contralateral side, cancellous-bone chips are deposited between the occiput, atlas, and axis.

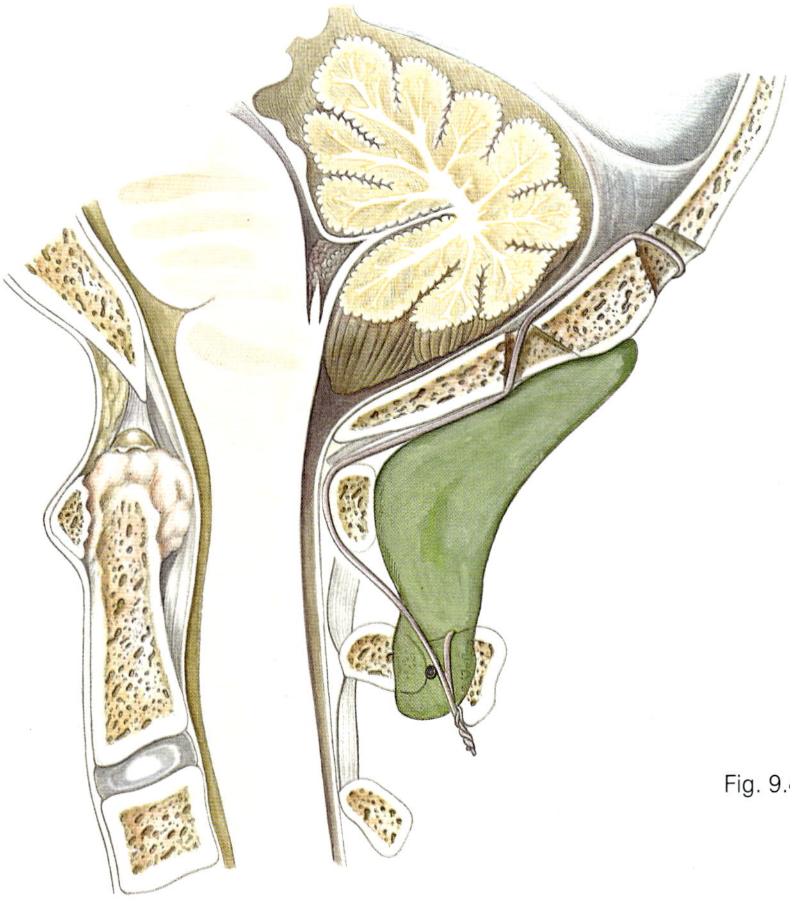

Fig. 9.**41** Brattström fusion in the sagittal plane.

Fusion Using Plates

This method is recommended for cases in which a posterior decompression becomes necessary because of transverse cord lesions, so that a sublaminar wire fixation is out of the question. Occipitocervical instability with basilar invagination and high-grade atrophy of the posterior arch of the atlas may also be indications for this operation.

The spine and the occiput are exposed, as are the vertebral joints C2–C4. The interspinal ligaments are left intact. With the aid of lateral image-intensifier control, the occiput is now fixed in the desired reduced position. Small, flexible lead plates are placed as a template between the occiput and the articular masses of the cervical spine (Fig. 9.**42**). One-third tubular plates or Harms reconstruction plates are bent as required. Roy–Camille plates can also be used. The reconstruction plate is advantageous, since it allows a tilted screw position in the cervical spine, thus providing for improved screw support. Using this plate, the drill holes are made obliquely from caudal–medial to cranial–lateral at the level of C3 and C4 (Fig. 9.**43**). The drill enters at the lower edge of the lamina, in the middle of the vertebral joints. The drill bit pierces the cortical layer lateral to the articular mass, but posterior to the intervertebral foramen. The drilling direction is sagittal: the drill is inserted into the pedicle of C2 ascending from caudal to cranial. Perforation of the anterior cortical layer is not necessary. At this level, screws 14 mm long are sufficient (Fig. 9.**44**). The plate is now applied and screwed onto the vertebral arches C2, C3, and C4 (Fig. 9.**45**). Three drill holes are made in the occipital squama, and appropriately short screws are inserted. The use of calibrated drills helps to avoid injury to the dura mater (Fig. 9.**46**). The positions of the axis, atlas, and occiput are now checked by lateral radiography. After decortication of the laminae of C2, C3, and C4 and of the occipital squama, a corticocancellous graft and cancellous chips are harvested from the pelvis. The cancellous chips are placed in the midline over the laminae as far as the occipital squama (Fig. 9.**47**). At the end, a solid corticocancellous graft is placed in the center (Figs. 9.**48**, 9.**49**).

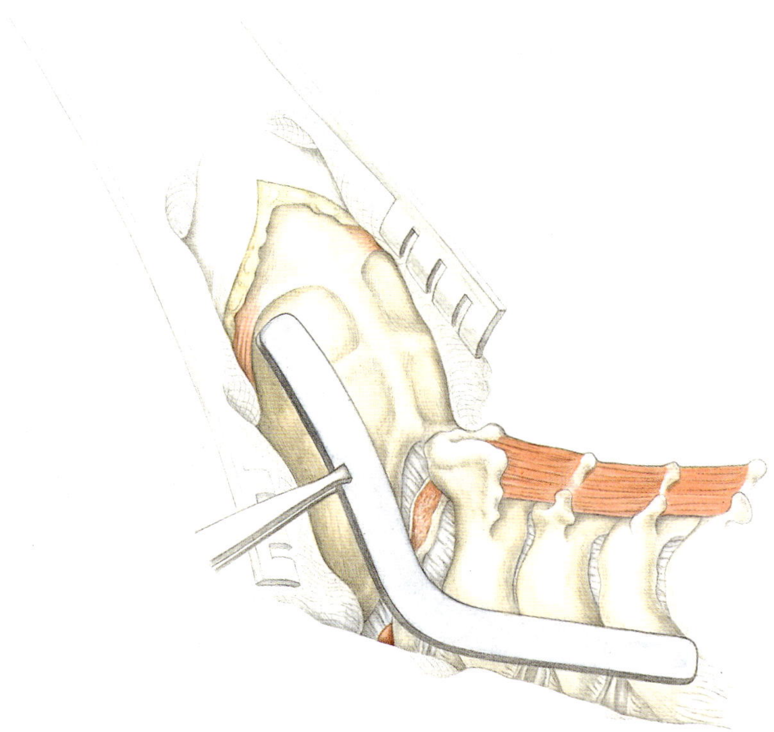

Fig. 9.**42** Application of flexible small lead plates as a template for the plates between the occiput and the posterior cervical spine.

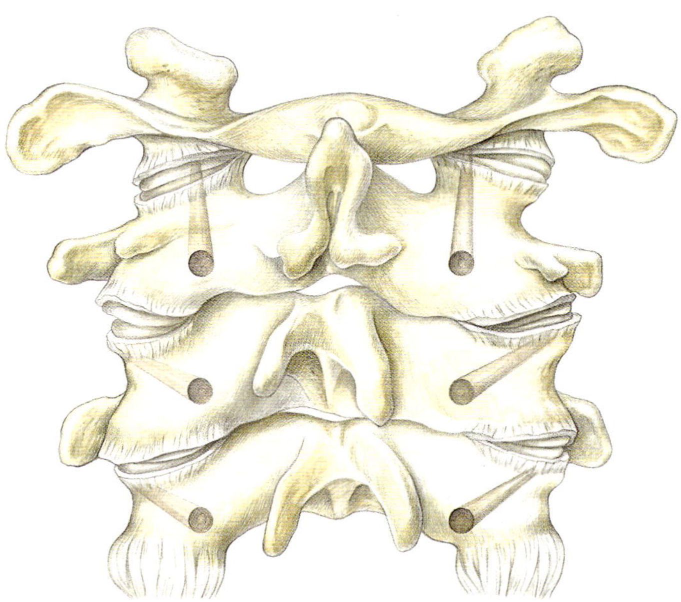

Fig. 9.**43** Drilling direction with the use of reconstruction plates. The drill bit enters at the lower edge of the lamina, in the middle of the vertebral joints, and is advanced laterally, posterior to the intervertebral foramen (exception: C1–C2).

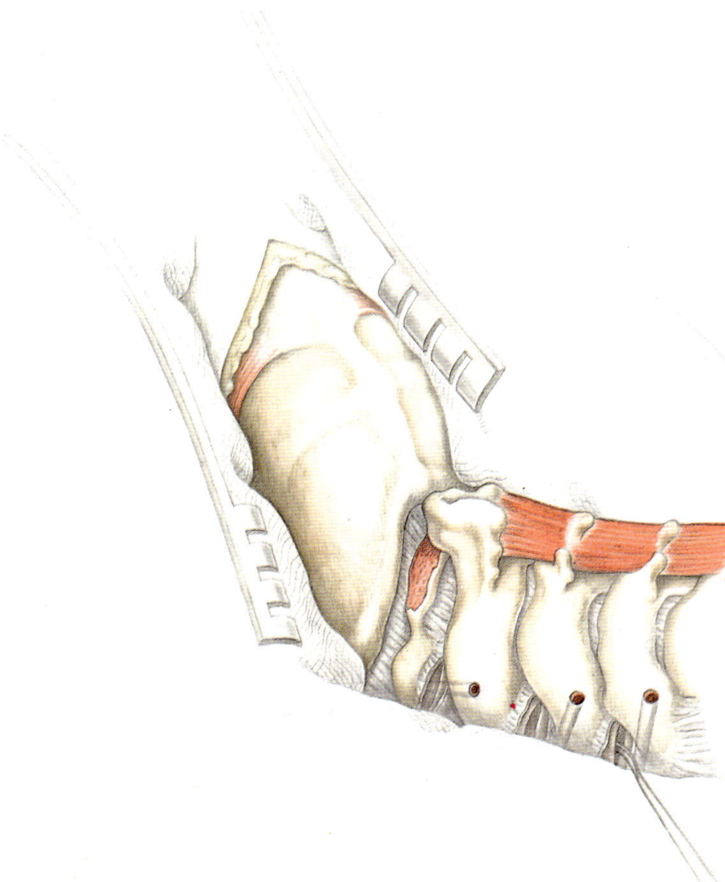

Fig. 9.**44** Drilling direction in the sagittal plane. In C2, the drill ascends from caudal to cranial into the pedicle of C2 (image-intensifier control). Perforation of the anterior cortical layer is not necessary.

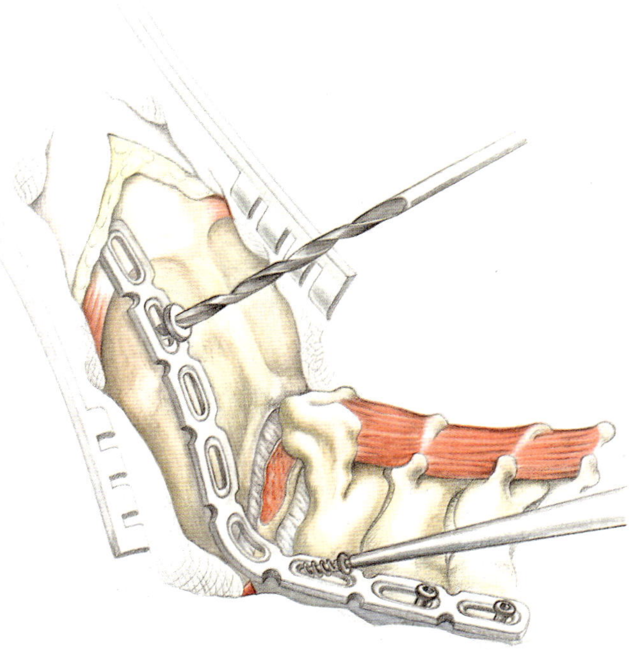

Fig. 9.**45** Application of the plate and attachment to vertebral arches C2, C3, and C4. With the plate in place, three drill holes are made in the occipital squama.

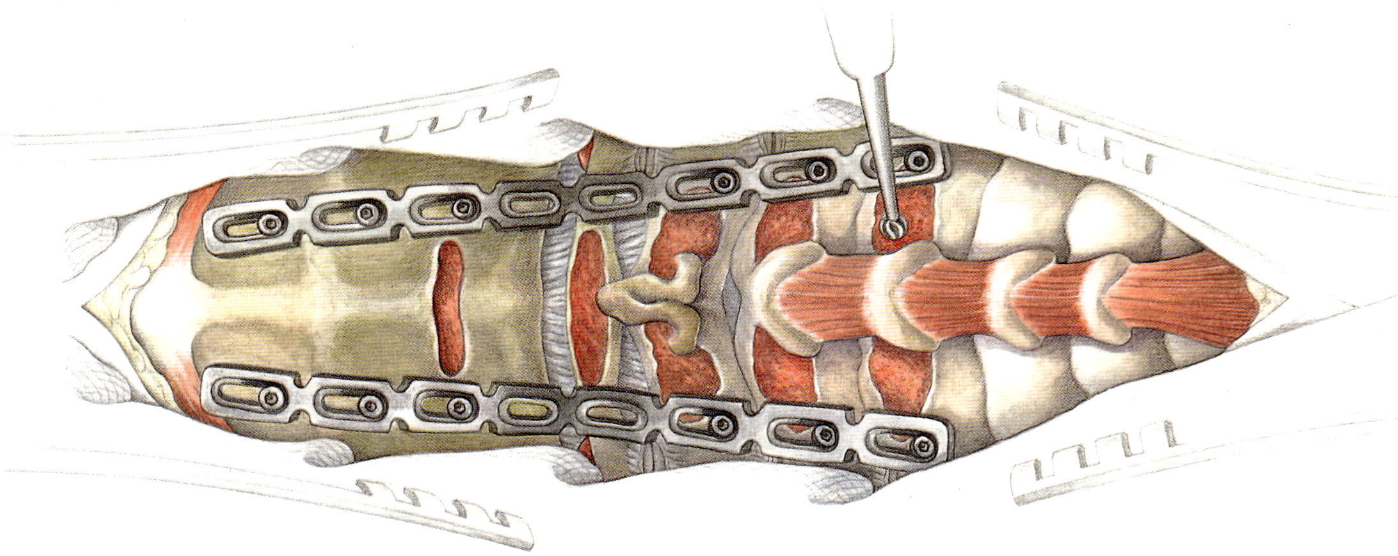

Fig. 9.**46** Fixation of the plates to the occiput with three screws each; decortication of the laminae.

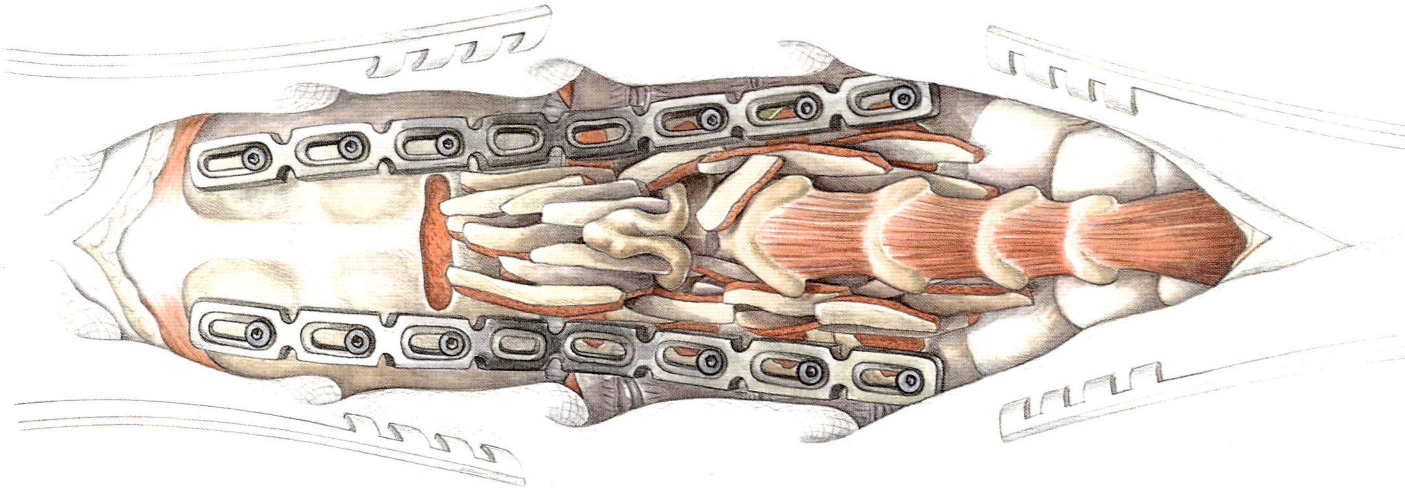

Fig. 9.**47** Cancellous chips are placed over the laminae.

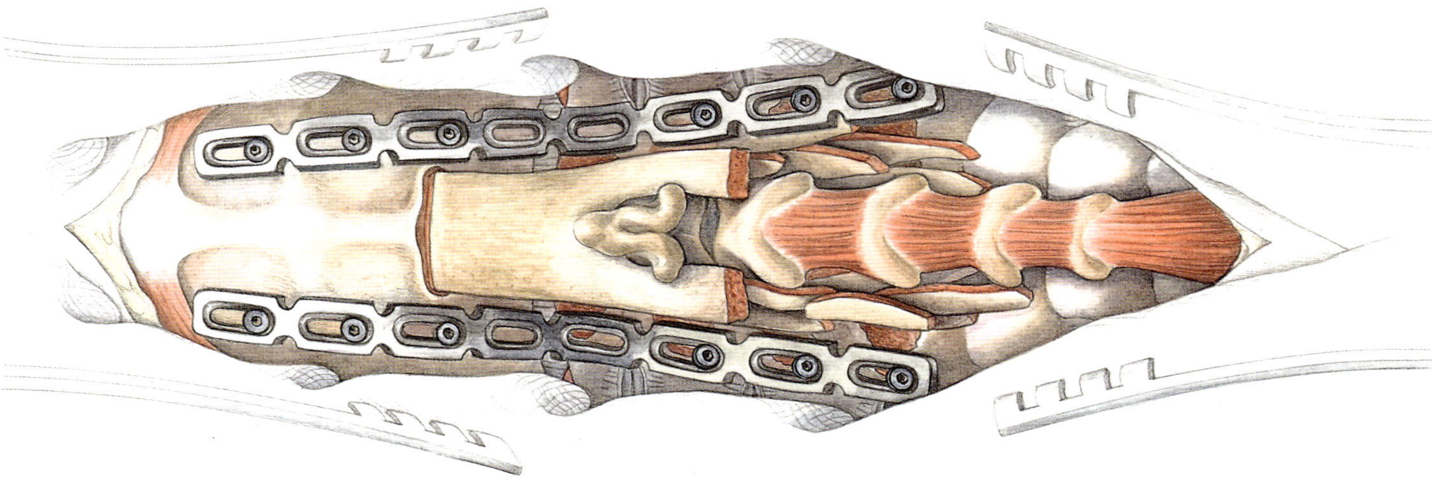

Fig. 9.**48** Application of a central corticocancellous graft.

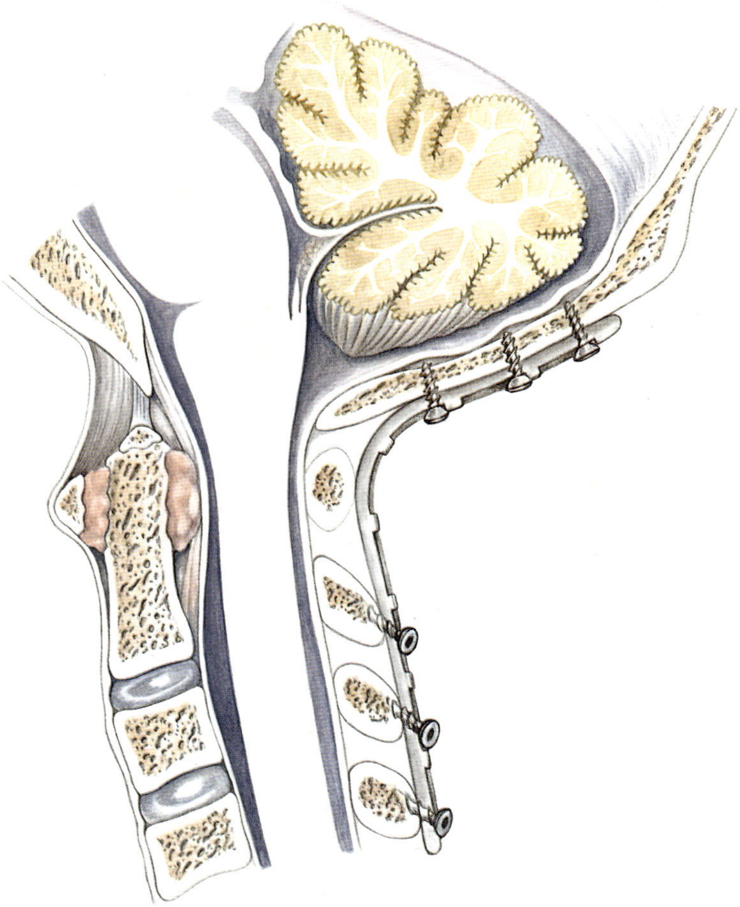

Fig. 9.**49** Status after plate fixation (sagittal plane).

Wound Closure

Following ample irrigation, the musculature is attached to the interspinal ligaments. In the second layer, the nuchal ligament is sutured to the spinous processes. Use of a Hemovac drain and perioperative antibiotic therapy are recommended.

Postoperative Treatment

Postoperatively, the traction device is removed under anesthesia, and a well-padded plaster collar is then applied. After removal of the sutures, the plaster collar can be replaced by plastic collars. Continued external support is recommended for a period of four months.

Pitfalls

Incorrect sublaminar dissection of the arch of the atlas entails a risk of injury to the dura or the cervical cord. Adequate reduction of the atlas should be verified using an image intensifier before the wires are tightened. In occipitocervical fusions, excessive tension on the wire and increased basilar impression must be avoided. In Magerl transarticular screw fixation, advancing the drill too far laterally could cause injury to the vertebral artery.

Anterior Transoral Operations

Marked secondary basilar impressions, as well as synovial proliferations in the area of the dens apex, occasionally lead to compression of the brain stem and the upper cervical cord. Only since MRI has come into routine use has it been possible to obtain clear images of these pathological processes. Posterior reduction and fusion may be inadequate in these cases, because sufficient decompression of the anterior spinal artery and of the cervical cord may not be accomplished. In such cases, anterior decompression in the first stage and posterior occipitocervical fusion in the second stage may be indicated. We agree with Harms that transoral resection alone, without any additional stabilization, is not effective, since the persistent instability is considered partly responsible for the development of cervical myelopathy. In rheumatoid arthritis, anterior fusion with the aid of a special plate is generally possible as well.

Approach

See Chapter 1, pp. 2–3.

Operative Technique

Expanded Approach and Technique of Transoral Operation (Harms and Schmelzle)

The operation starts with a midline incision of the soft palate and the mucosa of the hard palate (Fig. 9.**50**). Optionally, the hard palate can be resected using a U-shaped chisel cut. Resection appears indicated for extensive exposure of the clivus, particularly if a more extensive resection or osteosynthesis is planned in this bone segment. The posterior wall of the pharynx receives a window-

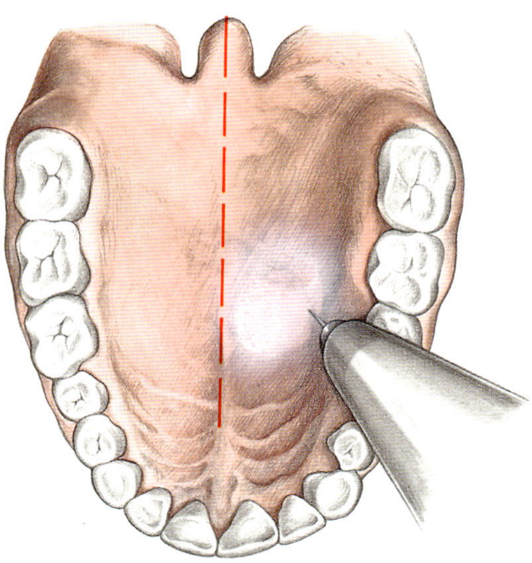

Fig. 9.**50** Median incision of the soft palate and of the mucosa of the hard palate following infiltration with epinephrine solution.

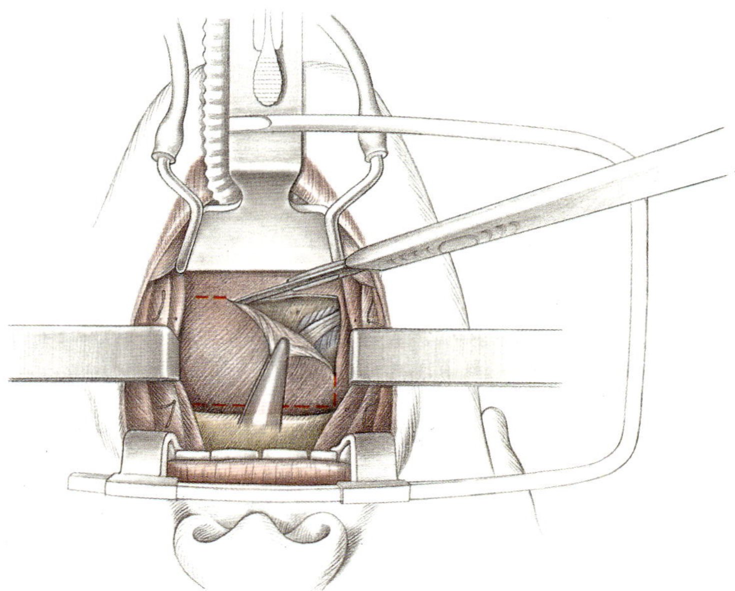

Fig. 9.**51** Incision of the posterior wall of the pharynx with the aid of a laterally-based flap.

shaped incision with a laterally-based flap (Fig. 9.**51**). This flap has to be carefully detached and dissected far enough to ensure a tension-free suture after the bone operation. The mucosal flaps are now temporarily fixed laterally with stay sutures. The longus colli muscle is divided in the middle; using an elevator, the soft tissues on the anterior side of C1 and C2 are retracted to the side. The clivus, the anterior arch of the atlas, the bodies of C2 and C3, as well as the lateral masses of C1 and C2 with the C0–C1 and C1–C2 joints are brought into view (Fig. 9.**52**).

The atlas can be exposed as much as 2 cm lateral to the midline. If dissection is carried too far laterally at the lower border of C2, there is a danger of injury to the vertebral artery. On the side of the lateral mass of the atlas, the elevator may penetrate the retromandibular fossa; this may lead to injuries of the cranial nerves IX and XII. Next, the anterior arch of the atlas and the pannus-like tissue behind the atlantal arch are removed, and the remainder of the dens apex is resected (Figs. 9.**53**, 9.**54**). Thickened scar tissue behind the dens apex is also resected to achieve decompression of the spinal cord. The joint surfaces in the area of the lateral mass of C1 and C2 are sparingly and carefully resected. Optionally, a special Harms plate connecting the lateral mass of C1 with the body of C2 can be inserted for added anterior security (Fig. 9.**55**). However, we prefer posterior fusion in the same or a second session.

Wound Closure

The wound is closed with nonabsorbable sutures. A two-layered closure of the soft palate is recommended (Figs. 9.**56**, 9.**57**).

Postoperative Treatment

Anterior resection of the dens is generally combined with a posterior stabilizing operation. Postoperatively, a collar of plastic material is applied which should be worn for four months. Additionally recommended are the following measures: antibiotic therapy for 12 days after the operation, disinfection of the oral mucosa twice a day, parenteral alimentation until the second postoperative day, liquid diet until the fourth day, a soft diet starting on postoperative day 6, and a normal diet after the third postoperative week.

Complications

Harms has reported a rate of infection of less than 1%. Nasopharyngeal fistulas were reported initially after partial resection of the hard palate. No such fistulas have been observed in the last two years.

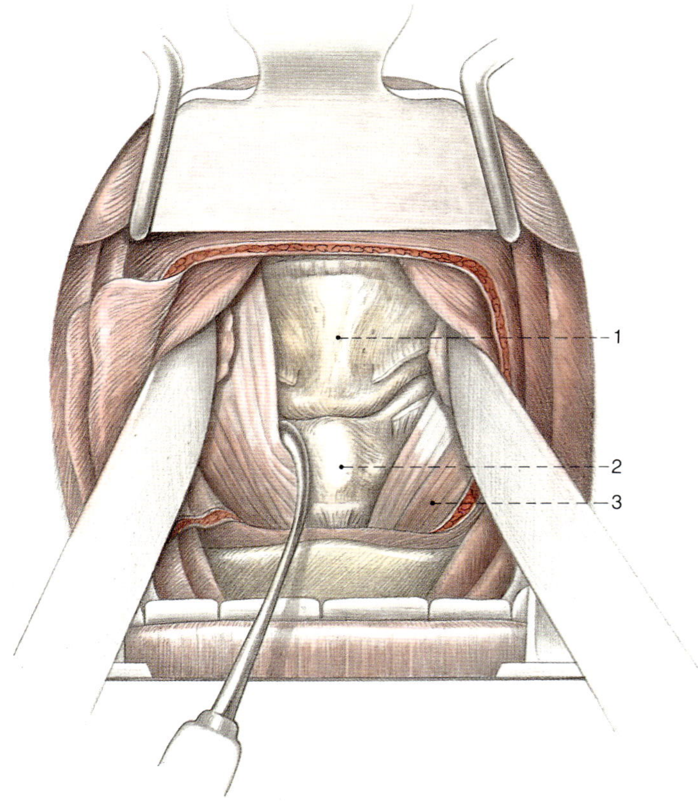

Fig. 9.**52** Exposure of the anterior atlantal arch, the body of the axis, and vertebral joints C1 and C2 by retraction of the soft tissues.

1 Body axis
2 Anterior tubercle of atlas
3 Longus capitis muscle

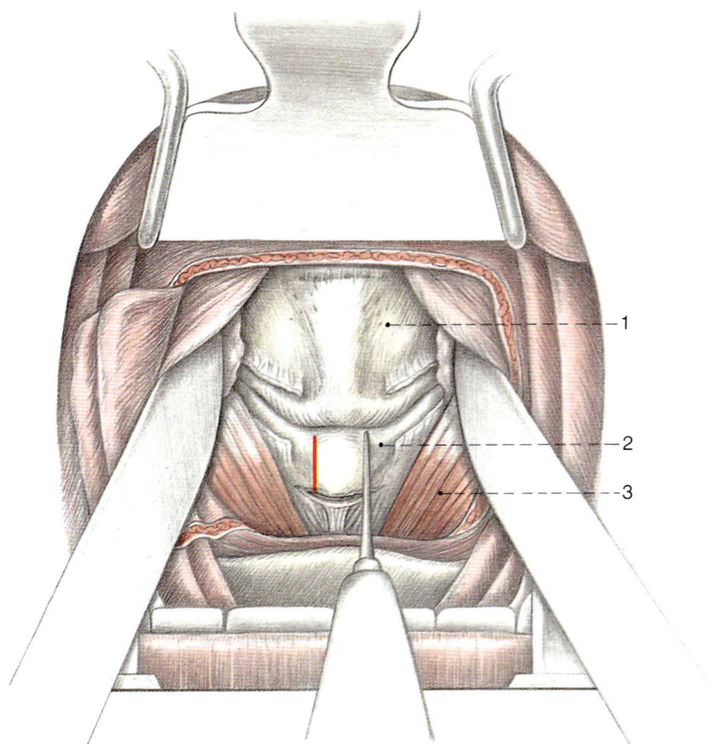

Fig. 9.**53** Resection of the anterior atlantal arch with a small oscillating saw.

1 Body axis
2 Anterior tubercle of atlas
3 Longus capitis muscle

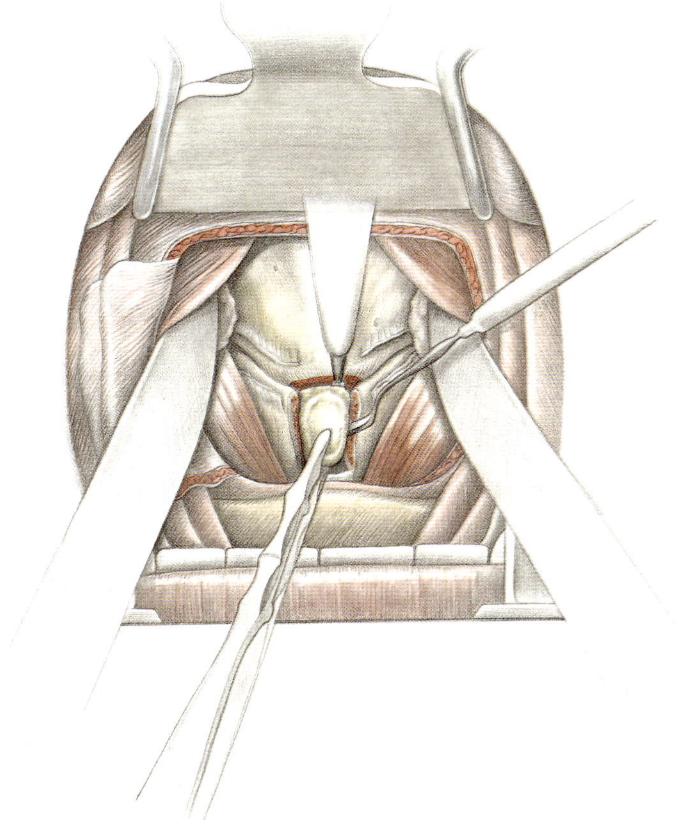

Fig. 9.**54** Resection of the remnants of the axial dens and of rheumatoid pannus tissue after careful detachment with an elevator. A small diamond-tipped drill is used for resection of the tip of the dens.

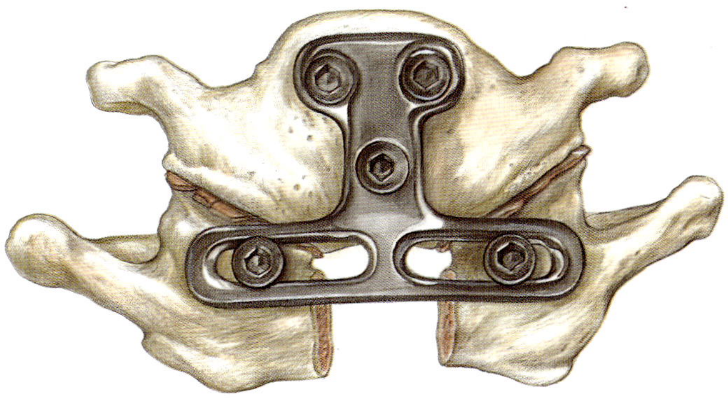

Fig. 9.**55** Optional anterior stabilization of C1 and C2 using a special Harms plate, and blocking of the C1–C2 articulations.

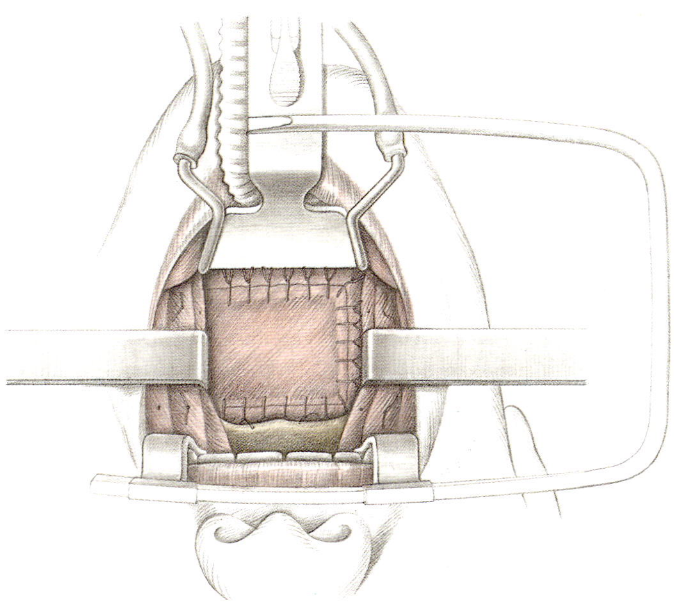

Fig. 9.**56** Closure of the posterior wall of the pharynx.

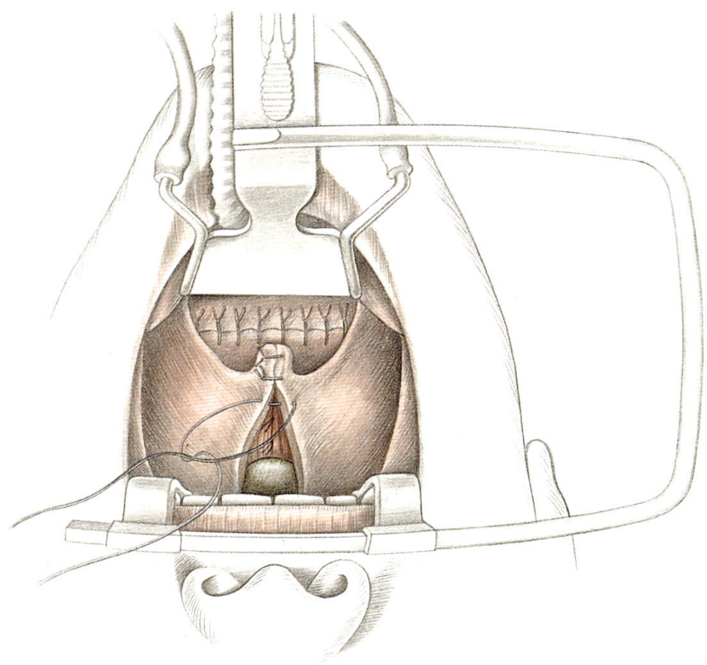

Fig. 9.**57** Two-layered closure of the soft palate.

Further Reading

Brattström H. Surgery in atlanto-axial dislocation in rheumatoid arthritis. Reconstr Surg Traumatol 1981;18:16–29.

Gschwend N, Scherer M, Munzinger V. Entzündliche Veränderungen der Wirbelsäule bei der chronischen Polyarthritis. Orthopäde 1981;10:155–68.

Johnson RM, Southwick WO. Surgical approaches to the spine. In: Rothman RH, Simeone FA, eds. The spine. Philadelphia: Saunders, 1982.

Magerl F, Seemann P. Stable posterior fusion of the atlas and axis by transarticular screw fixation. In: Kehr P, Weidner A, eds. Cervical Spine 1. Berlin: Springer, 1986.

Schmelzle R, Harms J. Indications and limits of the transoral entry by treatment of fractures, luxation and tumors of the vertebral column. Report on 7th Congress of the European Association for Maxillofacial Surgery, 1984.

10 Spondylitis

A. Härle

Active spondylitis is characterized by destruction of the intervertebral disk and adjoining parts of the vertebral body. Except in children, in whom a primary, isolated inflammation of the intervertebral disk may be observed, spondylitis begins in the vertebral body segments adjacent to the intervertebral disk and only secondarily spreads into the intervertebral disk (Fig. 10.**1**). The further course consists of bone destruction spreading to the two adjacent vertebral bodies, which may then lead to complete dissolution of the vertebral bodies; in about 10% of the cases, several motion segments are affected at the same time. The vertebral arches usually are not affected in hematogenous spondylitis and are even preserved when there is marked vertebral body destruction so that partial recovery will always result in a kyphotic deformity of the spine (Fig. 10.**2**). In the vertebral body itself, anterior destruction is slightly more pronounced than posterior destruction. In spondylitis, there is always a risk of posterior displacement of the destroyed intervertebral disk and bony tissue, leading to encroachment on the dural sac, but this is more commonly seen in spinal tuberculosis.

In one particular disease, sclerosing spondylitis, the inflammatory process in confined to the vertebral body, and the heights of the vertebral body and the intervertebral disk are not reduced.

Indications for Surgery

Generally, conservative and surgical treatment methods compete in cases of spondylitis. In the early phase and in children, systemic antibiotic therapy and immobilization in an extensive molded plaster cast can often control spondylitis, as monitored by laboratory parameters. In adults, and especially in the presence of osseous destruction, the chances of healing by mere drug therapy are slim, and protracted immobilization is required, though the prospects of success are uncertain.

Considering the pathogenetic and anatomical conditions, the surgical options are largely restricted to anterior operative procedures.

Approaches

According to the anatomical localization of the spondylitis, the following operative approaches can be recommended:

C1–C2 transoropharyngeal approach (p. 2)
C2–T2 anterior cervical approach (p. 4)
T2–T11 transthoracic approach (p. 13)
T11–L4 lateral thoracolumbar approaches (p. 24)
L3 –S1 pararectal approach (p. 46)

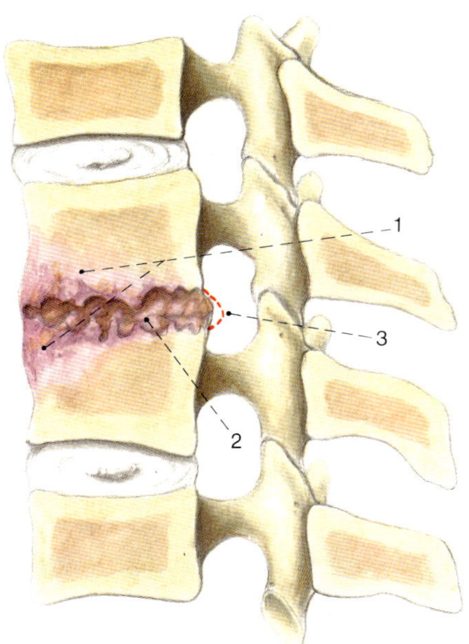

Fig. 10.**1** In acute spondylitis, the inflammation usually spreads secondarily to the intervertebral disk; spinal cord compression (dashed line) is not a rare entity in tuberculosis.

1 Inflamed parts of vertebral body
2 Intervertebral disk destroyed by infection
3 Threatened posterior protrusion of intervertebral disk tissue

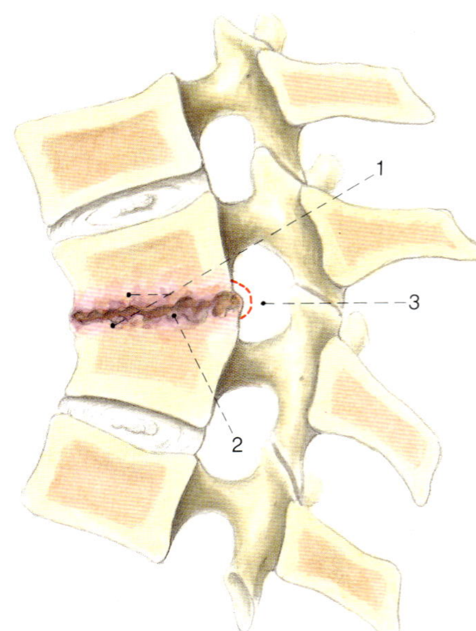

Fig. 10.**2** Kyphotic buckling due to spondylitis.

1 Anterior loss of vertebral height
2 Lowered disk space
3 Posterior displacement of intervertebral disk tissue

Transthoracic Approach

The operation is preferably performed with the table flexed and with use of a bolster, with the patient in the left lateral decubitus position and a double-lumen endotracheal tube permitting temporary isolated mechanical ventilation of the left lung (Fig. 1.**22**). To obtain a better overview, it is advisable to carry out the thoracotomy by rib resection:

T2–T4	Resection of the fourth rib
T5–T7	Resection of the fifth rib
T6–T8	Resection of the sixth rib
T8–T11	Resection of the eighth rib

If the spondylitis is located above T5, resection of the fourth rib requires partial separation of the scapula from the serratus anterior muscle and the greater rhomboid muscle (Fig. 10.**3**). However, in order to spare the lateral thoracic vessels and the long thoracic nerve, the anterior elevation of the serratus anterior muscle should be done approximately 5 cm more distally and in a caudoanterior direction.

In acute spondylitis, pleural effusion as well as an adhesion of the visceral pleura to the inflamed segment of the spinal column may be found (Fig. 10.**4**). These have to be separated with caution. After this, the visceral pleura in the inflammatory region on the right border of the vertebral body is carefully transected parallel to the axis of the body, so that the segmental vessels supplying the affected vertebrae can be identified.

Lateral Thoracolumbar Approaches

For extrapleural thoracolumbar approaches, a right lateral decubitus position, with the left side flexed convexly by angulating the table and bolstering, is recommended (Fig. 1.**60**). The following approaches may be considered:

T11–L2	Approach according to Mirbaha (p. 37)
L2 –L4	Retroperitoneal lumbar approach (p. 42).

Lumbosacral Localization

Exposure of the lumbosacral junction from a lateral approach is difficult. Due to the perivascular soft-tissue infiltration associated with spondylitis, there is a risk of injury to the large-volume iliac vessels. The anteriorly protruding iliac crest also impairs the approach and inspection. Transabdominal exposure, which has also been suggested for this unfavorable localization of spondylitis, theoretically provides a good view of the promontory; however, due to the inflammatory swelling or induration encountered in spondylitis, it is hardly possible to mobilize the vessels located anterior to the spine. Clear exposure of the vertebrae is therefore difficult. Finally, inflammatory material may be entrained into the abdominal cavity, and addi-

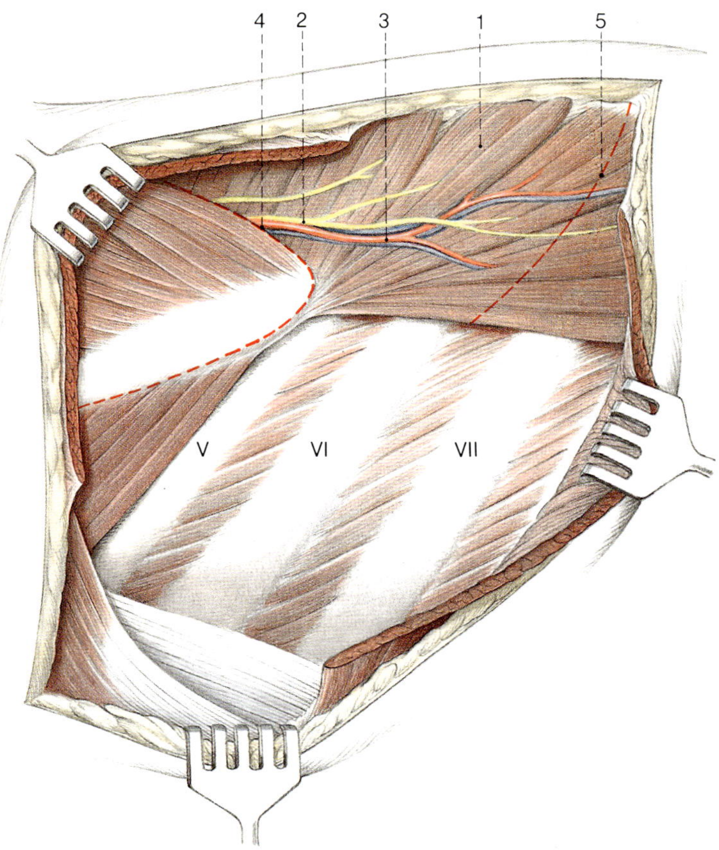

Fig. 10.**3** Anatomical exposure of operative site after division of the latissimus dorsi muscle and prior to incision of the serratus anterior muscle. The appropriate incision site is marked by a broken line.

1 Serratus anterior muscle
2 Long thoracic nerve
3 Lateral thoracic vessels
4 Detachment of scapula
5 Division of anterior serratus muscle
V–VII Ribs

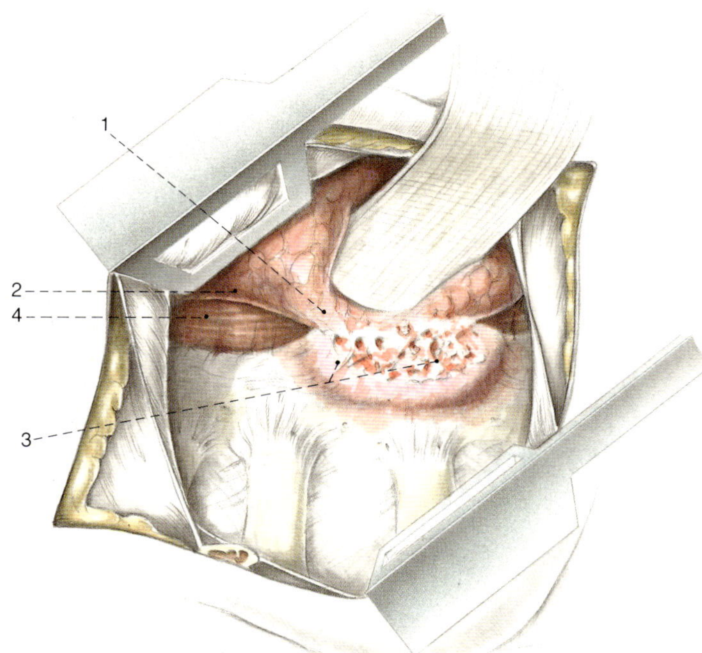

Fig. 10.**4** Adhesion of pleura to the inflamed spinal segment.

1 Adhesion of visceral pleura to inflammatory tumor
2 Visceral pleura
3 Inflamed spinal segment
4 Esophagus

tionally, intestinal dysfunction can easily result in decompensation in this occasionally severe disease.

We therefore basically select the *pararectal approach* when the spondylitis is localized below L 4.

Operative Procedure

Before debriding the zone of inflammatory and necrotic destruction, the segmental vessels of the affected vertebrae have to be isolated and ligated on the side of the approach. Becauses of the inflammatory edema usually present, and the increased susceptibility to injury, a twofold suture ligature proves to be advantageous; when carrying out the ligation, the position relative to the aorta must be taken into consideration (Fig. 10.**5**). In the presence of severe inflammation, the undermining and ligation not infrequently lead to ruptures, so that a primary suture ligature should be considered.

Identification of the pathogen and adequate resistance determination should always be attempted, so that specific systemic antibiotic therapy can be initiated after the operation. Collecting a smear merely on a cotton swab and then transporting it in a dry glass tube is not an appropriate practice, and often yields false-negative findings. Optimal microbiological results are obtained when several tissue samples are sent out for microbiological diagnosis in transport vessels containing a culture medium.

Surgical treatment has three goals:

- Prevention or correction of cord compression
- Control of the infection
- Stabilization of the damaged spinal segment

Whereas the first requirement is a painstaking debridement of necrotic and possibly posteriorly displaced intervertebral disk material and bony tissue, which should be the basic component of any operative procedure in this field, the two other goals may be reached by various methods.

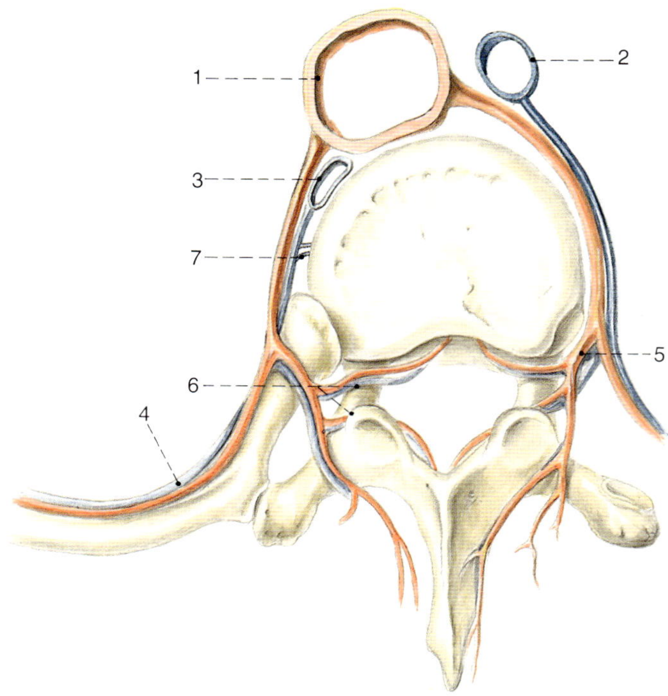

Fig. 10.**5** Topographic relation of vessels to thoracic vertebra.

1 Thoracic aorta
2 Azygos vein
3 Hemiazygos vein
4 Posterior intercostal vessels
5 Posterior branch
6 Spinal branches
7 Lateral vertebral veins

Abscess Drainage

Abscess drainage alone should be performed only in exceptional cases, as when the primary focus cannot be found or cannot be exposed. In tuberculous spondylitis, gravitation abscesses can become quite large and extend far caudally (Fig. 10.**6**). Drainage and digital debridement of the area of the abscess should be followed by careful curettage of the abscess membrane with a sharp curet. Resection of the abscess membrane is indicated and necessary only in callused areas; to avoid inadvertent damage to adjacent organs and structures, it can usually be omitted.

After repeated, intensive irrigation, a large-caliber Hemovac drain (16 Fr) or antiseptic irrigation–suction drainage can now be inserted. The exit drains should be placed in such a way that they allow drainage of the lowest areas of the abscess cavity in the supine patient, while the inlets should be placed as high as possible so as to use gravity to aid the circulation of the irrigation fluid (Fig. 10.**7**). Aspiration should be effected not with conventional Hemovac vacuum bottles, but either by the gravity principle or by the low-vacuum technique, so that a closure mechanism comparable to the lip valve can be avoided. In terms of technical execution and hygiene, irrigation–suction drainage remains problematic even when all rules of this procedure are observed and electronically controlled suction apparatus is used.

The insertion of Septopal chains (Merck, Darmstadt) is an alternative; in this case, of course, the same problems as those arising with antiseptic irrigation, also need to be taken into account, namely, appropriate positioning and the location of residual inflammatory tissue areas. Their removal, too, has to be borne in mind at the time of chain implantation. When we weighed the pros and cons of the two techniques, we decided in favor of using Septopal, since this permits better follow-up control and is less likely to be troublesome.

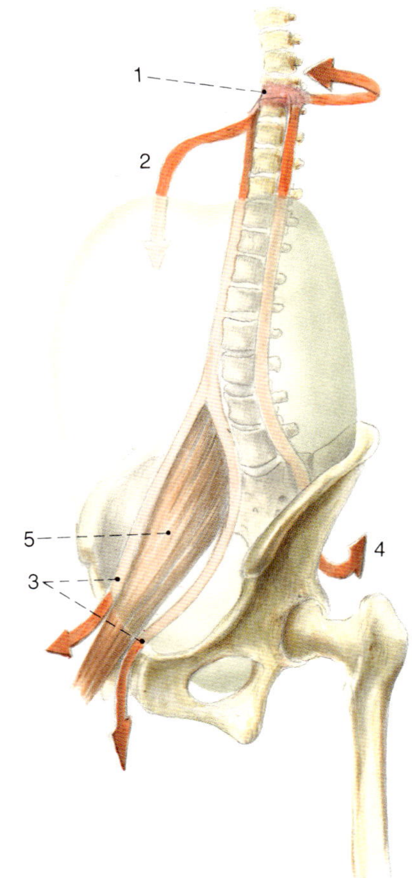

Fig. 10.**6** Spread of gravitation abscesses.

1 Primary focus of spondylitis
2 Retroperitoneal, posteriorly perforating spread of abscess
3 Retroperitoneal inguinal spread of abscess
4 Abscess perforation in the gluteal region
5 Greater psoas muscle

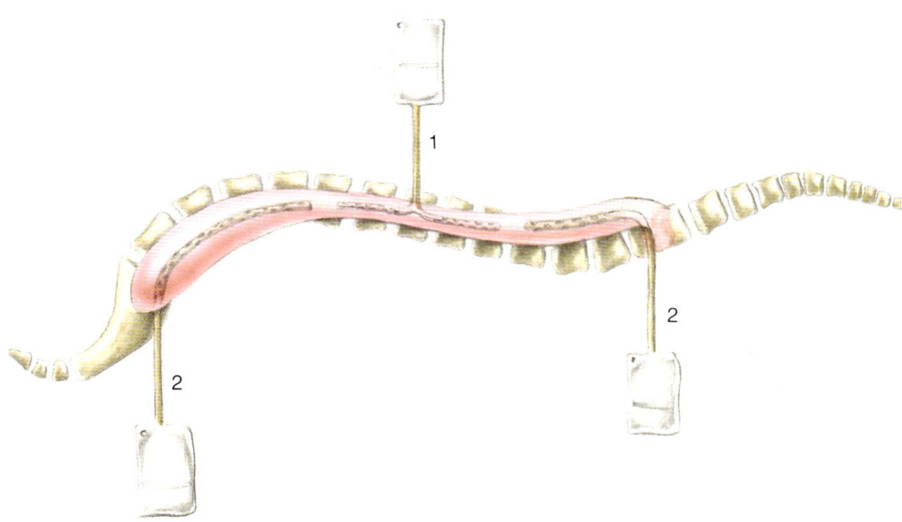

Fig. 10.**7** Placement of irrigation drains.

1 Inlet
2 Outlets

In an area of pronounced local inflammation, Septopal chains are inserted in a meandering line following careful debridement (Fig. 10.**8**). Depending on the susceptibility to injury of the surrounding structures, they are brought out percutaneously and then, after 6 days, either withdrawn or implanted more deeply; in the latter case, they have to be removed by a second procedure.

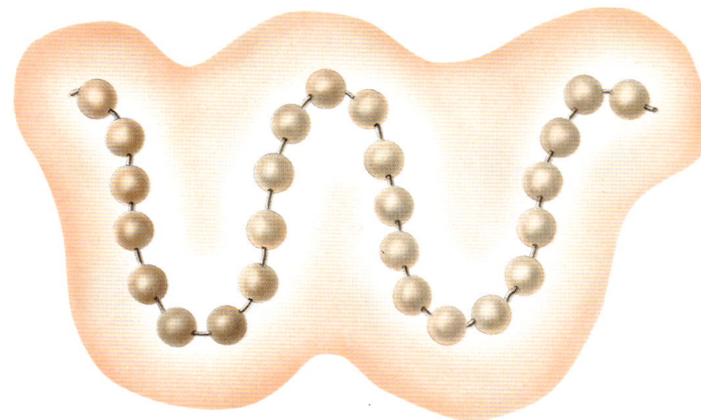

Fig. 10.**8** Meandering course of Septopal chains, designed to increase the area of exposure and to prevent entanglement of the chains.

Treatment of Presacral Abscesses

If there is extensive presacral abscess formation which cannot be approached adequately from the cranial side, a pararectal approach may be combined with a posterior one. In this case, a better view of the presacral cavity is obtained by resecting the coccygeal bone and the caudal portion of the sacrum as far as the third intervertebral foramen (Fig. 10.**9**).

Depending on individual factors, the exposure starts either posteriorly or anteriorly by the pararectal approach; other than in exceptional cases, the exposure is usually begun anteriorly, because the primary focus is found at a higher level in most cases. If it then turns out that adequate debridement cannot be accomplished from there, the anterior incision is dealt with and closed. After shifting the patient to a modified Hastings position (the buttocks being raised higher), the sacrum may, if necessary, be resected to the level of the third intervertebral foramen without any noticeable neural functional deficit. The nerves emerging in this segment are preserved, of course. Now the presacral space can be inspected, and the abscess located in the sacral curvature can be aspirated and curetted up to the caudal boundary of the promontory. The abscess formation generally causes considerable anterior displacement of the rectum, so that there is no risk of intestinal injury at the level of the sacral curvature if the procedure is performed prudently. We then place Septopal chains in the presacral cavity (Fig. 10.**10**). Because of their proximity to the intestine they are not withdrawn percutaneously, but have to be removed in a second operation after about three weeks.

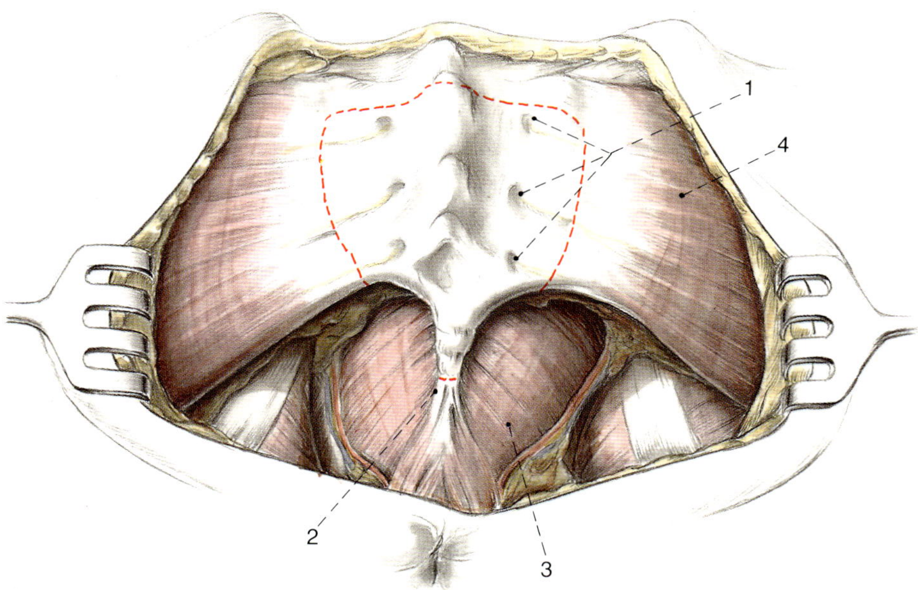

Fig. 10.**9** Caudal resection of sacrum (resection line dashed).

1 Posterior sacral foramina III–V
2 Anococcygeal ligament
3 Levator ani muscle
4 Greatest gluteal muscle

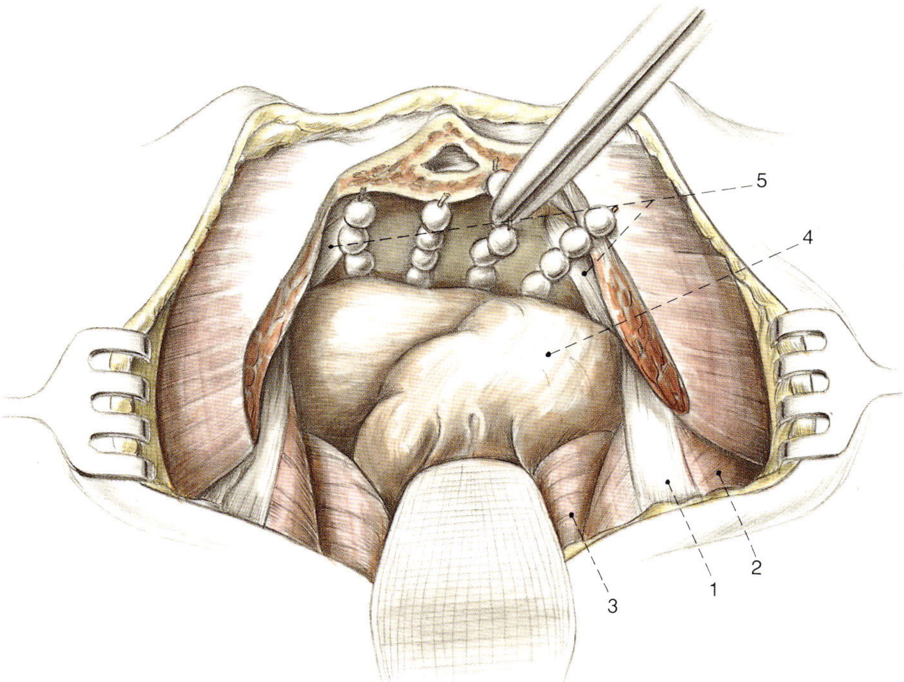

Fig. 10.**10** Treatment of presacral abscesses by posterior implantation of Septopal chains into the sacral curvature.

1 Sacrotuberal ligament
2 Internal obturator muscle
3 Levator ani muscle
4 Rectum
5 Branches of the sacral plexus

Debridement of Intervertebral Disks

Once the affected vertebrae have been exposed and the segmental vessels ligated, the inflammatory tumor is incised from lateral, and the central abscess is aspirated (Fig. 10.**11**). If the inflamed segment cannot be identified, lateral transillumination usually helps. A wider cannula inserted into an intervertebral disk space and used for localization. The inflammatory soft-tissue swelling around the vertebral body can be carefully removed with a sharp curet or a rongeur, to obtain a better overview of the bony destruction. The destroyed part of the intervertebral disk is then removed precisely under direct vision with a rongeur and a sharp curet to make contact with vital, i.e., bleeding, and structurally resistent cancellous bone (Fig. 10.**12**). Using a vertebral spreader is not recommended, since the likelihood that the cancellous bone, weakened by inflammation, will fracture is greater than the chance of achieving distraction of the intervertebral disk space. However, the visibility and evaluation of the quality of the debridement is significantly improved by using an angulated cold light rod from the Ossoscope set (Effner, Berlin), which makes visual control of the procedure possible (Fig. 10.**13**). In tuberculous spondylitis in particular, painstaking palpation and inspection, if necessary using an image intensifier, is required to make certain that posteriorly displaced intervertebral disk tissue has been completely removed. If there is appreciable bleeding from the destroyed vertebrae, a temporary tamponade with hemostatic materials is advisable; bone wax ought not to be introduced into the infected vertebra.

There are several options for subsequent procedures.

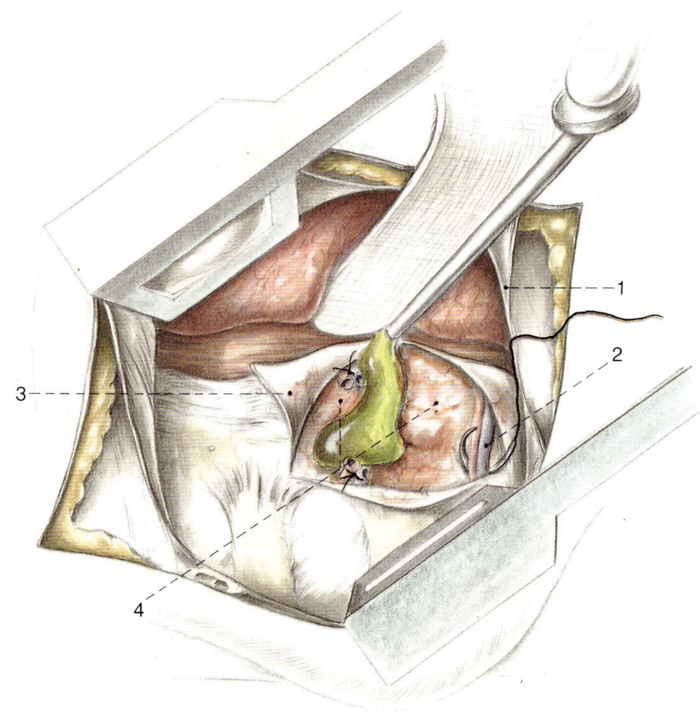

Fig. 10.**11** Opening of inflammatory tumor.

1 Costal pleura
2 Intercostal vessels, suture-ligated
3 T-shaped incision of mediastinal pleura
4 Inflamed vertebrae

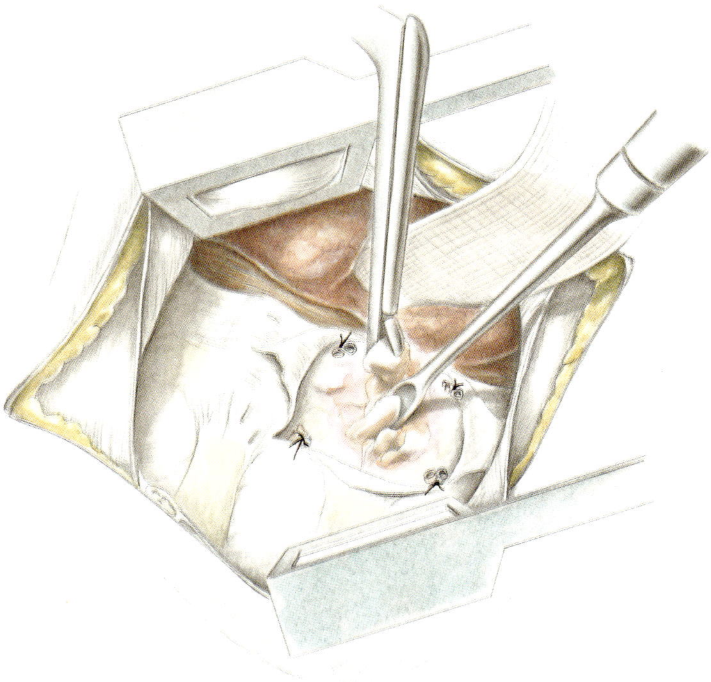

Fig. 10.**12** Curettage of abscess with sharp curet and rongeur.

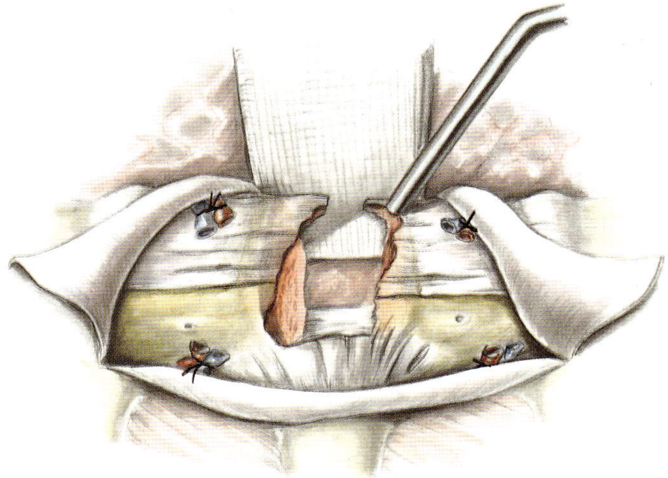

Fig. 10.**13** Illumination of the area of inflammation with the aid of an Ossoscope rod angulated cold light.

Bridging by Graft

Careful disk debridement, even when it is done sparingly, leaves a considerable bony substance defect which often results in healing with a residual kyphotic deformity if it is not filled. In the absence of a primary anterior support, fibular segments, tibial chips, fragments of resected ribs, or sufficiently thick bicortical iliac crest grafts can be considered for use as adequate anterior stabilizers. In selecting an appropriate graft, we are guided by the size of the defect, using iliac crest grafts or rib fragments for smaller defects and, as a rule, fibular segments for larger ones; the latter have good primary stability, and are more rapidly incorporated than cortical tibial chips. To anchor the fibular segments, they are sawed off to the desired length and implanted into grooves in the two adjacent vertebral bodies, so that they are firmly seated and solidly wedged in, and cannot become dislodged when the body is straightened (Fig. 10.**14**). For this reason, lateral insertion with preferably anterior and posterior support for the contact zones should be attempted. The final step is placement of a deep drainage tube of 10–12 Fr that reaches into the area of dissection. Graft bridging and irrigation–suction drainage may be combined, but we have done so only in a few selected cases, and then usually in tuberculous conditions, or because of persistent infection at the time of revision.

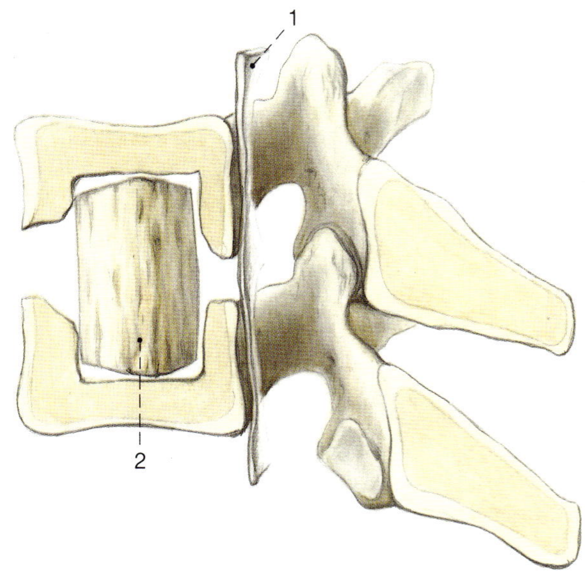

Fig. 10.**14** Strut with a fibular segment that is sunk into grooves in the adjacent vertebrae.

1 Posterior longitudinal ligament
2 Fibula segment

Septopal Implantation

The use of gentamicin-releasing Septopal chains in the debrided intervertebral disk space permits a more sparing resection of the bone, since a highly bactericidal drug level for most of the organisms found in spondylitis is provided in a spherical zone, about 1 cm in size, around the particles, allowing inflamed but viable bone tissue to be partially preserved (Fig. 10.**15**). The implantation of Septopal also serves as a spacer for smaller and medium-sized bony defects, and may make stabilization by graft dispensable. The hematoma between the beads is rapidly transformed into cencellous bone via reactive granulation tissue, and so provides a partial load-bearing capacity to the axial organ within two months.

When implanting Septopal, it is necessary, however, to check intraoperatively that the beads are not, or cannot be, displaced posteriorly in the direction of the spinal cord. In the presence of a sizable posterior osteolysis, the posterior longitudinal ligament should by all means be preserved as a barrier, and the chains of beads should be inserted somewhat anteriorly in a bunch, the free ends of the chains always being brought to the lateral exposure site. If there is a substantial posterior loss of bone, so that the beads might be displaced in the direction of the cord, the passageway can be bolted by inserting a bony plate, from a rib, for example (Fig. 10.**16**).

Although the Septopal chains in soft tissues and long bones are generally removed once the bacterial tissue infection has been brought under control, in spondylodiskitis we leave them in place after anterior debridement, since their removal may create problems and would, above all, lead to renewed destabilization of the spine. Also, the spacer function, and therefore the early load-bearing capacity, would be forfeited again. In five years of use, we have observed no adverse effects from Septopal beads osseously incorporated into vertebrae.

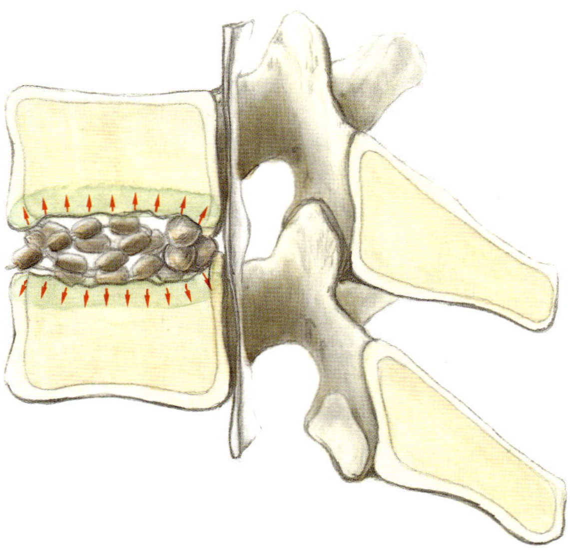

Fig. 10.**15** Insertion of gentamicin–PMMA beads into the debrided disk space. A bactericidal antibiotic concentration is built up in a space about 1 cm wide around the beads.

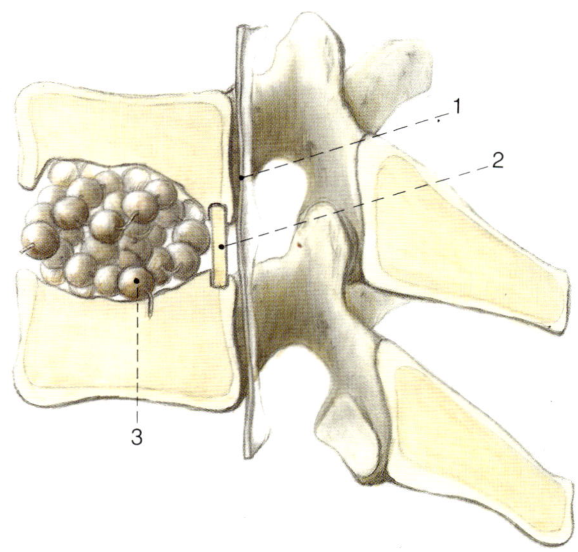

Fig. 10.**16** Sizable bony defects are filled with large gentamicin–PMMA beads, and the posterior gap is closed with a bone chip that is sunk into grooves.

1 Posterior longitudinal ligament
2 Bone chip for protection of the spinal cord
3 Laterally placed chain end

Combination of Graft Bridging and Mini-Septopal Implantation

We only implant minichains of Septopal for small bony defects in the areas of the cervical and lumbar spine, but ribs grafts with Septopal minichains inserted in between are used as additional graft material for medium-sized defects in the thoracic region.

For larger bony defects, we combine bridging by fibular chips with the implantation of Septopal minichains in order to create optimal conditions for lasting eradication of the infection. The minichains are placed between and around the fibular strut grafts, but not in the superior and inferior contact zones between the graft and the vertebra (Fig. 10.**17**). No chains should be placed posteriorly, in order to avoid irritating the spinal cord. Here again, the final step is the insertion of a deep drainage tube, which will act for 24 hours as an overflow drain so that there will be no unnecessary removal of wound secretions with a high gentamicin level; the system can be switched to suction drainage on the second day, when the wound secretion has almost completely subsided.

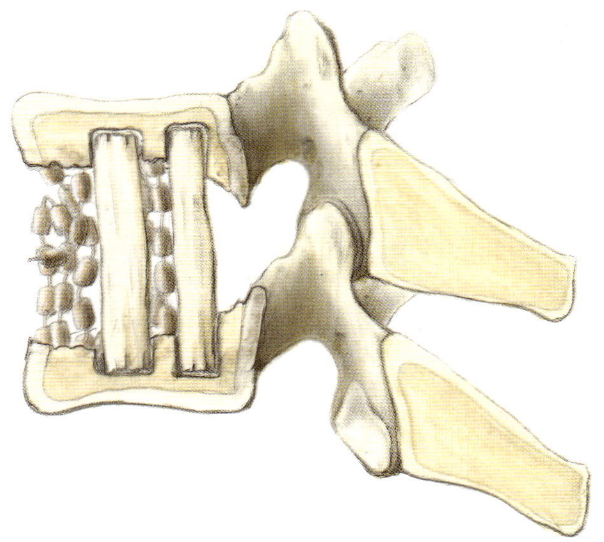

Fig. 10.**17** Combination of graft bridging and mini-Septopal implantation.

Drilling the Vertebral Body

In sclerosing spondylitis, which is rarely encountered, the inflammatory process confined to the vertebral body cannot be controlled by operations in the area of the intervertebral disk or by spondylodesis. As in other sclerosing bone infections, removal of the inflammatory focus is required; if the sclerosis involves the entire vertebra, a vertebrectomy may be required. By means of Septopal implantation, however, the vertebral debridement could be reduced, meeting the requirements for eradication of the infection in this way, and at the same time ensuring the preservation of a vertebra with sufficient, i.e., weight-bearing stability.

A window is drilled or chiseled into the sclerosed vertebral body from anterolateral (Fig. 10.**18**); this is followed by continuous drilling with ball-tip reamers until contact is made with soft cancellous bone, or until the remaining marginal vertebra shell has a thickness of less than 10 mm (Fig. 10.**19**). The hollow space is then packed as tightly as possible with Septopal minichains which, in addition to their antibacterial effect, also perform a mechanical load-bearing function (Fig. 10.**20**). Full load-bearing capacity is usually restored after about two months due to metaplastic transformation of the hematoma located between the beads.

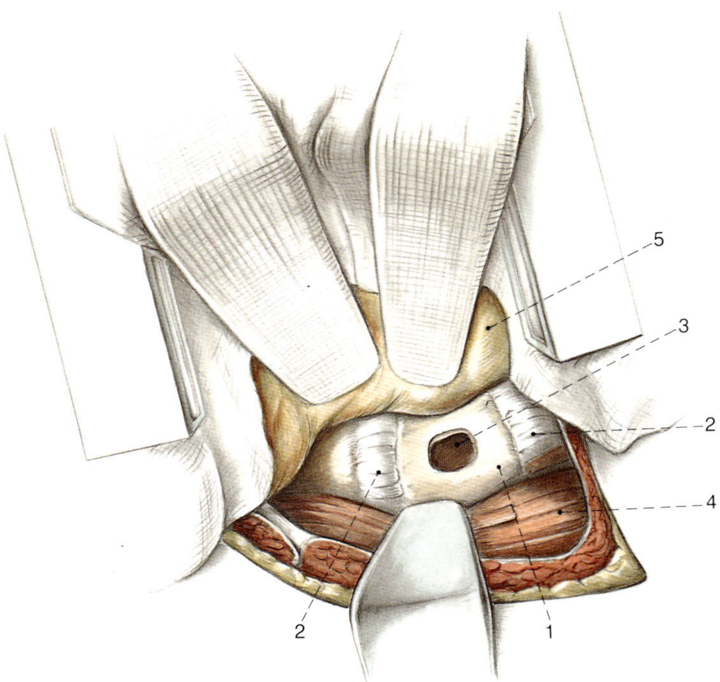

Fig. 10.**18** Anterolateral vertebral body fenestration in the lumbar spine region.

1 Sclerosed vertebra
2 Adjoining intervertebral disk
3 Window in sclerosed vertebra
4 Parietal peritoneum

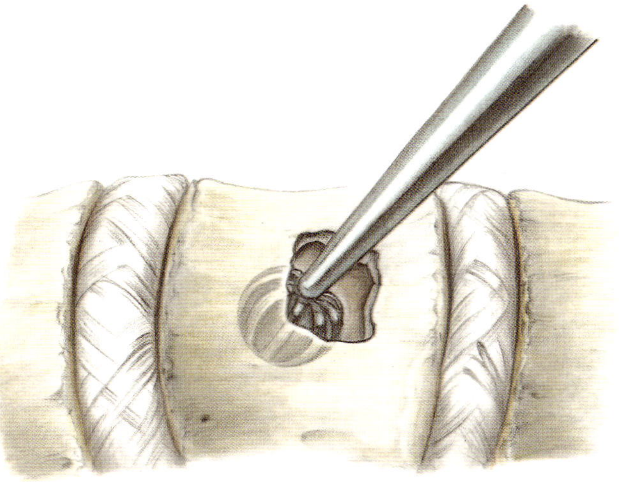

Fig. 10.**19** Central drilling of a sclerosed vertebral body.

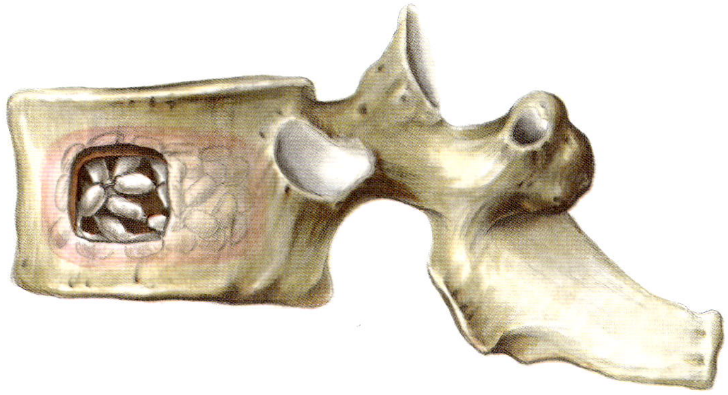

Fig. 10.**20** Packing of the opened vertebral body with Septopal minichains. Marked in red: area reached by diffusion.

Posterior Stabilization

If the stability resulting from the anterior procedures is not sufficient, or if there has been graft fracture or graft resorption, the instability can be restored by posterior instrumentation. If the objective is only to provide additional stability until sufficient bony incorporation develops anteriorly over a period of months, a posterior spondylodesis is not indicated. This can be achieved by posterior stabilization. For small pedicles (transverse diameter of less than 5 mm), we use the clamps or screws of the Cotrel–Dubousset system, placing them above and below the previous area of inflammation. This technique is described in detail in Chapter 2, Scoliosis (pp. 131–146) and Chapter 3, Kyphosis (pp. 220–221). For pedicles of normal transverse diameters and below T7, we carry out posterior stabilization with the aid of VOT plates (Varotec, Hamburg) which, because of the long hole and the lateral recesses, permit a transpedicular fixation that can easily be adapted to the existing anatomy (Fig. 10.**21**). If the residual height of the anteriorly debrided vertebral bodies, is sufficient, the posterior instrumentation can be restricted to the motion segment affected.

In patients with more extensive bone destruction, and if two adjacent motion segments are affected and anterior debridement has produced a sizable substance defect that is bridged by a long graft, we invariably perform posterior stabilization in a second intervention. The transpedicular fixation is then restricted to the cranial and caudal vertebrae of the spondylodesis zone.

If the previously implanted Septopal chains appear to be displaced posteriorly, this approach allows them to be removed in the posterior spondylodesis session and replaced by bone chips.

For biomechanical reasons, these posterior displacements are only possible—assuming the operation has been carefully planned and carried out—at the thoracolumbar junction, or in case of a premature loading, when, for example,

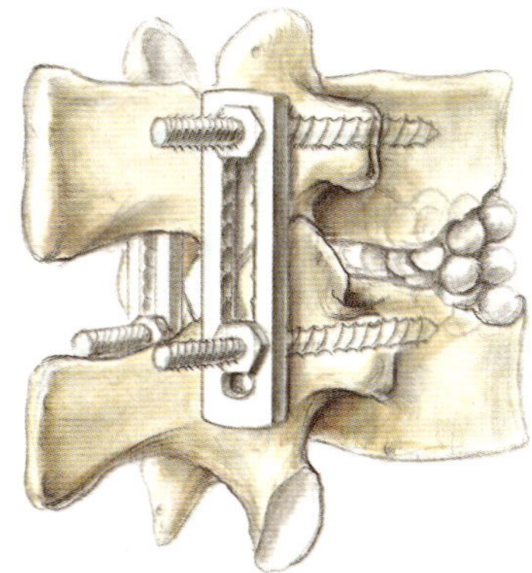

Fig. 10.**21** Posterior stabilization after anterior debridement of vertebral body and implantation of a Septopal chain with a VOT plate and transpedicular fixation. If at all possible, the screws should not touch the chains.

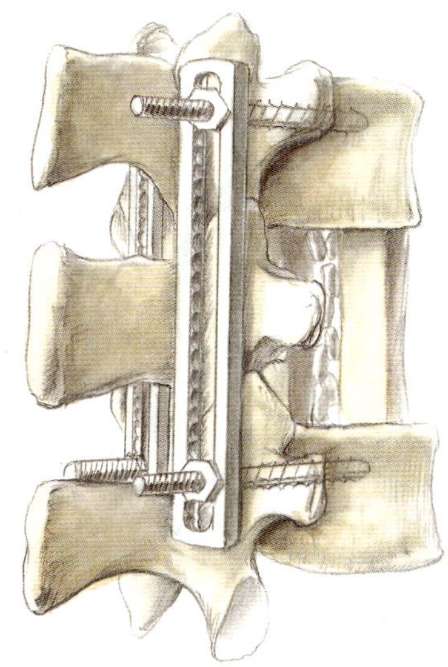

Fig. 10.**22** Posterior stabilization for sizable anterior substance defects and graft bridging. The transpedicular screw fixation is confined to the end vertebrae; dislocation of the chips should be prevented by appropriate placement of the screws.

a patient stresses the spinal column by getting up or sitting in the postoperative phase.

If the initial side of approach is raised into an oblique Relton frame position, a combined posterolateral and posterior operation can be performed, so that chain removal, anterior graft blockage, and posterior stabilization can be accomplished in one and the same stage (Fig. 10.**22**).

Treatment of Postoperative Infection

Postoperative infections after spinal surgery, as in other locations, call for early diagnosis and quick operative revision, with thorough debridement. We shall discuss here the treatment plan to be followed in case of infection after posterior operations, which account for more than two-thirds of all spinal procedures that require revision.

If no metal implants have been introduced in the first session, the infection can generally be controlled without difficulty. On reopening the wound, the infected hematoma or pus, from which material for preoperative staining and culture was obtained by puncture before the operation, is aspirated, and the wound is carefully irrigated. In posterior spondylodeses, the superficial layer of bone chips permeated with granulation tissue has to be removed, but usually enough graft material can be retained to form a stable spondylodesis later; we then implant Septopal chains on the debrided wound bed and densely pack the cavity with them, taking care to obtain good coverage of the soft tissues.

If metal implants were used in the first operation, the prospects for rapid control of the infection are less favorable, and implant-specific factors may also play a role. An attempt should, and can, be made in the majority of cases to control the infection with the implant in place. Particular care should be taken to ensure that the debridement includes the granulation tissue under the rods and hooks and on the screw heads. In the implantation, Septopal minichains should be deposited on or below the metal parts (Fig. 10.**23**), while the remaining cavity can be filled with regular Septopal chains. Painstaking debridement and postoperative drainage are the keys to successful treatment. Any secretion from the wound may be a first sign of failure. On the other hand, drainage has to continue as long as wound secretions are being produced. We use the wound secretions to evaluate the status of the wound infection, which can be reliably determined on the basis of the leukocyte count in the wound secretion.

If the first or second revision does not achieve control of the infection, temporary removal of the implant is unavoidable. It is our impression that the chances of success are poorer after a preceding CD instrumentation than with the use of other implants, such as Harrington or Luque rods, for example; this may be due to the different surface characteristics, but also to the massiveness of the CD implants. After removal of the metal, the previous hook and screw sites, in particular, have to be thoroughly debrided. Using curved sharp curettes and small rongeurs, all the granulation tissue has to be carefully removed as far as the spinal cord. The channels of the transpedicular screws are meticulously scraped out, and are widened sufficiently to allow implantation of Septopal minichains (Fig. 10.**24**).

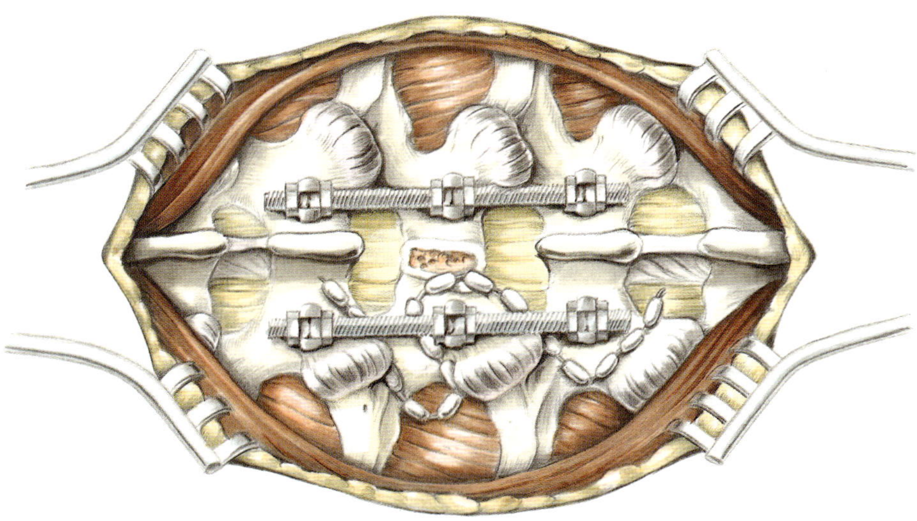

Fig. 10.**23** Deposition of Septopal minichains on implants in postoperative infections. The implants should be enclosed by minichains on all sides, also anteriorly.

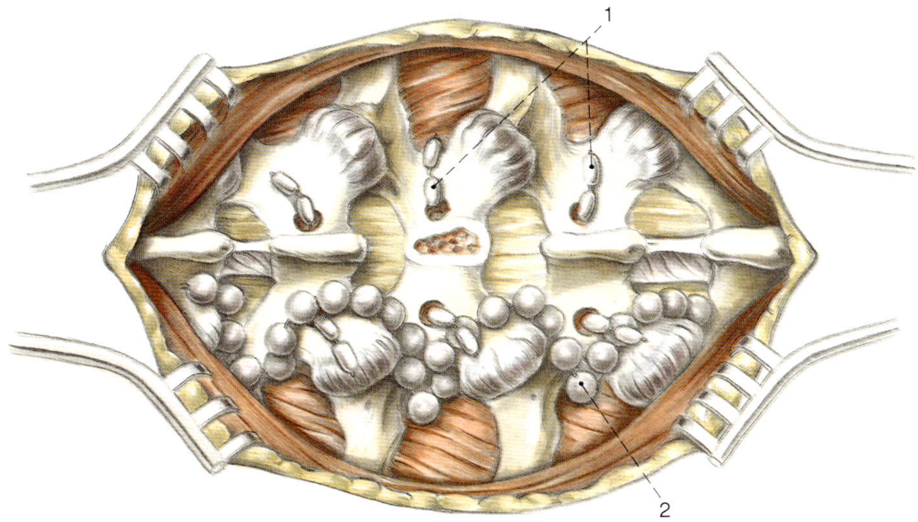

Fig. 10.**24** Implantation of Septopal after removal of transpedicular fixation devices.

1 Minichains implanted in screw channels
2 Regular Septopal chains used to fill empty spaces.

Wound Closure

Wound closure is performed in accordance with the general rules for wound care, in transthoracic operations obviously requiring chest tubes. The drain is left in place for at least three days, and is withdrawn once the 24-hour volume of wound secretion has decreased to less than 100 mL.

Postoperative Treatment

On the day before the operation, an extensive plaster cast is molded for patients in whom the pain is not severe enough to preclude this, and the patient is positioned in this cast immediately after the operation. In patients in whom no posterior stabilization is performed, we aim for immobilization in the molded cast for two months, and obtain control radiographs four and eight weeks after the operation. In case increasing incorporation is seen, measurements are taken for fabrication of a polyethylene trunk orthosis, which is then worn for another three months; after this, no further orthotic treatment is generally required.

In order to shorten the postoperative immobilization phase, we now usually carry out a secondary posterior stabilization, so that the patient is able to begin walking with an orthosis after 4–6 weeks.

Chemotherapy

Systemic antibiotic therapy is initiated intraoperatively with an antibiotic that has proved effective when tested—a cephalosporin sensitive against staphylococci is used if the causative organism has not been identified—and it is continued according to the intraoperative microbiological results until the end of the third postoperative month, or until the erythrocyte sedimentation rate is normal again. Patients with tuberculous spondylitis receive a 12-month course of a combination of tuberculostatic agents, with the treatment being started intraoperatively with streptomycin, which is replaced by another agent after ten days of administration. Because of possible drug-induced functional disorders, regular medical examinations of the eyes, and inner ear function are indicated during treatment with tuberculostatic drugs.

Further Reading

Albee FH. Transplantation of a portion of the tibia into the spine for Pott's disease. J Am Med Assoc 1911;57:885.

Bösch P, Chiari K, Dorn U. Erfahrungen mit der Vertebrotomie bei der Spondylitis tuberculosa. Z Orthop 1983;121:458.

Brussatis F, Blümlein H, Wunderlich T. Ergebnisse nach Ausräumung und ventraler Fusion bei Spondylitiden. Z Orthop 1983;121:458–459.

Collert S. Osteomyelitis of the spine. Acta Orthop Scand 1977;48:283.

Digby JM, Kersley JB. Pyogenic non-tuberculous spinal infection—an analysis of 30 cases. J Bone Jt Surg 1979;61-B:47.

Eismont FJ, Bohlman HH, Soni PL, Goldberg VM, Freehafer A. Pyogenic and fungal vertebral osteomyelitis with paralysis. J Bone Jt Surg 1983;65-A:19.

Göb A. Entzündliche Erkrankungen der Wirbelsäule. Chirurg 1982;53:299.

Härle A, Ritzerfeld W. The release of gentamicin into wound secretions from polymethylmethacrylate beads. Arch Orthop Traum Surg 1979;95:65.

Härle A. Die Bedeutung des postoperativen Verlaufs der Blutsenkungsreaktion. Orthop Prax 1979;15:695.

Härle A. Die optisch kontrollierte Markausräumung bei der Osteomyelitis-Behandlung. Z Orthop 1985;123:257.

Heine J, Immenkamp M, Matthiass HH. Ergebnisse der operativen Behandlung der Spondylitis tuberculosa. Z Orthop 1983;121:457.

Hodgson AR, Stock FE. Anterior spine fusion for the treatment of tuberculosis of the spine. J Bone Jt Surg 1960;42-A:295.

Jabbari B, Pierce JF. Spinal cord compression due to *Pseudomonas* in a heroin addict. Neurology 1977;27:1034.

Jäger M, Springer HH. Die entzündlichen Erkrankungen der Wirbelsäule. Orthopäde 1981;10:106.

Kemp HBS, Jackson JW, Jeremiah JD, Cook J. Anterior fusion of the spine for infective lesions in adults. J Bone Jt Surg 1973;55-B:715.

Kemp HBS, Jackson JW, Shaw NS. Laminectomy in paraplegia due to infective spondylosis. Br J Surg 1974;61:66.

Kessler P, Leibe H. Die Behandlung der Spondylitis tuberculosa unter besonderer Berücksichtigung der Indikation zur operativen Ausräumung. Beitr Orthop Traumatol 1982;29:188.

Krödel A, Stürz H. Differenzierte operative und konservative Therapie der Spondylitis und Spondylodiscitis. Z Orthop 1989;127:587.

Leventen EO. Closed irrigation–suction of spine infections. J Am Med Assoc 1966;196:81.

Martin NS. Tuberculosis of the spine. J Bone Jt Surg 1960;52-B:613.

Schmitt O, Biehl G. Operative Behandlung bei Entzündungen im Bereich der Wirbelsäule vom ventralen Zugang. Z Orthop 1983;121:459.

Thibodeau AA. Closed space infection following removal of lumbar intervertebral disc. J Bone Jt Surg 1950;50-A:400.

11 Tumors of the Spine

R. Bauer
R. Kotz

Indication for Surgery

Whether or not an operation is indicated depends, first of all, on the nature of the tumor. Generally speaking, the following types of tumor of the spine can be distinguished:

- Tumorlike diseases
- Benign tumors of the spine
- Primary malignant spinal tumors
- Secondary malignant spinal tumors (metastases)

The indications and operative techniques are further influenced by the patient's life expectancy and the location of the tumor. With spinal metastases, it is necessary to determine whether the lesions are isolated or multilocular. Additionally, the initial neurological status (unremarkable findings, radicular lesion, transverse cord lesion) is of critical importance.

Positioning and Incision

An anterior approach is generally required for lesions in the area of the spinal column. The operative technique is dictated by the level of the lesion (see Chapter 1, pp. 2–55).

If the tumor extends to both anterior and posterior vertebral elements, a combined single-stage or multistage procedure from the anterior and the posterior approach is necessary.

For tumors in the posterior segments of the spine, a posterior approach through a midline incision (Chapter 1, pp. 56–69) is used.

Operative Technique

It is very difficult to standardize the operative technique, since the location, extent, and virulence of the tumor are widely variable. Generally, however, the following treatment program can be formulated:

- *Benign spinal tumor or tumorlike diseases.* Resection of the tumor and reconstruction with cancellous bone. For tumors in the vertebral region, only a partial resection of the vertebral body is performed; with larger tumors, this should be followed by a block fusion of the vertebra (see Fig. 11.**41**).
- *Solitary, malignant spinal tumor, unfavorable prognosis.* Vertebral resection, possibly anterior decompression of the spinal cord. Stabilization: combined osteosynthesis (bone cement and plate), vertebral prosthesis (Polster) or bone cement.
- *Solitary benign or malignant spinal tumors, when the patient has good life expectancy.* Vertebral resection, block fusion of vertebra, anterior and posterior osteosynthesis (USIS).
- *Malignant spinal tumors, multilocular.* Posterior approach; possibly decompressive laminectomy in case of neurologic deficits; essentially, polysegmental stabilization of various types by the posterior approach: bilateral Harrington distraction, Harrington–Luque, Luque operation, transpedicular fixation with plate osteosynthesis (see Chapters 2 and 3).

Transpedicular Tumor Biopsy

If the diagnosis is not confirmed, a tumor biopsy is required prior to invasive spinal procedures. As a rule, a posterior approach is used. Posteriorly localized tumors are biopsied via a midline incision. However, transpedicular tumor biopsy also allows specimens to be obtained from the vertebral body (Figs. 11.**1**, 11.**2**).

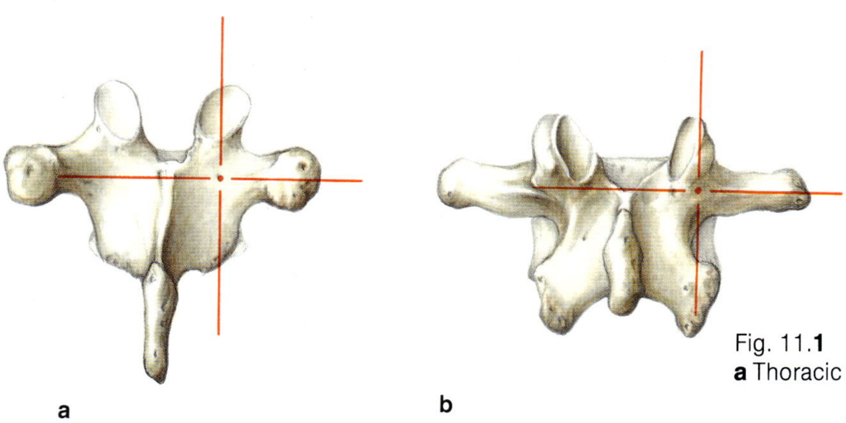

Fig. 11.**1** Orientation points for identification of the pedicle. **a** Thoracic spine, **b** lumbar spine.

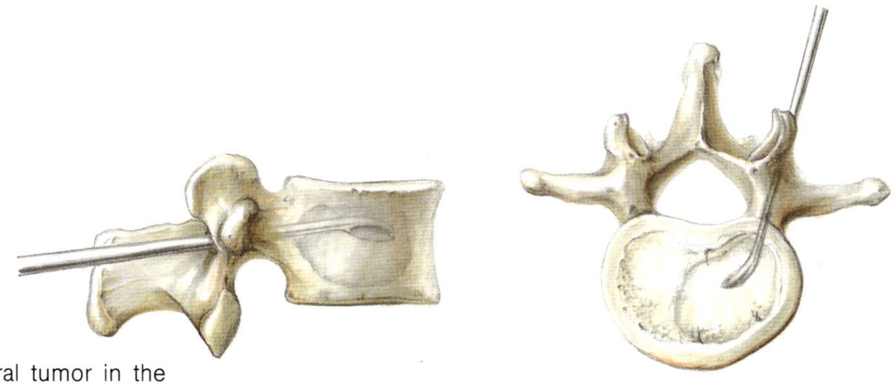

Fig. 11.**2** Transpedicular curettage of a vertebral tumor in the thoracic and the lumbar spine.

Thoracic Vertebral Body Replacement (Implant)

(Figs. 11.**3**, 11.**4**)

When the tumor is located in the area of the medial thoracic spine, the approach is made by a right-sided thoracotomy (Chapter 1, pp. 13–16). The affected vertebral body is resected as far as the posterior longitudinal ligament following ligation of the segmental vessels. An anterior decompression of the spinal cord can be now carried out if there are neurologic lesions. After anchoring holes have been produced in the end plates of the adjacent vertebrae, a vertebral body prosthesis (Polster) of appropriate size is applied. If there is a tumor-induced kyphotic deformity, the implant can be lengthened by counterclockwise rotation. It should be lengthened until the distance measures the length of the resected vertebra as well as that of the two adjacent intervertebral disk spaces (Fig. 11.**4**). The prosthesis is then incorporated into bone cement. Heat and pressure damage to the neural structures is prevented by applying Gelfoam to the posterior longitudinal ligament. A chest tube is then introduced, and the wound is closed in layers. In the area of the thoracic spine, it is not necessary to stabilize the implant by compression osteosynthesis.

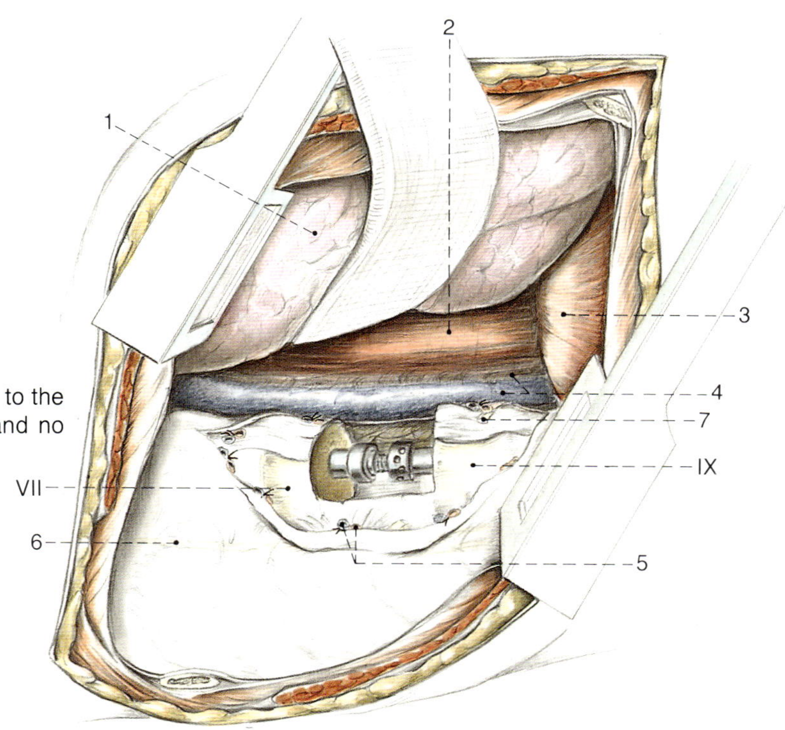

Fig. 11.**3** Replacement of T8 by a Polster prosthesis; due to the rigidity of the thoracic spine this is generally adequate, and no added osteosynthesis is required.

1 Right lung
2 Esophagus
3 Thoracic diaphragm
4 Azygos vein
5 Intercostal vessels
6 Sympathetic trunk
7 Greater splanchnic nerve
VII Body of thoracic vertebra
IX Body of thoracic vertebra

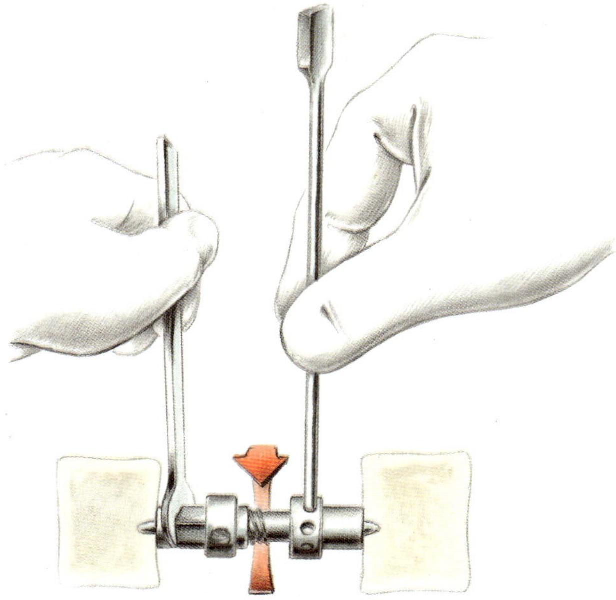

Fig. 11.**4** In many cases, a kyphosis is associated with a vertebral tumor. The Polster implant can be lengthened, correcting the kyphosis, by counterclockwise rotation.

Thoracolumbar and Lumbar Vertebral Body Replacement (Implant)

(Figs. 11.**5**–11.**7**)

For resection of a vertebra at the thoracolumbar junction, a Hodgson thoracophrenolumbotomy is carried out; for locations from L2 to L4, a retroperitoneal approach, usually from the left side, is chosen, while a transperitoneal approach is recommended for an L5 location (Chapter 1, pp. 24, 42, 52). After ligation of the segmental vessels, the vertebra is resected together with the adjacent intervertebral disks, and neural structures are decompressed if required. The implant (Polster) is then inserted and cut to the appropriate length (vertebra plus twice the height of the intervertebral disk) (Fig. 11.**5**). In the lumbar spine region, it is necessary to fix the implant by compression osteosynthesis with rectangular stability; the USI system (Zielke) is recommended (Fig. 11.**6**). The neural structures are protected by implantation of Gelfoam and insertion of a plastic retractor; after this, the implant is locked in with bone cement. If the posterior vertebral elements are intact, a second, posterior operation is unnecessary.

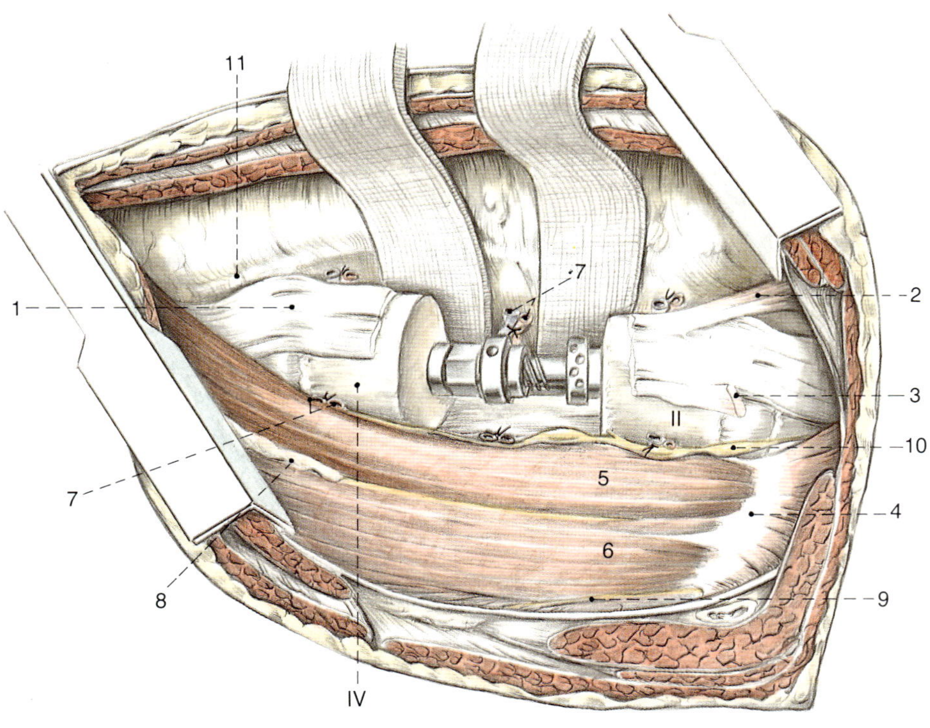

Fig. 11.**5** Resection of the third lumbar vertebra and replacement with a Polster implant; restoration of the physiological length (vertebral body plus two intervertebral disks)

1 Anterior longitudinal ligament
2 Right medial crus
3 Left medial crus
4 Left lateral crus
5 Greater psoas muscle
6 Quadratus lumborum muscle
7 Lumbar vessels
8 Ilioinguinal nerve
9 Subcostal nerve
10 Sympathetic trunk
11 Ureter
II Lumbar vertebral body
V Lumbar vertebral body

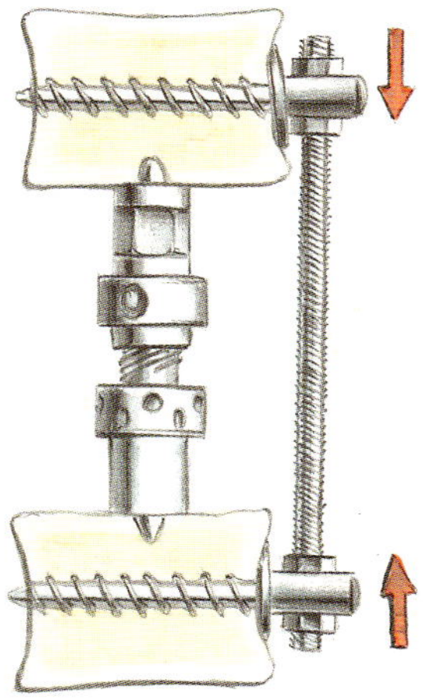

Fig. 11.**6** As a safeguard against hyperextension, a compression system with rectanguIar stability (USIS) is introduced laterally. Since the posterior vertebral elements are intact, no additional posterior instrumentation is necessary.

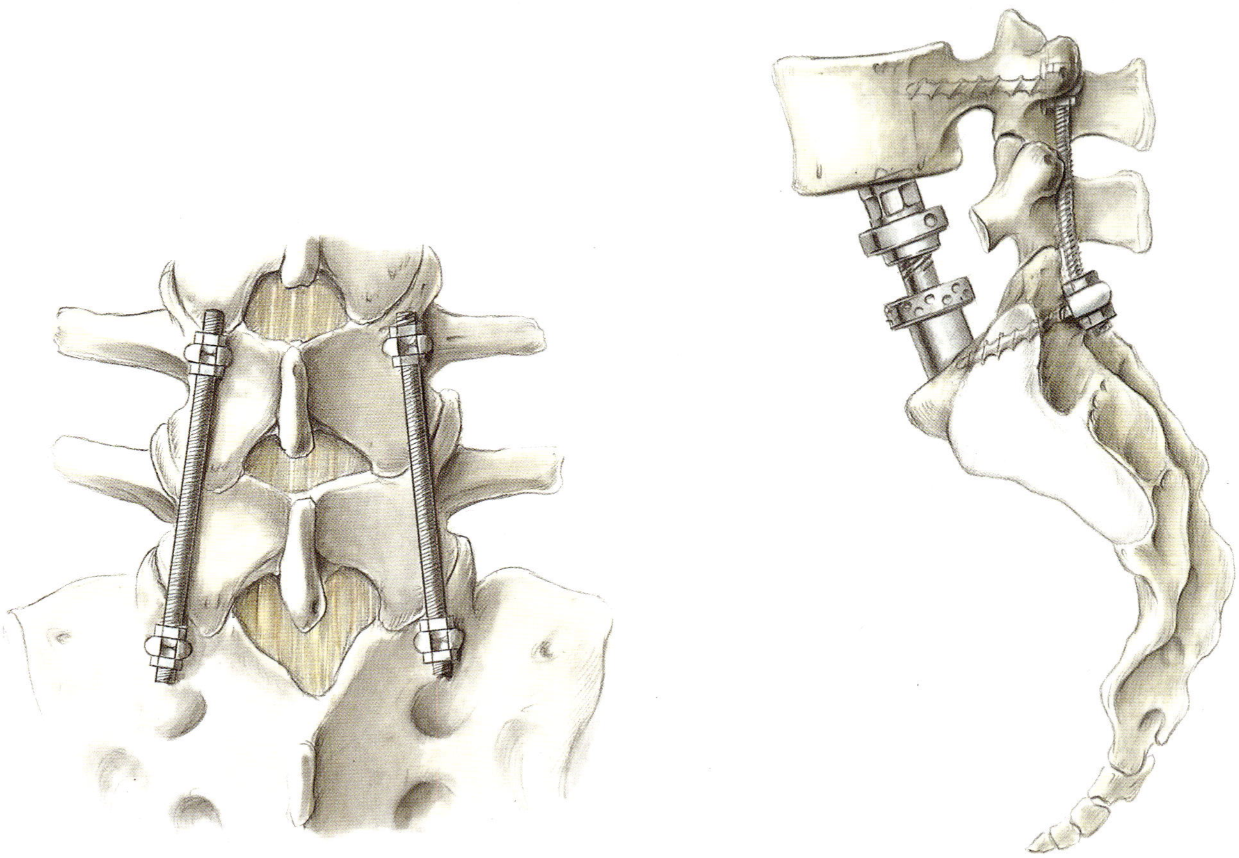

a

b

Fig. 11.**7** When L5 is replaced by a Polster implant and bone cement, added posterior transpedicular stabilization (e.g., USIS or fixateur interne) is essential, since the implant may otherwise become displaced. **a** Posterior view, **b** lateral view.

Replacement of Vertebral Body by Cement and Plate Osteosynthesis

(Fig. 11.**8**)

As a general rule, a vertebra can also be replaced, particularly in the lumbar spinal column, by a combination of bone cement enforcement and a plate osteosynthesis. The plate is applied to the vertebra laterally, with screw fixation in the area of the vertebra adjacent to the resection site.

Osteoplastic Replacement of Vertebral Body

(Benign tumors, malignant tumors with good prognosis; Figs. 11.**9**–11.**13**)

Depending on the level of the lesion, the approach is made by thoracotomy, by the Hodgson operation, or by retroperitoneal exposure of the lumbar spine. After ligation of the segmental vessels, the vertebral tumor is resected in the usual way as far as the posterior longitudinal

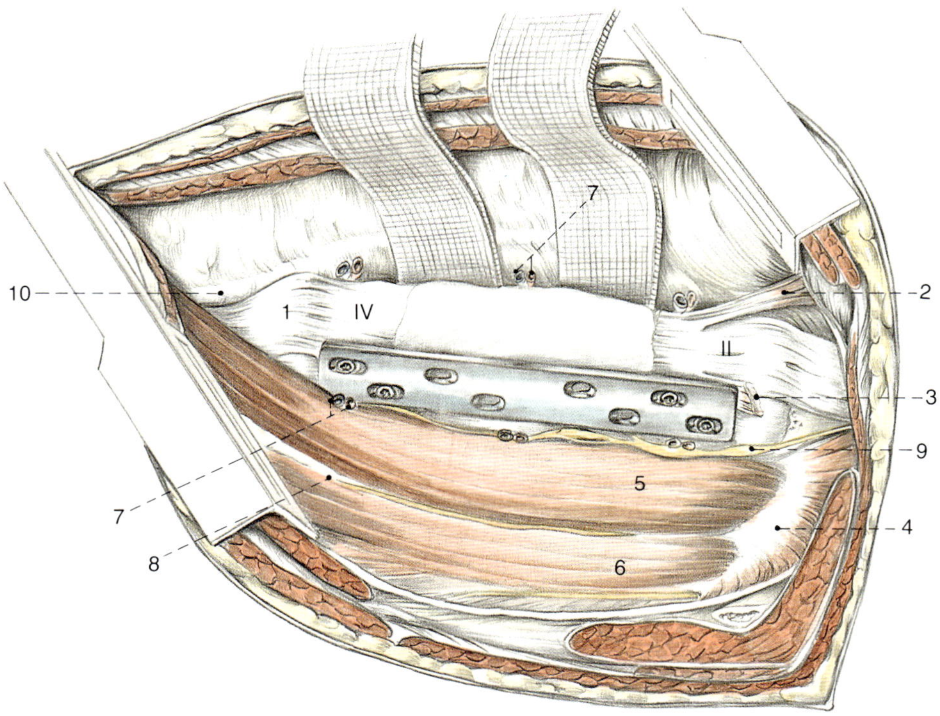

Fig. 11.**8** Status after resection of L3. Stabilization by compound osteosynthesis with bone cement and a plate for L2–L4.

1 Anterior longitudinal ligament
2 Right medial crus
3 Left medial crus
4 Left lateral crus
5 Greater psoas muscle
6 Quadratus lumborum muscle
7 Lumbar vessels
8 Ilioinguinal nerve
9 Sympathetic trunk
10 Ureter
II Lumbar vertebral body
IV Lumbar vertebral body

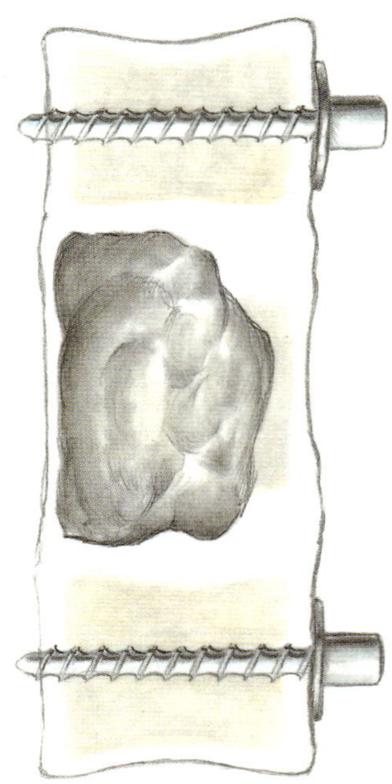

Fig. 11.**9** Osteoplastic replacement of vertebra. Following an anterior approach to the spine and exposure and removal of the tumor, DCS screws are inserted into the adjacent vertebrae. They are placed in the middle of the vertebral body or caudally to it (bearing in mind subsequent posterior transpedicular fixation).

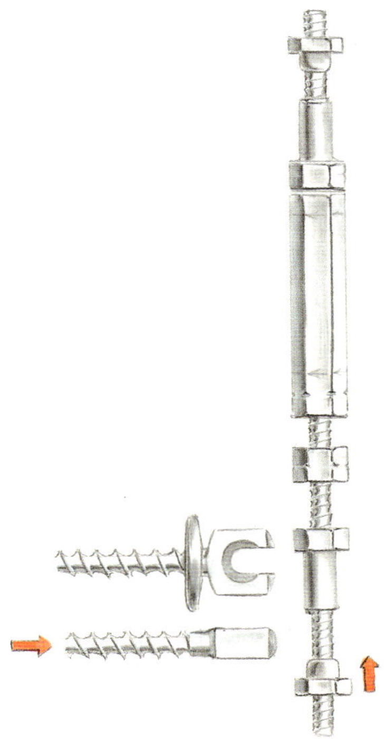

Fig. 11.**10** Zielke–Askani system. With the rod-extending system, both compression and distraction (or elongation and shortening) are possible. However, the threaded rod first has to be connected to the DCS screws to ensure rectangular stability.

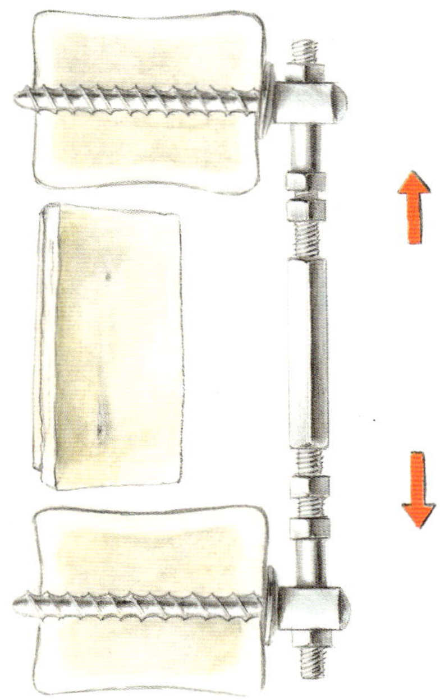

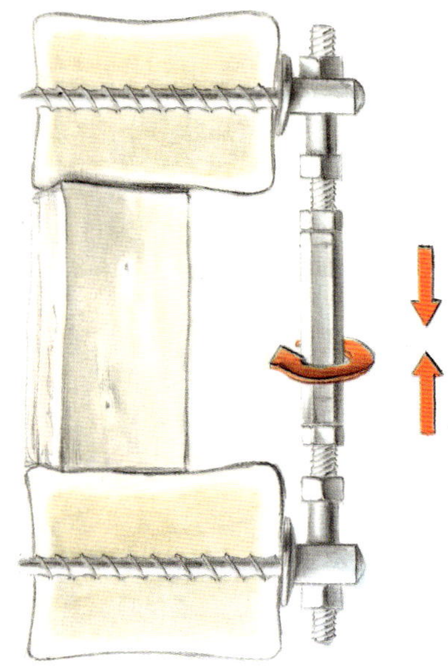

Fig. 11.**11** After removal of the vertebral tumor, the threaded rod is extended to physiological dimensions (vertebral body height plus twice the intervertebral disk). The defect is bridged by implantation of autologous corticocancellous bone chips.

Fig. 11.**12** The bone grafts are fixed and stabilized by shortening the threaded rod.

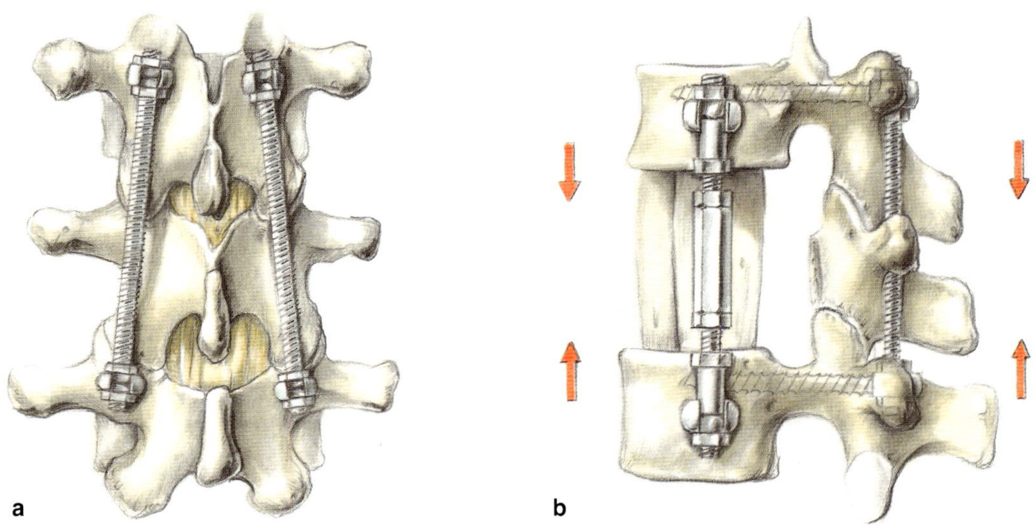

a **b**

Fig. 11.**13** In a second session, transpedicular stabilization is performed with DCS. In the course of this procedure, posterior vertebral elements affected by the tumor may be resected and replaced by autograft reconstruction. **a** Posterior view, **b** lateral view.

ligament. The adjacent intervertebral disks are removed, and the facing end plates of the two adjoining vertebrae are dechondrified. From the side of the approach, VDS screws are inserted transversely through the two adjacent vertebrae. After this, the Zielke–Askani system is assembled. To begin with, rectangular stability is produced between the distraction device and the vertebral screws. A distraction to normal length (vertebral body plus two disk spaces) is brought about by turning the thread in the central area. Next, the appropriately prepared corticocancellous bone chips are implanted, after which fixation of the grafts is accomplished by using the system to apply compression (Fig. 11.**12**). The graft should be inserted in such a way that no compression of neural structures will result posteriorly. Graft material that provides axial load-bearing capacity should be chosen. The VDS screws should be inserted in the middle of the vertebral body or caudally to it, so as to permit a transpedicular fixation by the posterior approach should this prove desirable.

In a second session, a transpedicular fixation is carried out by the posterior approach, using the DCS system with fusion of the vertebral joints (Fig. 11.**13**).

Tumor of the Cervical Spine, Compound Osteosynthesis

(demonstrated with C5, Figs. 11.**14**–11.**21**)

An anterior approach to the cervical spine (Chapter 1, pp. 4–6) is selected. The spine is approached in the usual way between the laterally situated neurovascular bundle and the medially situated visceral structures (Fig. 11.**14**). Cloward retractors are applied. The affected fifth cervical vertebra, together with the two adjacent intervertebral disks, is now resected as far posterior as the posterior longitudinal ligament. The two adjacent end plates are debrided, and meticulous hemostasis is carried out. For tumors with an unfavorable prognosis, bone cement is used for the replacement. When introducing the bone cement, care must be taken not to exert pressure on the spinal cord. If the prognosis is favorable, the defect is bridged by a corticocancellous graft from the iliac crest. In either case, the stabilization is effected with the use of an Orozko plate. With regard to the screw exit site, it should be borne in mind that in the cervical spine, the end plates ascend in a posterior direction, so that the screw for the cortical layer should not be inserted more caudally than in the middle of the anterior wall (Fig. 11.**20**). The screws should pass straight through the posterior vertebral cortex. To avoid injury to the dura lying behind it or to the cervical cord, it is necessary to use a drill with an adjustable drill stop. The drill length needed depends on the vertebral diameter as measured by a lateral radiograph (Fig. 11.**21**).

In principle, fixation with an osteolysis plate is also possible (Chapter 5). Apart from the angular stability, this fixation technique has the advantage of not requiring engagement of the posterior cortical substance.

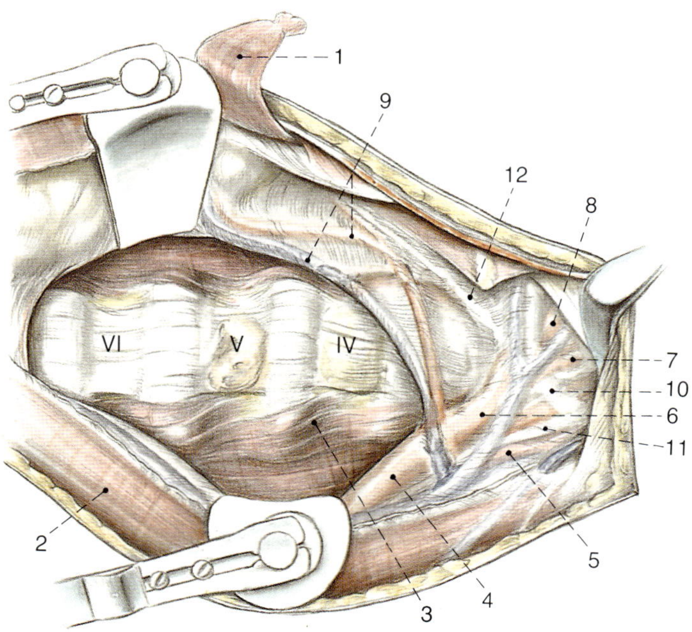

Fig. 11.**14** Exposure of affected cervical vertebra (C5) from the anterior approach.

1 Omohyoid muscle
2 Sternocleidomastoid muscle
3 Longus colli muscle
4 Common carotid artery
5 Internal carotid artery
6 External carotid artery
7 Facial artery
8 Lingual artery
9 Superior thyroid vessels
10 Hypoglossal nerve
11 Ansa cervicalis profunda
12 Superior laryngeal nerve
IV Cervical vertebra
V Cervical vertebra
VI Cervical vertebra

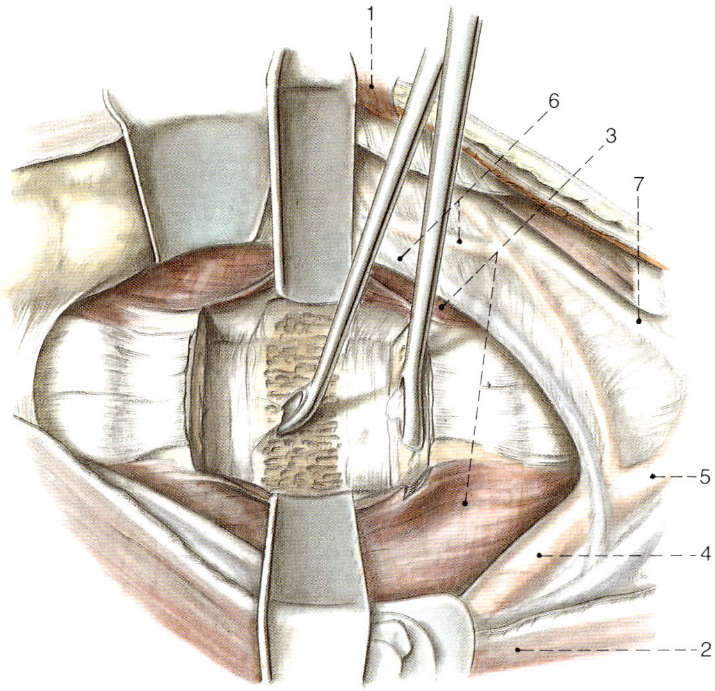

Fig. 11.**15** Excision of tumor with rongeur and sharp curet. The intervertebral disks are excised; the end plate is debrided with a curet.

1 Omohyoid muscle
2 Sternocleidomastoid muscle
3 Longus colli muscle
4 Common carotid artery
5 External carotid artery
6 Superior thyroid vessels
7 Superior laryngeal nerve

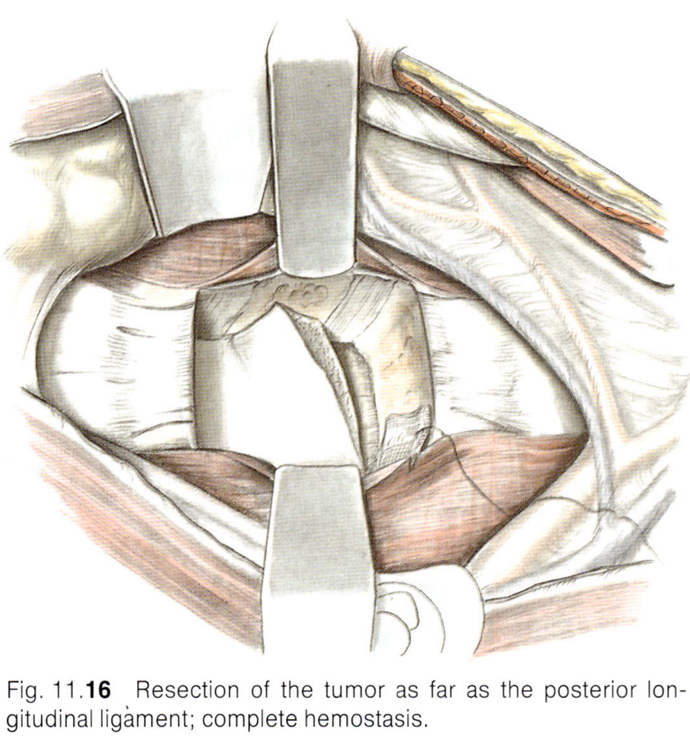

Fig. 11.**16** Resection of the tumor as far as the posterior longitudinal ligament; complete hemostasis.

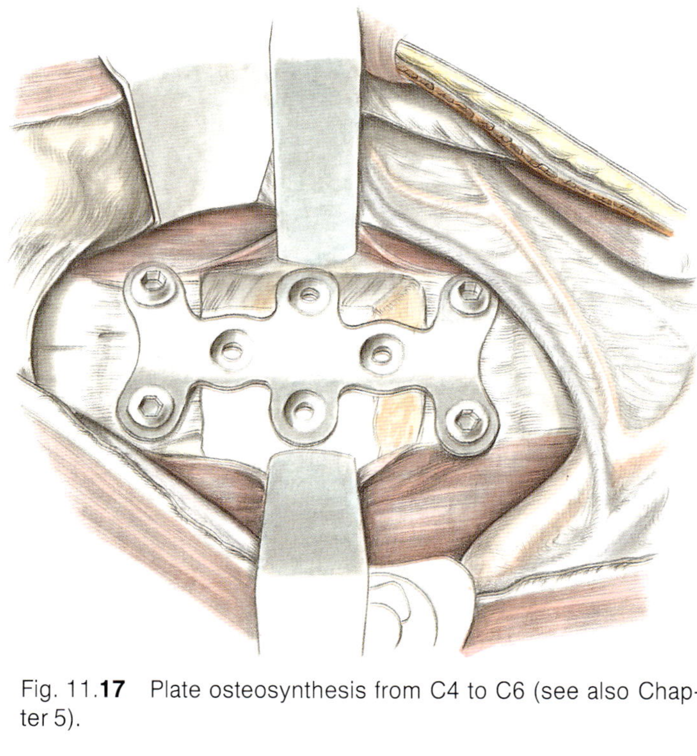

Fig. 11.**17** Plate osteosynthesis from C4 to C6 (see also Chapter 5).

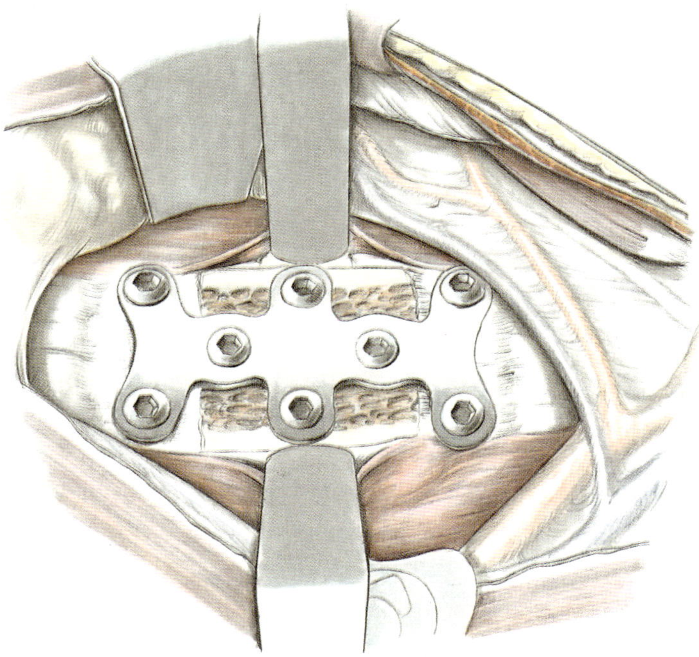

Fig. 11.**18** Bridging of the defect with autograft, in tumors with a good prognosis.

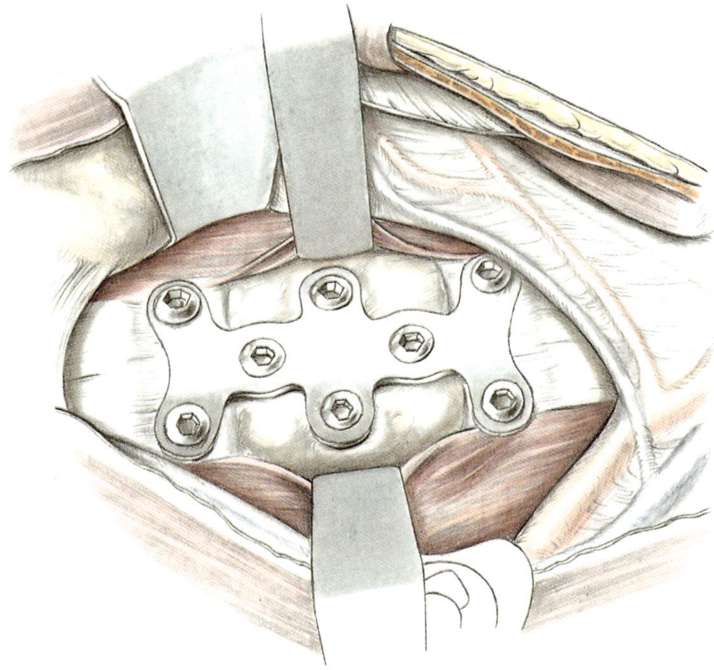

Fig. 11.**19** Bridging of the defect with bone cement by way of compound osteosynthesis, in malignant tumors.

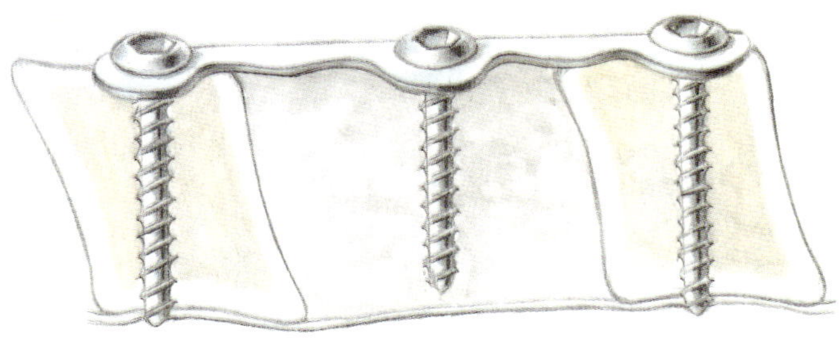

Fig. 11.**20** Compound osteosynthesis in the cervical spine; position of screws in bone and cement. *Note:* The end plates ascend posteriorly. The screw entry site should therefore not be farther caudal than the middle of the anterior wall of the vertebral body.

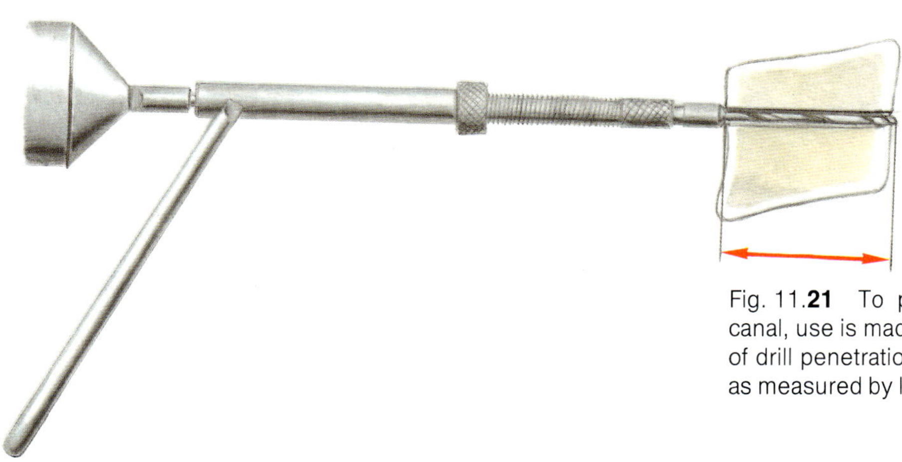

Fig. 11.**21** To prevent penetration of the drill into the spinal canal, use is made of a drill with an adjustable drill stop. The depth of drill penetration depends on the orthograde vertebral diameter as measured by lateral radiography.

Replacement of the Fourth Lumbar Vertebra by Compound Osteosynthesis L3–L5

(Figs. 11.**22**–11.**30**)

Retroperitoneal exposure of the medial and lower lumbar spine is effected via a left-sided flank incision (Chapter 1, pp. 42–45; Fig. 11.**22**). The segmental vessels are ligated from L3 to L5, and the tumor is exposed. The two adjacent intervertebral disks and the tumor are excised (Figs. 11.**23**, 11.**24**). The tumor is removed, primarily with a rongeur and a curet (Figs. 11.**24**, 11.**26**); the dissection is carried as far as the posterior longitudinal ligament, and this also allows decompression of neural structures if required. Following careful hemostasis, an osteosynthesis plate is fixed with screws in the area of L3 and L5. Posteriorly, Gelfoam is implanted, and a plastic retractor is inserted for direct protection of neural structures. Finally, the defect is bridged with bone cement.

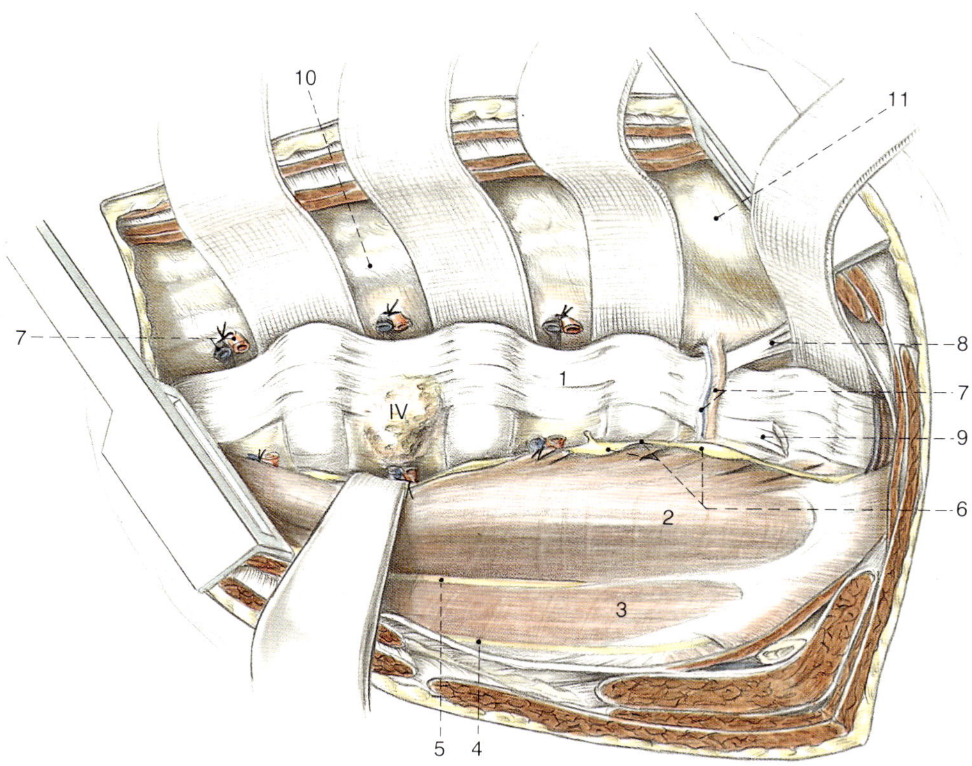

Fig. 11.**22** Exposure of a tumor in L4 using a left-sided retroperitoneal approach.

1 Anterior longitudinal ligament
2 Greater psoas muscle
3 Quadratus lumborum muscle
4 Subcostal nerve
5 Ilioinguinal nerve
6 Sympathetic trunk
7 Lumbar vessels
8 Right medial crus
9 Left medial crus
10 Left ureter
11 Left kidney
IV Tumor of the lumbar vertebra

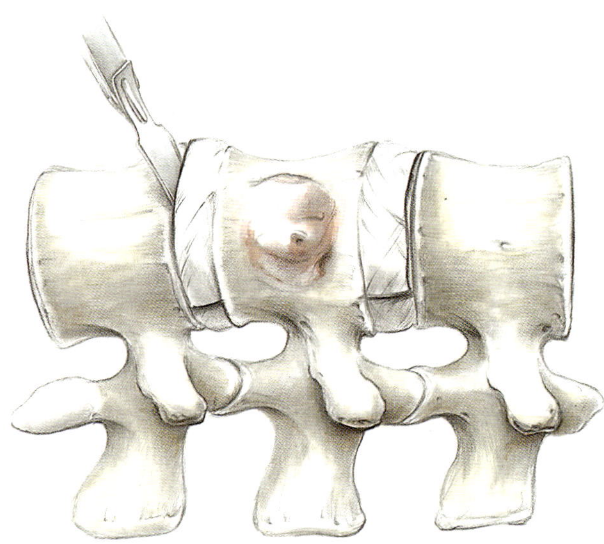

Fig. 11.**23** Excision of the tumor together with the adjacent intervertebral disks.

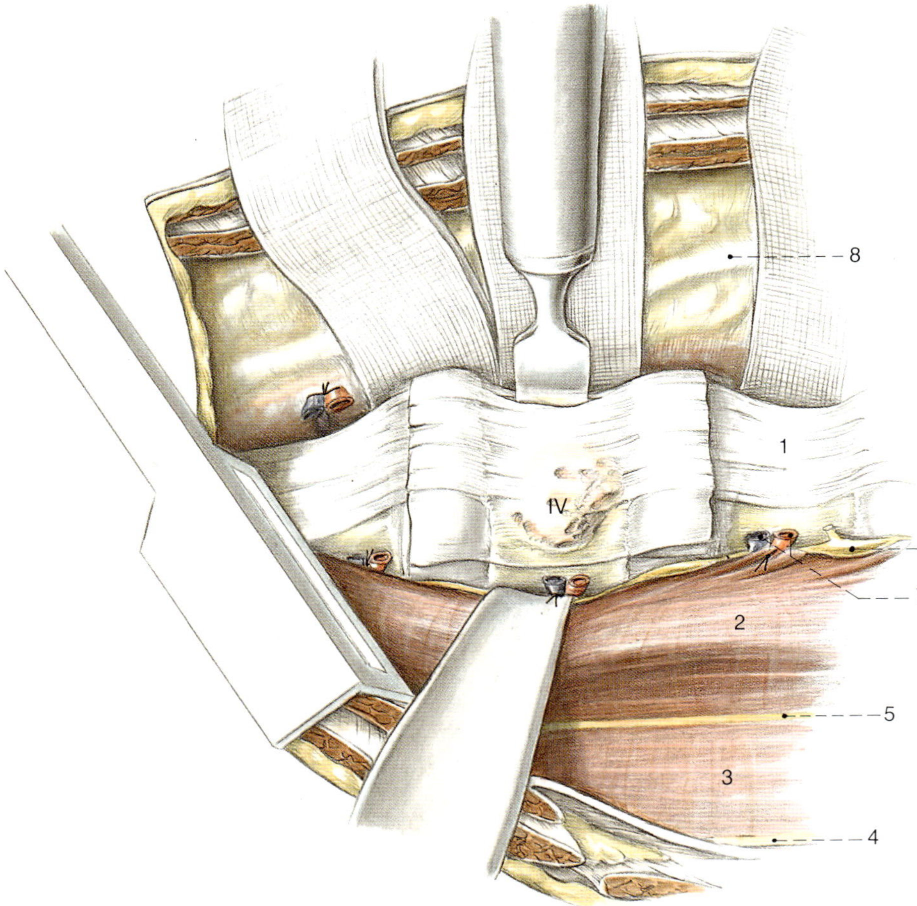

Fig. 11.**24** Bony portions of the vertebral body have to be partly divided with a chisel

1 Anterior longitudinal ligament
2 Greater psoas muscle
3 Quadratus lumborum muscle
4 Subcostal nerve
5 Ilioinguinal nerve
6 Sympathetic trunk
7 Lumbar vessels
8 Left ureter
IV Tumor of the lumbar vertebra

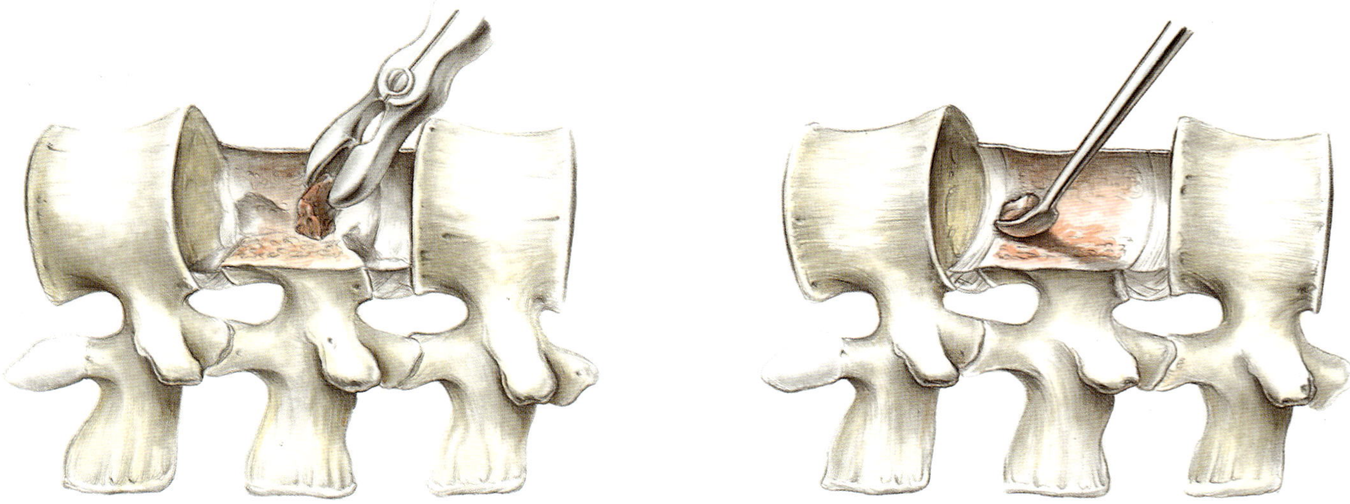

a

b

Fig. 11.**25** Removal of the bulk of the tumorous tissue is followed by further dissection using a rongeur (**a**) or a sharp curet (**b**).

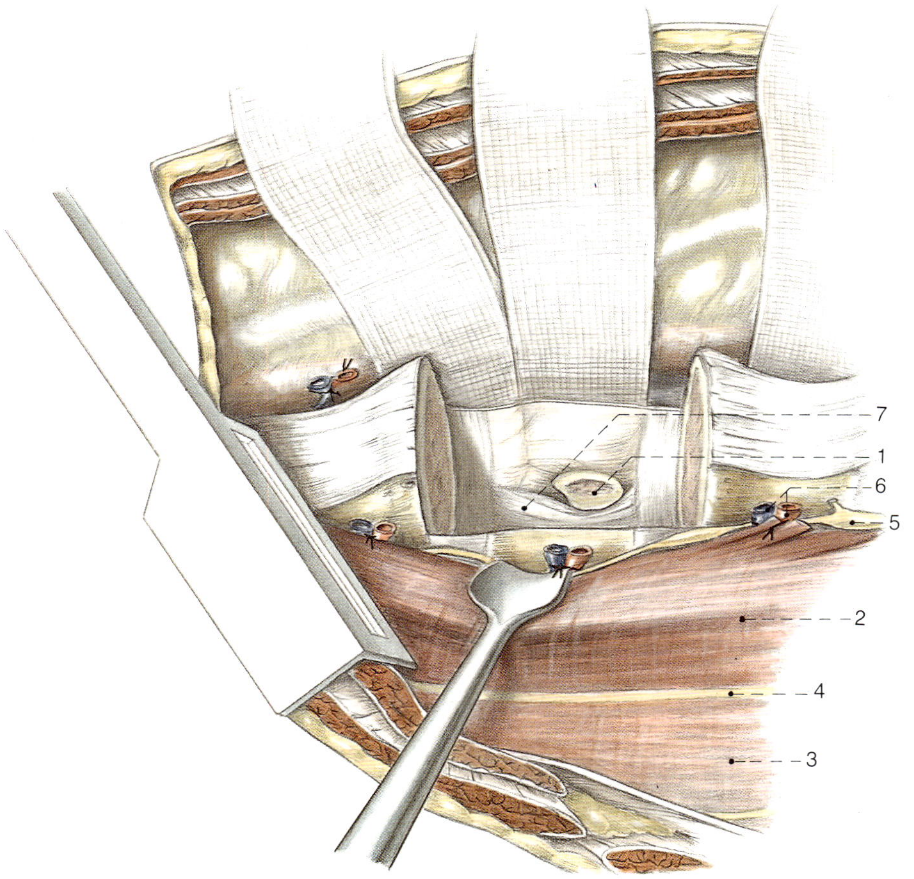

Fig. 11.**26** Status after removal of L4 including the two adjacent intervertebral disks.

1 Pedicle of the vertebral arch
2 Greater psoas muscle
3 Quadratus lumborum muscle
4 Ilioinguinal nerve
5 Sympathetic trunk
6 Intercostal vessels
7 Posterior longitudinal ligament

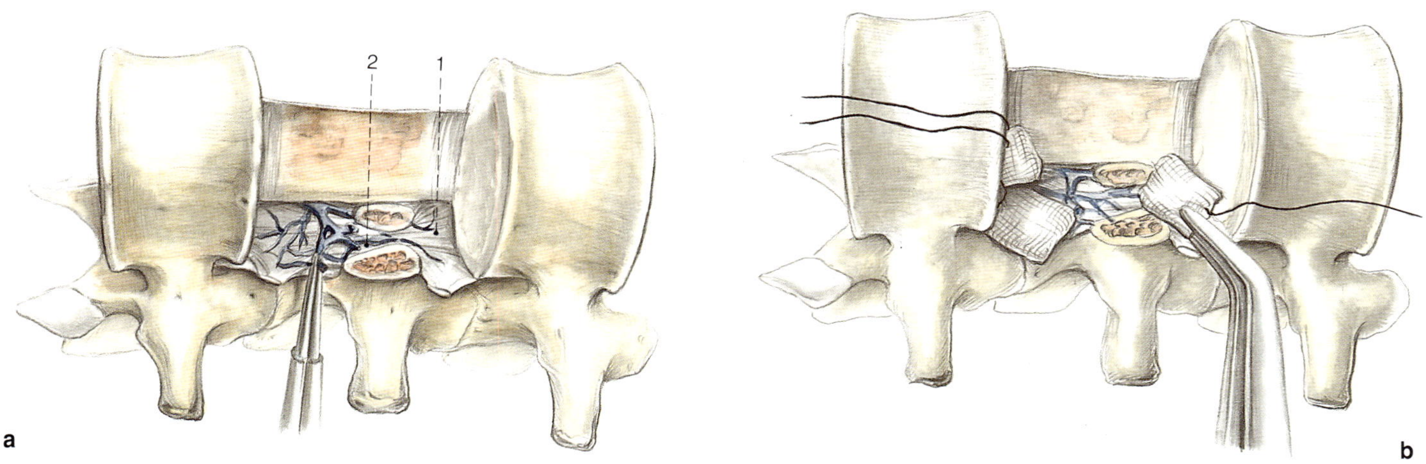

a **b**

Fig. 11.**27** Careful hemostasis in the area of the posterior longitudinal ligament or the dura, **a** by bipolar coagulation, **b** by insertion of Gelfoam, Surgicel, and paddies.

1 Posterior longitudinal ligament
2 Posterior internal vertebral venous plexus

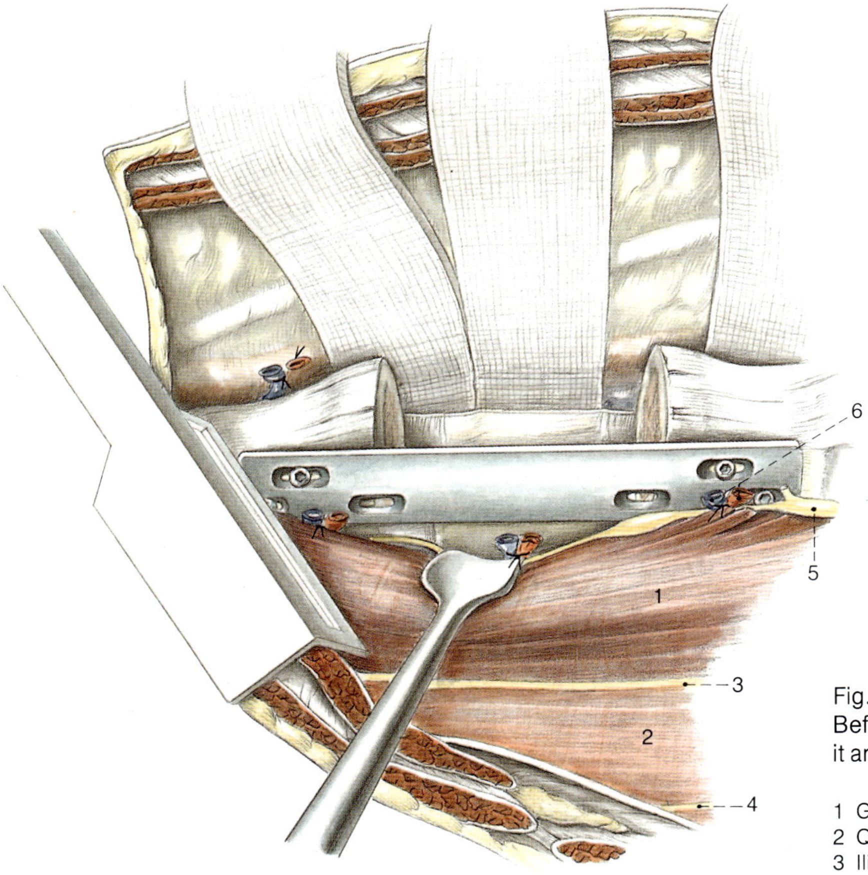

Fig. 11.**28** Status after L3–L5 plate osteosynthesis. Before cementing, Gelfoam with a plastic retractor over it are applied for protection of neural structures.

1 Greater psoas muscle
2 Quadratus lumborum muscle
3 Ilioinguinal nerve
4 Subcostal nerve
5 Sympathetic trunk
6 Lumbar vessels

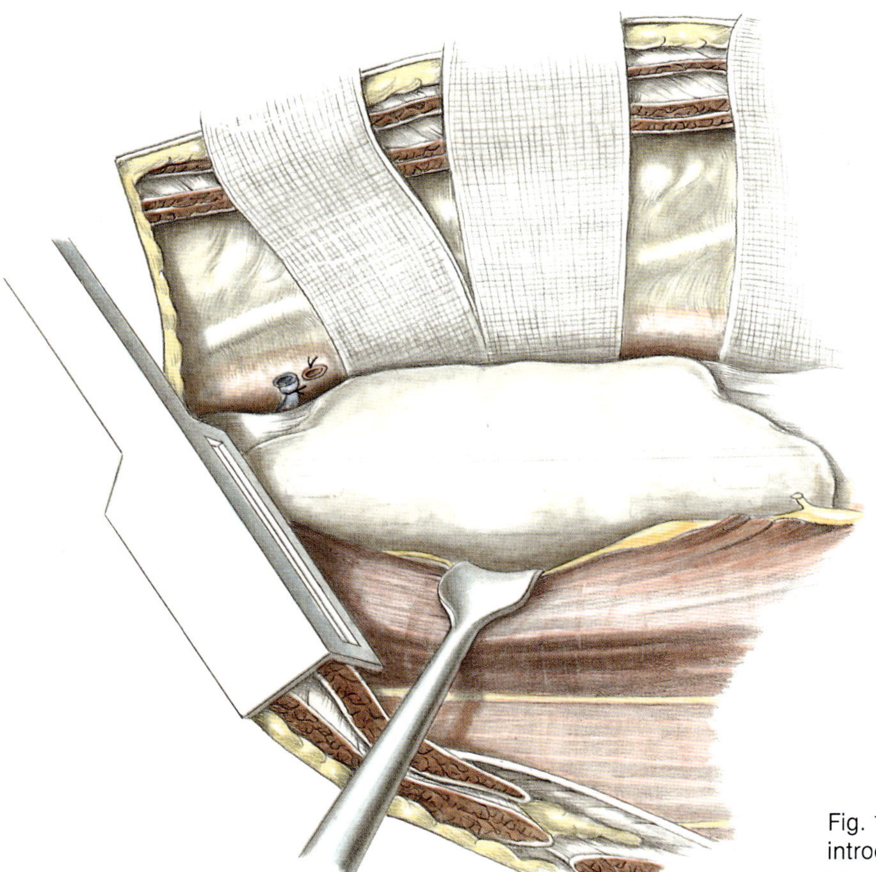

Fig. 11.**29** Completed compound osteosynthesis after introduction of bone cement. *Note:* no posterior compression.

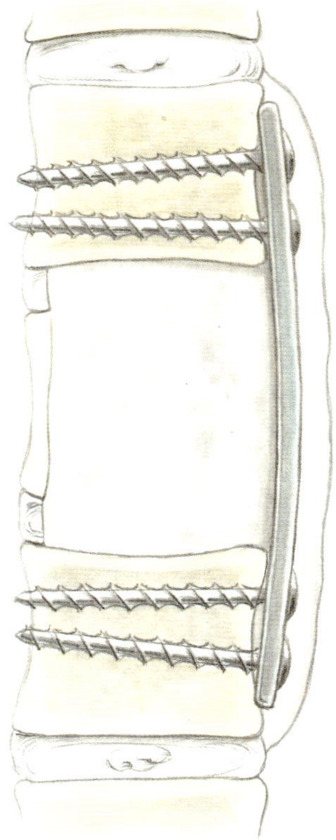

Fig. 11.**30** Representation of compound osteosynthesis in frontal section.

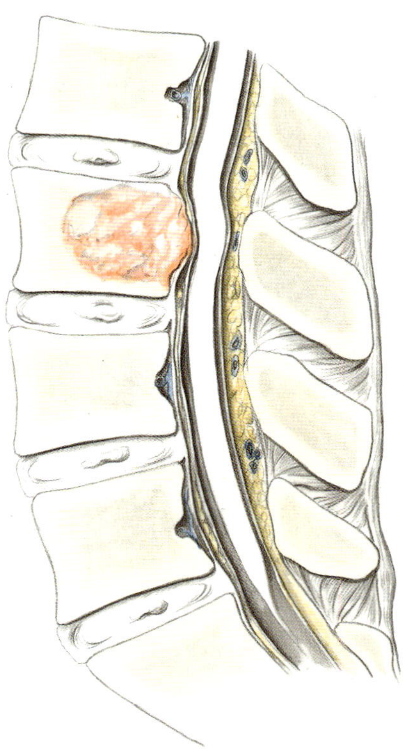

Fig. 11.**31** Benign tumor of L3 with constriction of spinal canal.

Osteoplastic Blockage of Vertebra, Benign Tumor of the L3 Vertebra

(Figs. 11.**31**–11.**41**)

If the nature of the tumor is such that an oncologically radical resection is not necessary, the vertebra can be partially resected from the anterior approach. For more extensive lesions of the vertebra, fusion of the adjacent vertebral segments is required. Whether or not an operation is indicated depends in part on the absence or presence of compression of the neural structures (Fig. 11.**31**). A left-sided flank incision is made for retroperitoneal exposure of the medial lumbar spine (Chapter 1, pp. 42–45). The segmental vessels in the proposed fusion zone are ligated and divided. The psoas muscle is retracted laterally; if necessary, it can be medially notched or transected entirely. Care should be taken to spare the subjacent nerve roots (Fig. 11.**33**).

The adjacent intervertebral disks are excised with a knife, and the portion of the vertebra affected by the tumor is resected with a chisel. Further removal of the tumorous bone portions is effected with a rongeur or sharp curet. If necessary, decompression of neural structures can now be carried out. Meticulous control of any hemorrhage from the vertebral venous plexus is important.

In preparation for blockage of the vertebra, the end plates of the adjacent vertebrae are debrided, and a groove is created.

After measurements with a caliper, a chip of suitable size is harvested from the ilium and dovetailed for bridging of L2–L4 (Figs. 11.**37**, 11.**38**).

For further stabilization, a cortical bone graft is harvested from the tibia, and is then prepared with a drill and a countersink for receiving cortical screws. The tibial graft is fixed to the spine laterally with two cortical screws which, in the usual way, should sparingly pierce the contralateral cortical layer. The remaining space is packed with cancellous bone graft from the iliac bone. Finally, fibrin glue can also be applied for further fixation of the graft (Fig. 11.**41**).

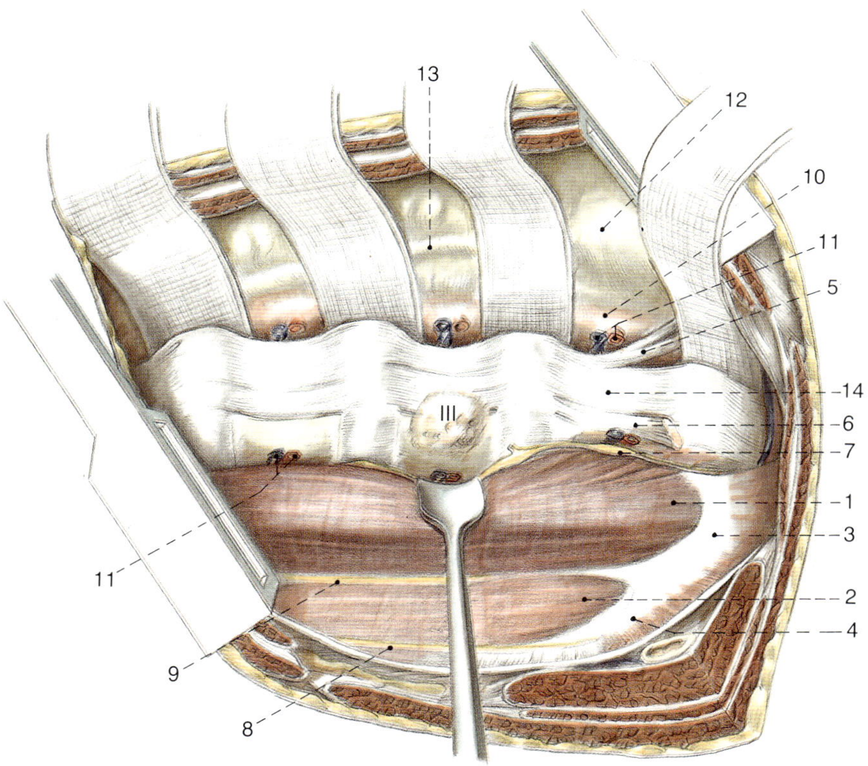

Fig. 11.**32** Exposure of tumor in L3 by left-sided retroperitoneal approach.

1 Greater psoas muscle
2 Quadratus lumborum muscle
3 Medial arcuate ligament
4 Lateral arcuate ligament
5 Right medial crus
6 Left medial crus
7 Sympathetic trunk
8 Subcostal nerve
9 Ilioinguinal nerve
10 Abdominal aorta
11 Lumbar vessels
12 Left kidney
13 Left ureter
14 Anterior longitudinal ligament
III Tumor of the lumbar vertebra

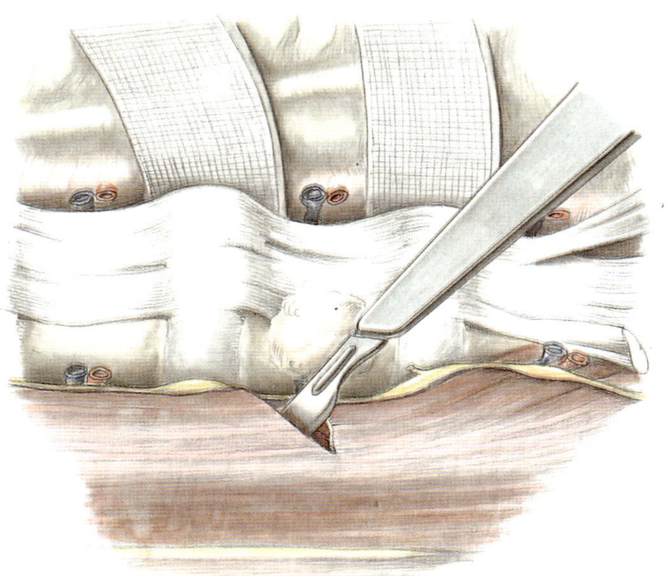

Fig. 11.**33** The psoas muscle is retracted or transversely incised (watch for spinal nerves!).

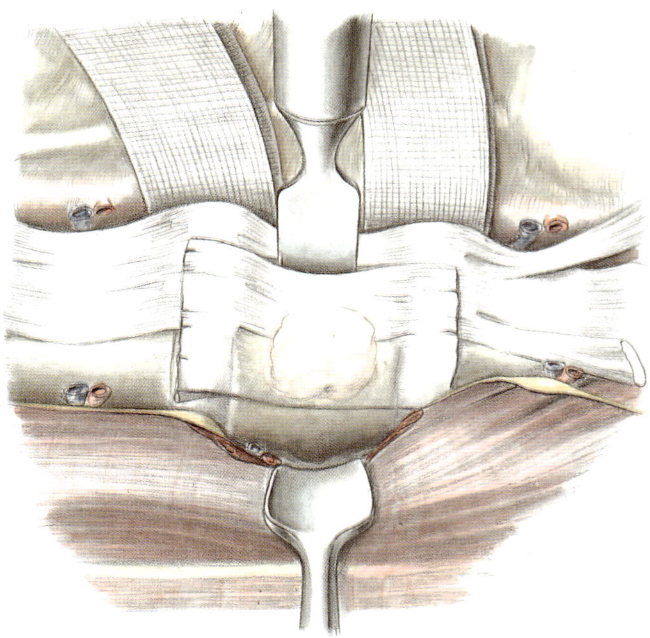

Fig. 11.**34** Excision of the intervertebral disk with a knife; removal of bony structures with a chisel.

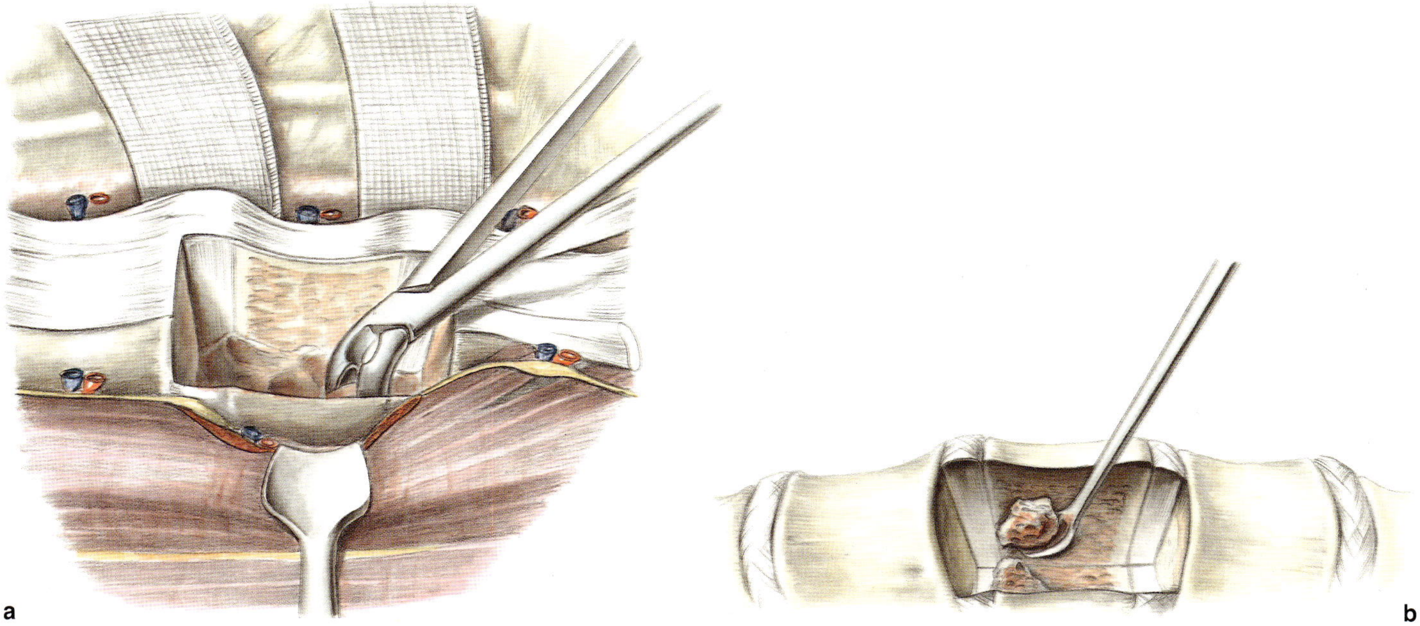

a b

Fig. 11.**35** Further resection of the tumor down to healthy cancellous bone is done with a rongeur (**a**) or a sharp curet (**b**).

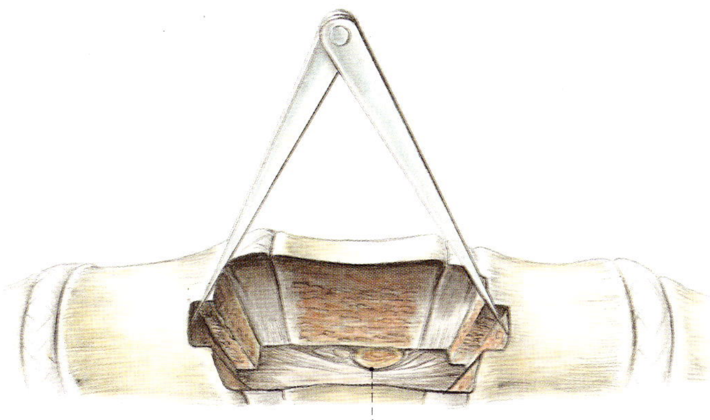

Fig. 11.**36** Status after partial resection of L3 for tumor removal. An osteoplastic block for L2–L4 is being prepared. After caliper measurements, an appropriately-sized corticocancellous graft is harvested from the iliac bone.

1 Pedicle of vertebral arch

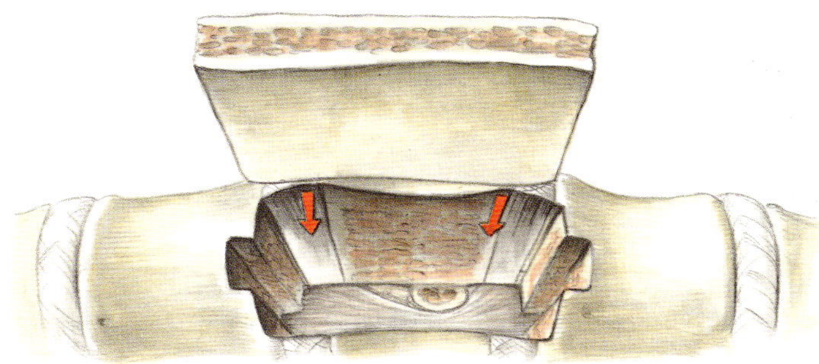

Fig. 11.**37** Dovetailing of the corticocancellous autograft.

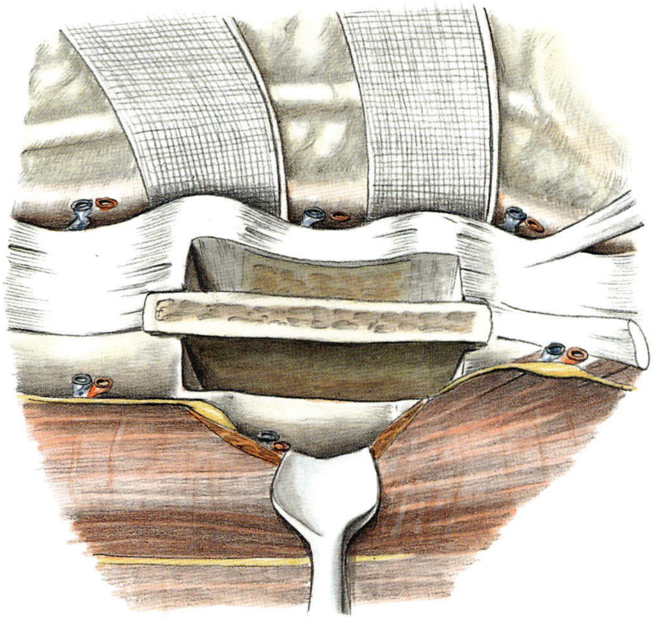

Fig. 11.**38** Osteoplastic blocking of the L2–L4 vertebrae; operative site.

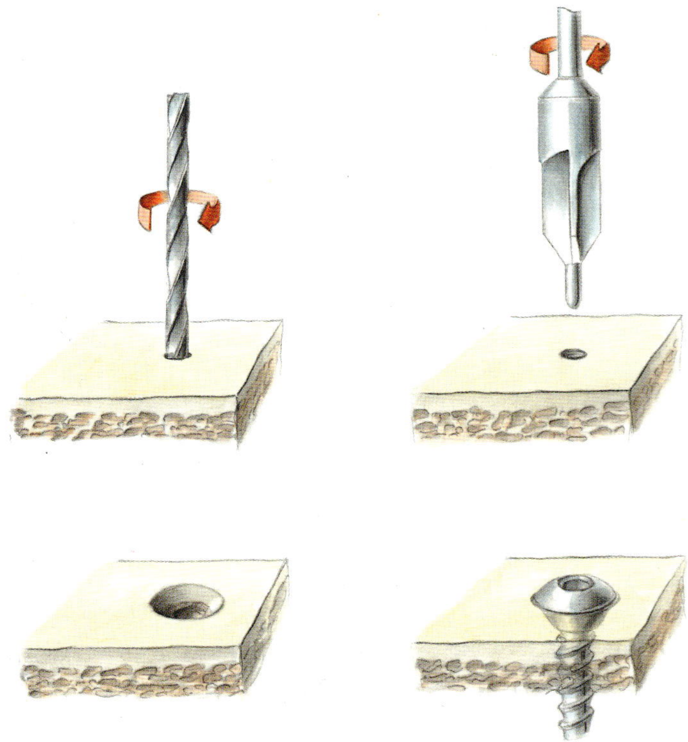

Fig. 11.**39** A cortical chip taken from the tibia, appropriately sized, is prepared for screw fixation with a drill and a countersink.

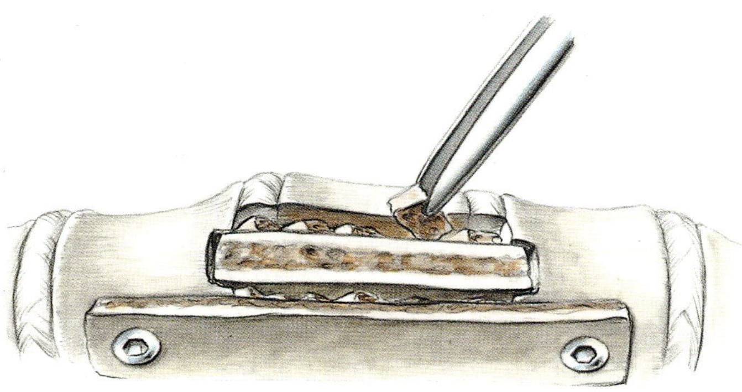

Fig. 11.**40** Status after osteoplastic blocking of the L2–L4 vertebrae. Residual hollow spaces are packed with cancellous bone.

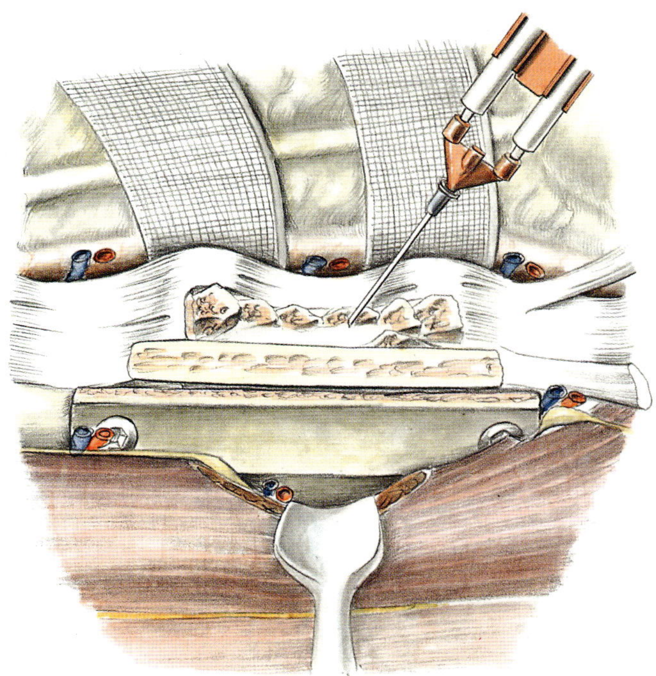

Fig. 11.**41** Osteoplastic blockage of the vertebrae; operative site. The final step is application of fibrin glue.

Further Reading

Bauer R, Achammer T. Concept for operative stabilisation after intralesional vertebrectomy. Combined Meeting SRS/ESDS, Amsterdam, September 1989; Abstracts:79.

Bauer R, Russe W. Die operative Behandlung von primären und sekundären Wirbelsäulentumoren. SICOT Munich, 1987; Abstracts:312.

Bauer R, Russe W. Operative Zugangswege zur Wirbelsäule und operationstechnische Prinzipien. In: Gradinger R, Optiz G, eds. Wirbelsäulentumoren. Gräfelfing: Demeter, 1989.

Dewald R, Bridwell KH, Prodromas C, Rodts MF. Reconstructive spinal surgery as palliation for metastatic malignancies of the spine. Spine 1985;10:21.

Lack W, Eyb R, Ramach W, et al. Erfahrungen mit der ventralen Stabilisierung bei Wirbelkörpermetastasen im Brust- und Lendenwirbelsäulenbereich. Z Orthop 1987;125:233–346.

Manabe S, Tateishi A, Abe M, Ohno T. Surgical treatment of metastatic tumors of the spine. Spine 1989;14:41.

Onimus M, Schraub S, Bertin D, Bosset JF, Guidet M. Surgical treatment of vertebral metastasis. Spine 1986;11:883.

Polster J, Brinckmann P. Ein Wirbelkörperimplant zur Verwendung bei Palliativoperationen an der Wirbelsäule. Z Orthop 1977;115:118.

Ritschl P, Eyb R, Samec P, Lack W, Kotz R. Behandlungsstrategie maligner Knochentumoren der Wirbelsäule. Orthopäde 1987;16:379.

Salzer M, Salzer G, Denck H, Brenner H. Operative Behandlung „solitärer" Metastasen der Brust- und Lendenwirbelkörper. Arch Orthop Unfall-Chir 1973;75:249.

Simmons EH, Light KI. Metastatic disease of the spine. American Orthopedic Association, Hot Springs, 1988; Abstracts.

12 Tumors of the Chest Wall

R. Kotz

Rib Resections

Indications

Principal indications

- *Secondary tumors* (metastasis by direct extension or lymphatic).
- *Primary* malignant bone tumors (fibrosarcoma, malignant fibrous histiocytoma, chondrosarcoma) or malignant soft-tissue tumors of the chest wall (1% of chest wall tumors, according to Atkins 1983).

Secondary indications

- Hematogenous metastases of the ribs (solitary, or, in case of instability and pain, with a good prognosis using chemotherapy)
- Benign tumors, such as neurinomas, lipomas, and neurofibromas (ratio of benign to malignant chest wall tumors 3:1, according to Merkle et al. 1988).

Positioning and Incision

The patient is positioned on the unaffected side (Fig. 12.**1**). The arm is elevated with a support, or placed above the head. The skin incision is made at a considerable distance from the site of the biopsy. The skin is pulled up, and the subcutis is divided (Fig. 12.**2**).

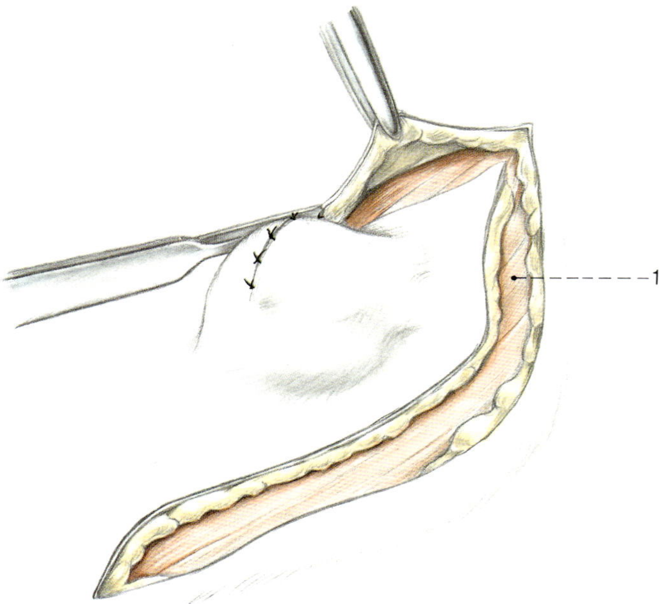

Fig. 12.**2** The incision around the lesion with the biopsy wound is made far off in healthy tissue, that is, at least 3 cm away from the cutis–subcutis affected by the tumor and the underlying structure.

1 Anterior serratus muscle

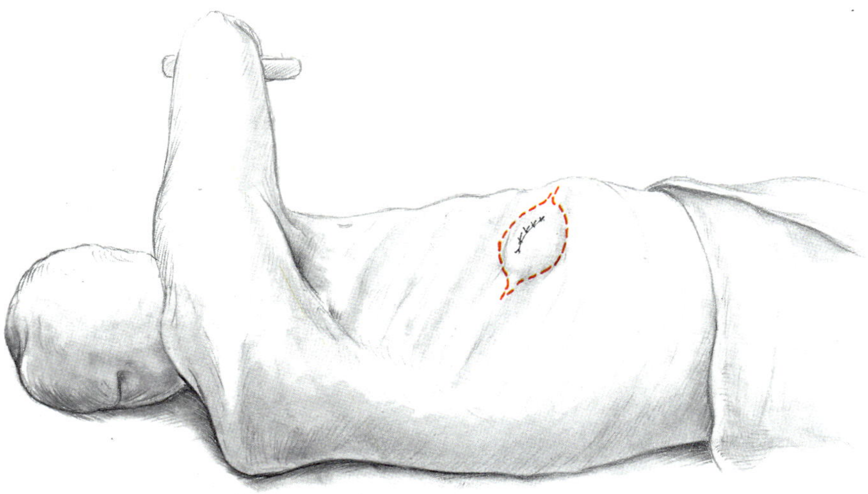

Fig. 12.**1** Positioning the patient on the unaffected side, and elevating the site of the lesion. The arm is raised to allow better mobilization and lateral retraction of the scapula.

Operative Technique

Exposure of Ribs

The adjacent (cranial and caudal) unaffected ribs are exposed subperiosteally after division of the fascia and the musculature (Fig. 12.**3**). The periosteum is sharply incised and retracted to the unaffected side with an elevator.

Opening the Pleural Cavity

At the cranial border of the cranial rib, the parietal pleura is transected intercostally with a scalpel, opening the pleural cavity. The pleural space is then cautiously split anteriorly and posteriorly with scissors (Fig. 12.**4**), the ribs are forced apart, and the pleural space is inspected. If there is adhesion of the visceral pleura to the tumorous area, lung tissue has to be resected as well. The pleura can now also be divided at the inferior border of the caudal rib, and dissected free up to the resection margins of the rib, far from the tumor.

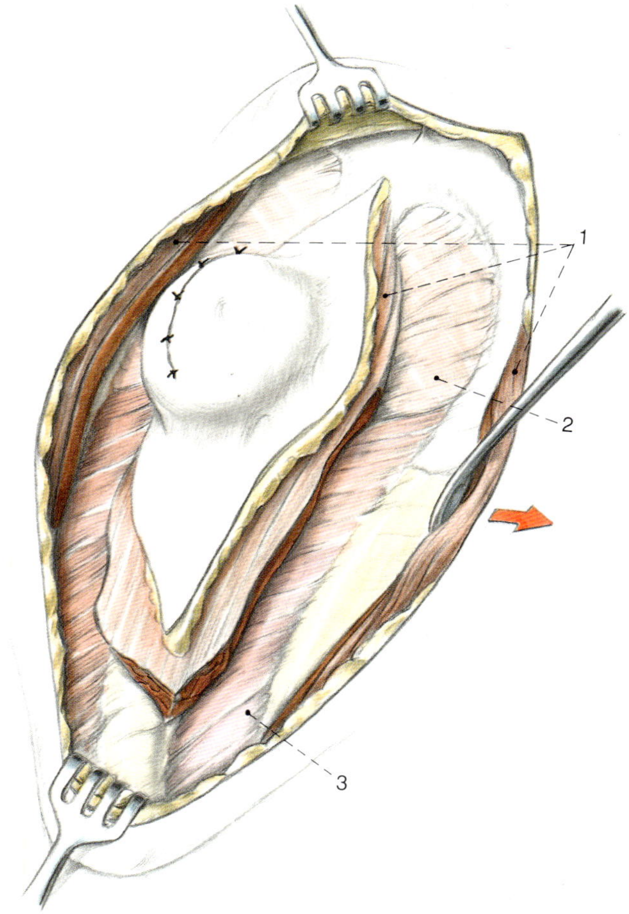

Fig. 12.**3** The ribs adjoining the tumor are subperiosteally exposed with an elevator on the side facing away from the tumor.

1 Anterior serratus muscle
2 External intercostal membrane
3 External intercostal muscle

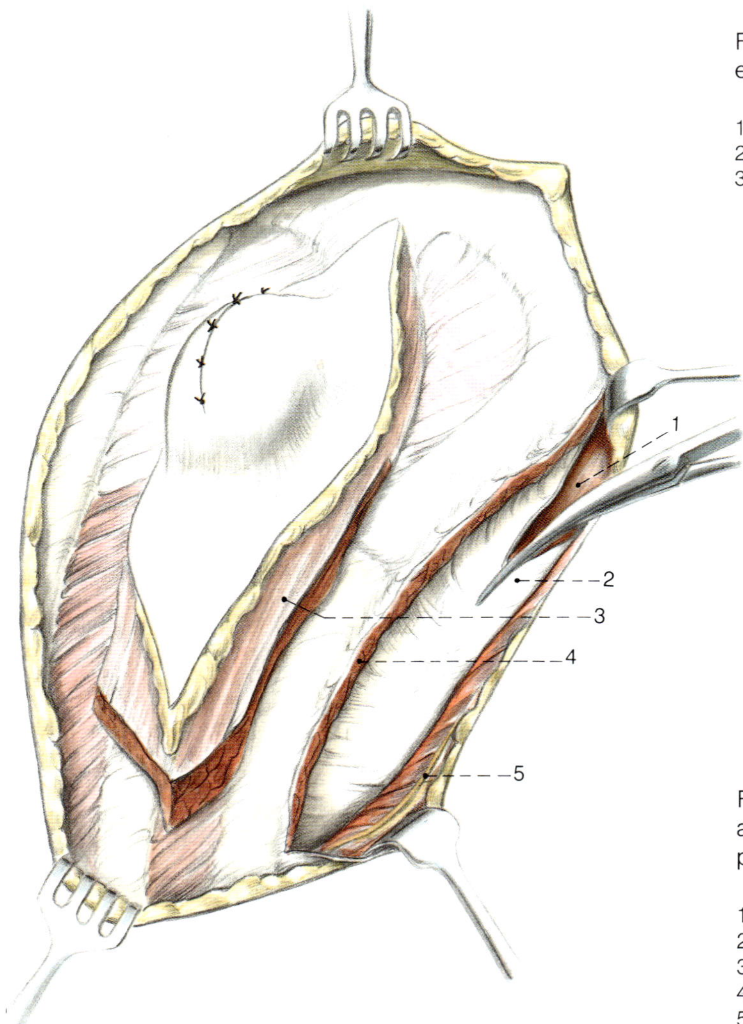

Fig. 12.**4** Division of the intercostal musculature between the rib adjacent to the tumor and the nearest healthy rib, opening the pleural cavity.

1 Thoracic diaphragm
2 Parietal pleura
3 Anterior serratus muscle
4 Intercostal muscles
5 Intercostal nerve

Exposure of Ribs and Resection of Tumor

The ribs are dissected free subperiosteally to the outer caudal end; the intercostal arteries and veins are exposed, clamped, transected, and ligated. The rib stripper is applied around the ribs (Fig. 12.**5**). After this, the ribs are cut off directly at the spine with rib cutters. The ribs can now be lifted (Fig. 12.**6**). The remainder of the pleura can be retracted (Fig. 12.**7**), or the visceral pleura, with a part of the lung, can be resected; this may be done by electrocautery, after which the cartilaginous portion of the ribs at the costal arch and the sternum can be exposed. The cartilaginous rib portions can be divided by electrocautery, or may also be transected with heavy scissors or rib cutters (Fig. 12.**8**). The tissue block can now be removed. The diaphragm begins in the area of the seventh rib and more distally, and it, too, has to be cut off with scissors. One or two chest tubes should be inserted prior to reconstruction.

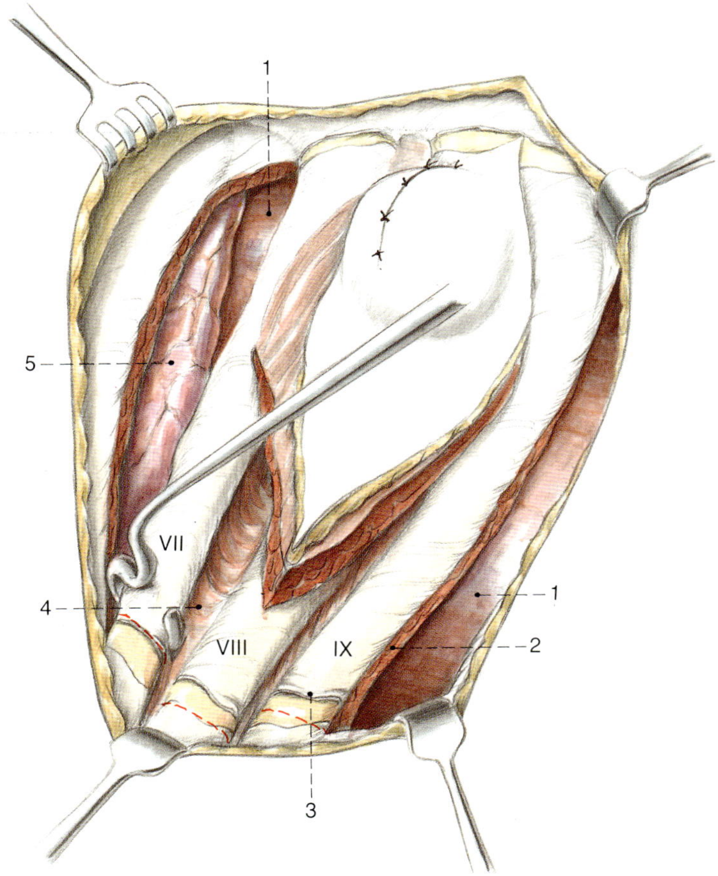

Fig. 12.**5** Circumvention of posterior portions of affected ribs with a rib stripper.

1 Thoracic diaphragm
2 Intercostal muscles
3 Periosteum
5 Intercostal artery
6 Right lung
7 Thoracic diaphragm

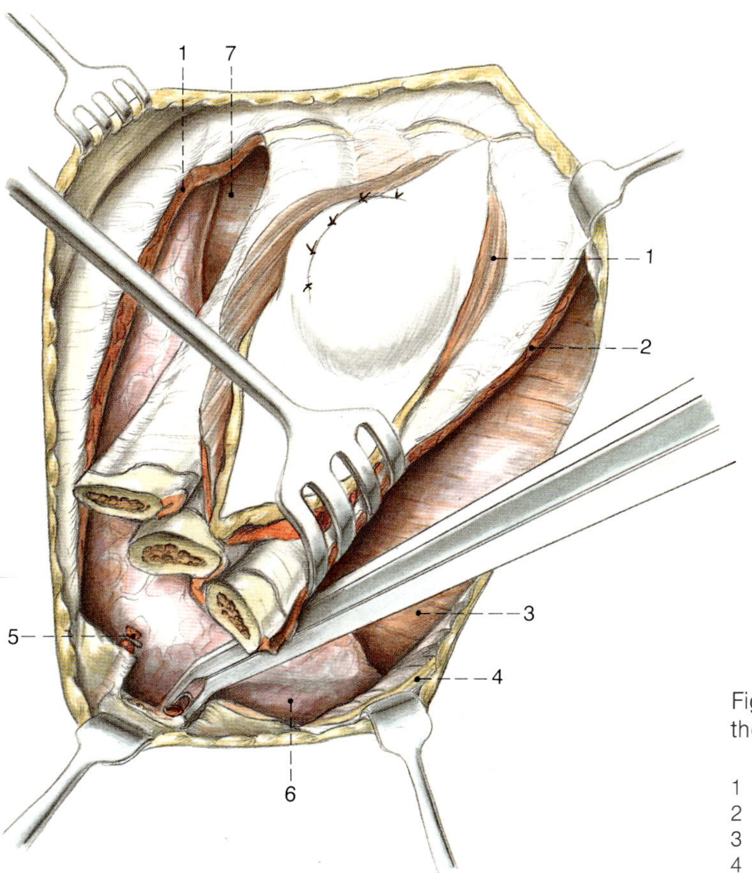

Fig. 12.**6** The ribs are separated from the spine with rib cutters at the extreme posterior end.

1 Intercostal muscles
2 Anterior serratus muscle
3 Thoracic diaphragm
4 Intercostal nerve
4 Internal intercostal muscle
5 Right lung
VII–IX Ribs

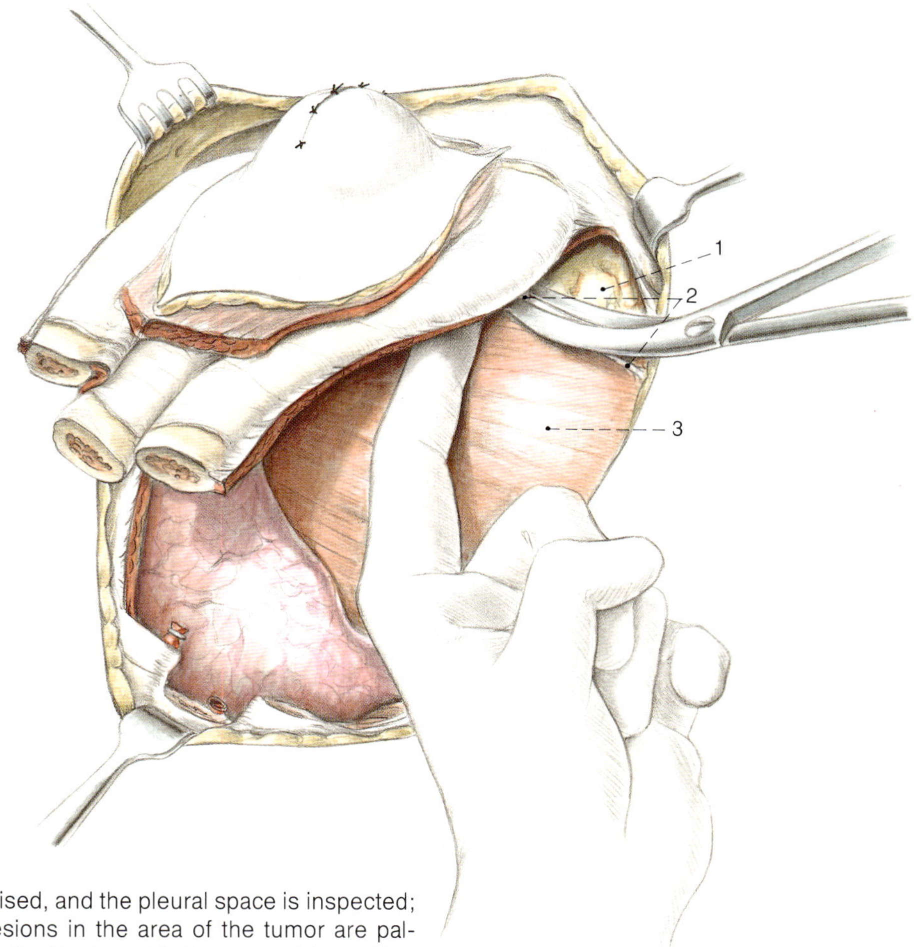

Fig. 12.**7** The ribs are raised, and the pleural space is inspected; possible pulmonary adhesions in the area of the tumor are palpated, and the diaphragmatic attachment in the musculature of the diaphragm is separated from the preparation.

1 Greater omentum
2 Origin of thoracic diaphragm
3 Thoracic diaphragm

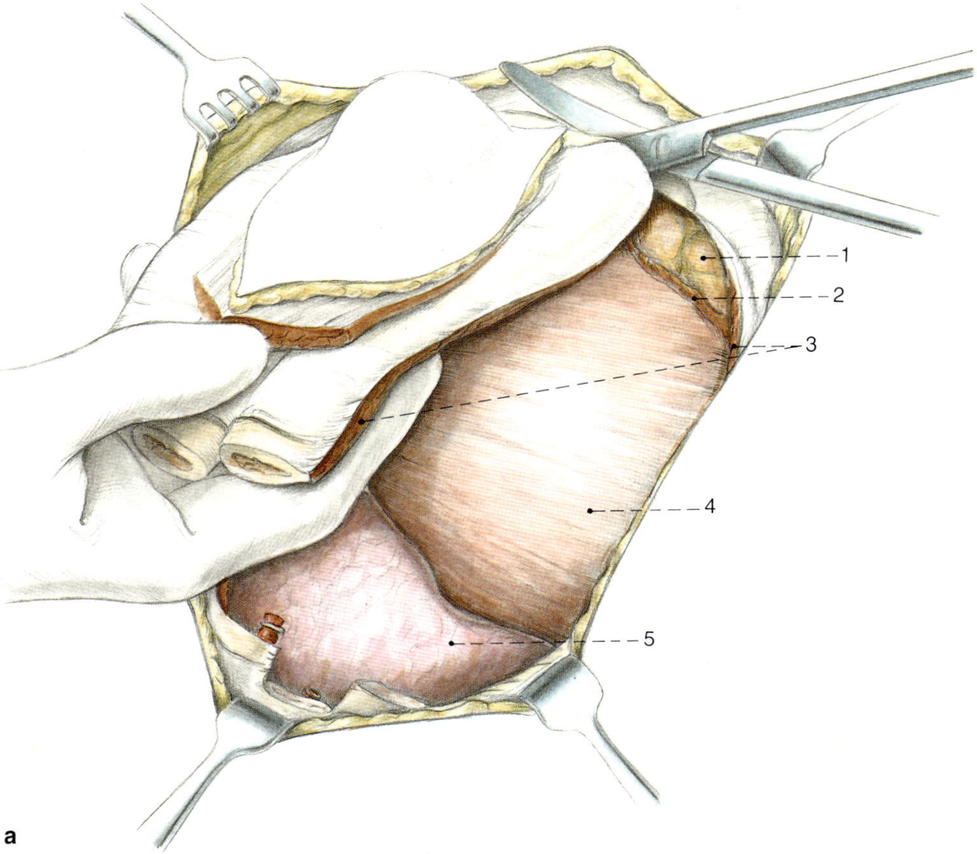

a

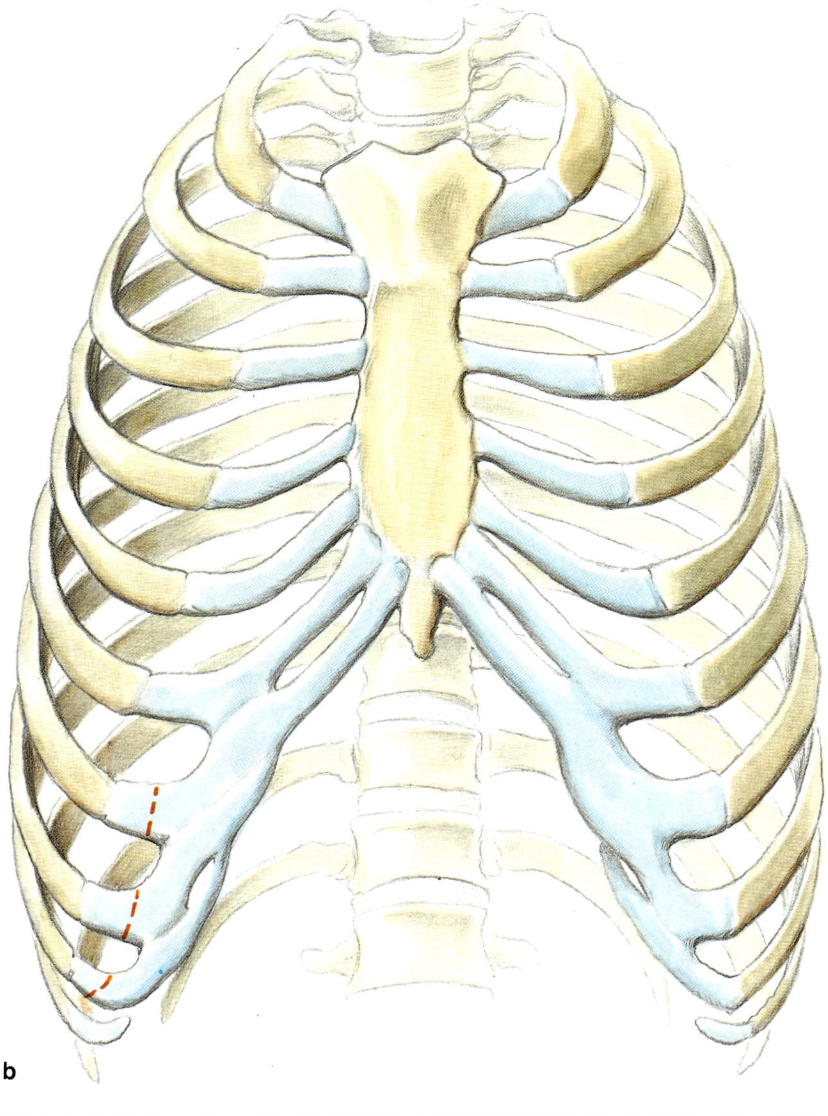

b

Fig. 12.**8a** The posteriorly-separated ribs are lifted out of the thoracic space. In the cartilaginous portion, the preparation is now divided with rib cutters at a good distance from the tumor area.

1 Greater omentum
2 Origin of the thoracic diaphragm
3 Intercostal muscles
4 Thoracic diaphragm
5 Right lung

b The dashed line marks the resection margin in the cartilaginous portion of the affected ribs.

Reconstructive Coverage

A stable chest wall reconstruction has to be provided, with the material for the reconstruction being osseously attached to the rib stumps and the suprajacent and subjacent ribs. Fascia, diaphragmatic ribs, the latissimus dorsi muscle, as well as plastics and metal mesh, have been used as graft material. A secure coverage is provided by dermis, which can be removed from the thigh by split-skin resection and sutured into the defect in strips.

Harvesting of Dermis

Two slices of a split-thickness skin graft, 20–30 cm long, are retracted from the anterior or lateral side of the thigh with a dermatome, and folded back. The dermis is now cut on all sides, lifted at the end, and carefully dissected from the thigh, leaving the subcutis intact (Fig. 12.**9**). This piece of corium should be large enough to cover the defect in the costal region. After removal of this piece of skin, the split skin is replaced on the subcutis of the thigh, and the thigh is covered with Adaptic or fat gauze (Fig. 12.**10**).

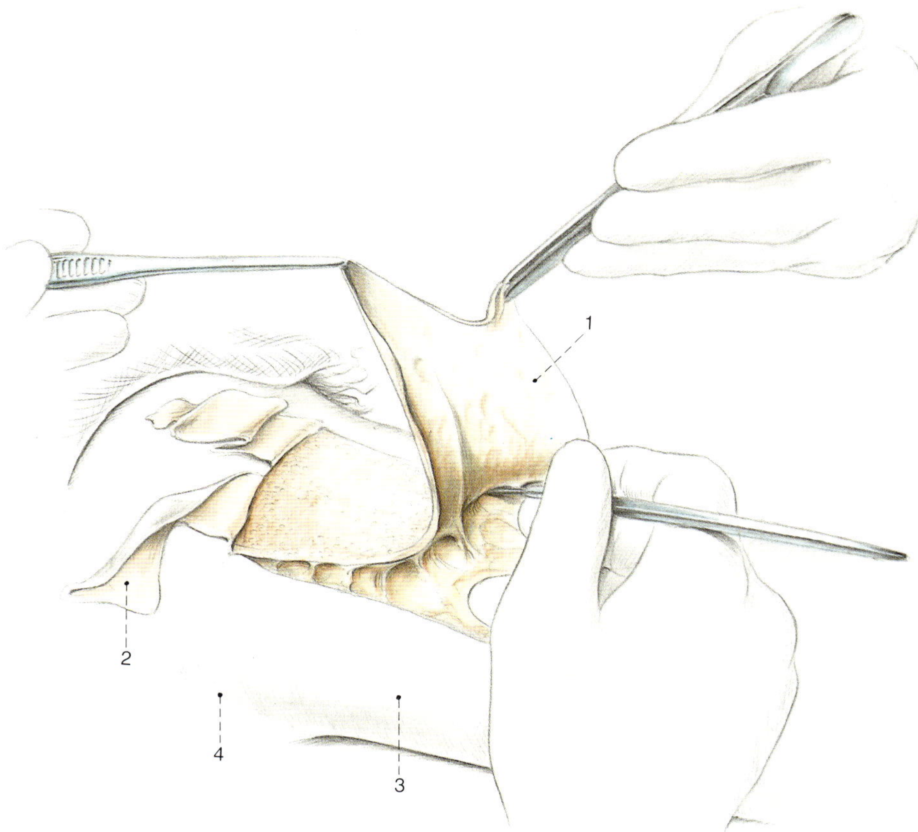

Fig. 12.**9** Removal of dermis from the thigh following split-skin resection.

1 Split-skin flap, dermis
2 Split-skin flap, epidermis
3 Femur
4 Gluteal region

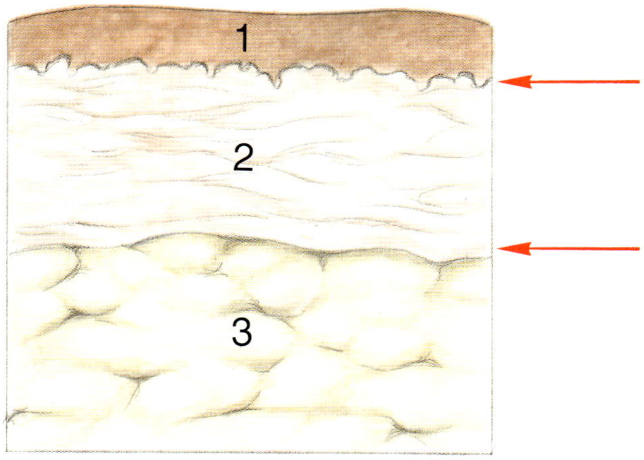

Fig. 12.**10** Composition of skin.

1 Epidermis
2 Dermis
3 Hypodermis

Stabilization of the Thorax

The piece of dermis is now fitted into the defect (Fig. 12.**11**) and sutured to the rib stumps in the posterior region with partly transosseous sutures, and to the borders of the adjacent unaffected ribs with periosteal sutures. The dermis is also used to cover the peritoneum if the diaphragmatic attachment has also been resected (Fig. 12.**12**), in order to separate the two cavities again.

Sliding Flap Coverage

Following complete implantation of the dermal flap (Fig. 12.**13**), the plastic reconstruction on the chest wall is carried out with a rotation flap (Fig. 12.**14**).

The defect itself is covered by direct wound closure of the cutis–subcutis flap if the resection has been small, and by skin flap rotation for larger resections, for which a large pectoral graft is best suited.

Postoperative Treatment

Chest wall defects covered in this manner are primarily stable, so that after 2–4 days, the chest tube can be withdrawn, and the patient can also be disconnected from continuous machine-assisted ventilation. The patient is discharged from the hospital after 7–10 days, and can resume physical exercise after six weeks.

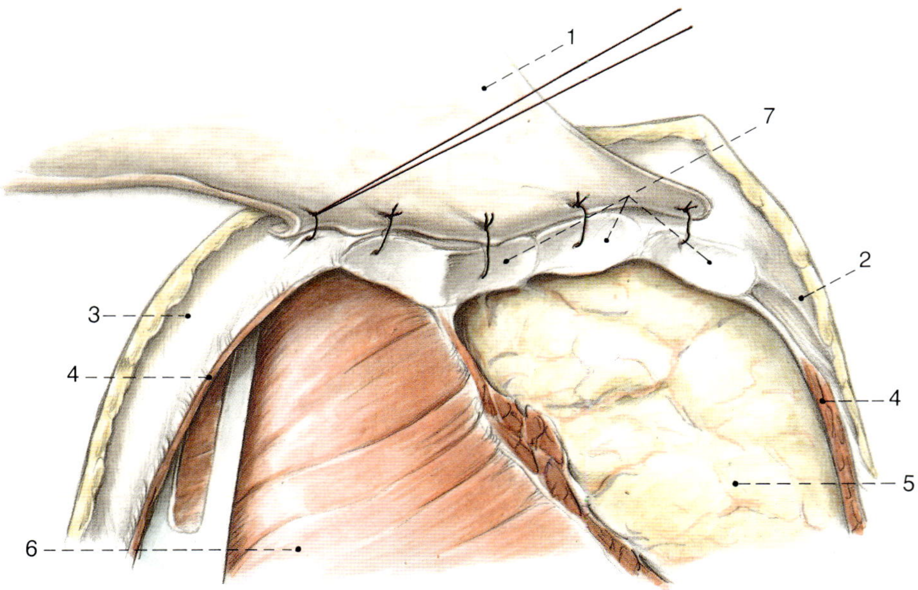

Fig. 12.**11** The dermis is fixed into the chest wall with sutures through the cartilaginous and bony ribs.

1 Split skin flap
2 Tenth rib
3 Sixth rib
4 Intercostal muscles
5 Greater omentum
6 Thoracic diaphragm
7 Costal cartilage

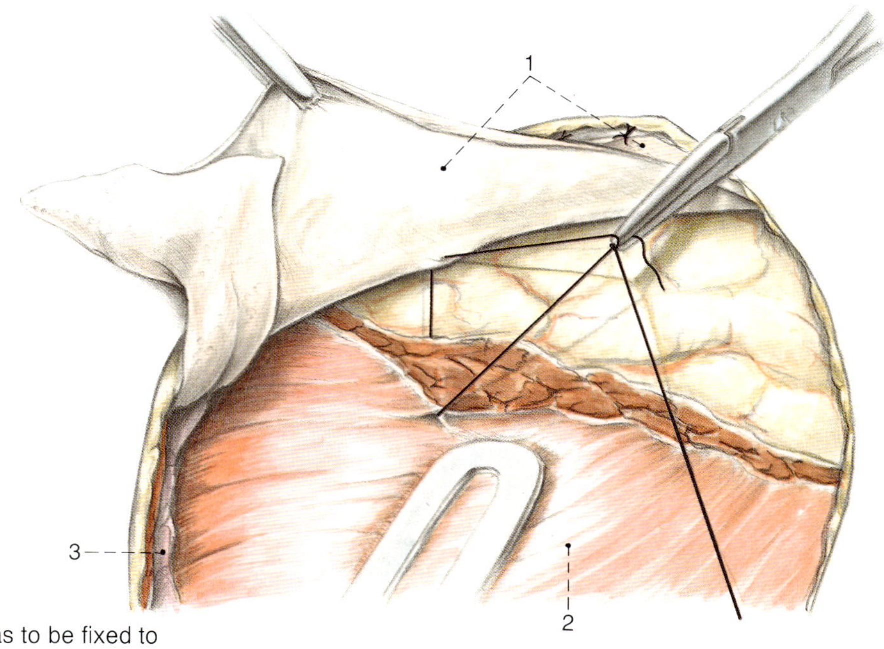

Fig. 12.**12** The diaphragmatic attachment also has to be fixed to the dermis, using interrupted sutures.

1 Dermis
2 Thoracic diaphragm
3 Right lung

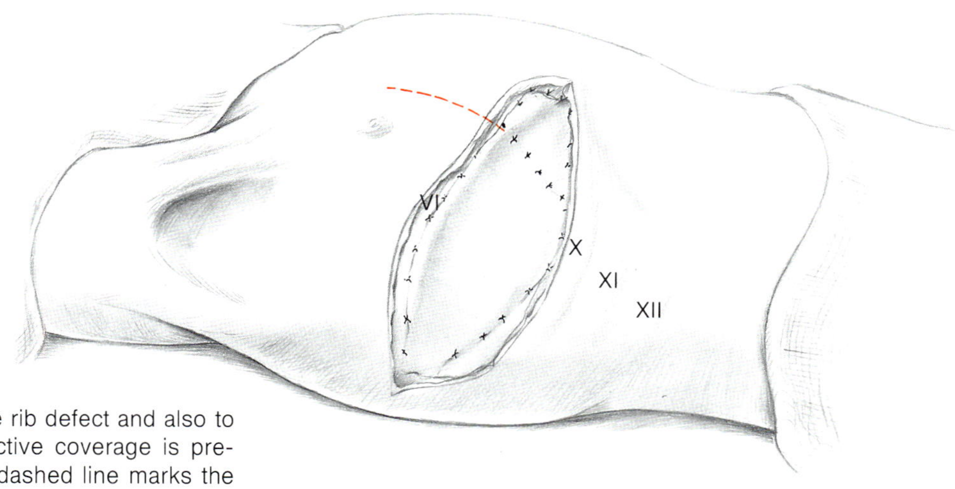

Fig. 12.**13** The dermis is now fixed in the rib defect and also to the diaphragmatic attachment. Reconstructive coverage is prepared with the use of a rotation flap (the dashed line marks the relief skin incision).

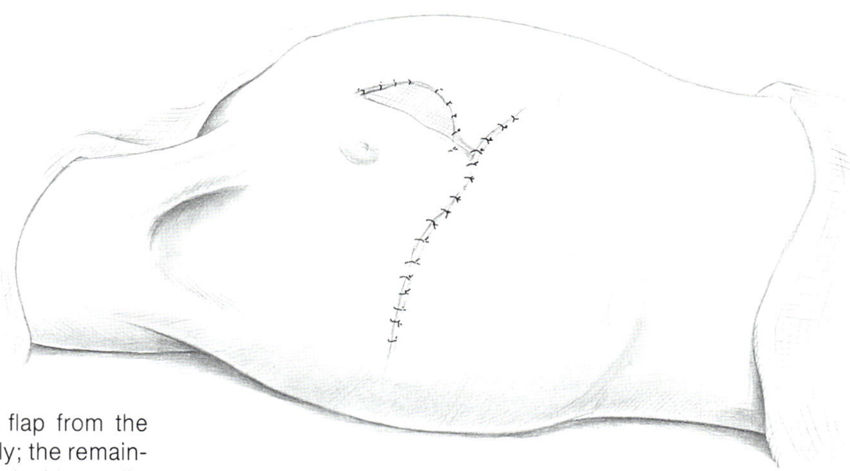

Fig. 12.**14** After rotation of a musculocutaneous flap from the pectoral region, the rib defect can be covered directly; the remaining skin defect on the anterior chest wall is covered with a split-thickness skin graft.

Further Reading

Atkins PC. Tumors of the chest wall. In: Shields TW, ed. General thoracic surgery. 2nd ed. Philadelphia: Lea and Febiger, 1983:453.

Biscard JD, Swenson SA. Tumors of the sternum: report of a case with special operative technic. Arch Surg 1984;56:570.

Boyd AD, Shaw WW, McCarthy JG. Immediate reconstruction of full-thickness chest wall defects. Ann Thorac Surg 1981;32:336.

Bruck H. Die Dermislappenplastik für den Verschluß von Körperhöhlen. Langenbecks Arch Klin Chir 1963;303:277.

Dingman RO, Argenta LC. Reconstruction of the chest wall. Ann Thorac Surg 1981;32:202.

Gingrass RR. Flaps for chest wall reconstruction. In: Grabb WC, Myers MB, eds. Skin flaps. Boston: Little, Brown, 1975.

Hubbard SG. Repair of chest wall defects with prosthetic material. Ann Thorac Surg 1979;27:440.

McCormack P, Bains MS, Beattie EJ, Martini N. New trends in skeletal reconstruction after resection of chest wall tumors. Ann Thorac Surg 1981;31:45.

McCraw JB, Penix JO, Baker JW. Repair of major defects of the chest wall and spine with the latissimus dorsi myocutaneous flap. Plast Reconstr Surg 1978;62:197.

Merkle NM, Isele G, Vogt-Moykopf I. Die chirurgische Therapie der Brustwandtumoren. Chirurg 1988;59:248–55.

Metheny D, Lundmark VO, Marcom T. The use of dermal graft to supply defects in the diaphragm. West J Surg 1962;60:156.

Piza-Katzer H, Appel WH, Kotz R, Wagner O. Funktionsgerechte Wiederherstellung eines kombinierten Bauch-, Thoraxwand- und Zwerchfelldefektes mit Corium nach Sternum-Tumorresektion. Chirurg 1983;54:157–60.

Ramming KP, Holmes EC, Zarem HA. Surgical management and reconstruction of extensive chest wall malignancies. Am J Surg 1982;144:146.

13 Deformities of the Chest Wall

H. Sauer

Funnel Chest

Indications

Initially, evaluation of a funnel chest was based only on the surface conditions. For function, however, the skeletal conditions are more important. The funnel chest indices provide objective criteria (Backer et al. 1961).

The frontosagittal index (Fig. 13.**1a**) is the ratio between the smallest sagittal diameter from the most posteriorly situated point of the sternum to the anterior surface of the vertebral body (at the same level), and the largest frontal diameter (inner surface of the ribs).

$$\text{Frontosagittal index} = \frac{\text{Sagittal diameter} \times 100}{\text{Frontal diameter}}$$

Normal values: 36–56, mean value 46; pathological values: below 36.

The vertebral index (Fig. 13.**1b**) is the ratio between the shortest sagittal diameter and the diameter of the vertebral body at the same level.

Normal values: 15–25, mean value 20; pathological values: above 25.

These indices also cover restrictive funnel chests that are characterized by high-grade flattening of one or both halves of the thorax, so that the excavation does not appear very deep.

Many surgeons also recognize the psychologic–cosmetic factor as an indication. The most favorable age for surgery is 2–6 years. Because of the anticipated increase in growth, some authors warn against an operation between ages 8 and 12 (von der Oelsnitz 1983), while others see no reason for such a restriction (Hecker et al. 1981).

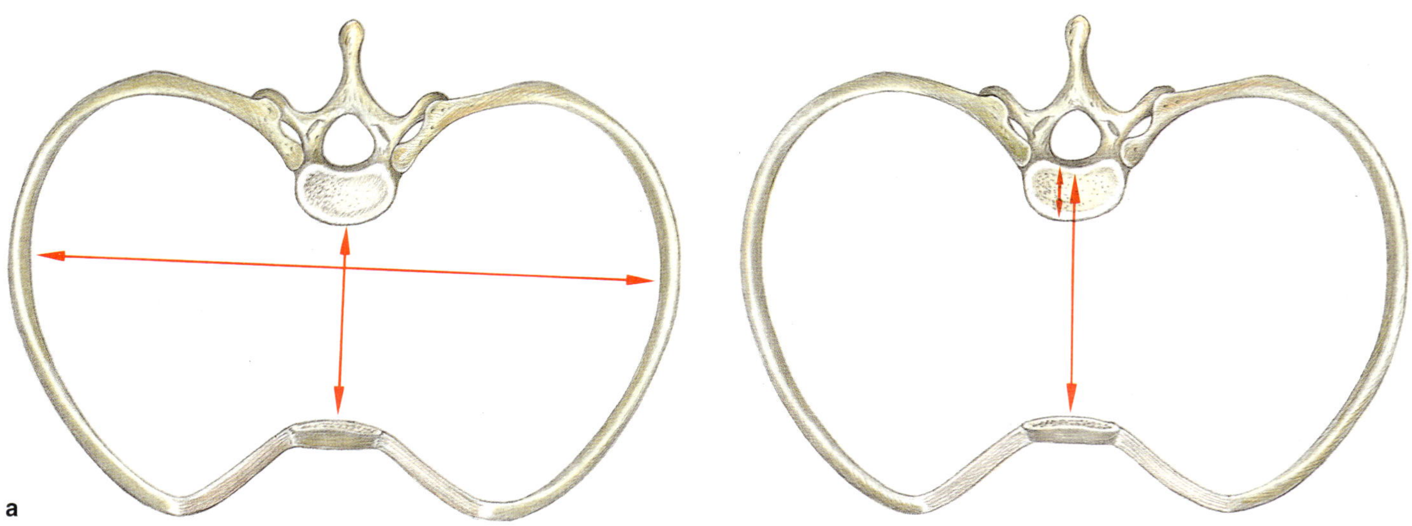

a

Fig. 13.**1** Measurements for determination of funnel chest indices.

Rehbein Operation

Principle

The sternum and the costal cartilage are sufficiently mobilized to be placed in the desired (slightly overcorrecting) position. The stabilization is effected by means of metal braces, which are left in place for three to five years and prevent renewed sagging. The plates can slide against each other.

Approach

The patient is positioned supine with the arms symmetrical, abducted or adducted.

The anterior chest wall has to be exposed beyond the excavation of the sternum and costal cartilage. This exposure is possible only from median to lateral (Fig. 13.**2**).

The midline incision from the manubrium sterni to the midpoint between the xiphoid process and the umbilicus allows the skin, subcutis, and musculature to be dissected from the bone en bloc.

The submammary incision necessitates cranial and caudal dissection of the skin, since the muscle complex, too, is dissected from medial to lateral in this approach. This incision, performed in women, causes the scar to disappear under the mammae, but is more frequently associated with wound healing complications, and in girls breast development may be impaired. This type of incision, therefore, is preferably used in postpubertal female patients.

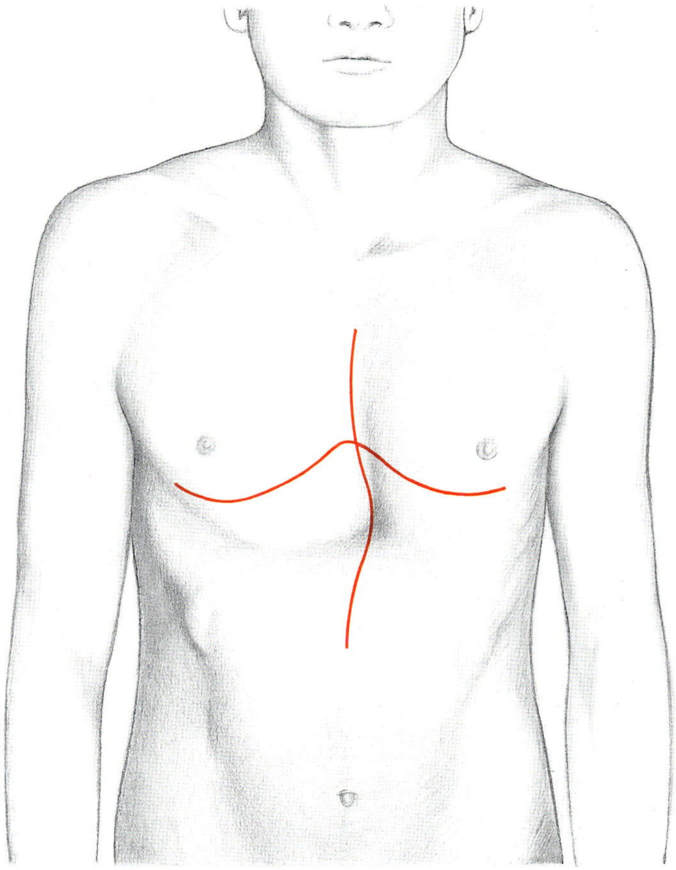

Fig. 13.**2** Median or submammary skin incision.

Operative Technique

Exposure of the Anterior Chest Wall

The sternal membrane and the linea alba are incised (Fig. 13.**3**). The sternal membrane is dissected free of the sternal periosteum, together with the pectoral musculature. At the lowest point of the excavation, at the lower end of the sternum, the fixation is particularly firm. Care should be taken that the membrane does not tear, as it is important to cover the implanted braces completely with the musculomembranous layer. The posterior leaf of the rectus abdominis muscle sheath is split in the midline (Fig. 13.**4**). The rectus abdominis muscle, with the anterior leaf of the rectus sheath, is freed from its thoracic origin and dissected free laterally, together with the sternal membrane and the pectoral musculature. The bony portion of the ribs is exposed for about 2–3 cm. In patients with an asymmetrical funnel chest, the ribs on the flattened side should be exposed laterally beyond the anterior axillary line (Fig. 13.**5**), and the same should be done bilaterally for a through-shaped, flat funnel chest. This also requires partial detachment of the origins of the serratus anterior muscle from the thorax. The vessels emerging from the chest wall, medial and lateral cutaneous branches, are carefully coagulated. The superior epigastric vessels can usually be spared; occasionally, however, they have to be ligated. Following exposure of the anterior thorax from one side, a large bowel towel is placed in the lateral wound angle, and the other side is dissected (Fig. 13.**6**).

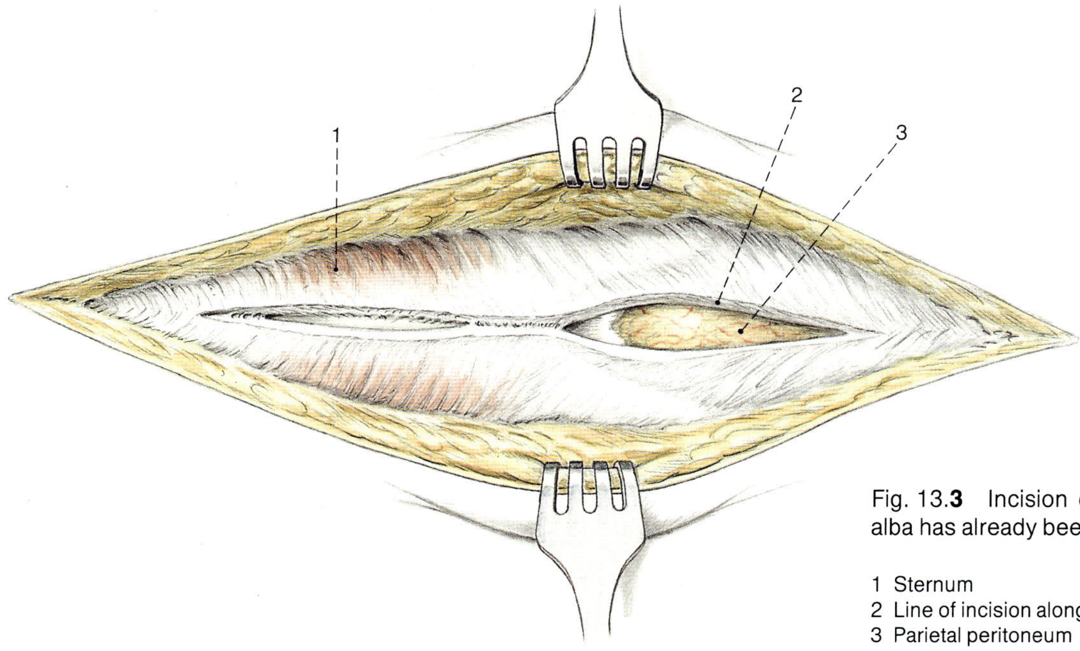

Fig. 13.**3** Incision of sternal membrane. The linea alba has already been incised.

1 Sternum
2 Line of incision along the linea alba
3 Parietal peritoneum

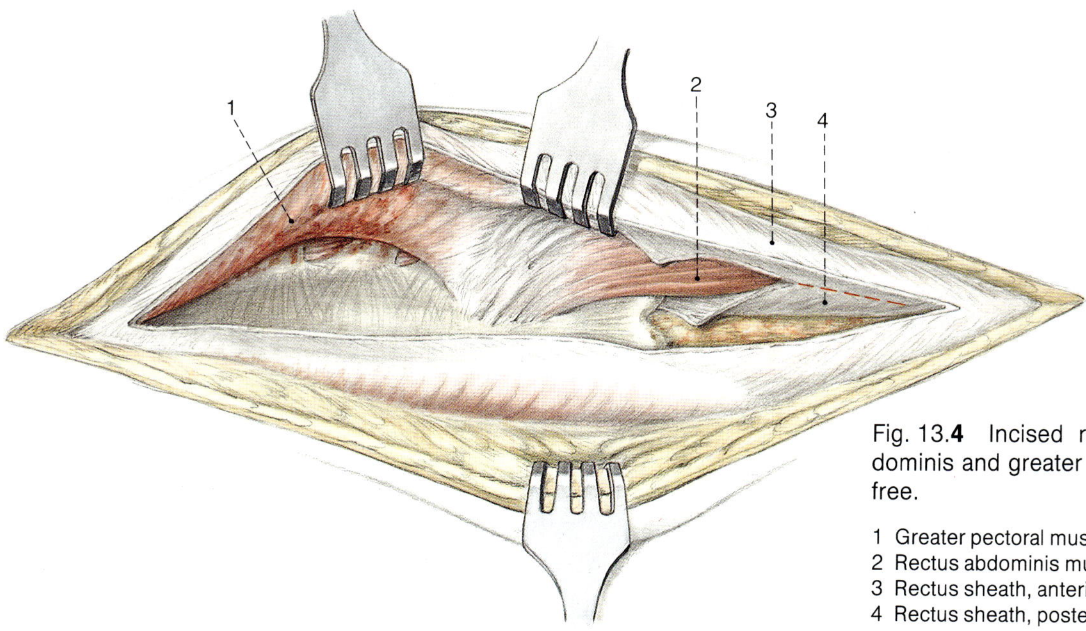

Fig. 13.**4** Incised rectus sheath. The rectus abdominis and greater pectoral muscles are dissected free.

1 Greater pectoral muscle
2 Rectus abdominis muscle
3 Rectus sheath, anterior leaf
4 Rectus sheath, posterior leaf

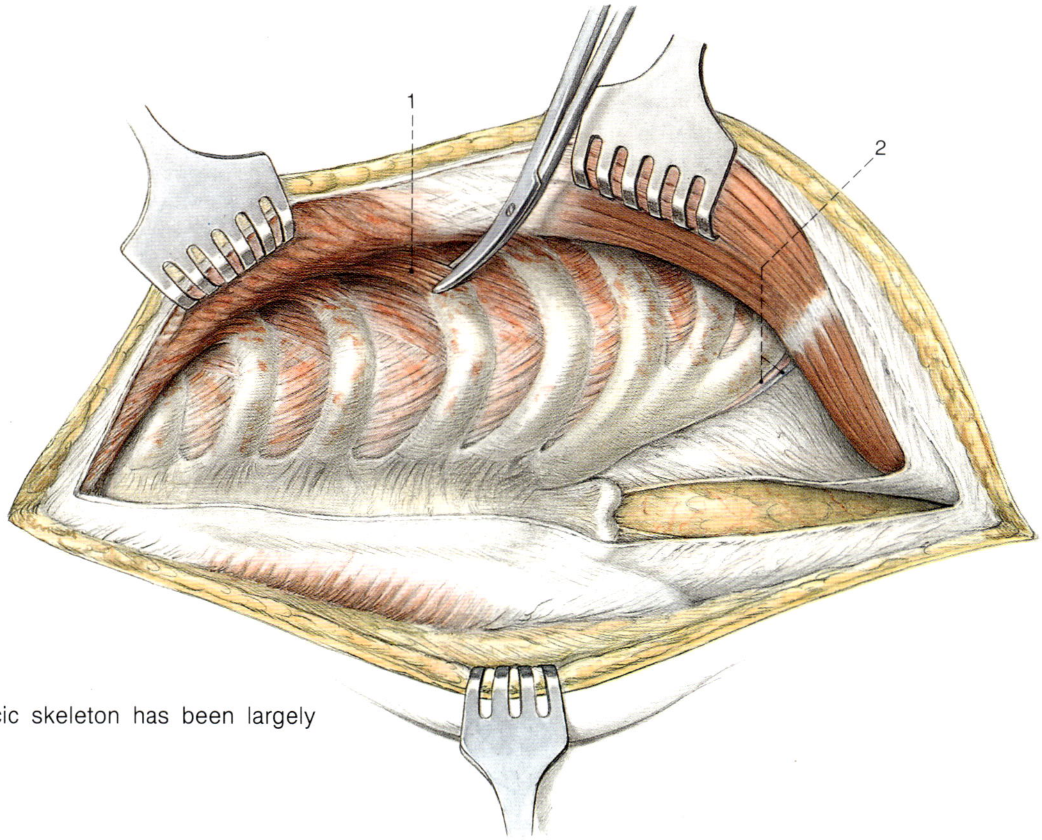

Fig. 13.**5** The left anterior thoracic skeleton has been largely exposed.

1 Anterior serratus muscle
2 Superior epigastric vessels

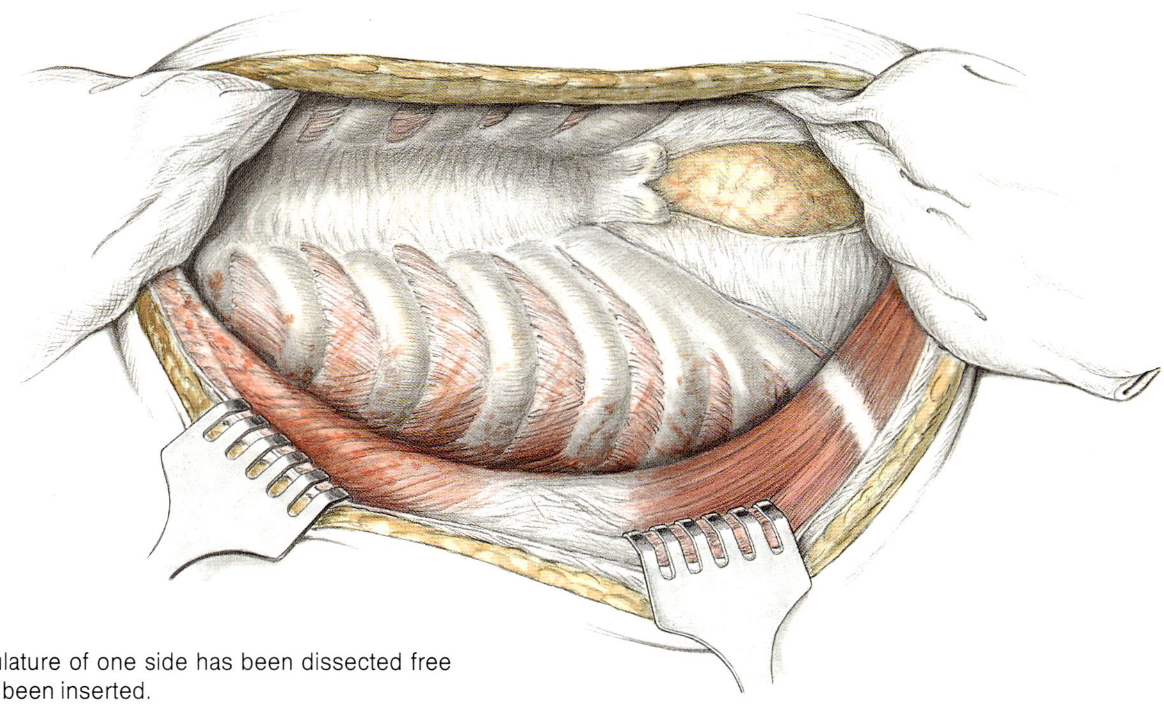

Fig. 13.**6** The musculature of one side has been dissected free and a bowel towel has been inserted.

Mobilization of Anterior Chest Wall

The xiphoid process is resected (Fig. 13.**7**), the sternum is lifted with a bone hook and the mediastinum is retracted from the sternum with the index finger (Fig. 13.**8a**). In addition, the pleura is bluntly detached bilaterally from the anterior chest wall. On the right side, in particular, the delicate costal pleura may easily tear during this step. If this happens, it is expedient to widen the opening, to insert a chest tube in the mediastinum before the end of the operation, and to bring it out over the linea alba. For mobilization of the costal arches, the rib attachments of the diaphragm are detached anteriorly, and the pleura is retracted further (Fig. 13.**8b**).

The perichondrium of ribs 3–10 is incised for about 1 cm in a winglike fashion at the sternal rib attachment (Fig. 13.**9a**), and retracted (Fig. 13.**9b**). After this, a portion of cartilage 3–5 mm wide is resected with a rongeur over the entire circumference of the cartilage (Fig. 13.**9c**). The same procedure is followed at the costochondral boundary lateral to the costal cartilages. With an asymmetrical excavation, it is expedient to notch the costal bone, too, further laterally on the flat side, so that it can be straightened from the mediastinal side by kinking of the inner cortical lamella (Fig. 13.**9d**). The mobilization is completed by notching the anterior sternal lamella with a rongeur and kinking the posterior lamella (Fig. 13.**10**). It should now be possible to move the sternum into the desired position without any significant resistance.

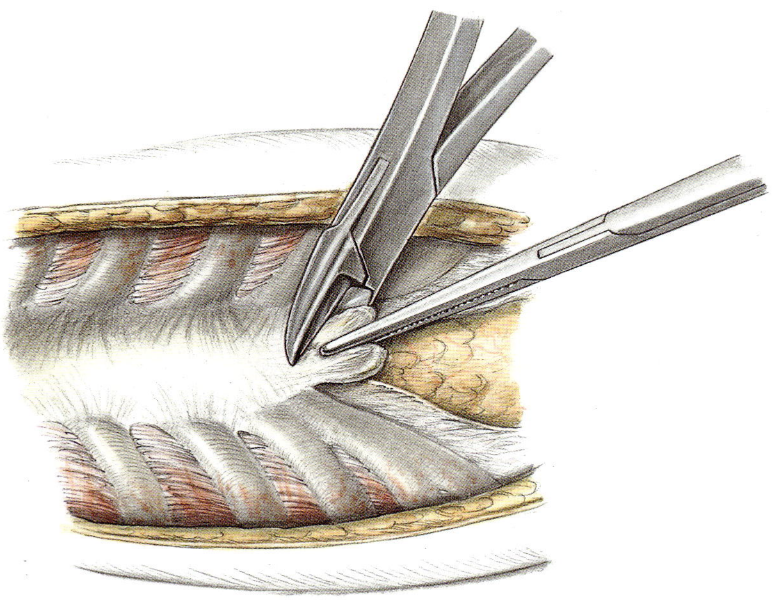

Fig. 13.**7** Resection of the xiphoid process.

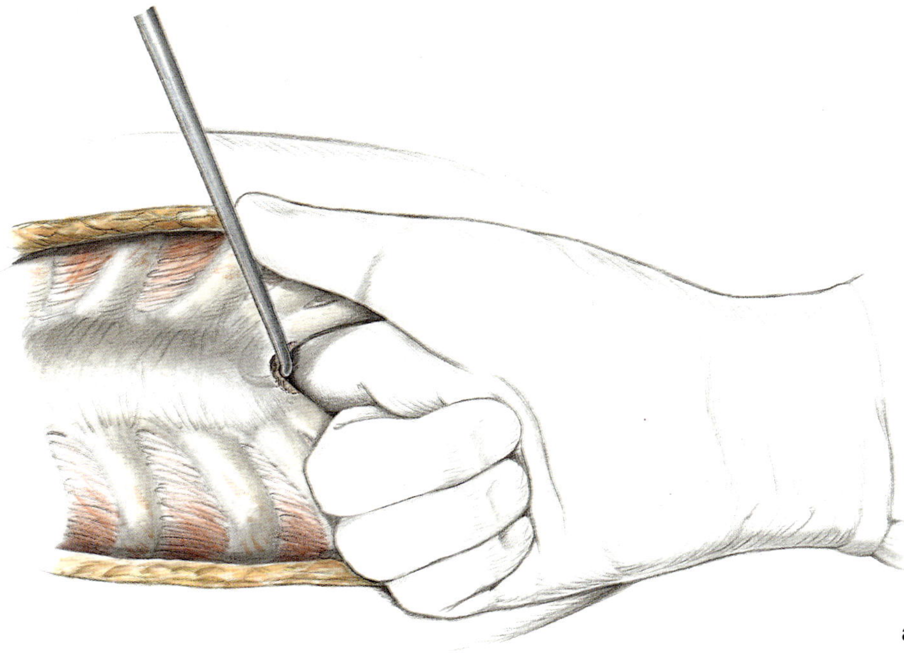

a

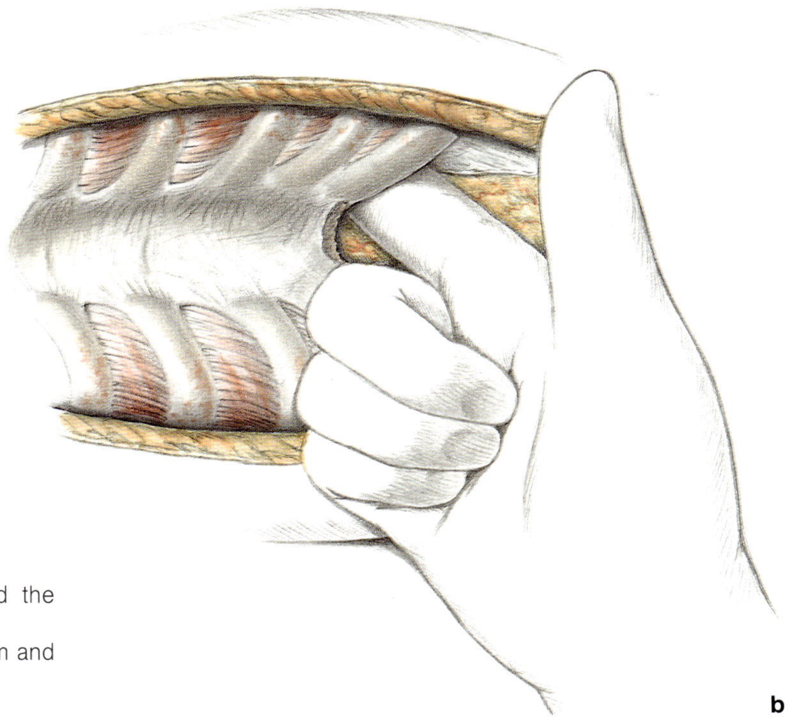

b

Fig. 13.**8a** The sternum is lifted with a bone hook, and the mediastinum is retracted with the index finger.
b Detachment of the anterior costal origins of the diaphragm and of the pleura.

Fig. 13.**9a** Winglike incision of the perichondrium at the medial and lateral ends of the costal cartilage.
b Detachment of the perichondrium.
c Resection of costal cartilage.
d Asymmetrical funnel chest. The cortical layer of the rib is notched on the flattened side.

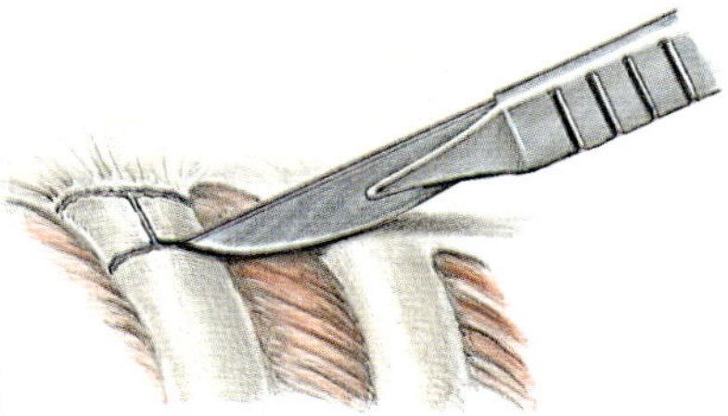

a

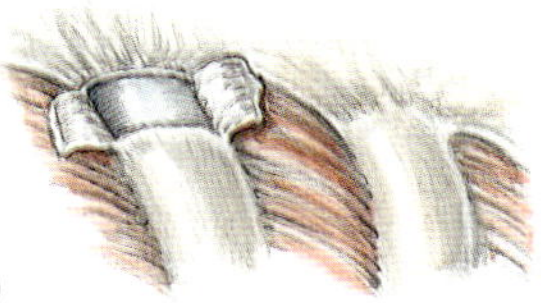

b

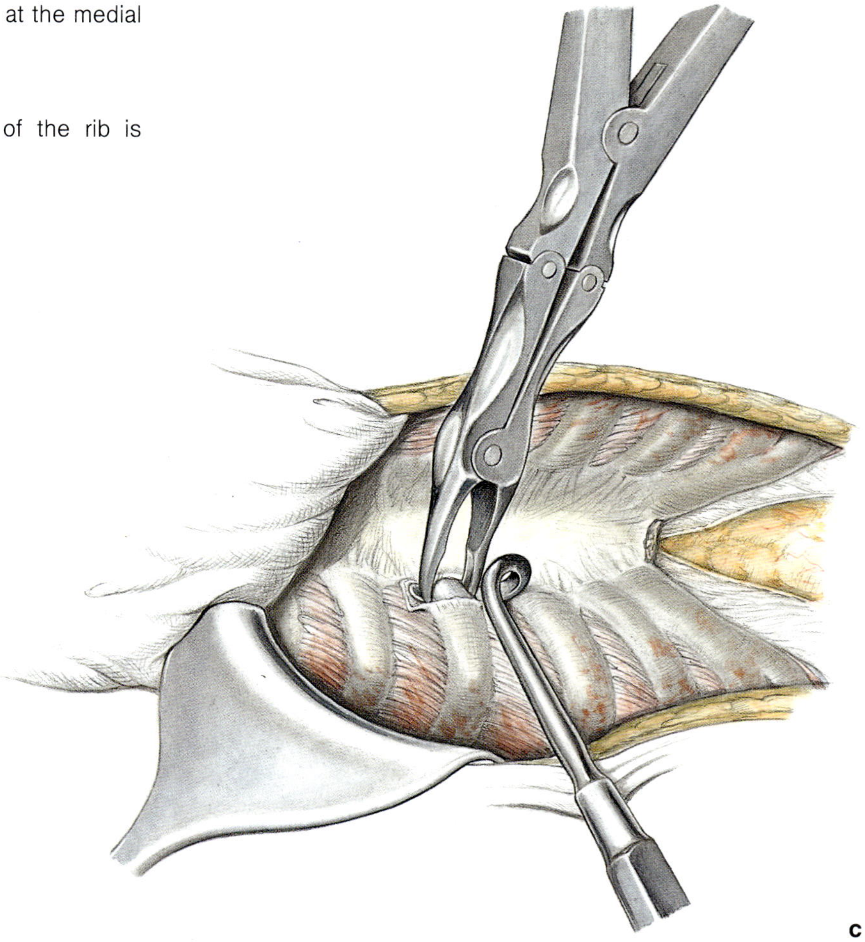

c

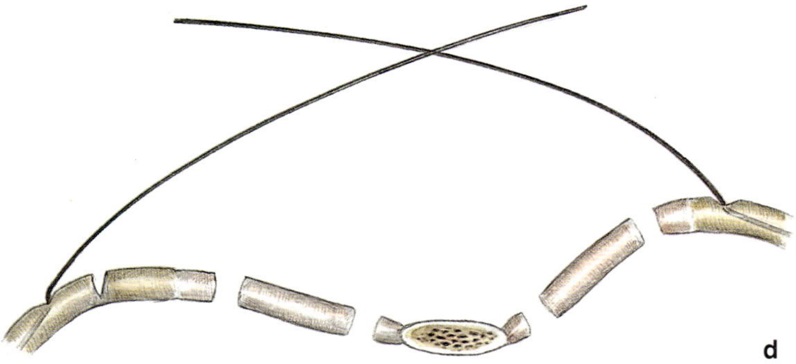

d

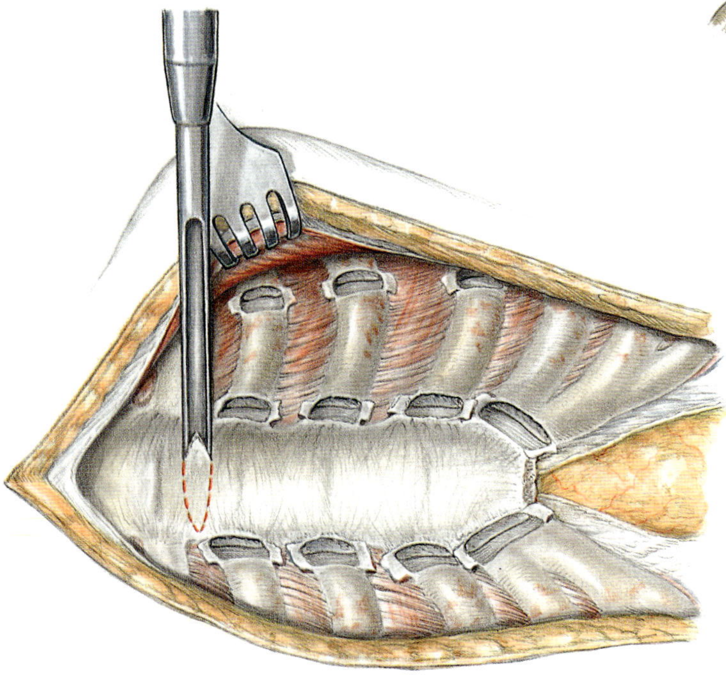

Fig. 13.**10** The anterior cortical layer of the sternum is notched approximately between the manubrium and the body.

Stabilization of Anterior Chest Wall

The mobilized anterior chest wall is attached to metal braces, the bases of which have been inserted into the medullary space of the ribs, and is stabilized by them. The Rehbein braces are available in four different sizes (Fig. 13.**11**). Usually, three pairs and, rarely, two or four are used. The braces are usually implanted into the medullary space of the third, fourth, and fifth ribs. For this purpose, the periosteum of the rib is cruciformly incised 1–2 cm lateral to the costochondral boundary (Fig. 13.**12**) and retracted from the rib. The outer cortical lamella of the rib is opened with a rongeur, special care being taken that the lamella does not splinter. Using a narrow dissector, the medullary space is then opened (Fig. 13.**12**), and the short limb of the brace is introduced. It should extend as far as the bend in the medullary space, if possible (Fig. 13.**13a**). A certain degree of overcorrection should be obtained. Should this turn out to be excessive, the angle between the stem of the brace and the arch has to be flattened. Occasionally, a brace may have to be shortened.

When the funnel chest is asymmetrical, the brace on the flat side occasionally forms a pair with the next lower one on the contralateral side, so that the braces slant.

The sternum is fixed to the braces with steel bands. The bands are pulled through with a wire passer, and tightened with the tensioning device (Fig. 13.**11c**). The mobilized costal cartilages, too, are attached to the braces with these steel bands; at the conclusion of the procedure, the bands are shortened to size.

A wide Hemovac drain is bilaterally introduced into the wound and brought out inferiorly; if necessary, a chest tube is placed in the mediastinum and brought out via the linea alba (Fig. 13.**14**).

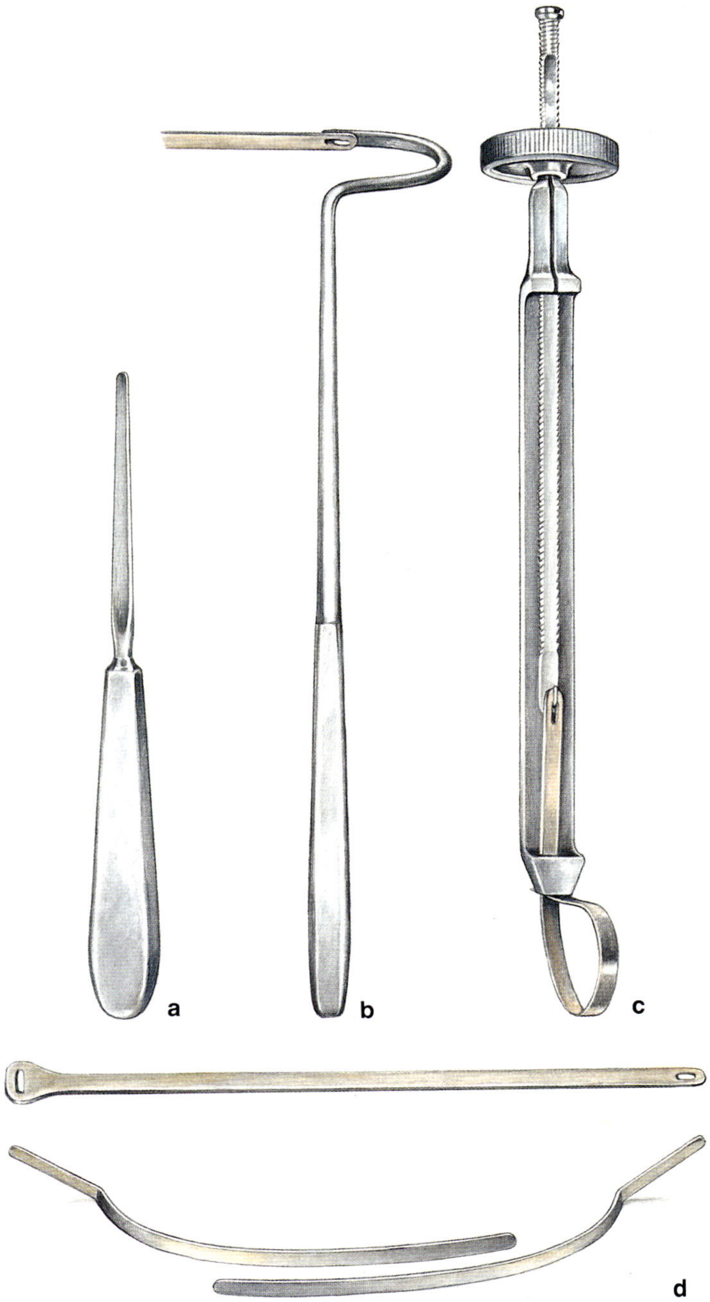

Fig. 13.**11a** Dissector.
b Wire passer for fixation bands.
c Tensioner with fixation band.
d Rehbein braces and fixation band.

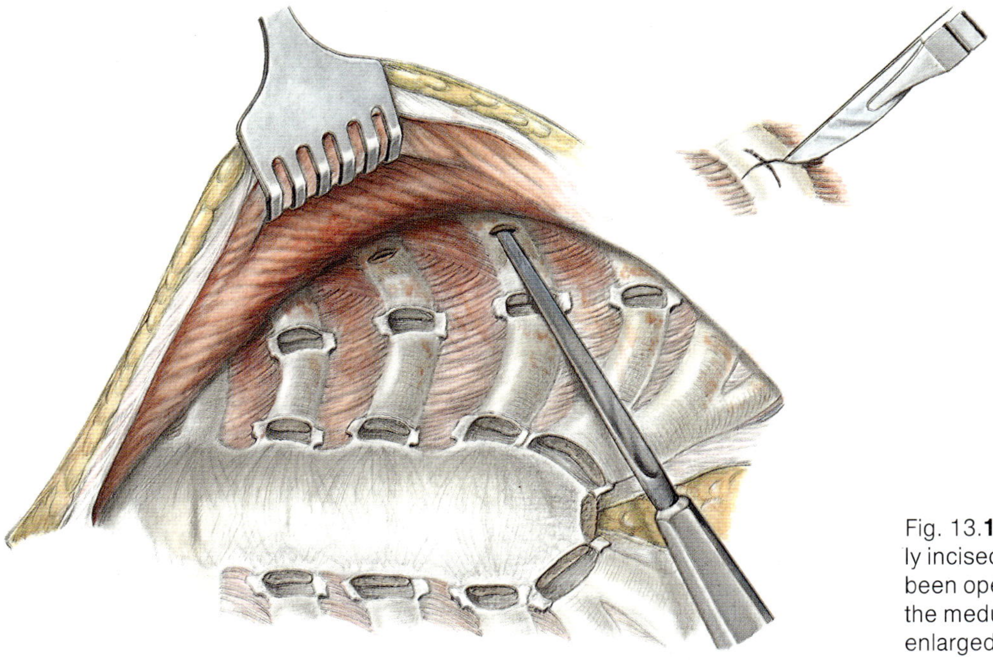

Fig. 13.**12** The periosteum has been cruciformly incised at the ribs; the medullary space has been opened with a rongeur. Using the dissector, the meduallary space of the rib is sufficiently enlarged to permit insertion of the stent base.

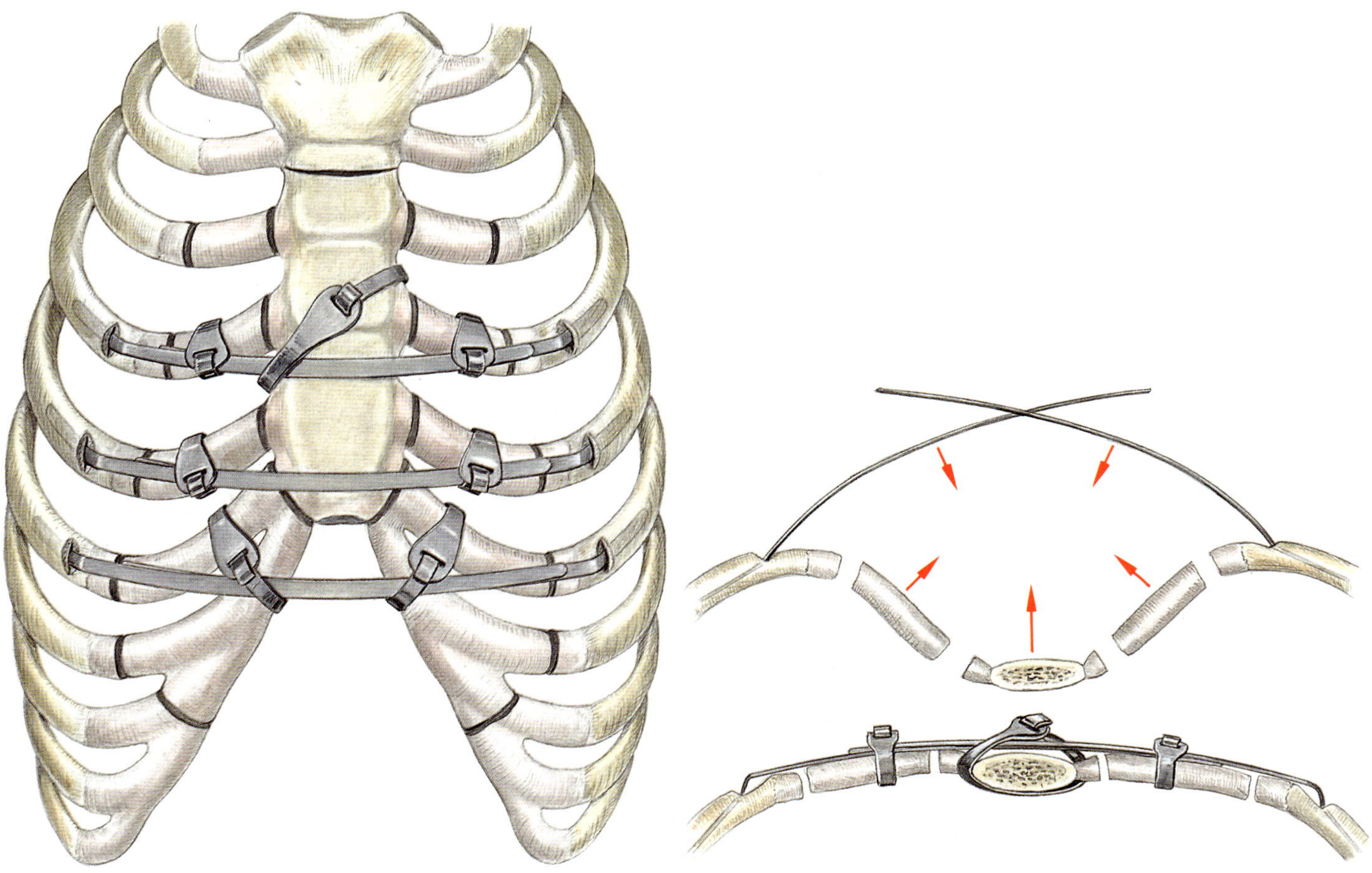

Fig. 13.**13** Stabilization of the anterior chest wall by means of Rehbein braces and fixation bands.

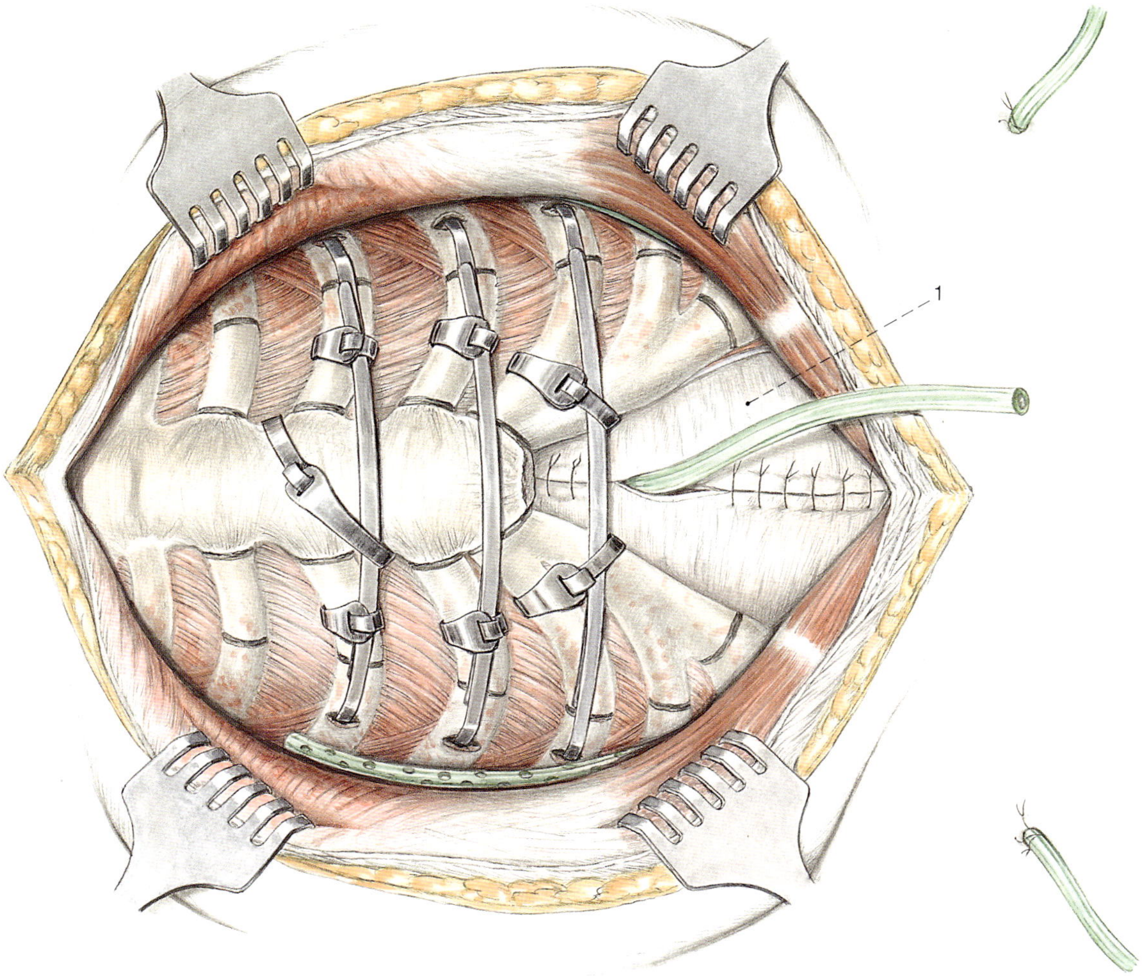

Fig. 13.**14** Position of braces and drains. The posterior rectus sheath (1) is already closed.

Wound Closure

Closure is begun by suture of the anterior and posterior leaves of the rectus sheath and of the sternal membrane, using 2–0 or 3–0 resorbable sutures and subcutaneous suturing. The skin is closed with a continuous intracutaneous wire suture.

Postoperative Treatment

Prophylactic antibiotic therapy should be started intraoperatively and continued for 3–5 days. The patients are positioned flat in bed; intensive care is not required. The drains are removed as soon as drainage ceases. The patients are then mobilized. Physical activities should be restricted during the first three months; after that, it is quite desirable for the patients to engage in exercise, such as swimming, for example. Breathing exercise and orthopedic calisthenics are recommended.

Removal of the Braces

The braces are left in place for at least three years, and up to five years in younger children. To remove them, the median scar is excised and the braces are exposed. The superficial brace is transected with a side cutter and pulled out in two parts; the gliding layer between the braces is split down to the fixation bands, and these are then removed. Finally, the deeper-lying brace, is also taken out. The skin is closed again with an intracutaneous wire suture.

Complications

Defective wound healing is the most important complication. Serious disturbances of wound healing have been prevented for many years now by the following measures:

- Postponement of the operation in the presence of infections, especially of the airways.
- Use of wide Hemovac drains.
- Intraoperative initiation of a short course of prophylactic antibiotic therapy.

Ravitch Operation

Principle

The deformed costal cartilage are completely resected. The body of the sternum is freed from all its lateral, caudal, and posterior connections, corrected posteriorly, and placed on the stumps of the second costal cartilage. The overcorrection is reduced by closure of the muscular layer.

Approach

Positioning and incision are the same as for the Rehbein operation (p. 423).

Operative Technique

Exposure of the Anterior Chest Wall

The sternal membrane and the pectoral musculature are dissected free laterally as far as the costochondral boundary. The costal cartilages are exposed by oblique incision of the anterior leaf of the rectus sheath and the rectus abdominis muscle (Fig. 13.**15**). A winglike opening is made across the entire perichondrium of the deformed costal cartilage, and the perichondrium is then retracted cranially and caudally with a raspatory. Subsequently, the cartilages are also detached from the perichondrium on the posterior side, using a rib stripper. The cartilage is then divided laterally, lifted and, after being completely freed, sepa-

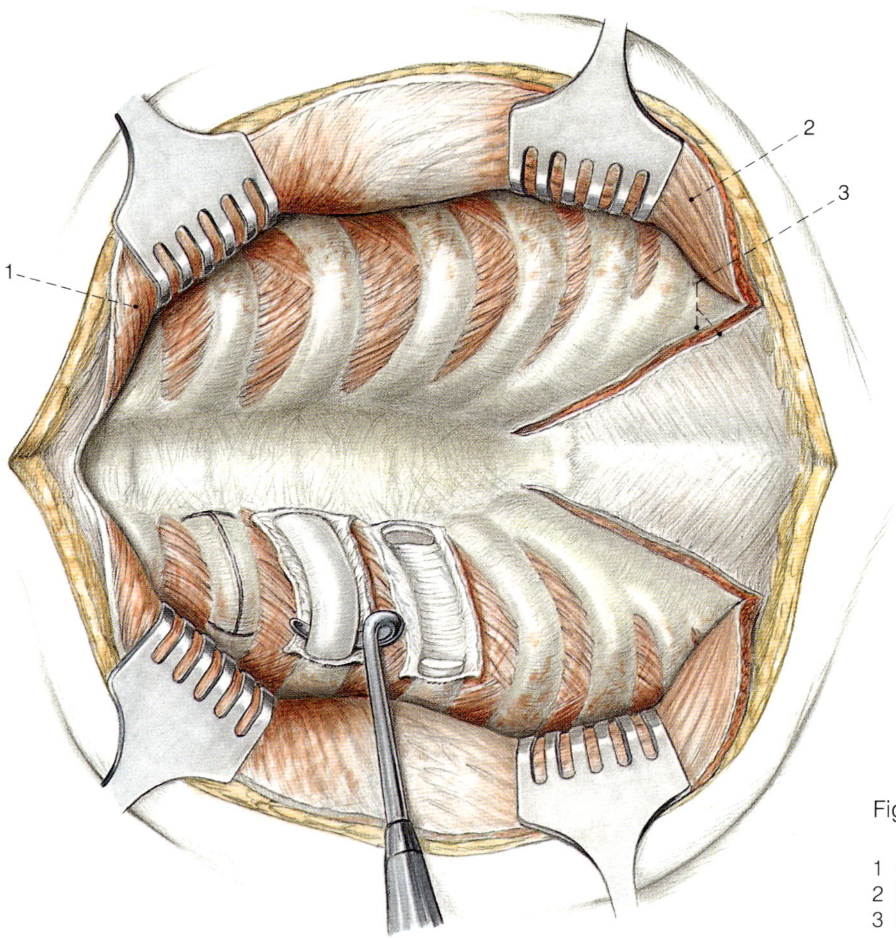

Fig. 13.**15** Resection of deformed costal cartilage.

1 Greater pectoral muscle
2 Rectus abdominis muscle
3 Rectus sheath

rated at the sternum. Occasionally, it is easier to grasp it in the middle with a Kocher clamp, divide it, and then remove the two halves of the cartilage individually. After resection of the costal cartilages, the xiphoid process is separated from the sternum with scissors. It remains connected to the rectus abdominis muscles. The caudal end of the sternum is lifted with a bone hook; using the index finger or a cotton-tipped tissue dissector, the mediastinum and the pleura of the costomediastinal sinus are retracted (Fig. 13.**8a**). Close to the lateral border of the sternum, the perichondrium, the intercostal musculature, and the endothoracic fascia are now divided with scissors. To spare the internal thoracic vessels, it is imperative to stay directly at the sternal border (Fig. 13.**16**). The first normal costal cartilage from the caudal side (generally the second, and occasionally the third) is divided with a scalpel near the sternum, going obliquely from medial–anterior to lateral–posterior (Fig. 13.**17**). After this, the sternum is raised, and the posterior cortical lamella is transversely notched along a guide wire. A narrow bone wedge taken from a rib is implanted into this notch and fixed in the manubrium with a mattress suture (Fig. 13.**18**). Elevation of the sternum has placed the lateral ends of the divided costal cartilage behind the medial ends; the two ends of the costal cartilage are attached to one another by sutures.

If the sternum shows a strong posterior curvature, the anterior cortical lamella is notched at the sharpest bend, and here, too, a bone wedge from the rib is implanted

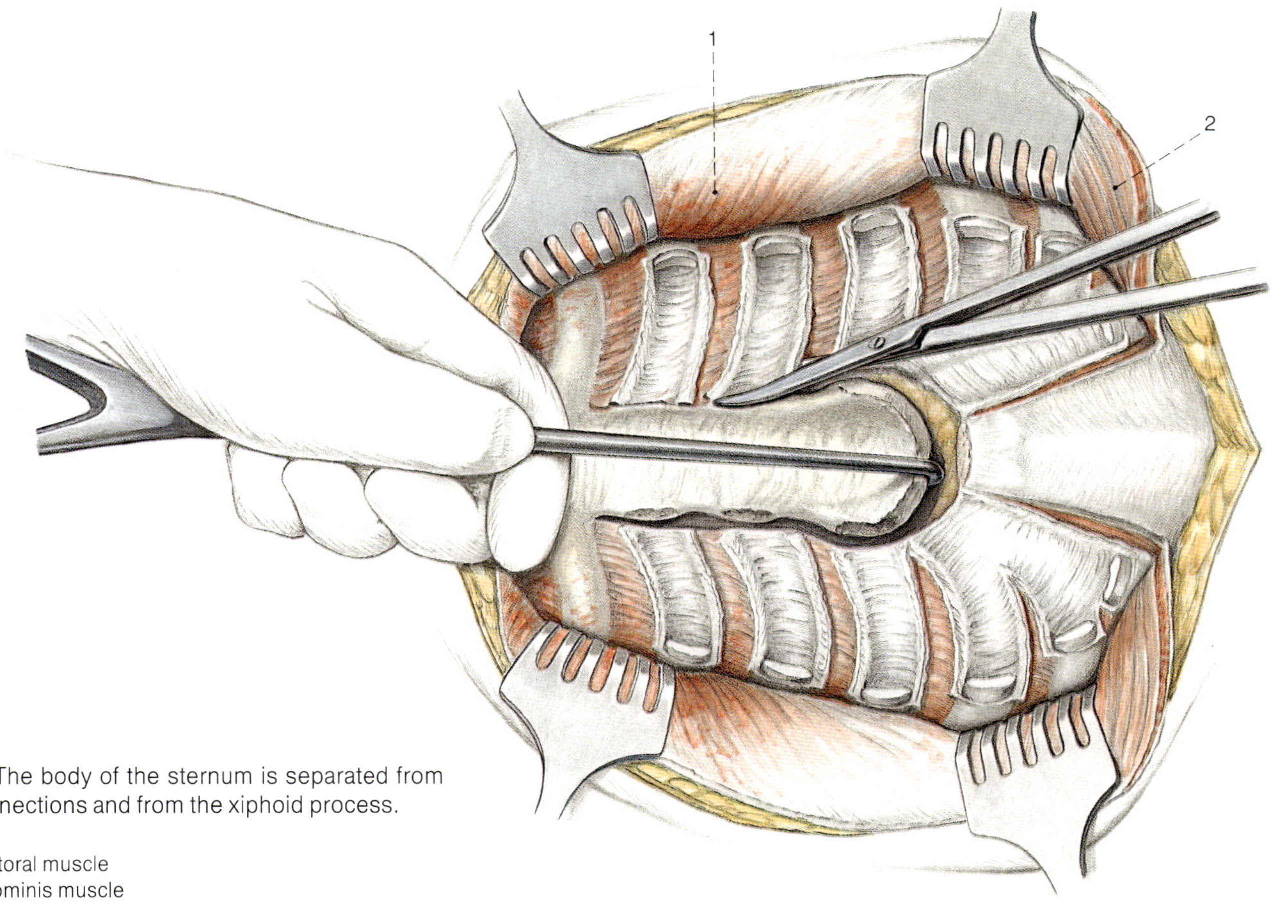

Fig. 13.**16** The body of the sternum is separated from all lateral connections and from the xiphoid process.

1 Greater pectoral muscle
2 Rectus abdominis muscle

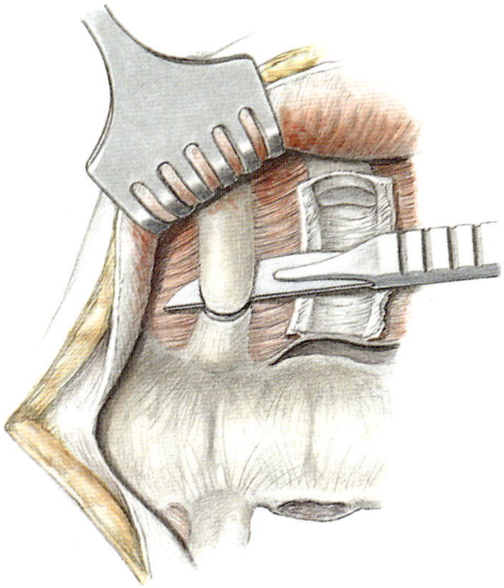

Fig. 13.**17** Bilateral oblique incision of the second costal cartilage.

In difficult cases, particularly in elderly patients, Ravitch fixes the sternum by running a Kirschner wire transversely through the medullary space. The ends are bent back (Fig. 13.**19**). The wire can be removed, after six months. Not invariably, but frequently, a suction drain is inserted into the mediastinum.

Wound Closure

The sternal membrane and the pectoral musculature are closed over the sternum, and so is the subcutis. The rectus sheath is sutured. The xiphoid process, the perichondrium, and the intercostal musculature are not fixed. The skin is closed with an intracutaneous wire suture.

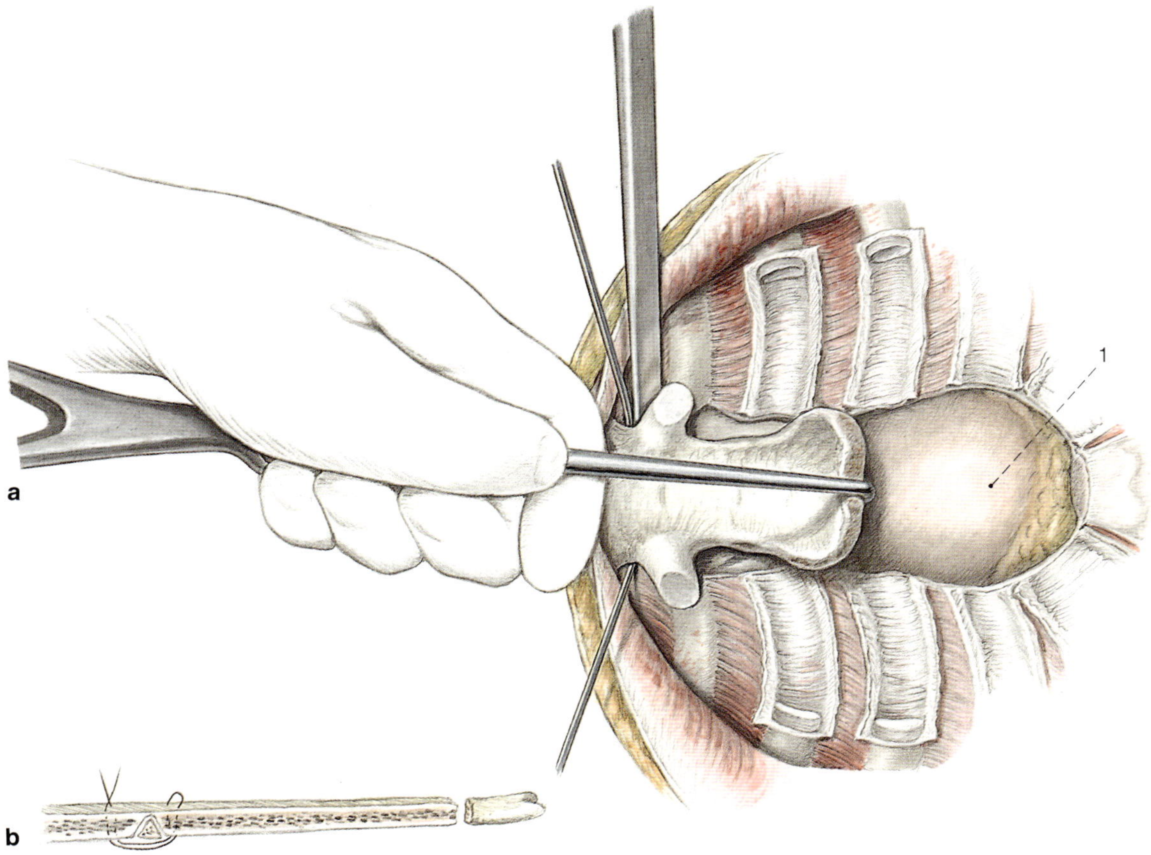

Fig. 13.**18a** The posterior cortical lamella of the sternum is notched along a guide wire.
b A bone wedge is fixed in the notch by mattress suture.

1 Pericardium

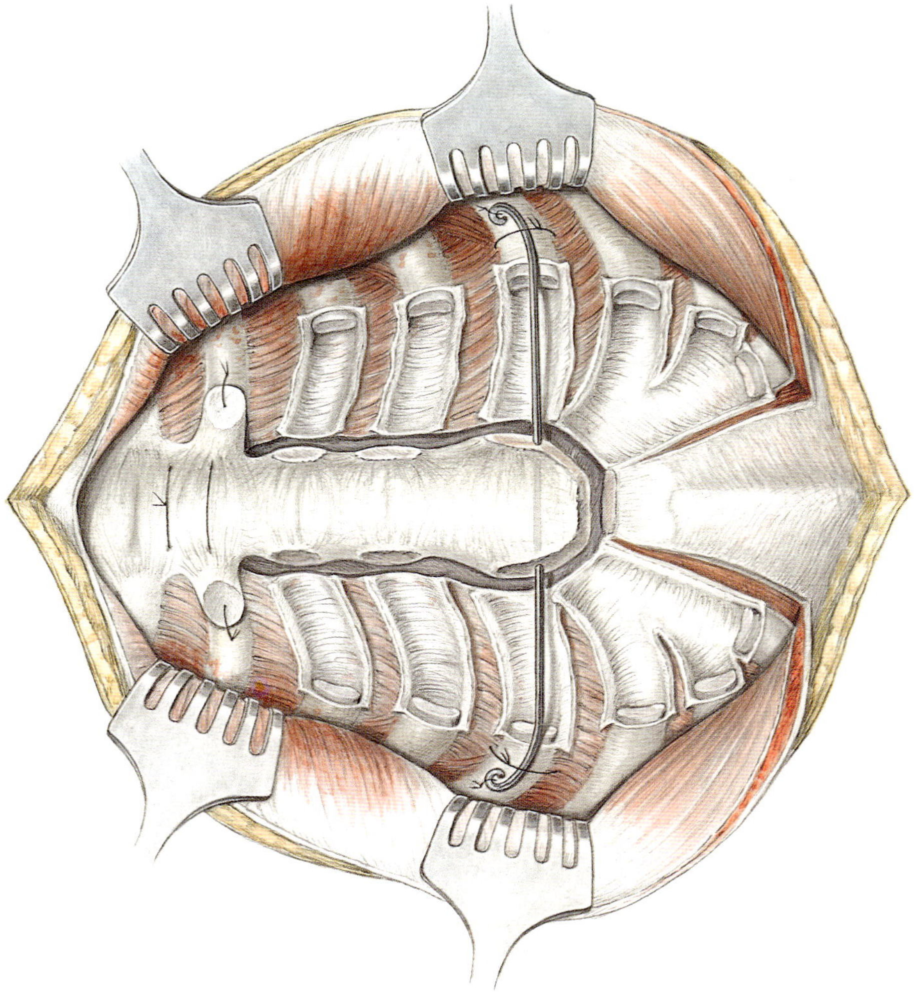

Fig. 13.**19** A bone wedge has been fitted into the sternal notch and fixed by mattress sutures. The sternal portion of the second costal cartilage overlies the lateral one and is fixed by suture. A Kirschner wire has been drilled transversely through the medullary space of the sternum. The ends have been bent back and fixed to the ribs.

Postoperative Treatment

This is similar to that after the Rehbein operation (p. 431).

Complications

In rare cases, the instability of the chest wall may necessitate mechanical ventilation postoperatively in adolescents.

Defective wound healing.

Alternative Methods

Brunner operation and the Wada turnover operation.

The Ravitch and Rehbein methods have been variously modified (Bettex, Hecker).

Pigeon Breast

Indications

In contrast to the funnel chest, pigeon chest is not associated with functional impairment of the cardiovascular system. The perceived psychological burden of the deformity is an indication for surgery.

The operation may be performed from the age of 12.

Ravitch Operation

Approach

The positioning, approach, and exposure of the anterior chest wall are the same as in the operation for funnel chest.

Operative Technique

In contrast to the funnel-chest operation, the rectus sheath and the muscles over the costal arch are not merely incised obliquely, but are dissected free en bloc in a caudal direction. The perichondrium of the deformed costal cartilages receives a winglike incision, and is detached from the cartilage with an elevator. The costal cartilages are resected. The perichondrium is longitudinally tightened by means of sutures (Fig. 13.**20**). If there is significant posterior angulation of the sternum, it is notched on the anterior side, and the distal portion is raised with mattress sutures.

The sternal membrane and the pectoral musculature, and the rectus muscles or the rectus sheath, are reunited (Fig. 13.**21**). Wire sutures are applied subcutaneously and intracutaneously.

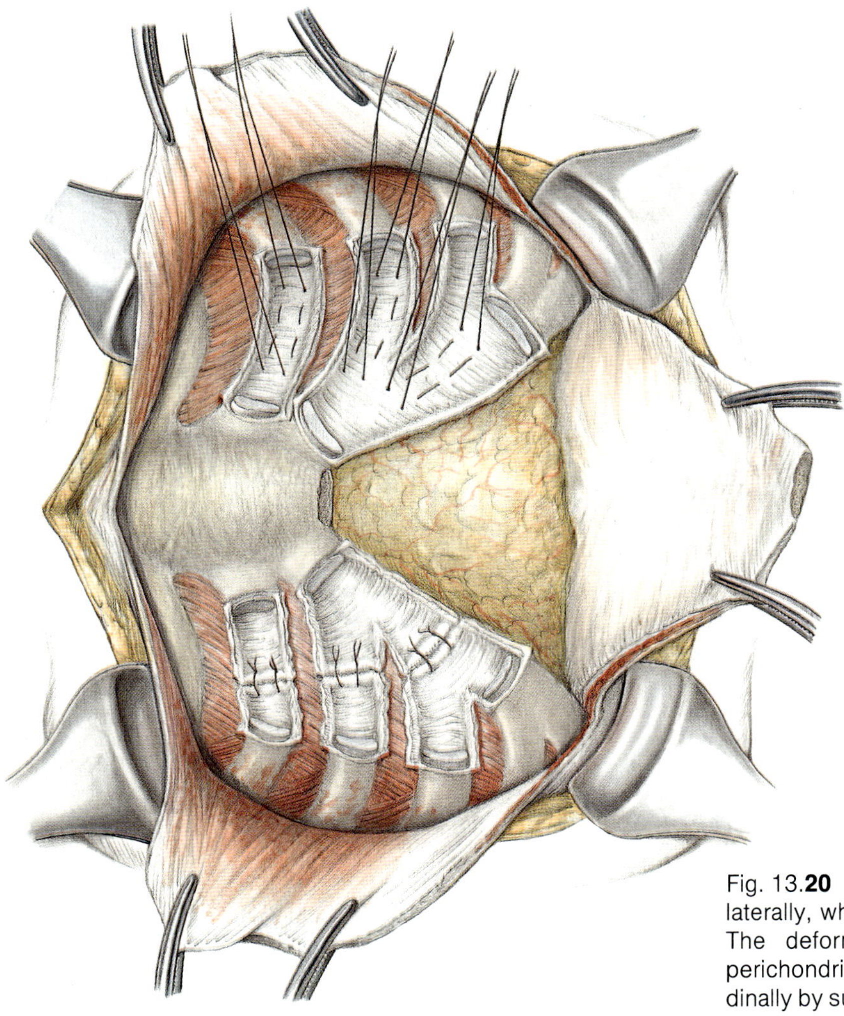

Fig. 13.**20** The pectoral musculature has been dissected free laterally, while the rectus muscles have been dissected caudally. The deformed costal cartilages have been resected subperichondrially. The perichondrium has been drawn tight longitudinally by sutures.

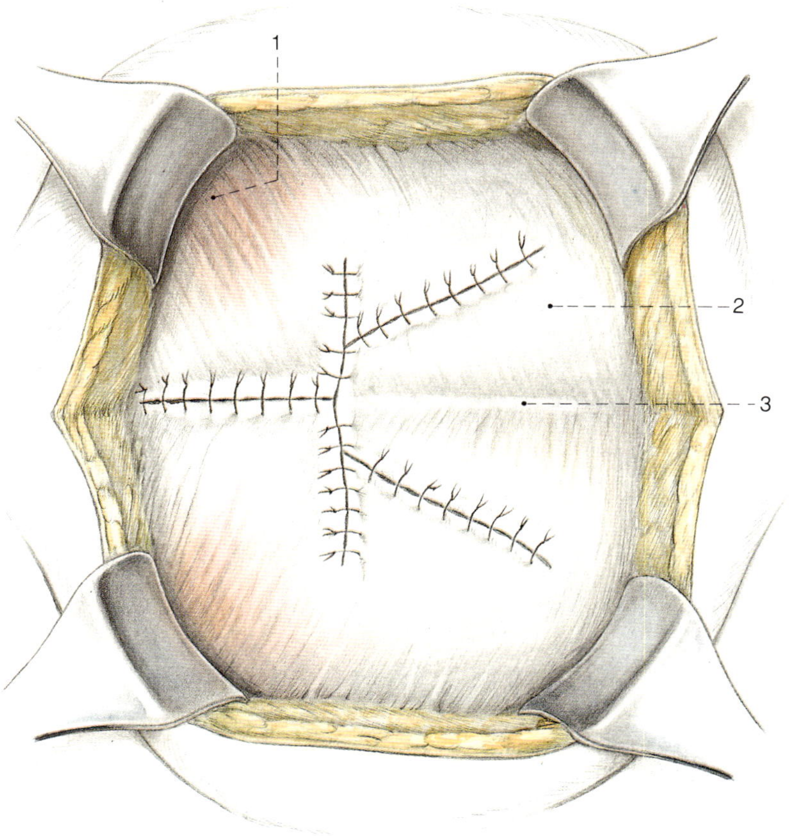

Fig. 13.**21** Suture closure of sternal membrane and of the musculature over the sternum.

1 Greater pectoral muscle
2 Rectus sheath, anterior leaf
3 Linea alba

Complications

The same as in funnel chest operations.

Postoperative Treatment

Not required.

Alternative Method

Cosmetic correction according to Ramsey.

Superior Sternoschisis

Sabiston Operation

Approach

An incision is made in the median plane, and the skin is dissected free of the pericardium. The greater pectoral muscle and the rectus abdominis muscle are dissected free laterally, to expose the costal cartilages.

Operative Technique

Closure of the Cleft

The periosteum is incised anteriorly on both sides of the sternum, and retracted posteriorly (Fig. 13.**22**). In the region of the united sternum, a bone wedge has to be excised. The perichondrium of ribs 1–4 is incised, and the costal cartilage is freed from the perichondrium and obliquely divided. The mobilized sternal plates are approximated by strong sutures, and the periosteum is sutured (Fig. 13.**23**).

Wound Closure

The origins of the pectoral muscles and the rectus sheath are united in the midline. Subcutaneous and intracutaneous sutures are applied.

Alternative Method

Closure by bone graft (Sauerbruch).

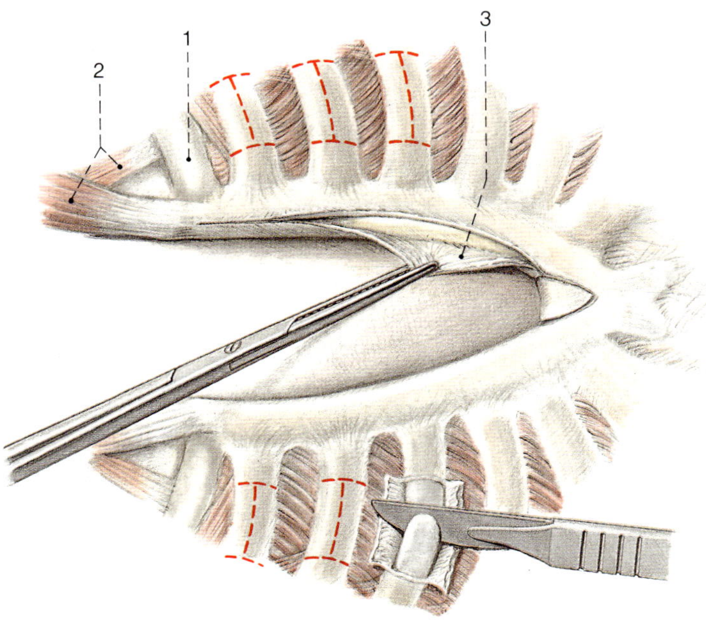

Fig. 13.**22** The periosteum is medially freed at the sternal plate, and a caudal wedge is resected. The perichondrium of the costal cartilage is opened and the costal cartilage is obliquely divided from medial to lateral. A wedge is removed from the caudal part of the sternum.

1 Clavicle
2 Sternocleidomastoid muscle
3 Periosteum

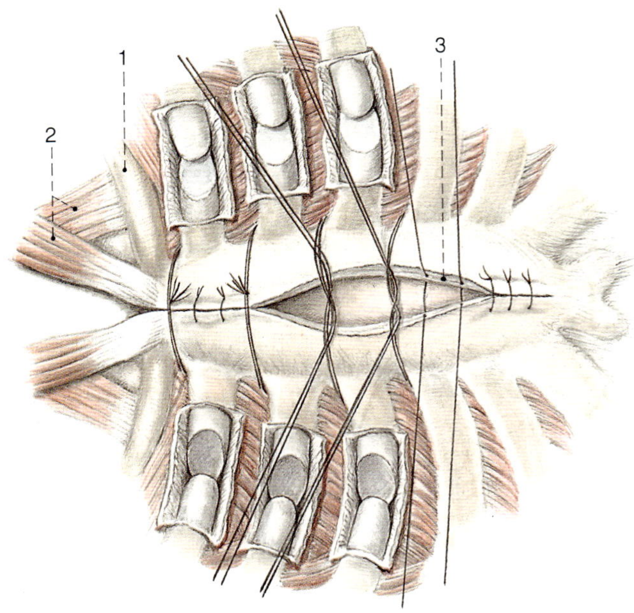

Fig. 13.**23** Union of the sternal plates and suture of the periosteum.

1 Clavicle
2 Sternocleidomastoid muscle
3 Periosteum

Poland's Syndrome

Indication

Paradoxical respiration due to costal cartilage defects and conversion of the pectoral muscles to connective tissue.

Haller Operation

Approach

The patient is placed in semilateral decubitus position on the unaffected side. A horizontal incision is made on the affected side of the chest and extended toward the back.

Operative Technique

The fascia replacing the pectoral musculature is dissected from the pleura, and the rib stumps are exposed. The sternum is mobilized.

A caudal rib on the same or the contralateral side is taken out subperiosteally, and split or divided with an oscillating saw. A bed for each graft is drilled into the lateral border of the sternum. After debridement of the rib stumps, the grafts are fitted into the sternal beds and connected to the rib stumps by sutures (Fig. 13.**24**). The latissimus dorsi muscle is freed from its origin and displaced anteriorly together with its neurovascular supply. It is fixed to the sternum. Hemovac drains are inserted; the wound is closed in layers.

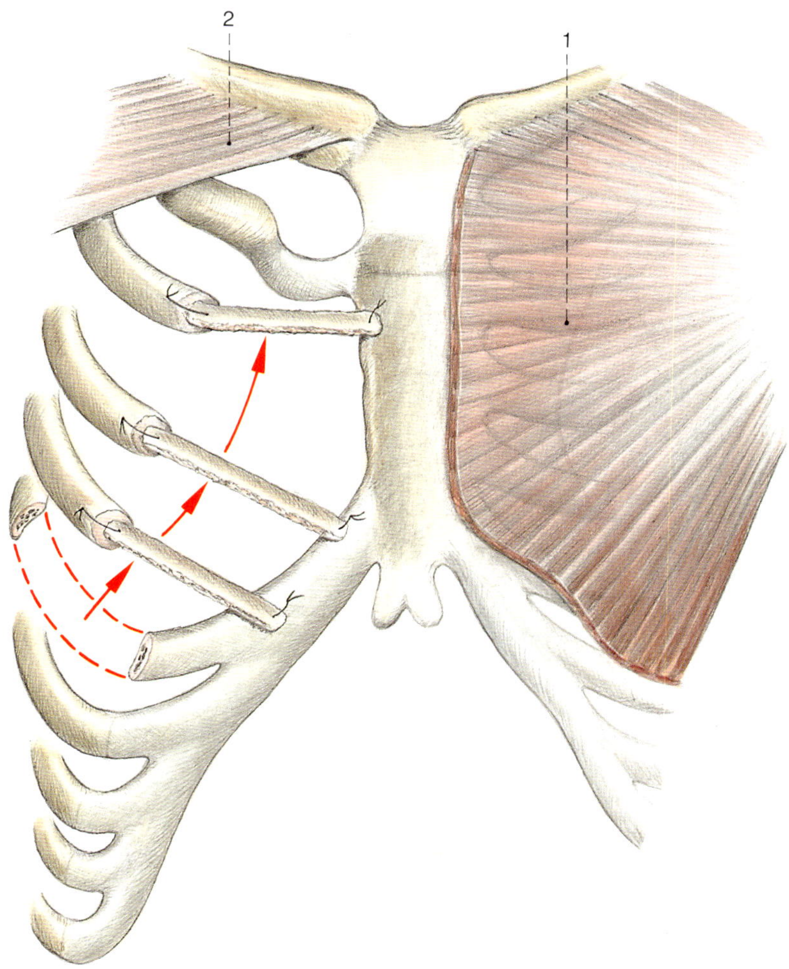

Fig. 13.**24** Implantation of rib grafts between the debrided rib stumps and the sternum.

1 Greater pectoral muscle
2 Greater pectoral muscle, clavicular part

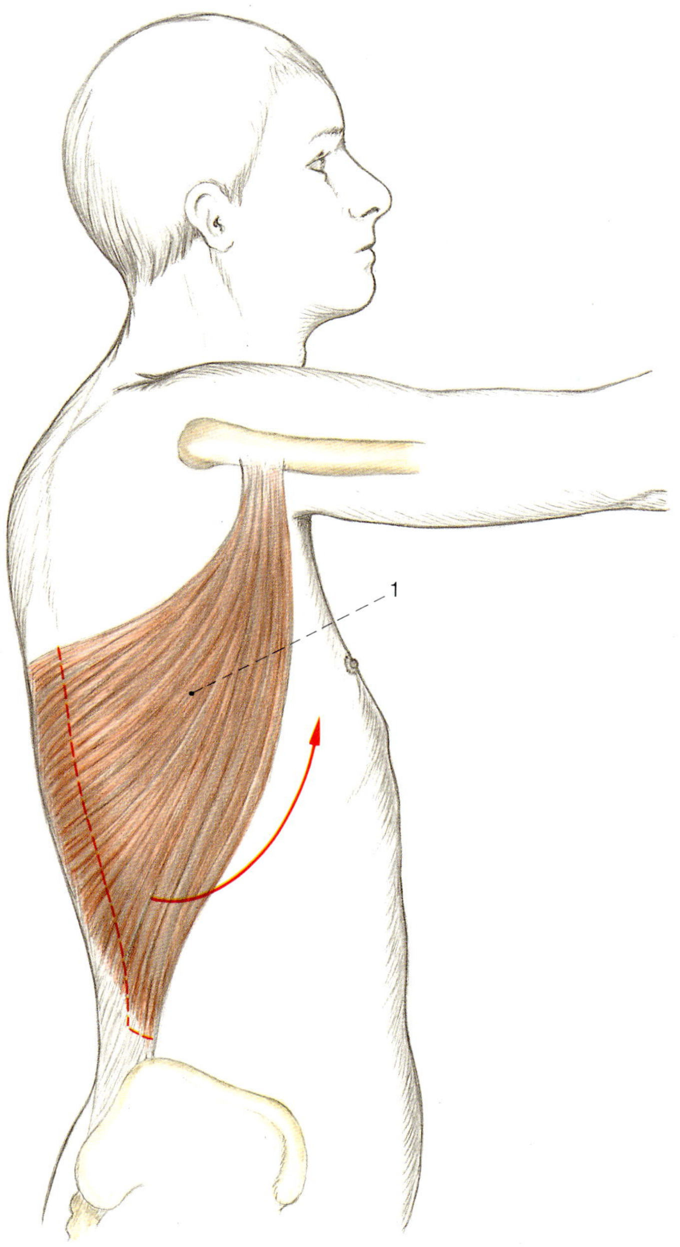

Fig. 13.**25** The latissimus dorsi muscle is posteriorly detached at its origin, transposed in an anterior direction with the thoracodorsal artery and vein and the thoracodorsal nerve, and fixed to the sternum.

1 Latissimus dorsi muscle

Postoperative Treatment and Complications

The same as with other chest wall deformities.

Further Reading

Backer O, Brünner S, Larsen V. Radiological evaluation of funnel chest. Acta Radiol Scand 1961;55:249.

Haller A Jr, Colombani PM, Miller D, Manson P. Early reconstruction of Poland's syndrome using autologous rib grafts combined with a latissimus muscle flap. J Pediat Surg 1984;19:423.

Oelsnit G von der. Die Trichter- und Kielbrust. Stuttgart: Hippokrates, 1983.

Hecker WC, Procher G, Dietz AG. Ergebnisse operativer Korrektur von Kiel- und Trichterbrust. Z Kinderchir 1981;34:220.

Ravitch MM. Congenital deformities of the chest wall and their operative correction. Philadelphia: Saunders, 1977.

14 Torticollis

C. J. With

Indications

General. Torticollis deformity due to a contracted sternocleidomastoid muscle which the patient or the parents find cosmetically unacceptable.

Specific. If the sternocleidomastoid hematoma persists beyond the fifth month of life and the wryneck deformity worsens, with or without the muscle hematoma, and persists beyond the first year of life, and the myographic activity of the contracted sternocleidomastoid muscle is markedly diminished.

Contraindications

Osseous anomalies that are partly responsible for the torticollis. Contractions of other muscles, such as the trapezius muscle, for example, which cause the torticollis.

Timing of the Operation

The best time is pre–school age, since active cooperation of the young patients in the highly important postoperative rehabilitation is required and there is a greater chance of remission of secondary changes such as facial asymmetry and spinal scoliosis. Operations are generally performed more frequently between the ages of 1 and 6.

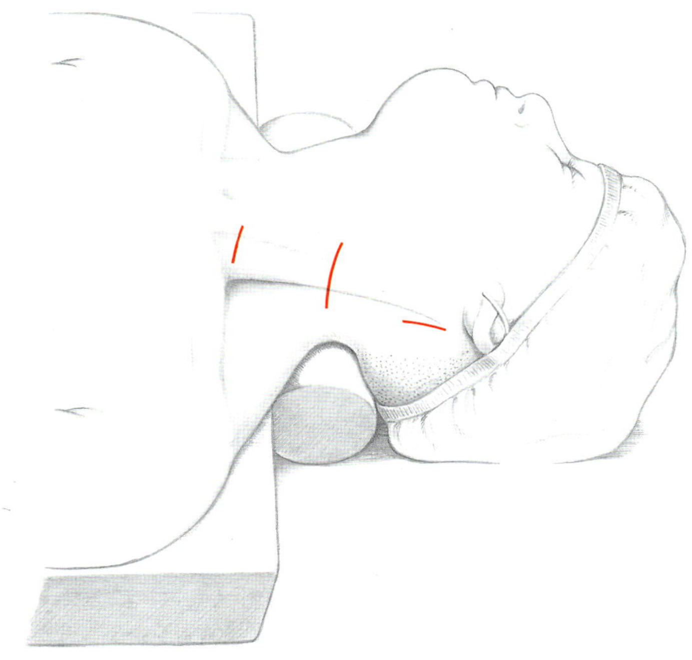

Fig. 14.**1** Positioning for torticollis operation. Semilateral position. The side of the body with the affected portion of the neck is raised. The head, resting on a neck roll, is turned toward the healthy side, and the neck is slightly hyperextended. The contracted sternocleidomastoid muscle is distinctly prominent. Shown here are the skin incisions for caudal and mastoidal tenotomy, and the transverse skin incision for extirpation of the sternocleidomastoid muscle.

The scope of the operation is proportional to the age. In young children, subcutaneous caudal tenotomy of the sternocleidomastoid muscle is often sufficient for correction; in children of pre–school age, added division of the deep, contracted cervical fascia is often needed together with open tenotomy. In late cases, it is always necessary to carry out open caudal and cranial tenotomy with division of the fascia, or to remove the whole contracted muscle.

Positioning

The patient is placed in a semilateral position, the torso with the affected side of the neck being raised. the neck is moderately hyperextended over a neck roll. The head is turned to the healthy side. In this position, the contracted sternocleidomastoid muscle is under maximal traction, and juts out most prominently with its tendinous insertions (Fig. 14.**1**).

Caudal Sternoclavicular Subcutaneous Tenotomy of the Sternocleidomastoid Muscle (Strohmeyer, König)

Indication

Torticollis in young children.

Operative Technique

To begin with, the index finger is passed around the taut tendinous fibers of the clavicular portion of the muscle from a medial direction, in order to sweep aside and so protect the posteriorly situated vessels (external and internal jugular vein, subclavian artery and vein).

Approximately 15 mm cranial to the bony insertion at the clavicle, again to protect the jugular veins, the curved tenotome is transcutaneously entered at the tendon from the lateral side. The knife is driven hard toward the invaginating index finger around the posterior border of the tendon. The tendon is then divided from the inside outward (Fig. 14.**2**).

Not infrequently, the sternal tendinous portion, too, needs to be cut for adequate relaxation of the contracted muscle. This produces a lasting change in the outline of the neck, and the necessity for this maneuver should always be weighed up for this reason. After invagination of the skin from a medial direction, the sternal tendon is grasped with the index finger. The tenotome that has been inserted 15 mm cranial to the clavicle from lateral transects the tendon from the inside outward.

The transverse stab incisions may gap after extensive correction; if so, they should each be closed with an interrupted suture. Dressing of the wound follows.

Complications

Hemorrhage is the main complication. If the bleeding cannot be reduced or stopped by compression for several minutes, the site has to be opened and the injured vessel, which usually is the external jugular vein, has to be ligated. Also at risk are, in the depth, the subclavian vein and the internal jugular vein, in addition to the common carotid artery with the vagus nerve and the subclavian artery. The calculated rate of injury to the external jugular vein is 3.3%.

Postoperative Treatment

See p. 448.

Caudal Sternoclavicular Open Tenotomy (von Volkmann)

Indication

Torticollis in pre–school age children.

Operative Technique

A transverse skin incision 2 cm long is made between the caudal tendons of the sternocleidomastoid muscle, about 1 cm cranial to the clavicle. Incisions over the clavicle should be avoided because of disfiguring scar formation.

The platysma is separated at the clavicle. After this, the skin incision is initially carried over the clavicular tendon of the sternocleidomastoid muscle (Fig. 14.**3**). The latter is

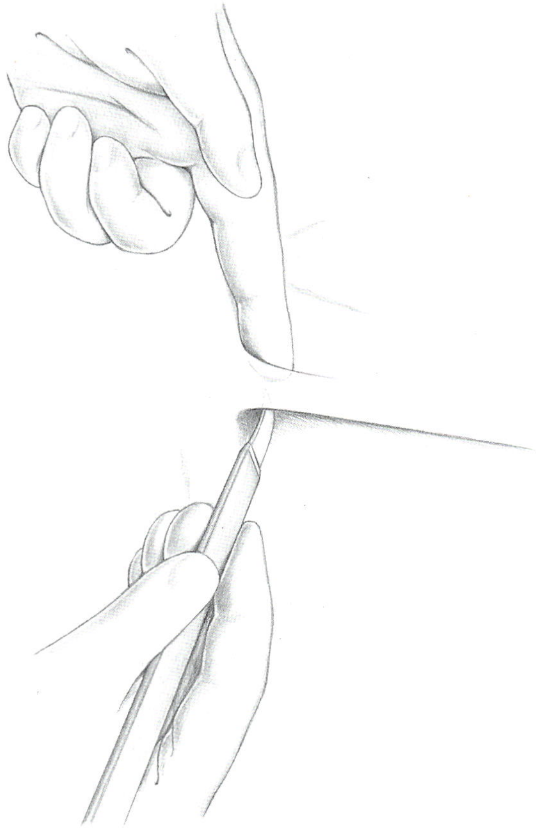

Fig. 14.**2** The index finger is passed around the tightened muscle insertion, and the tenotome is applied for a closed tenotomy.

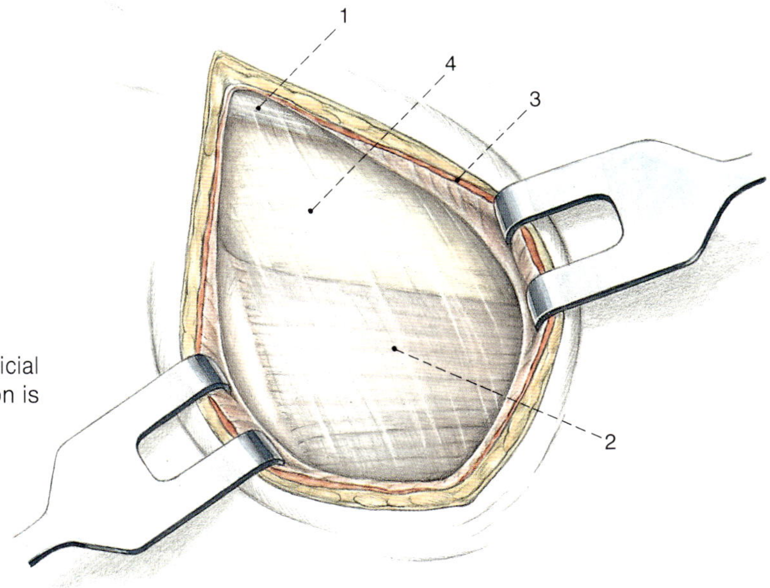

Fig. 14.**3** After separation of the platysma and the superficial cervical fascia from the clavicle, the clavicular muscle insertion is exposed first.

1 Sternocleidomastoid muscle (pars sternalis)
2 Sternocleidomastoid muscle (pars clavicularis)
3 Platysma
4 Cervical fascia, superficial lamina

exposed after division of the superficial cervical fascia, and a grooved director is passed around it. The tendon is transected over the grooved director (Fig. 14.**4**). The muscle retracts spontaneously. It is advisable nonetheless to resect a portion of at least 5 mm of the tendon to prevent bridging by scar tissue. It often proves necessary to transect the medial cervical fascia as well since it, too, is contracted, and may prevent the correction (Fig. 14.**5**).

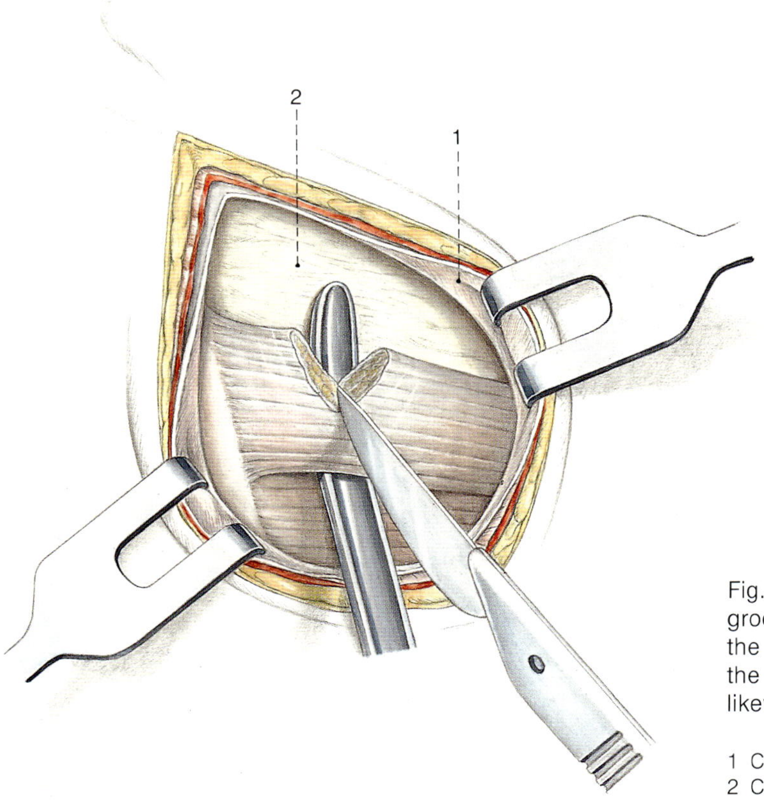

Fig. 14.**4** The tendon insertion is closely undermined with a grooved director approximately 15 mm cranial to the clavicle, and the tendon surface is transected. Additional tightened portions of the tendon are identified by lateral and deep palpation, and are likewise sharply divided.

1 Cervical fascia, superficial lamina
2 Cervical fascia, pretracheal lamina

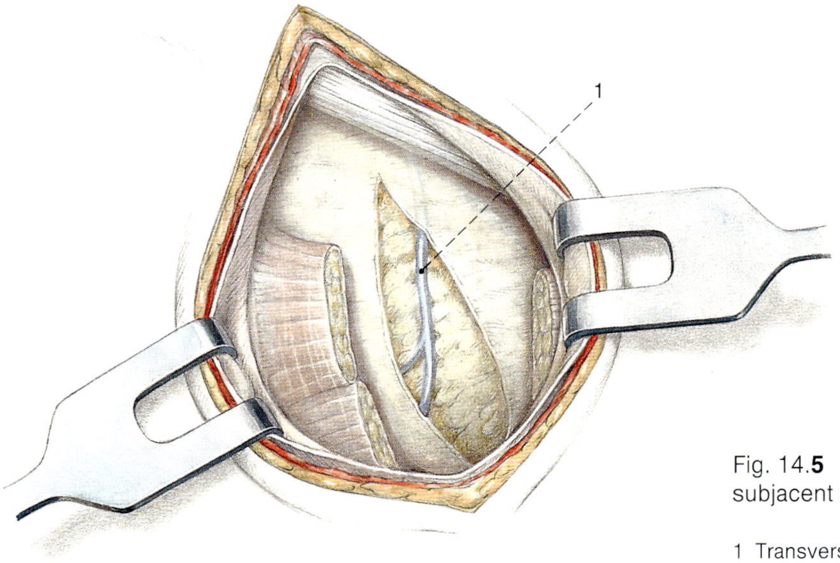

Fig. 14.**5** Transection of the deep cervical fascia, sparing the subjacent neurovascular bundle.

1 Transverse cervical vein

Since the range of variation of the clavicular muscle insertion is extremely wide, careful palpation and a possible re-resection are required to optimize the result of the correction.

If the correction has been inadequate, the skin incision is extended over the sternal muscle insertion. The tendon is also undermined and divided (Figs. 14.**6**, 14.**7**).

Following meticulous hemostasis, the skin alone is sutured.

Complications

As in subcutaneous tenotomy, the external jugular vein is susceptible to injury, and its individual course should be determined preoperatively through congestion. Under the medial cervical fascia, it is again necessary to watch for the internal jugular vein, the common carotid artery, the superficial ansa cervicalis, and the vagus nerve.

Postoperative Treatment

See p. 448.

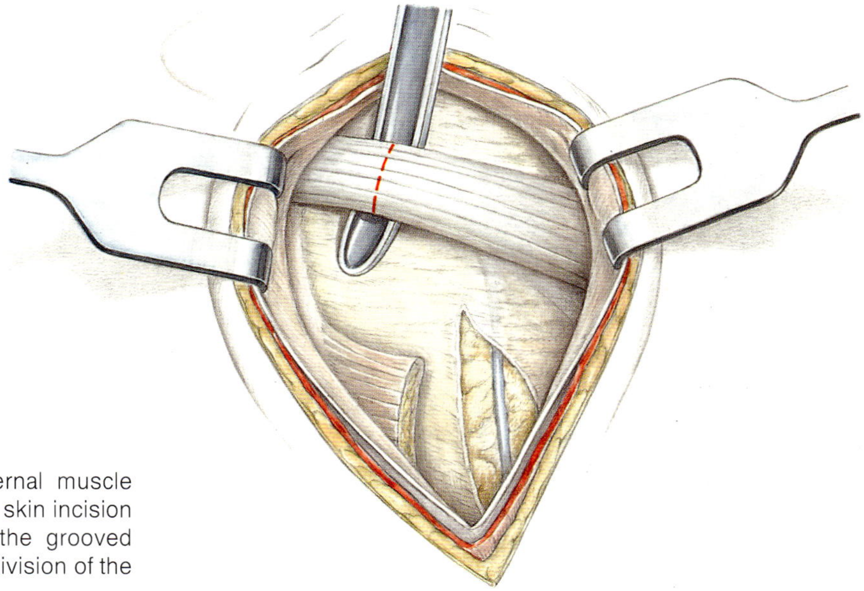

Fig. 14.**6** If the correction is inadequate, the sternal muscle insertion, too, is exposed by medial distraction of the skin incision and undermining of the tendinous insertion with the grooved disector. Shown here is the level of the incision for division of the tendon.

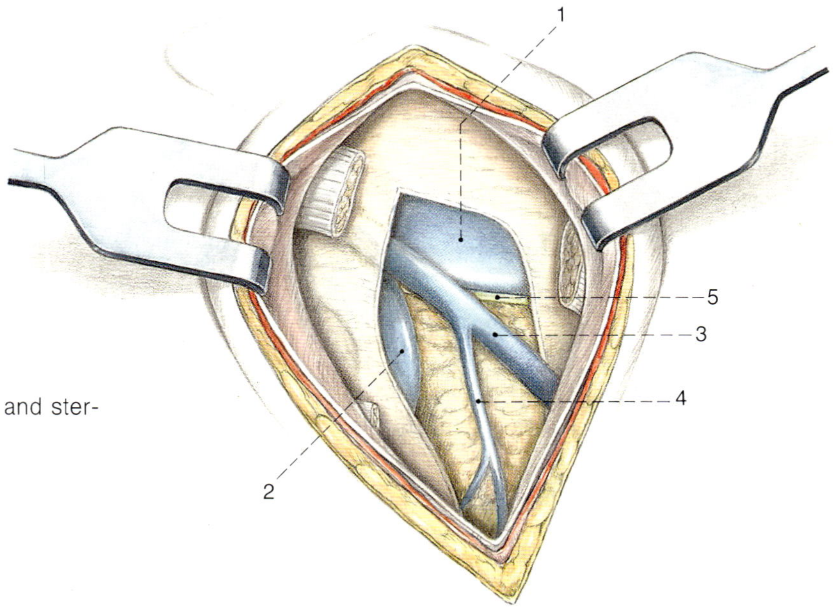

Fig. 14.**7** Operative site after division of the clavicular and sternal tendinous insertions and the deep cervical fascia.

1 Internal jugular vein
2 Subclavian vein
3 External jugular vein
4 Transverse cervical vein
5 Superficial ansa cervicalis

Cranial Mastoidal Open Tenotomy (Tillaux, F. Lange)

Indication

Torticollis in pre–school age children.

Operative Technique

The hair around the ear is shaved. After insertion of a swab into the auricular canal, the auricle is reflected toward the face by traction with adhesive tape. The operative site is square-draped, so that only the muscle cord with the mastoid and the caudal attachments remains free.

A transverse or longitudinal incision is possible. The incision, 3 cm in length, runs from the mastoid to the muscle belly. It should not be made at the anterior border of the sternocleidomastoid muscle, since even the skin incision risks injuring the facial nerve. The transverse incision is made directly below the mastoid process. After division of the superficial cervical fascia, the tendinous insertion of the contracted muscle is exposed close to the mastoid with a dissecting swab stick by anterior and posterior retraction of the soft tissues, and is closely undermined with a grooved disector (Fig. 14.**8**). Even at this point, the anesthetist should be called to watch the patient's expression in the affected half of the face (facial nerve). Cautious, step-by-step division of the wide tendon from the outside inward, down to the last fiber, then follows (Fig. 14.**9**). Again, it is advisable to resect a portion of the tendon at least 5 mm wide to prevent premature, tight bridging by scar formation. The middle cervical fascia is notched; this is necessary to bring about noticeable relaxation of the muscle (Fig. 14.**10**).

The subcutis and the skin are sutured, and the wound is dressed. Cranial tenotomy has advantages over caudal tenotomy. The resultant scar can be concealed by the ear and hair. The outline of the neck is not altered. The position of the head can be corrected even if the muscle is adherent within its fascial compartment. The operation is a comparatively minor one, and is brief. In contrast to caudal tenotomy, however, there is a risk of nerve injury.

Complications

Particularly at risk are branches of the facial nerve that appear at the anterior border of the mastoidal insertion of the sternocleidomastoid muscle. The incidence of injury recorded in the literature data is 3.4%. The nerves are crossed by the posterior auricular artery, and travel over the internal jugular vein and the external carotid artery. These vessels, like the occipital artery, may be damaged. The accessory nerve is hardly vulnerable if the tenotomy is performed directly at the mastoid.

Postoperative Treatment

See p. 448. The facial nerve is tested (whistling, pursing of lips) immediately after the operation.

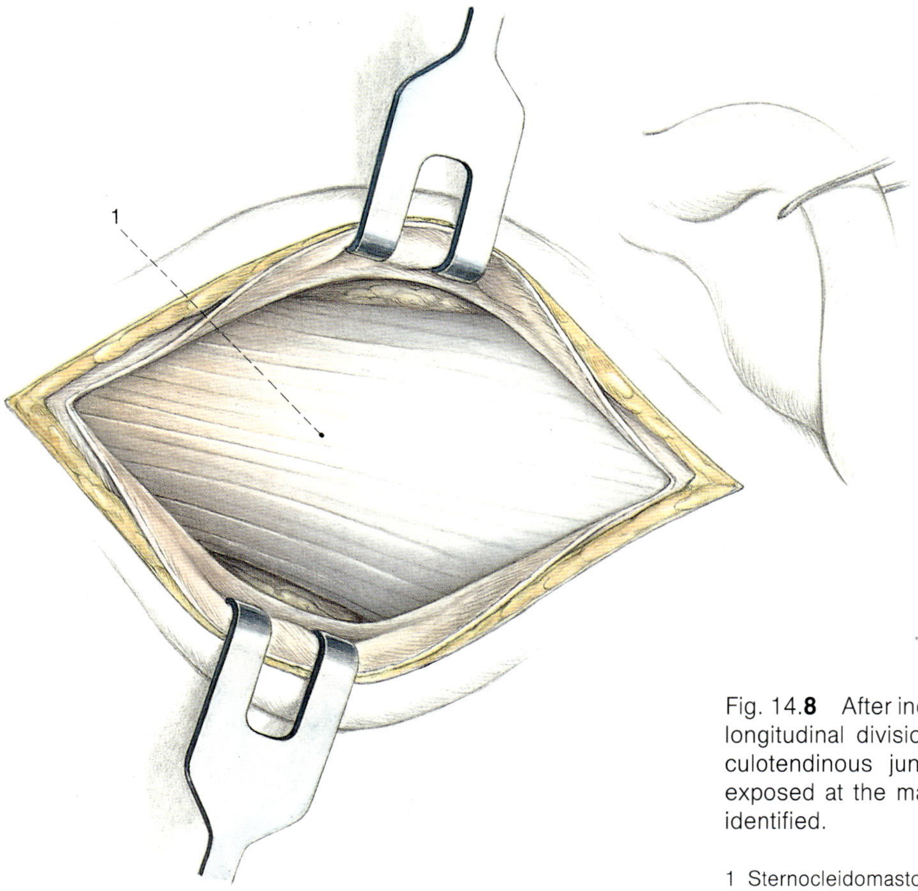

Fig. 14.**8** After incision of the skin in a craniocaudal direction and longitudinal division of the superficial cervical fascia, the musculotendinous junction of the sternocleidomastoid muscle is exposed at the mastoid. The anterior and posterior borders are identified.

1 Sternocleidomastoid muscle

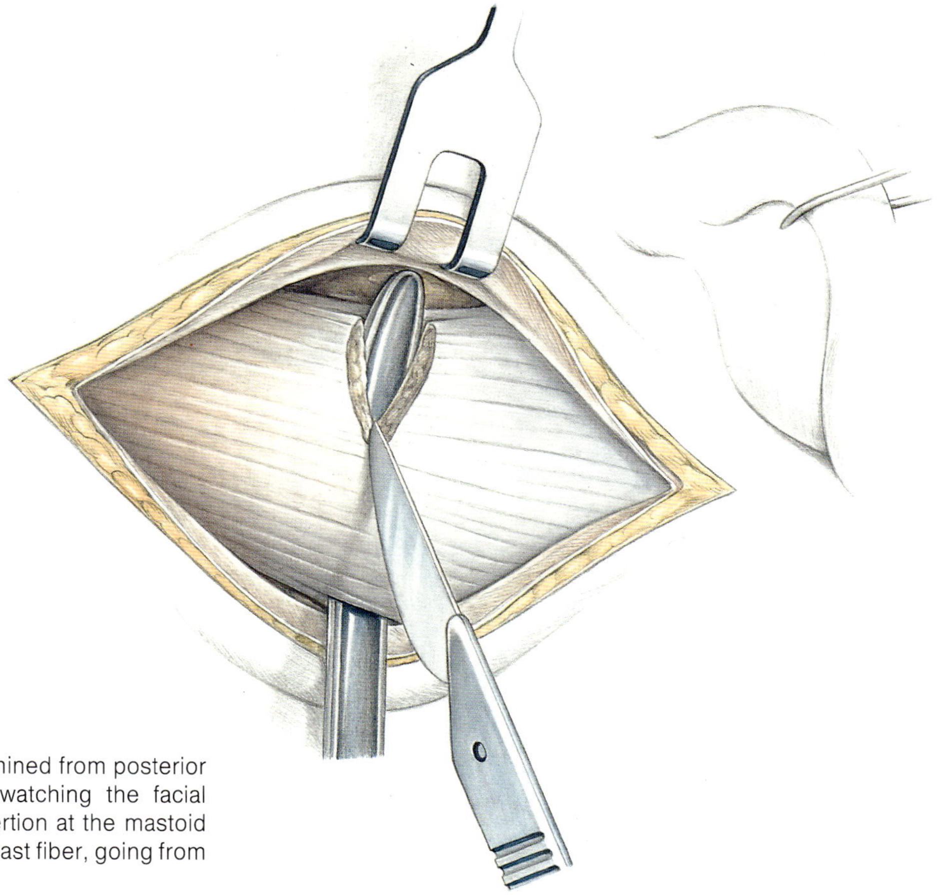

Fig. 14.**9** The aponeurosis is closely undermined from posterior to anterior, directly at the mastoid, while watching the facial expression (facial nerve). The tendinous insertion at the mastoid is carefully resected step by step down to the last fiber, going from the outside inward.

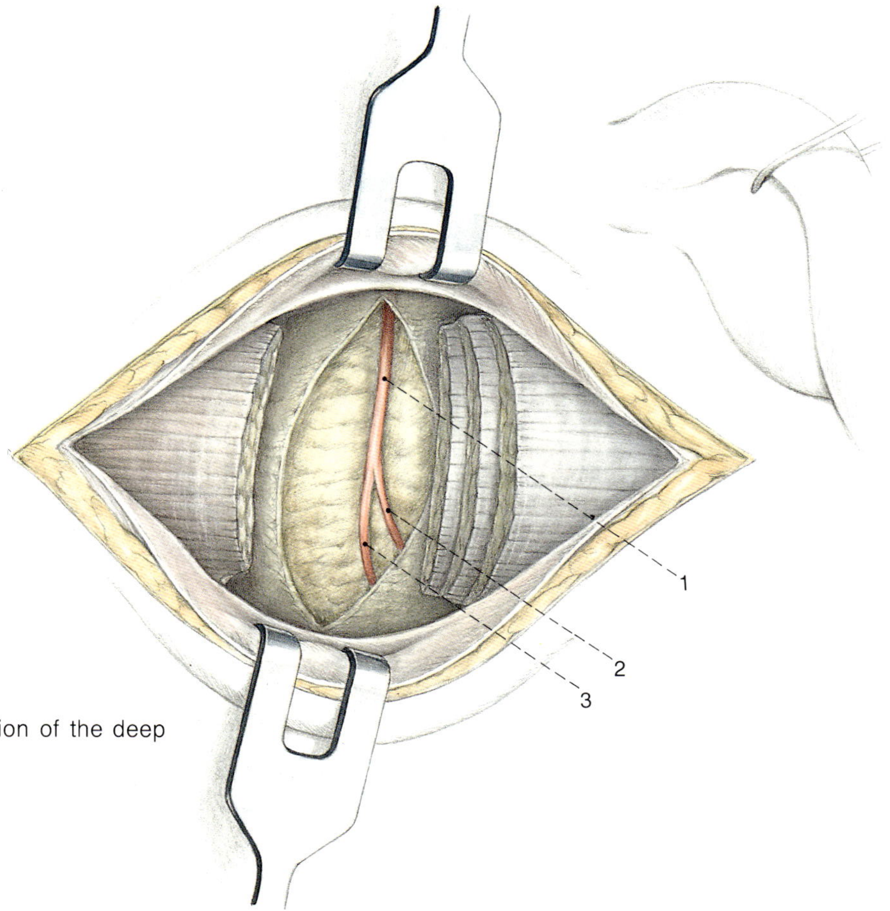

Fig. 14.**10** Operative site after transverse division of the deep cervical fascia.

1 Great auricular artery
2 Auricular branch
3 Occipital branch

Biterminal Tenotomy (Hellstadius, Putti)

Indication

Torticollis in schoolchildren; late cases.

Operative Technique

This is a combination of caudal and cranial tenotomy, and includes division of the deep cervical fascia. See caudal and cranial tenotomy for the operative technique.

Complications

The rate of complications is no higher than with cranial or caudal tenotomy alone.

Postoperative Treatment

See p. 448.

Total Extirpation of the Sternocleidomastoid Muscle (Mikulicz)

Indication

Extremely severe contraction of the sternocleidomastoid muscle. Recurrences of torticollis.

Operative Technique

A transverse incision is made in the middle of the muscle. The platysma is split longitudinally, as is the superficial cervical fascia. After distraction of the skin incision, the muscle is bluntly freed from its fascial sheath, beginning caudally and as far as the mastoid process, on its anterior side (Fig. 14.**11**). After this, again after caudal distraction of the skin incision, the sternal and clavicular muscle insertions are tenotomized. The contracted muscle is now also developed, under vision, on its lower surface as far as the mastoid, where it is resected. This surgical step endangers the accessory nerve, which passes obliquely along the posterior surface of the muscle, or even perforates the deep muscle layer (Fig. 14.**12**). The motor branch to the sternocleidomastoid muscle has to be transected. To complete correction of the torticollis, additional division of the deep cervical fascia may become necessary. The subcutis and the skin are sutured after insertion of a drain.

Complications

At risk are the common carotid artery, the internal jugular vein, the vagus nerve, the accessory nerve and, finally, the motor cervical branches of the facial nerve and the origins of the carotid coursing toward the ear and the occiput. The rate of injury to the accessory nerve alone, with consequent partial paralysis of the trapezius muscle, generally amounts to 13.6%.

Postoperative Treatment

Postoperative care is essentially the same for all torticollis surgery, with the exception of the Mikulicz total extirpation.

Satisfactory results are obtained in patients up to six years of age with a body cast incorporating a ring enclosure for the head at the level of the forehead (diadem cast). The cast is applied postoperatively with the patient recumbent and still under anesthesia, and is replaced 14 days after the operation with the patient standing. Attention must be paid to the correct head position; the head should lean toward the healthy side and be slightly hyperextended, while the chin is turned toward the side of the operation. One should avoid overcorrection, particularly under anesthesia, because of the risk of overstretching the cervical plexus.

At school age and later, a soft collar is sufficient, and allows early functional treatment. This dressing can also be recommended after total extirpation, although Mikulicz himself did not consider postoperative external support necessary.

Physiotherapy should continue for about six months after removal of the plaster cast. Passive stretching exercises by inclination of the head to the healthy side and turning of the chin to the side of the operation are appropriate. Similar active exercises and holding exercises in front of a mirror should be added.

Further Reading

Helstadius A. Torticollis congenita. Acta Chir Scand 1927;62:570–98.
König F. Subcutane Tenotomie des muskulären Schiefhalses. Zbl Chir 1907;34:812.
Lange F. Zur Behandlung des Schiefhalses. Z Orthop Chir 1910;27:440.
Mikulicz J. Über die Exstirpation des Kopfnickers beim muskulären Schiefhals. Zbl Chir 1895;22:1.
Strohmeyer GF. Beiträge zur operativen Orthopädik oder Erfahrungen über die subcutane Durchschneidung verkürzter Muskeln und deren Sehnen. Hannover: Helwig, 1838.
Tillaux F. Sur deux observations de torticolis. Bull Soc Chir 1890;16:481.
Volkmann R von. Das sogenannte Caput obstipum und die offene Durchschneidung des Sternocleidomastoideus. Zbl Chir 1885;12:233.
Wirth CJ, Hegena FW. Der muskuläre Schiefhals. In: C. Burri, Ch. Herfarth, M. Jäger, ed. Aktuelle Probleme in Chirurgie und Orthopädie. Vol. 27. Berne: Huber, 1983.

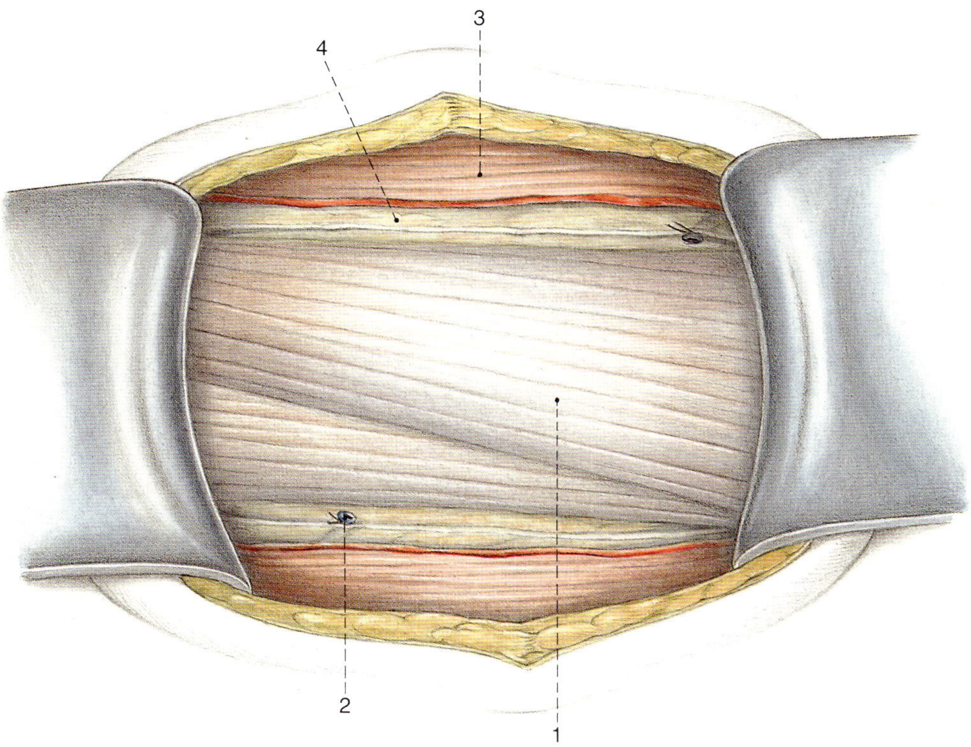

Fig. 14.**11** By proximal and distal distraction of the transverse skin incision, the platysma and the superficial cervical fascia have been longitudinally divided over the entire length of the muscle. The anterior and posterior borders of the muscle belly are exposed.

1 Sternocleidomastoid muscle
2 External jugular vein
3 Platysma
4 Cervical fascia, superficial lamina

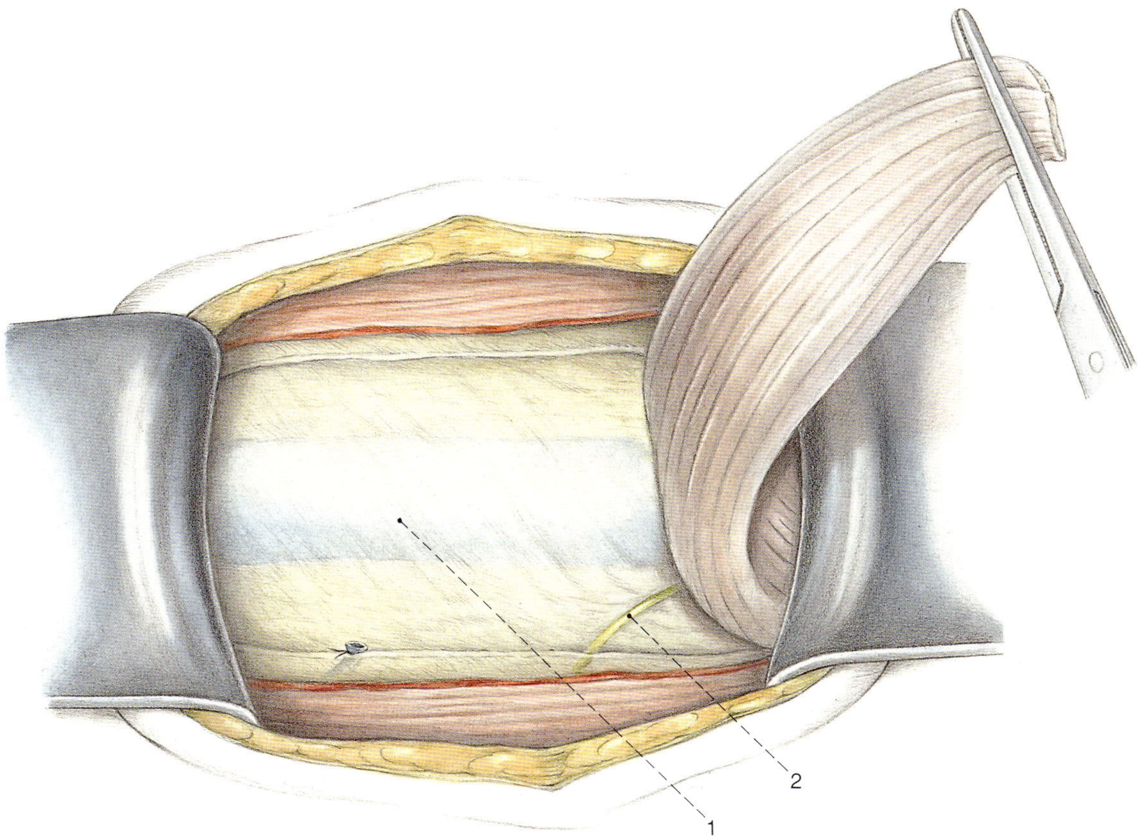

Fig. 14.**12** The sternal and clavicular muscle insertions have been resected. The muscle belly has been developed cranially, and is subsequently resected at the mastoid from the inside outward. The accessory nerve is exposed.

1 Internal jugular vein
2 Accessory nerve

Index

A

Abdominal wall, anterior, nerve supply 25
Abscess
  costotransversectomy 60–63
  drainage 381–382
  presacral 382–383
Adamkiewicz artery, blood supply of spinal cord 20–21
Andersson lesion (spondylodiskitis) 228, 248
Ankylosing spondylitis 227–249
  operation for fractures 248
  operations for kyphotic deformity 228–235
    Hsu–Yau–Leong technique 236–240
    Mason–Urist technique 241–247
    Zielke technique 228–235
  operations for spondylodiskitis (Andersson lesion) 228, 248
  see also Spondylodiskitis
Annulus fibrosus 270, 272, 304, 320
Anterior strut grafting 189–190
Antibiotics, in spondylitis 389
Approaches 2–72
  anterior approaches 2–55
    cervical spine and cervicothoracic junction 2–12
    lumbar spine and lumbosacral junction 24–41
    thoracic spine 13–15
    thoracolumbar junction 24–41
  posterior approaches 56–71
    cervical spine 56–59
    costotransversectomy 60–63
    lumbar spine 68–69
    lumbosacral junction 70–72
    thoracic spine 64–67
Atlantoaxial anterior instability 348–360
  cord compression 349
  insufficiency of atlantal transverse ligament 348
  posterior operations 351–360
    Brooks–Southwick fusion 352–357
    Gallie fusion 358
    Magerl (transarticular screw fixation) method 359–360
Atlas vertebra
  subluxation 348
  transoral approach 2, 312, 373–375
Axis vertebra
  dens elevation
    anterior resection 373–375
    transoral approach 310–313
  transoral approach 2, 312, 373–375
Azygos vein, positional variants 18
Azygos–hemiazygos venous system, variants 19

B

Basilar impression
  dens elevation 310–313
  secondary (pseudobasilar) impression 350
    anterior transoral operations 373–375
    Harms–Schmelzle method 373–375
Brace
  Rehbein brace 429
  Stagnara brace 235
Bradford's technique, replacement of vertebral body with vascularized rib graft 196–197
Brain stem compression 373–375
Brattstrom method, posterior fusion, occipitocervical junction 367–368
Brooks–Southwick fusion, posterior operation for atlantoaxial anterior instability 352–357

C

Caspar spreader 252
Cauda equina compression
  evaluation 342
  see also Spinal cord compression
Cement and plate osteosynthesis
  cervical spine 398–400
  replacement (implant) of vertebral body 396
Cervical lordosation spondylodesis, monosegmental 241–247
Cervical myelopathy, in spondylosis 314–316
Cervical spine
  anatomical site 6–9
  anterior approaches 2–12
    transoropharyngeal approach 2–3
  cross-sectional anatomy
    C3 level 8
    C6 level 9
  fusion 251–268
    anterior fusion (Robinson) 252–255
    interbody fusion with anterior plate 256–259
    plate fixation 260–263
    posterior fusion 263–268
  lateral, right side anatomy 7
  lower
    anatomy 9
    C3 to T2 11
    C6 to T2 9
    left side anatomy 10
  posterior approaches 56–59
  tumor excision and compound osteosynthesis 398–400
  upper, left side anatomy 7
Cervicothoracic junction
  anatomy 9–12
  anterior approaches 2–12
    transoropharyngeal approach 2–3
  left side anatomy 10
Chassaignac's tubercle 11
Chest wall deformities 421–440
  funnel chest 422–435
  pigeon chest 436–437
  Poland's syndrome, Haller operation 439–440
  superior sternoschisis, Sabiston operation 438
Chest wall tumors, rib resection 411–420
  indications 412
  operative technique 413–416
  reconstructive coverage 417–419
Children
  congenital kyphosis 205–206
  epiphysiodesis 99
  Harrington operation for scoliosis 97–102
    subcutaneous instrumentation 100–102
  see also Scoliosis
Cobb angle 152
Cobb elevator, Harrington instrumentarium 81
Corticocancellous graft, atlantoaxial anterior instability 358
Costotransversectomy 60–63
Cotrel rod 131
Cotrel–Dubousset technique
  mobile thoracic lordosis 223–224
  Scheuermann's kyphosis 220
  scoliosis 131–146
    implants 131
    instrumentarium 131–133
    lumbar kyphoscoliosis 145–146
    mobile thoracic lordoscoliosis 135–142
    operative technique 131–146
    rigid thoracolumbar scoliosis 143–144
Crutchfield tongs 348

D

Daniaux funnel 283
DCS screws 396–398
Dens
  anterior resection 373–375
  elevation, transoral approach 310–313
Device for transverse traction *see* DTT stabilization system
Diaphragm, anatomical exposure 32
Disk *see* Intervertebral disk
Disk herniation *see* Lumbar disk herniation; Thoracic disk herniation
Dollar method, scoliosis 84
Drainage methods 381–382
DTT stabilization system 220–222
  Cotrel–Dubousset technique 142
Dwyer operation
  scoliosis 163–177
    alternatives 169
    fixation of pelvic obliquity 168–177
    instrumentarium 163–164
    operative technique 164–177
Dwyer screws 163

E

Epiphysiodesis 160–162
  children's operations 99

F

Facet joints
  multiple osteotomies 104–105
  resection, Hall technique 91
  superior facet syndrome 340
Fixateur interne
  Swiss model 284
  USIS 248

Flexibility index, scoliosis, defined 82
Frontosagittal index 422
Funnel chest 422–435
  Ravitch operation 432–435
  Rehbein operation 422–431

G

Gallie corticocancellous graft, atlantoaxial anterior instability 358
Galveston technique
  Luque operation 126
  pelvic fixation 209, 210
  pelvic obliquity 127–128
Gentamicin–PMMA beads *see* Septopal chains
Genufacial position 325
Genupectoral position 325
Geschwend method, posterior fusion, occipitocervical junction 361–366
Grafts
  anterior strut grafting 189–190
  Bradford's technique 196–197
  combined graft bridging and Septopal chains 386
  Gallie corticocancellous graft 358
  lumbar spine 272
  vascularized rib graft 196–197, 199

H

Haller operation, Poland's syndrome 439–440
Hall's sacral anchor 163, 169
Hall's two-hole clamp 163
Halo traction techniques, scoliosis 74–79
  halo–femoral traction 76
  halo–gravity traction, wheelchair 76
  halo–pelvic traction 77
Halo vest 246
Harms reconstruction plates 369
Harms–Schmelzle method, secondary (pseudobasilar) impression 373–375
Harrington compression system, Scheuermann's kyphosis 218
Harrington operation
  instrumentarium 80–81
  scoliosis 80–96
    blood-saving procedures 96
    children's operations, subcutaneous instrumentation 100–102
    fusion 91–96
    instrumentation 89–90
    mobilizing spinal osteotomy 104–107
    one-stage operation 103–104
    operative technique 110–113
    with sublaminar Luque wires 129–130
Harrington stable zone 85, 86
Harrington–Luque system 129–130, 224
Hellstadius' operation, biterminal tenotomy of sternocleidomastoid muscle 448–449
Hematomas, prevention 235
Hemivertebra, resection 100
  in children 97
  wedge resection 151–155
Herbert method, osteotomies 235
Hodgson approach, replacement of vertebral body with vascularized rib graft 196–197, 199
Hodgson's operation
  thoracolumbar junction 24–36
  thoracolumbar vertebral body replacement (implant) 394–395
Hohmann elevators 51
Horner's syndrome 316
Hsu–Yau–Leong technique, ankylosing spondylitis 236–240
Hypogastric plexus, protection 51

I

Image intensification, monitoring spondylolisthesis 304
Intercostal neurovascular bundles 63
Intercostal thoracotomy 16
  closure 23
    with rib resection 22
  scoliosis 21–22
Interlaminar windows, anatomy 329
Internal jugular vein, tributary variations 8
Intervertebral disk
  bridging by graft 384
  debridement 383
  graft bridging and Septopal chains, combined 386
  removal
    in cervical myelopathy 315
    and laminotomy 71–72
  sclerosing spondylitis 386
  see also Lumbar disk herniation; Thoracic disk herniation
Intervertebral space, stenosis 340–343
Isthmus, reconstruction of isthmus (pars interarticularis) 294–297

J

Judet screw 304
Jugular vein, internal, tributary variations 8

K

Kerrison rongeur 319
King classification, scoliosis 82–87
Kirschner wires 279–288, 302
  removal 288
König's operation, caudal sternoclavicular open tenotomy of sternocleidomastoid muscle 443–445
Kyphoscoliosis, with very severe rotatory component 203–204
Kyphosis 187–225
  congenital kyphosis 205–206
  long-arc kyphosis (Scheuermann's) 215–222
  management
    anterior strut grafting 189–190
    fusion in situ 191–193
    intraoperative correction followed by fusion 194–193
    mobilizing spinal osteotomy 188
    myelomeningocele 207–211
    principles of treatment 188
    spinal cord, ventral decompression 198–204
    vascularized rib graft 194–197
  scoliotic component and vertebral torsion 203
  short-arc kyphosis 212–214
Kyphotic buckling, caused by spondylodiskitis 378

L

Laminotomy
  interlaminar windows 329
  and intervertebral disk removal 71–72
  opening ligamentum flavum 328
Langenbeck probes 327
Lange's operation, caudal mastoidal open tenotomy of sternocleidomastoid muscle 446–447
Lindseth operation, myelomeningocele 207–211
Lumbar disk herniation 325–336
  anatomical variations 335
    conjoined root 335
    high origin of root 335
    rectantgular origin of root 335
  bipolar coagulation 338
  complications 335–336
    neurological deficits 336
    spondylodiskitis 335–336
    ventral perforation of anulus fibrosus 335
  epidural fibrosis 334
  extracanalicular disk herniation 337–339
  injury of vertebral joint 334
  medial herniations 334
  mediolateral herniations 330–333
  postoperative treatment 335
  principles 334
  root-sheath fibrosis 334
Lumbar spinal canal, stenoses 340–345
Lumbar spine
  anterior approaches 24–41
    pararectal retroperitoneal approach 46–51
    retroperitoneal approach 42–45
    transperitoneal approach 52–55
  fusion 269–292
    anterior monosegmental fusion, other segments 275–278
    anterior monosegmental fusion L5–S1 270–274
    posterior transpedicular stabilization techniques 279–290
  kyphoscoliosis, Cotrel–Dubousset instrumentation 145–146
  L2, cross-sectional anatomy 28
  L3, tumor excision and osteoplastic blockage 405–409
  L4, tumor excision and compound osteosynthesis 401–405
  lordosation spondylodesis 241
    monosegmental, Hsu–Yau–Leong technique 236–240
    polysegmental, Zielke technique 228–235
  posterior approaches 64–69
    laminotomy and intervertebral disk removal 71–72
    paraspinal approach (Wiltse) 70–72
  spondylodiskitis 379
  vertebral body replacement (implant) 394–395
    of fourth vertebral body by osteosynthesis 401–405
Lumbosacral junction
  approaches *see* Lumbar spine, approaches
  fixation (Dunn) 210, 211
  fusion, posterolateral fusion (Wiltse) 291–292
  pararectal retroperitoneal approach 46–51
    advantages 51
  spondylodiskitis 379
Lumbosacral plate, spondylolisthesis 306
Lumbosacral stabilization (Dunn) 209
Luque operation
  myelomeningocele 208–209
  scoliosis 114–130
    Galveston technique 126–128
    Harrington operation with sublaminar Luque wires 129–130
    neurologic risk 125
    operative technique 114–124
Luque system
  Luque wires, with Harrington operation 129–130
  Scheuermann's long-arc kyphosis 219

M

Magerl hooks 264
Magerl (transarticular screw fixation) method
  fusion of the cervical spine 265–268, 279
  posterior operation for atlantoaxial anterior instability 359–360
Malignant progressive scoliosis, children 100
Mason–Urist technique, ankylosing spondylitis 241–247
Mediastinum, anatomy *see* Posterior mediastinum
Medulla oblongata, dens compression 310
Mikulicz' operation, total extirpation of sternocleidomastoid muscle 448–449
Mirbaha's operation, thoracolumbar spine 37–41
Mobilizing osteotomies *see* Osteotomies
Moe hook, Harrington operation 80
Moe technique, fusion 91
Myelomeningocele
  kyphosis 207–211
  Luque technique 208–209
  Stelzer operation 207–211
Myelopathy
  cervical, in spondylosis 314–316
  see also Neurosurgical operations

N

Neurosurgical operations 309–345
  dens elevation, transoral approach 310–313
  see also Atlas subluxation; Basilar impression; Spinal cord compression
Nuchal muscles, anatomical site 59

O

Occipitocervical junction
  posterior approach 56–59
    anatomy 58
  posterior fusion
    Brattstrom method 367–368
    Geschwend method 361–366
    plate application method 369–372
  vertical instability, with pseudobasilar impression 350
Oral approach
  cervical spine and cervicothoracic junction 2–12
  secondary (pseudobasilar) impression 373–375
Orozko plate, indications 398
Osteolysis plate, indications 398
Osteoplastic blockage, lumbar vertebra L3, and tumor excision 405–409
Osteosynthesis
  replacement (implant) of vertebral body 396
    cervical spine 398–400
    lumbar spine (L4) 401–405
Osteotomies
  ankylosing spondylitis, Zielke technique 231–234
  for anterior segmentation failures 149–150
  Herbert method 235
  mobilizing spinal osteotomy 104–107
  mobilizing ventral osteotomy 147–150
  multiple
    facet joints 104–105
    posterior 106–107
    rib resection 108–109
  Smith–Petersen monosegmental arch osteotomy 236

P

Pelvic fixation (Dunn, Galveston) 208, 209
Pelvic obliquity
  complete vs partial 168
  fixation 169–177
Pelvic–halo traction 77–79
Pigeon chest, Ravitch operation 436–437
Plate osteosynthesis
  cervical spine 398–400
  posterior fusion, occipitocervical junction 369–372
  replacement (implant) of vertebral body 396
Poland's syndrome 439–440
Ponseti classification, scoliosis 82–83
Posterior mediastinum
  anatomical site
    left half 18
    right half 17
Promontory, exposure technique 50
Pseudobasilar (secondary) impression 350, 373–375
Putti's operation, biterminal tenotomy of sternocleidomastoid muscle 448–449

R

Ravitch operation
  funnel chest 432–435
  pigeon chest 436–437
Recessotomy 341
Recurrent laryngeal nerve, course 10
Rehbein braces 429
Rehbein operation, funnel chest 422–431
Relton–Hall frame 64
Respiration, paradoxical, Poland's syndrome 439–440
Retropleural space, anatomical site 17
Rheumatoid instability 347–376
  see also Atlantoaxial anterior instability; Occipitocervical junction
Rib approximator 22
Rib grafts, kyphosis 194–197
Rib resection, choice of ribs 13
Risser frame 235
Risser–Hibbs technique, spondylodesis 234
Robinson's fusion, cervical spine 252–255
Rongeurs
  Kerrison rongeur 319
  Luer bone rongeur 60
  opening angle 336
Roy–Camille reconstruction plates 369

S

Sabiston operation, superior sternoschisis 438
Sacral anchor, Dwyer operation 163, 169
Sacral cavity
  exposure technique 50
  pararectal retroperitoneal anterior approach 46–51
Sacrum, ventral aspect, anatomy 51
Schanz screws 213–214
Scheuermann's long-arc kyphosis 215–222
  Cotrel–Dubousset technique 220
  Harrington compression system 218
  Luque system 219
  Zielke technique 228
Scoliosis 73–185
  adult operations 103–113
    mobilizing spinal osteotomy 104–107
    patient groups 103
    rib resection
      concave side 108
      convex side 109–113
  children's operations 97–102
    convex-side epiphysiodesis 99
    Harrington operation (subcutaneous) 100
    hemivertebra resection 100
    idiopathic malignant progressive scoliosis 100
    posterior fusion with instrumentation 98
    posterior fusion in situ 98
  classification
    combined 167
    dorsal 82
    dorsolumbar 82
    idiopathic 82–87
    lumbar 82, 88
    thoracic curves 83–87
    thoracolumbar 88
  congenital, neurological risks 97, 98
  dorsal operations 80–146
    Cotrel–Dubousset instrumentation 131–146
    Harrington operation 80–96
  Dwyer operation 163–177
  epiphysiodesis 160–162
  flexibility index 82
  fusion area
    choice 84–88
    dollar method 84
    Dwyer operation 164–165
  halo traction techniques 74–79
  Harrington operation
    adults 103–113
    children 97–102
  idiopathic, classification 82–87
  intercostal thoracotomy 21–22
  Luque operation 114–130
  ventral derotation spondylodesis (Zielke) 178–185
    fusion area 164–165
  ventral scoliosis operations 147–185
    mobilizing ventral osteotomy 147–185
  vertebrectomy 156–169
  see also specific techniques
Screws
  DCS screws 396–398
  Dwyer screws 163
  Judet screw 304
  Magerl (transarticular screw fixation) method 359–360
  Schanz screws 213–214
  VDS screws 179
  Zielke pedicular screws 236–238
Septopal chains
  drainage methods 382, 383, 386
  implantation 385–386
  osseous incorporation 385
Skeletal traction, checklist 78
Smith–Petersen monosegmental arch osteotomy 236
Spinal canal
  stenoses 340–345
    complications 345
    postoperative treatment 344
Spinal compensation, available methods 166–168
Spinal cord
  blood supply 20–21
    segmental arterial tributaries 20
  compression
    acquired 343
    tuberculous spondylodiskitis 378
    ventral decompression 198–204
  segmental arteries, "critical supply zones" 20
  and vertebral canal, blood supply 20
Spinal tumors *see* Tumors of the spine
Spondylodesis
  anterior interbody 248
  lumbar spine 274
  Risser–Hibbs technique 234
Spondylodiskitis 377–390
  abscess drainage 381–382
  Andersson lesion 228, 248

Spondylodiskitis, approaches
lateral thoracolumbar approach 379
lumbosacral localization 379
pararectal approach 380
transoropharyngeal approach 378
transthoracic approach 378, 379
posterior stabilization 387–388
postoperative infection
chemotherapy
revisions 388
postoperative treatment 389
see also Ankylosing spondylitis
Spondylolisthesis 293–306
posterior decompression with/without arthrodesis 307
reconstruction of isthmus 294–297
reduction combined with fusion 298–306
Spondylophytes, formation, lateral recess 340
Spondylosis, cervical myelopathy 314–316
Stagnara brace 235
Steinmann nails 76, 300, 304
Stelzer operation, myelomeningocele 207–211
Stenotic syndromes
lumbar spinal canal 342–345
stenosis of lateral spinal recess 340–341
Sternocleidomastoid muscle, torticollis deformities 441–449
Sternum
in funnel chest 422–435
Sabiston operation, superior sternoschisis 438
Strohmeyer's operation, sternocleidomastoid muscle, caudal sternoclavicular subcutaneous tenotomy 442
Superior facet syndrome 340–341

T

Thoracic aorta, positional variants 18
Thoracic disk herniation 317–324
anterolateral transthoracic approach 318–321
approaches evaluated 317
posterolateral approach after costotransversectomy 321–324
see also Lumbar disk herniation
Thoracic duct, positional variants 18
Thoracic spine
anterior approaches 13–15
closure of intercostal thoracotomy 23
closure of thoracotomy with rib resection 22
dorsolateral thoracotomy with rib resection 13–15
intercostal thoracotomy 16–23
site in scoliosis 21
cross-sectional anatomy 66
lordoscoliosis, mobile, Cotrel–Dubousset instrumentation 135–142
lordosis, Cotrel–Dubousset technique 223–224
posterior approach 60–67
costotransversectomy 60–63
posterior mediastinum
anatomical site 17
and right retropleural space 17
scoliosis, rigid, Cotrel–Dubousset instrumentation 143–144
vertebral body replacement (implant) 393–394
Thoracolumbar junction
anterior approaches
choice of rib for resection 24
retroperitoneal–extrapleural (Mirbaha) 37–41
transpleural–retroperitoneal (Hodgson) 24–36
dorsal view 38
rigid scoliosis, Cotrel–Dubousset instrumentation 143–144
vertebral body replacement (implant) 394–395
Thoracotomy *see* Intercostal thoracotomy
Thyroid artery, ligation and transection 9
Tillaux operation, caudal mastoidal open tenotomy of sternocleidomastoid muscle 446–447
Torticollis deformity 441–449
indications and contraindications for operation 442
sternocleidomastoid muscle
biterminal tenotomy 448–449
caudal mastoidal open tenotomy 446–447
caudal sternoclavicular open tenotomy 443–445
caudal sternoclavicular subcutaneous tenotomy 442–443
total extirpation 448–449
Traction
checklist 78
device for transverse traction *see* DTT system
Hohmann elevators 51
skeletal, checklist 78
see also Halo traction
Tuberculous spondylodiskitis
antibiotics 389
cord compression 378
Tumors of the chest wall *see* Chest wall, tumors
Tumors of the spine 391–409
transpedicular tumor biopsy 392
vertebral body replacement (implant)
lumbar 394–395
thoracic 393–394
thoracolumbar 394–395

U

USIS (universal spinal instrumentation system) 220–222
fixateur interne 248

V

Vascularized rib graft 194–197
replacement of vertebral body 196–197
VDS *see* Ventral derotation spondylodesis
Ventral derotation spondylodesis (Zielke)
instrumentation 180–185
scoliosis 178–185
fusion area 164–167
VDS screws 179
Ventral scoliosis operations 147–185
mobilizing ventral osteotomy 147–150
Vertebrae, strategic, Cotrel–Dubousset instrumentation 134
Vertebral body
disorders of formation 97
osteoplastic replacement (Zielke–Askani) 396–398
replacement (implant)
cement and plate osteosynthesis 396
lumbar 394–395
thoracic 393–394
thoracolumbar 394–395
replacement with vascularized rib graft 196–197
Vertebral canal, blood supply 20–21
Vertebral rotation, Nash and Moe method 81
Vertebral venous plexus 66
Vertebrectomy, complete, in scoliosis 156–159
von Volkmann's operation, caudal sternoclavicular open tenotomy of sternocleidomastoid muscle 443–445

W

Wake-up test, defined 96
Wheelchair, halo–gravity traction, scoliosis 76
Wiltse's operation
lumbosacral junction 70–72
posterolateral fusion of lumbosacral junction 291–292
Wisconsin compression system, Harrington operation 80, 92

Z

Zielke
pedicular screws 236
implantation 238
USIS (universal spinal instrumentation system) 220–222
implant 230
Zielke–Askani system
lumbar vertebral body replacement (implant), osteoplastic replacement 396–398
short-arc kyphosis 212–214
Zielke's operation
ankylosing spondylitis 228–235
lumbar vertebral body replacement (implant) 394–395
ventral derotation spondylodesis 178–185